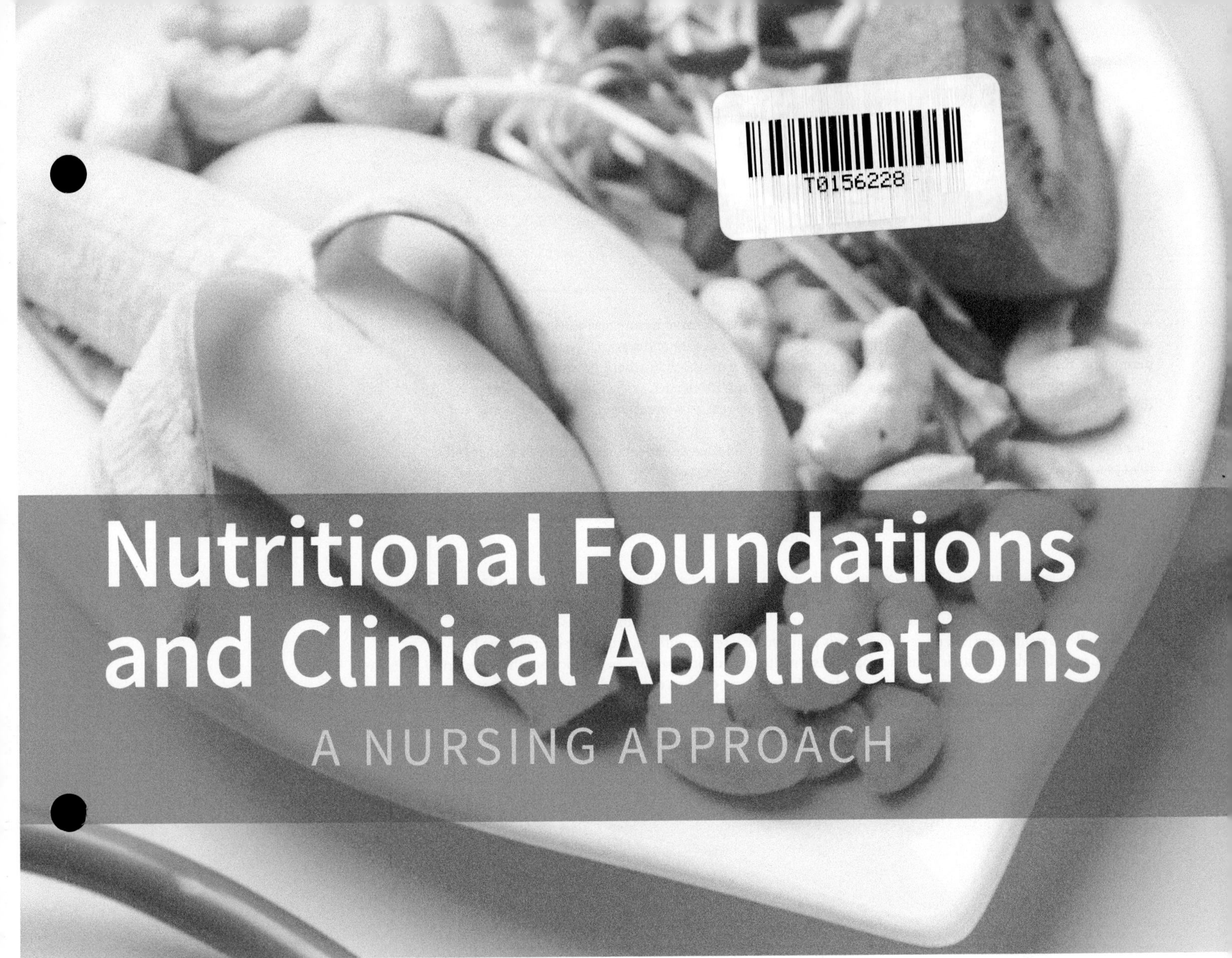

Nutritional Foundations and Clinical Applications

A NURSING APPROACH

8th Edition

Michele Grodner, EdD, CHES
Professor
Department of Public Health
William Paterson University
Wayne, New Jersey

Sylvia Escott-Stump, MA, RDN, LDN, FAND
Faculty Associate
University of Wisconsin
Madison, Wisconsin

Suzanne Dorner, MSN, RN, CCRN
Assistant Manager
Medical Intensive Care Unit
Tampa General Hospital
Tampa, Florida

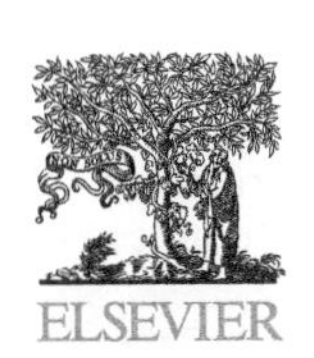

Elsevier
3251 Riverport Lane
St. Louis, Missouri 63043

NUTRITIONAL FOUNDATIONS AND CLINICAL APPLICATIONS:
A NURSING APPROACH, EIGHTH EDITION

ISBN: 978-0-323-81024-1

Copyright © 2023 by Elsevier, Inc. All rights reserved.

No part of this publication may be reproduced or transmitted in any form or by any means, electronic or mechanical, including photocopying, recording, or any information storage and retrieval system, without permission in writing from the publisher. Details on how to seek permission, further information about the Publisher's permissions policies and our arrangements with organizations such as the Copyright Clearance Center and the Copyright Licensing Agency, can be found at our website: www.elsevier.com/permissions.

This book and the individual contributions contained in it are protected under copyright by the Publisher (other than as may be noted herein).

Notice

Practitioners and researchers must always rely on their own experience and knowledge in evaluating and using any information, methods, compounds or experiments described herein. Because of rapid advances in the medical sciences, in particular, independent verification of diagnoses and drug dosages should be made. To the fullest extent of the law, no responsibility is assumed by Elsevier, authors, editors or contributors for any injury and/or damage to persons or property as a matter of products liability, negligence or otherwise, or from any use or operation of any methods, products, instructions, or ideas contained in the material herein.

Previous editions copyrighted 2020, 2016, 2012, 2007, 2004, 2000, and 1996.

Library of Congress Control Number: 2021946990

Senior Content Strategist: Sandra Clark
Senior Content Development Manager: Lisa P. Newton
Publishing Services Manager: Deepthi Unni
Senior Project Manager: Manchu Mohan
Design Direction: Brian Salisbury

Printed in the United States of America

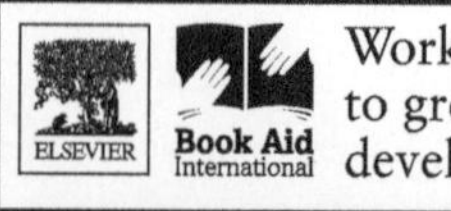

Working together
to grow libraries in
developing countries
www.elsevier.com • www.bookaid.org

Last digit is the print number: 9 8 7 6 5 4 3 2 1

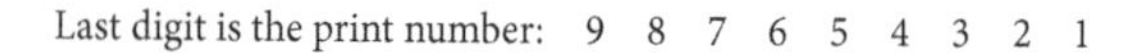

To all my children Adam, Jared, Judith and especially my granddaughters Ruby and Lily whose enthusiasm for life nourishes me.

Michele Grodner

I wish to dedicate this text to my husband, my children, and their families (Russ; Matt, Katie and children; Lindsay and Zac) and the wonderful nurses in my family and network of friends.

Sylvia Escott-Stump

CONTRIBUTORS

Bethany Hawes Sykes, EdD, RN, CEN, CCRN (retired)
Retired Adjunct Faculty
Department of Nursing
Salve Regina University
Newport, Rhode Island
Nursing Approach Boxes - Next-Generation NCLEX® Examination-Style Questions

Hailey Morris, MS
Division of Nutrition
College of Health
University of Utah
Salt Lake City, Utah
Next-Generation NCLEX® Examination-Style Questions

Ancillary Writers

Charla K. Hollin, RN, BSN
Allied Health Division Chair
University of Arkansas Rich Mountain
Mena, Arkansas
TEACH for Nurses, PowerPoint Slides

PREFACE

That our personal behavior patterns and our level of health are interrelated is no longer questionable as knowledge continues to support the linkage. But which study results, or "healthiest" dietary patterns and behaviors, should be adopted for ourselves, and more so for our patients? As health professionals, we need to be aware of our own dietary patterns as well as those of our patients. Changing food behavior patterns can be difficult even if we are knowledgeable of the benefits to be accrued. So many distractions of contemporary life keep us from achieving our goals. *Nutritional Foundations and Clinical Applications*, 8th edition continues to recognize the role of nurses in nutritional healing and wellness.

This nutrition text considers the personal nutrition needs of nurses to nourish themselves and their families as well as their demanding professional responsibilities to educate patients, clients, and family members to follow prescribed therapeutic nutrition to maintain or improve health. This approach unites the worlds of nutrition and nursing. Indeed, the first dietitians were nurses!

The role of nurses expands from the medical clinic into the community, thereby having a significant influence on the health promotion of individuals and the communities in which they work. Consequently, the need for nurses to have a thorough background in both personal and clinical nutrition applications becomes paramount.

This edition continues the modernization of *Nutritional Foundations and Clinical Applications: A Nursing Approach* as The Nursing Approach feature of all chapters have been modified to reflect changes in nursing preparation. The nursing licensure examination (NCLEX®) has traditionally used the nursing process to determine clinical decisions, to reflect the recognition that, to determine the most efficacious clinical decisions, nursing students need the ability to apply knowledge into actions. To do so requires an additional focus on developing nursing cognitive skills for effective clinical judgment to be implemented. Consequently, NCLEX® is incorporating assessment of these clinical judgment cognitive skills into the licensure examination resulting in Next-Generation NCLEX® (NGN). These skills are best developed through contextual case studies that require knowledge application within real-world situations. Clinical judgment is necessary to determine which cues from a case study can be used to develop hypotheses and then generate and implement clinical solutions. All The Nursing Approach features of *Nutritional Foundations and Clinical Applications, 8th edition* are now revised to reflect the NGN assessment of clinical judgment.

Michele Grodner, EdD, CHES, Professor, Department of Public Health, William Paterson University, continues as the author of nutrition and health content (Chapters 1–10). **Sylvia Escott-Stump, MA, RD, LDN**, Faculty Associate, University of Wisconsin-Madison and a former President, Academy of Nutrition and Dietetics, has updated the nutrition therapy content (Chapters 11–20). **Bethany Sykes** edited The Nursing Approach feature of all chapters. This approach engages the reader in both wellness and medical nutrition content while implementing the new Next Generation NCLEX® (NGN) approach to nursing clinical judgment.

AUDIENCE

Nursing students are the primary audience for this book as they explore and apply basic and therapeutic nutrition concepts with their patients. Secondary audiences include public health and health science majors. Useful in a variety of health care settings, the text provides an excellent reference for nurses, nurse practitioners, and other health care professionals.

The book consists of four parts, allowing for selective use within a one-semester course. For instance, Part I, *Wellness, Nutrition, and the Nursing Role;* Part II, *Nutrients, Food, and Health;* and Part III, *Health Promotion Through Nutrition and Nursing Practice*, can be used for a basic, one-semester nutrition course, whereas Part IV, *Overview of Nutrition Therapy*, may be used as a future course or reference related to applications of nutrition therapy. Or all parts may be covered within a one-semester course.

APPROACH

Our focus is on the nursing professional, concentrating on the nutrition skills applicable to nursing practice. This text tailors normal and therapeutic nutrition in the unique perspective of the nursing profession. Most other nutrition texts attempt to meet the needs of dietetic and nutrition majors in addition to nursing majors. Here, information needed by nurses is presented. We appreciate that nurses do not prescribe or develop nutrition interventions. Instead, skills essential for nursing professionals are emphasized for implementation of diet orders and education of patients and clients about their prescribed dietary patterns.

FEATURES AND CONTENT

The nursing profession is multifaceted. Although health promotion and clinical care are primary concerns, nurses have other factors to consider when providing care. These are addressed in every chapter of this edition of *Nutritional Foundations and Clinical Applications*. Consider these features:

- **Cultural diversity of populations served**
  Food and health customs and concerns are analyzed specific to an array of ethnic groups. Students become sensitized and respectful of culturally defined food differences and are then able to approach, interview, and assess patients from diverse backgrounds. Each **CULTURAL CONSIDERATIONS** box includes a section called "Application to Nursing," to highlight

how to use the knowledge in daily practice. As an added resource, Chapter 12, Food-Related Issues, provides resources about cultural dietary patterns of different ethnic and religious groups, allowing nurses to focus on the specific population with whom they work.

- **Controversial health issue explorations**
  Health care professionals and the public at large have access to an abundance of health-related information through many forms of media. Consequently, differing opinions or controversies about food, nutrition, and health concerns emerge. Students are encouraged to develop their own beliefs, based on the current evidence. As applicable, some chapters have **HEALTH DEBATE** boxes.
- **Awareness of the personal perspective of individuals**
  Content throughout this text is expressed in a human, personalized way. This approach, which underlies the philosophy of this text, is reflected by firsthand accounts of the ways in which nutrition affects the lives of both nursing professionals and everyday people. Powerful images of patients and their families emerge as individuals describe in their own words their experiences pursuing health and healing. Each chapter offers a **PERSONAL PERSPECTIVE** box on a relevant experience.
- **Comprehension of societal issues that impact health status**
  SOCIAL ISSUES boxes emphasize ethical, social, and community concerns to reveal the various influences on health and wellness, from local to international. It is imperative for nursing and health care professionals to understand the potential effects of societal issues on the lives and health status of the populations they serve.
- **Recognition of the educational role of nursing**
  Nursing professionals have a primary role in supporting clients as they strive to achieve compliance of prescribed therapeutic dietary modifications or just attempt to improve their nutrient intake. **TEACHING TOOL** boxes in every chapter provide strategies for teaching clients about optimum dietary patterns and therapeutic nutrition recommendations. When appropriate, specific issues of literacy, such as strategies for enhancing patient education for those with low literacy skills, are also presented in these boxes.
- **Recognition of psychosocial strategies for behavior change to achieve wellness**
  The **TOWARD A POSITIVE NUTRITION LIFESTYLE** section in each chapter within Parts I, II, and III presents psychosocial strategies to support health behavioral changes for individuals wishing to adopt healthier lifestyles. This section recognizes the multidisciplinary skills needed to apply lifestyle changes for oneself and one's clients/patients.
- **Focus on the Cognitive Skills for Clinical Judgment in Nursing**
  THE NURSING APPROACH boxes analyze a realistic nutrition case study according to cognitive skills for clinical judgment in nursing. By describing situations that may be encountered in clinical practice, each chapter's subject matter is aligned with a nursing perspective. Discussion questions based on the case study enhance critical thinking and application of knowledge skills. These can be used for class discussions or as homework assignments. Responses are included for instructors. They are written from a professional nursing perspective. The case studies have been updated by Bethany Sykes, who brings her relevant perspective and experiences in nursing and patient education.

TEACHING AND LEARNING RESOURCES

For Instructors

Instructor Resources on Evolve, available at http://evolve.elsevier.com/Grodner/foundations, provides a wealth of material to help you make your nutrition instruction a success. In addition to all of the Student Resources, the following are provided for Faculty:

- **TEACH for Nurses Lesson Plans**, based on textbook chapter Learning Objectives, serve as ready-made, modifiable lesson plans and a complete road map to link all parts of the educational package. These concise and straightforward lesson plans can be modified or combined to meet your scheduling and teaching needs.
- **PowerPoint Presentations** are organized by chapter with approximately 30 slides per chapter for in-class lectures. These are detailed and include customizable text and image lecture slides to enhance learning in the classroom or in Web-based course modules. If you share them with students, they can use the note feature to help them with each lecture.
- **Audience Response Questions** are provided with one to three multiple-answer questions per chapter to stimulate class discussion and assess student understanding of key concepts.
- The **Test Bank** has more than 650 test items, complete with the correct answer, rationale, cognitive level of each question, corresponding step of the nursing process, appropriate NCLEX®, Client Needs label, and text page reference(s).
- **Image Collection** Over 100 illustrations and photos that can be used in a presentation or as visual aids.
- **Next-Generation NCLEX® (NGN)–Style Case Studies** for Nutritional Foundations and Clinical Applications: Six NGN-style case studies focused on nutritional care.
- **Answers to Applying Content Knowledge Boxes**
- **Answers to Critical Thinking/Clinical Application Boxes**
- **Answers to Nursing Approach Boxes**

For Students

Student Resources on Evolve, available at http://evolve.elsevier.com/Grodner/foundations.

Students will find a wealth of valuable learning resources on Evolve. The Evolve Resources page in the front of the book gives login instructions and a description of each resource.

- **Virtual Case Studies:** Video clips of six fictitious patients—including one with type 2 diabetes mellitus, one with a respiratory infection, and one with HIV/AIDS wasting syndrome—are accompanied by written case studies; short-answer and essay questions; NCLEX®-formatted, multiple-choice, examination-style questions; and Internet assignments. This exciting feature provides students with realistic clinical practice.

- **Applying Content Knowledge Questions:** One case and question per chapter are provided online, in addition to the cases and questions contained within the foundation and life span chapters of the textbook (Chapters 1–10).
- **Critical Thinking: Clinical Applications Questions:** One case study with accompanying application questions is provided online for each of the clinical chapters (Chapters 11–20), in addition to the cases and questions contained within those same textbook chapters.
- **NCLEX® Style Questions:** Questions for each chapter are provided to help in preparation for the NCLEX® Examination.
- **Review Questions:** Approximately 5 to 10 short-answer questions per chapter are supplied online.
- **Answers to Nursing Approach Boxes.**

ACKNOWLEDGMENTS

To the individuals who shared their stories with us in the *Personal Perspective* boxes, our gratitude for your willingness to educate nursing professionals through your experiences. We acknowledge Veronica Soperanes and Yetta Kaemmer.

SPECIAL ACKNOWLEDGMENTS

We appreciate and acknowledge the support and direction from the staff of Elsevier. Under the guidance of Sandra Clark, Senior Content Strategist, we prepared the eighth edition to fine-tune and update the organizational structure and content. Lisa Newton, Senior Content Development Manager, cheerily assisted our revisions for the Nursing Approach organization. Manchu Mohan, Senior Project Manager, meticulously led us through the maze of proofing and production. Brian Salisbury, Design Director, provided the revised and updated design content for this edition. We were delighted to have new art drawn by Rose Boul at Graphic World for many of our figures.

And finally, as always, we greatly appreciate the Nursing Marketing Department for ongoing efforts communicating the unique aspects of our concept to instructors in North America and internationally.

Writing a textbook that is regularly revised such as *Nutritional Foundations and Clinical Applications* keeps the next edition in mind as soon as the latest is printed. Is there a new health, nutrition, or nursing trend that could be incorporated into the next edition? With projects such as this continually revised textbook, the process becomes a private aspect of self that cannot be shared. To family, friends, and colleagues who are unavoidably inconvenienced by this lengthy process, our thanks.

As a collaboration of expertise in nutrition education, dietetics, and nursing, we represent interconnective health care. As we become more sensitized to the always increasing complex responsibilities of nursing, we continue to fine-tune our answers to the questions of "What do nurses need to know about nutrition?" and "How would they apply this knowledge to their patients and clients?" Not only do we want to include the "need to know" content but the "nice to know" as well. This new edition continues our ever-evolving responses to these questions.

Michele Grodner
Sylvia Escott-Stump

CONTENTS

Nutritional Foundations and Clinical Applications

A NURSING APPROACH

1

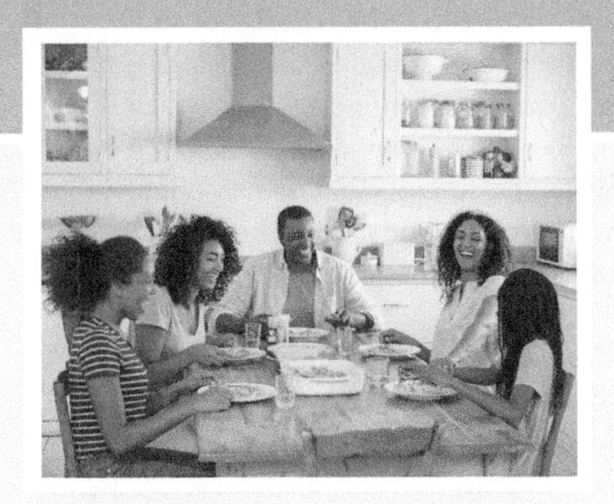

Wellness Nutrition

"Wellness nutrition" approaches food consumption as a positive way to nourish the body. This approach focuses on ways to organize our lives so we can more easily follow an eating pattern designed to enhance health status. Consuming a diet based on beneficial fat and dietary fiber (increase in plant-based foods such as fruits, vegetables, and whole grains) as well as moderate caloric consumption is then not a chore but rather an affirmation of our competency to care for ourselves.

http://evolve.elsevier.com/GRODNER/FOUNDATIONS

LEARNING OBJECTIVES

- Define health and wellness.
- Describe health promotion.
- State the purpose of *Healthy People 2030 (HP2030)*.
- Discuss health literacy.
- Identify the six nutrient categories.
- List the functions of essential nutrients.

ROLE IN WELLNESS

Nourishing our bodies seems so simple. Just eat food. But which food? How much food? How prepared? Foods to promote or maintain health? Which foods are "best" during illness or trauma? Who shops for food? How much should we spend on food or, rather, nourishment? Should we buy ready-made (or "order in"), purchase a meal delivery service, or cook from scratch? Who cooks? Who should we eat with or do we eat alone? Who cleans the kitchen? Not so simple after all.

The intent of this nutrition textbook is twofold. The first is to educate about the nutrients, foods, and related issues for our personal health and wellness goals. The second is to prepare nursing health professionals who understand the function and context of prescribed care for nutritional intervention for the prevention and treatment of diseases and conditions that may be alleviated or treated through specific dietary recommendations. Nutrition care is diagnosed and prescribed by registered dietitian/nutritionists (RDNs) as part of multidisciplinary health care teams. Although nurses do not develop dietary treatment regimens, nurses often educate patients about prescribed dietary treatment. Nurses may reinforce the dietary recommendations within the context of an overall nursing care plan. Therefore, in every chapter *The Nursing Approach* box addresses related issues of implementation of dietary therapy and case management.

This chapter starts by considering the question, what are the concepts of health and wellness for which we strive?

DEFINITION OF WELLNESS

In the past, health was defined as the absence of disease or illness. Modern medicine conquered many life-threatening diseases, such as smallpox and polio. Public health measures, such as pasteurization and sanitation, reduced the risk of foodborne and environmental hazards. As concern about the physical status of the human body lessened, we have been able to consider other aspects of the qualities of health.

One of the first expanded definitions of health was provided by the World Health Organization (WHO, 1946): "Health is a state of complete physical, mental, and social well-being and not merely the absence of disease and infirmity." Although this definition addresses the concern that health is more than just the absence of disease, health is presented as a static concept that individuals achieve.

A more expanded definition of health was presented by Rene Dubos (1968), biologist and philosopher, who wrote, "Health is a quality of life involving social, emotional, mental, spiritual, and biologic fitness on the part of the individual, which results from adaptations to the environment." This view leads to our present understanding of health as a complex concept best represented by physical and psychological dimensions, as follows:

1. ***Physical health:*** The efficiency of the body to function appropriately, to maintain immunity to disease, and to meet daily energy requirements
2. ***Intellectual health:*** The use of intellectual abilities to learn and to adapt to changes in one's environment
3. ***Emotional health:*** The capacity to easily express or suppress emotions appropriately
4. ***Social health:*** The ability to interact with people in an acceptable manner and sustain relationships with family members, friends, and colleagues
5. ***Spiritual health:*** The cultural beliefs that give purpose to human existence, found through faith in the teachings of organized religions, in an understanding of nature or science, or in an acceptance of the humanistic view of life
6. ***Environmental health:*** The external factors that affect our health and well-being, including the physical context within which one lives and works as affected by determinants of ethnicity, education, income, and occupation, and extending to the larger environment of safeguarding natural resources to reduce exposure to preventable hazards

This holistic view incorporates many aspects of human existence. Using this definition of health allows more individualized assessment of health status. As our own health and the health of our clients are evaluated in relation to each dimension, some dimensions will be stronger than others (see the *Teaching Tool* box Dimensions of Health).

TEACHING TOOL

Dimensions of Health

To broaden a patient's understanding of health, use the six dimensions of health. Describe the dimensions and then discuss with the patient each that pertains to his or her nutrition and health situation. By exploring aspects of health other than physical health, a person can then use all resources to restore the overall level of well-being.

Wellness Through the Six Dimensions of Health

- Physical health: Efficient body functioning
- Intellectual health: Use of intellectual abilities
- Emotional health: Ability to control emotions
- Social health: Interactions and relationships with others
- Spiritual health: Cultural beliefs about the purpose of life
- Environmental health: External factors that impact living and work settings

Role of Nutrition

Nutrition is the study of nutrients and the processes by which they are used by the body. **Nutrients** are substances in foods required by the body for energy, growth, maintenance, and repair. Some nutrients are essential; they cannot be made by the human body and must be provided by foods.

Because the primary role of nutrients is to provide the building blocks for efficient functioning and maintenance of the body, nutrition may appear to belong only within the physical health dimension. However, the effects of nutrients and their sources on the other health dimensions are far-reaching. Nutrition is the cornerstone of each health dimension.

Physical health depends on the quantity and quality of nutrients available to the body. The human body, from skeletal bones to minute amounts of hormones, is composed of nutrients in various combinations.

Intellectual health relies on a well-functioning brain and central nervous system. Nutritional imbalances can affect intellectual health, as occurs with iron-deficiency anemia. Although milk is an excellent source of protein, calcium, and phosphorus, it provides a negligible amount of iron. Some young children drink so much dairy milk (from baby bottles or sippy cups) that it diminishes their appetite for other foods, such as meats, chicken, legumes, and leafy green vegetables, all of which are good sources of iron. As a result, iron deficiency may occur in children with nutritional imbalances. The cognitive abilities of iron-deficient children may be affected, which could lead to possible learning problems.

Emotional health may be affected by poor eating habits, resulting in hypoglycemia or low blood glucose levels. Low blood glucose occurs normally in anyone who is physically hungry. When the body's need for food is ignored (e.g., when we miss meals because of poor planning or are too busy to eat), feelings of anxiety and confusion and trembling may occur. Emotions may be harder to control when we feel this way. Although blood glucose levels may affect our emotions, there are, of course, other factors that influence emotional health.

Social health situations often center on food-related occasions, ranging from holiday feasts to everyday meals. Nutritional status is sometimes affected by the quality of our relationships with family and friends. Are family meals an enjoyable experience or a tense ordeal? How might this issue affect a person's dietary intake?

Spiritual health often has ties to food. Several religions prohibit the consumption of specific foods. Many followers of Islam and Judaism adhere to the dietary laws of their religions. Both forbid consumption of pork products. Seventh Day Adventists follow an ovo-lacto vegetarian diet in which they consume only plant foods and dairy products. In India cows are viewed as sacred, not to be eaten but to be revered as a source of sustenance (milk), fuel (burning of feces), power (as a work animal), and fertilizer (manure).

Environmental health includes access to adequate meal-preparation facilities, knowledge about preparation, and financial and physical access to food stores within one's community. In major cities as well as in rural areas of the United States, some residents may live in "food deserts" within which large grocery stores are not easily accessible, thereby limiting access to fresh and reasonably priced foods. The environmental health of such a community is compromised.

DEFINITION OF WELLNESS

Wellness is a lifestyle (pattern of behaviors) that enhances our level of health. It occurs through development of each of the six dimensions of health. Individuals engaged in wellness lifestyles feel a sense of competency and achievement in their ability to modify their behaviors to increase or maintain positive levels of health.

Hectic contemporary schedules may seem to interfere with efforts to achieve wellness. The aim is to strive for wellness even if the path may seem more like a roller coaster than a smooth uphill climb (Fig. 1.1). At times, clients may falter in their efforts, but the key is to renew positive behaviors as soon as possible.

Role of Nutrition

"Wellness nutrition" approaches food consumption as a positive way to nourish the body. This approach focuses on ways to organize our lives so we can more easily follow an eating pattern designed to enhance health status. Consuming a diet based on beneficial fat and higher fiber (increase in plant-based foods such as fruits, vegetables, and whole grains) as well as moderate caloric consumption is then not a chore but rather an affirmation of our competency to care for ourselves. Conveying this approach to clients is a nursing challenge (see the *Personal Perspectives* box Control Ourselves and Not Live in Fear).

PERSONAL PERSPECTIVES

Control Ourselves and Not Live in Fear

This section in each chapter features an individual's viewpoint about a nutrition or health issue. Sometimes the viewpoint may represent a composite of opinions on a topic. Here's how Veronica adapted to cope with living through the COVID-19 pandemic.

The past six months, living through the COVID-19 pandemic was a challenge. What I experienced was division between people and that each person was on their own to survive. Entering a store to buy essentials for my household did not look the same. Instead of seeing discount signs and specials, I was greeted by social distancing signs and a sign on how to wear a facemask properly.

This pandemic did not pick a race, a socioeconomic status, or a certain age. I saw people trying to survive and losing their humility. Fear, wariness, and depression ate me up for the first months. Fear of losing my job that provided my family and me with health insurance, in a time when health was my priority. Wariness of leaving the house and being attacked by this illness. Depression about not seeing or hugging my loved ones, being told not to leave your house unless necessary. I felt like I did not have power over my life or feelings.

As humans we are made to adapt to different situations and environments. After establishing a work area and how to carry out my work from home, I started to have extra time. Before the pandemic, I had no time to do certain things like cook, clean, and/or do hobbies. With my extra time staying home, I started to cook more home meals for my family and improved my meals. I cleaned every corner of my house and organized as much as I could. I decluttered years of hoarding and donated things I was not using. I had time to do things I loved, like exercise each morning, dancing with my husband, and doing scrapbooking.

I do not want to live my life in fear any more. Health experts communicated what we need to do to lower our risk of infection, and, as a family, we adopted these procedures in our daily lives. The most import thing I learned from this pandemic is that we cannot control other's actions or thoughts, but we can control ourselves and not live in fear.

Veronica Soperanes
Pompton Lakes, NJ

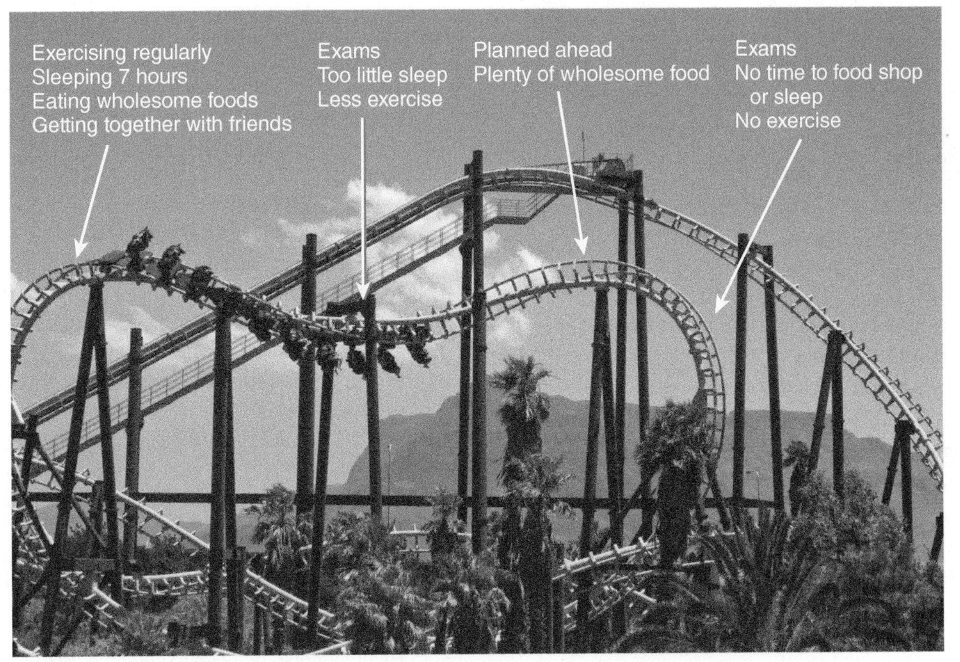
Exercising regularly
Sleeping 7 hours
Eating wholesome foods
Getting together with friends
Exams
Too little sleep
Less exercise
Planned ahead
Plenty of wholesome food
Exams
No time to food shop or sleep
No exercise

Fig. 1.1 Wellness effort roller coaster. (Modified from www.thinkstockphotos.com.)

HEALTH PROMOTION

Health promotion consists of strategies used to raise the level of the health of individuals, families, groups, and communities. In community and occupational health settings, health-promotion strategies implemented by nurses often focus on lifestyle changes that will lead to new, positive health behaviors. Development of positive behaviors may depend on knowledge, techniques, and community supports, as follows (see the *Teaching Tool* box Literacy and Health later in the chapter):

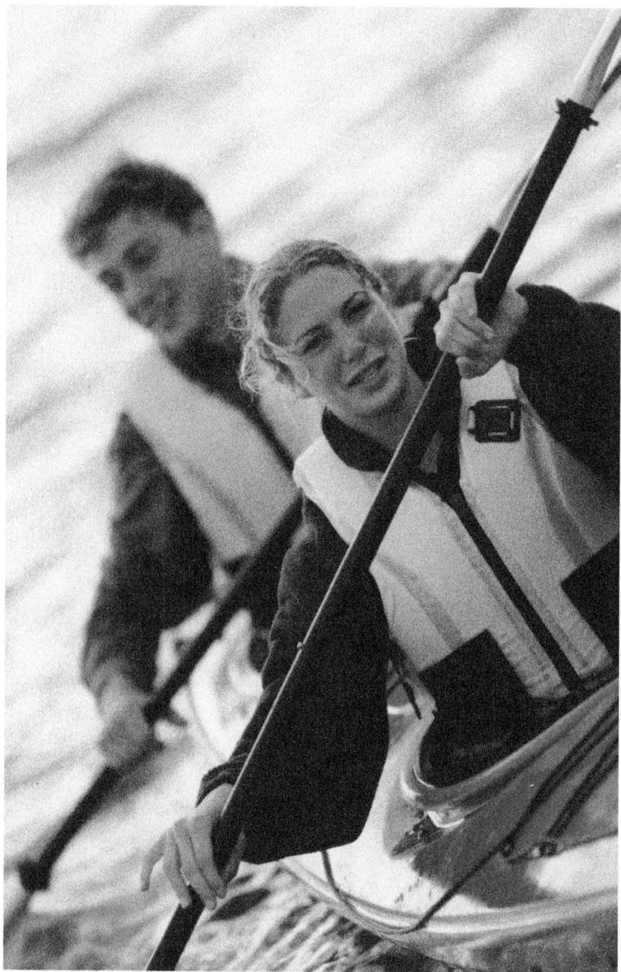

Physical health benefits from a good diet. (From www.thinkstockphoto.com)

1. ***Knowledge:*** Learning new information about the benefits or risks of health-related behaviors
2. ***Techniques:*** Applying new knowledge to everyday activities; developing ways to modify current lifestyles
3. ***Community supports:*** Availability of environmental or regulatory measures to support new health-promoting behaviors within a social context

Role of Nutrition

For over 40 years, national health targets have been set. The first initiative, the Surgeon General's report titled *Healthy People*, laid out life-stage targets that continue to be tracked today. Since then, health targets have been updated every 10 years through collaboration among the government, voluntary and professional health associations, businesses, and individuals under the direction of the secretary of the U.S. Department of Health and Human Services (USDHHS, n.d.). The objectives focus on the decisions and policies that affect prevention efforts and create a standard against which to later assess the performance of meeting these goals. In addition, the interrelatedness of the health of communities and individuals is emphasized. The health status of an individual depends on the health supports accessible within the community. (This is also discussed in Chapter 2 under the heading Community Nutrition.)

This decade's *Healthy People 2030* (*HP2030*) is guided by a framework based on the vision of "a society in which all people can achieve their full potential for health and well-being across the lifespan" (USDHHS, n.d.).

The mission is "to promote, strengthen, and evaluate the nation's efforts" to realize this vision. Five overarching goals present pathways by which mission may be achieved. To provide further support for the mission, the newest goal entails "engaging leadership, key constituents, and the public across multiple sectors to take action and design policies" to fulfill national goals. Details of the *HP2030* framework are listed in Box 1.1.

To accomplish these goals, *HP2030* focuses on a group of 355 core objectives created with more precise data standards to enable the federal government and *HP2030* partners to achieve positive outcomes within the decade. Compared to previous *Healthy People* initiatives, *HP2030* includes new objectives associated with social determinants of health, as well as goals for decreasing youth e-cigarette use, and an emphasis on decreasing

BOX 1.1 Healthy People 2030 Framework

Vision

A society in which all people can achieve their full potential for health and well-being across the lifespan.

Mission

To promote, strengthen, and evaluate the nation's efforts to improve the health and well-being of all people.

Overarching Goals

Achieving these broad and ambitious goals requires setting, working toward, and achieving a wide variety of much more specific goals. *Healthy People 2030*'s overarching goals are to:

- Attain healthy, thriving lives and well-being free of preventable disease, disability, injury, and premature death.
- Eliminate health disparities, achieve health equity, and attain health literacy to improve the health and well-being of all.
- Create social, physical, and economic environments that promote attaining the full potential for health and well-being for all.
- Promote healthy development, healthy behaviors, and well-being across all life stages.
- Engage leadership, key constituents, and the public across multiple sectors to take action and design policies that improve the health and well-being of all.

(From HealthyPeople.gov *Healthy People 2030 Framework*, n.d. Accessed October 3, 2020 from www.health.gov/healthypeople/about/healthy-people-2030-framework.)

How can I use Healthy People 2030 in my work?

Healthy People addresses public health priorities by setting national objectives and tracking them over the decade. Join us as we work to improve health and well-being nationwide.

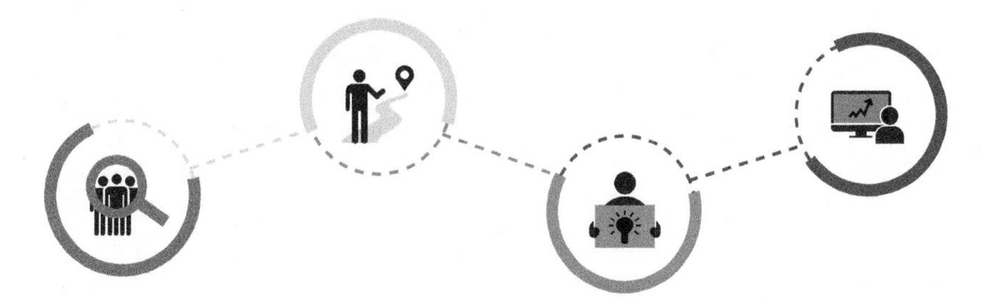

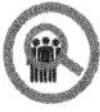 **1. Identify needs and priority populations**

- Browse objectives to learn about national goals to improve health
- See how national goals align with your priorities
- Consider focusing on groups affected by health disparities

Use this information to make the case for your program, secure resources, and build partnerships.

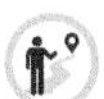 **2. Set your own targets**

- Find data related to your work
- Use national data to set goals for your program

Healthy People 2030 establishes objectives and targets for the entire United States, but setting local targets contributes to national success.

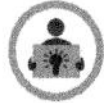 **3. Find inspiration and practical tools**

- Explore critical public health topics relevant to your work
- Learn about successful programs, policies, and interventions
- Look for evidence-based resources and tools your community, state, or organization can use

 **4. Monitor national progress — and use our data as a benchmark**

- Check for updates on progress toward achieving national objectives
- Use our data to inform your policy and program planning
- See how your progress compares to national data

Visit **health.gov/healthypeople/tools-action** to get started using Healthy People 2030 — and use **#HP2030** to share your successes on social media!

Fig. 1.2 How can I use *Healthy People 2030* in my work? https://health.gov/sites/default/files/2020-08/ODPHP_HP2030_HowtoUseHP.pdf

opioid use disorder. Resources are also included for adjusting *HP2030* to evolving public health threats, such as the COVID-19 pandemic, while supporting ongoing efforts to concentrate on issues of health disparities, health equity, and health literacy.

Leading Health Indicators will guide efforts. This translates into focusing on risk factors and behaviors, rather than disease consequences. The ability to adapt to urgent public health concerns, such as COVID-19, is emphasized through action interventions based on confirmed data on the national, state, local, and community levels. Each of us can improve health and well-being within our own professional sphere of influence (Fig. 1.2).

Nutrition Monitoring

The nutritional status of the American population is monitored through several ongoing surveys. The National Nutrition Monitoring Act of 1990 provides for partnerships among government organizations that conduct national surveys of the nation's health and nutritional status. This collaboration supports the use of similar standards and research methods so the surveys' findings can be compared.

The National Health and Nutrition Examination Survey (NHANES) is a series of studies created to evaluate the health and nutritional status of adults and children in the United States. The survey is unusual because the protocol includes both interviews and physical examinations (Centers for Disease Control and Prevention/National Center for Health Statistics [CDC/NCHS], 2021). The survey focuses on data from the dietary intake, medical history, biochemical evaluation, physical examinations, and measurements of American population groups who are carefully chosen to represent the total population. The dietary intake portion of the

NHANES is called What We Eat in America (WWEIA). Records of food intake for 2 days are kept. These nutrient values are then compared with recommended dietary standards. Researchers are able to discover relationships between dietary intakes and health status as the WWEIA food intake data can be compared with health status data from other NHANES sections (CDC/NCHS, 2015).

WWEIA is conducted as a partnership between the U.S. Department of Agriculture (USDA) and the USDHHS. NHANES and WWEIA are conducted as a collaboration between the USDA, USDHHS, and the National Center for Health Statistics at the CDC (USDA et al, 2017).

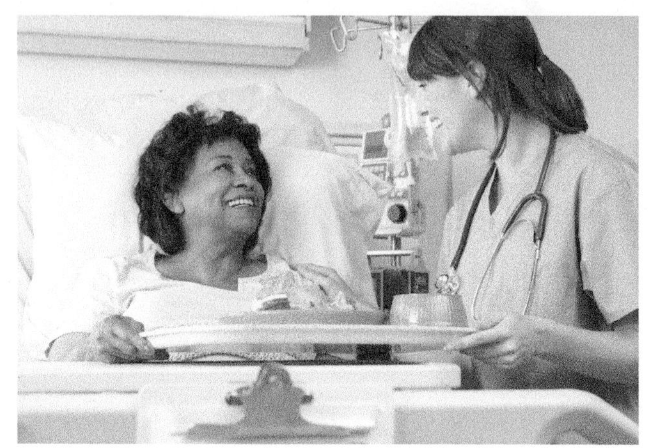

Nutrition is an integral part of health care education. (From www.thinkstockphoto.com)

DISEASE PREVENTION THROUGH NUTRITION

Disease prevention is the recognition of a danger to health that could be reduced or alleviated through specific actions or changes in lifestyle behaviors. The hazard may be caused by disease, lifestyle, or genetic factors or by an environmental threat. The three classifications of disease prevention are primary, secondary, and tertiary. Disease prevention has strong ties to nutrition (see the *Cultural Diversity and Nutrition* box Culturally Competent Care and *Healthy People*).

Primary prevention consists of activities to avert the initial development of a disease or poor health. A primary disease prevention approach is to eat a variety of foods to avert nutrient deficiencies. Adopting a low-fat, high-fiber (plant-based) eating style before diet-related health problems develop is a form of primary prevention.

Secondary prevention involves early detection to halt or reduce the effects of a disease or illness. Some diseases cannot be prevented, but early detection can minimize negative health effects. Secondary prevention strategies are useful to reduce the effects of chronic diet-related diseases. Controlling the intake of certain nutrients can decrease the severity of some disorders. Some individuals with high blood pressure (hypertension) are sodium sensitive, and simply reducing the amount of sodium they consume can decrease their blood pressure levels and thus bring the disorder under control. Because hypertension is a risk factor for coronary artery disease, stroke, and renal disease, reduction of blood pressure through decreased sodium consumption is a secondary prevention strategy.

Tertiary prevention occurs after a disorder develops. The purpose is to minimize further complications or to assist in the restoration of health. These efforts may involve continued medical care. Often, learning more about the disorder is helpful for patients and their families. Tertiary prevention often involves diet therapy. Direct treatments of many disorders have a dietary component. Some of these disorders are ulcers, diverticulitis, and coronary artery disease; they usually occur during the middle and older years of adulthood. Other disorders may

CULTURAL DIVERSITY AND NUTRITION

Culturally Competent Care and Healthy People

Culture can be considered a blend of shared knowledge, acceptance of communal principles, beliefs, and behaviors. Many factors influence cultural groups, such as language, group identifications, traditions, values, and special organizations that may be unique to racial, ethnic, geographic, or spiritual or religious communities (National Institutes of Health [NIH], 2017).

The approach of cultural respect—accepting diversity—that forms our perceptions creates a positive effect on patient care by preparing health providers to offer care that is respectful of and receptive to patients with diverse cultural, ethnic, and racial backgrounds (NIH, 2017). For nurses, as providers of health care and health information, those cultural factors guide the understanding and acceptance of belief systems encompassing wellness, health, illness, and provision of health services.

Lifestyle and behavior are central to the maintenance of health and wellness. To influence lifestyle and behavior, health professionals can take into consideration the values, attitudes, culture, and life circumstances of individuals. Changes in health status, particularly those of minority populations, require professionals to take into account the increasing ethnic and cultural diversity of Americans. Major minority groups in the United States include Asian, Pacific Islander, Black, Latina, and Native Americans. A growing number of Americans are a mix of several racial and ethnic identification and beliefs.

Healthy People reports that premature and excess deaths of ethnic and racial minority populations far outweigh those of White majority groups. Research shows that the factors contributing to this difference are complex and have multiple elements. Socioeconomic status among minority groups is generally lower than among the majority groups. Socioeconomic status is measured by the combination of occupation, income, and educational attainment. A second major factor is the use of and access to health care programs by diverse populations. Many of the available health programs may not be culturally relevant or sensitive to the minority populations they serve. There is a paucity of bilingual and bicultural health professionals, and health education materials are generally not culturally or ethnically specific.

Application to Nursing

Diet and nutrition assessment are imperative to provide culturally competent and respectful care. Efforts to understand dietary patterns of clients need to go beyond relying on their "membership" in a defined group. For example, by learning the assimilative practices of an individual, nurses can assist dietitians in developing the most effective and culturally sensitive nutrition recommendations. Together they can develop a treatment regimen that does not significantly conflict with the cultural food practices of the client but will enhance the journey to wellness.

(From National Institutes of Health (NIH): *Cultural respect*, 2017. Accessed January 9, 2021, from www.nih.gov/institutes-nih/nih-office-director/office-communications-public-liaison/clear-communication/cultural-respect.)

affect food intake and the ability of the body to absorb nutrients. For example, chemotherapy for cancer may have the side effects nausea and loss of appetite. Nutrition counseling during and after these treatments is necessary so patients are as well-nourished as possible to aid the healing process. The six dimensions of health can be an excellent teaching tool in promoting health and preventing diseases related to nutrition.

HEALTH LITERACY

Health literacy is the ability to acquire, comprehend, communicate, and apply basic health information and services, such as nutrition, and apply them to one's own health decisions (CDC, 2016).

So how does health literacy develop? It is not the same as literacy of the printed word, although it is related. Health literacy develops through education on topics related to health promotion and illness. This process of education occurs in three different forms: formal, nonformal, and informal. Formal education is purposefully planned for implementation in an educational setting. Nonformal education takes place through organized teaching and learning events in hospitals, clinics, and community centers. Informal education encompasses a variety of educational experiences that occur through daily activities. The informal experiences include watching television news and other programs, reading newspapers and magazines, browsing the Internet, and conversing with other people. Health information from many sources becomes part of an individual's database of knowledge. Some information may be valid, some may be partially true, and some may be completely false. Our goal is to ensure that health decisions are based on accurate information (see the *Teaching Tool* box Literacy and Health).

Health literacy allows for education to be most effective, resulting in behavior changes. Nurses, through formal, nonformal, and informal educational interactions, can introduce knowledge and strategies for personal lifestyle choices that consider the health context of patients' lives. Health context takes into account the influence of cultural, social, and individual factors on the acquisition of health literacy. Cultural factors may encompass ethnic, religious, and racial traditions surrounding health issues. Social factors create the settings in which members of a community receive support or lack support for health-promoting behaviors. Individual factors reflect on the choices people make regarding willingness to acquire and then apply health knowledge. Health literacy actualization means being able to use acquired health knowledge and skills. The extent to which this occurs within health care settings is influenced by the level to which health care providers are supportive of literate

TEACHING TOOL

Literacy and Health

Although health professionals may take their high level of literacy for granted, many clients do not have a command of basic literacy skills. Limited literacy skills often equate with even more limited health literacy (the ability to use health information to make appropriate health decisions) and with limited numeracy (the ability to understand simple math concepts and apply them in everyday life situations). In fact, low reading skills are associated with poor health and greater use of health services. The implications of these limitations are important because they may limit the effectiveness of a nurse's efforts to educate clients to improve their knowledge and compliance. (Fig. 1.3)

Health literacy affects patient care in many ways; only a few are mentioned here. Simply filling out medical history and consent forms can leave patients struggling. Patients may also have difficulty explaining their symptoms because of limited vocabulary. They may not understand the medical terminology health care providers use to discuss health conditions but may be too uncomfortable to ask for clarification. Even if understood, the recommendations given to clients may be difficult to implement because their ability to decode or understand food labels is limited. Following cooking directions may be hard and serving sizes may be misinterpreted. If clients are to track carbohydrate or sodium consumption, their reading literacy level and numeracy limitations may hinder accuracy and may foster discouragement or worsening of symptoms.

Throughout this textbook, strategies are provided for working with low-literacy clients, discussing the cultural connection, and evaluating and writing health education materials—all with the goal of enhancing health outcomes.

Patients with low
HEALTH LITERACY...

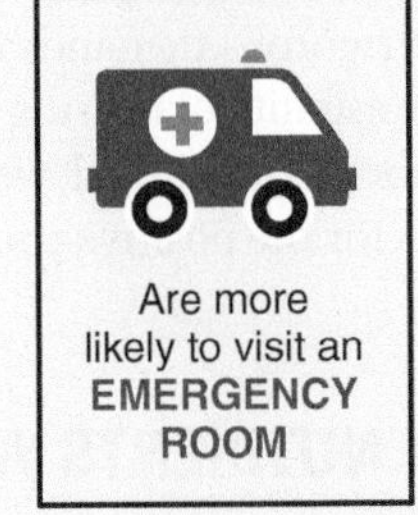
Are more
likely to visit an
EMERGENCY
ROOM

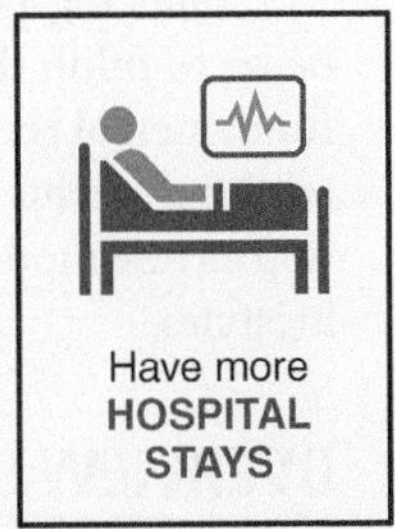
Have more
HOSPITAL
STAYS

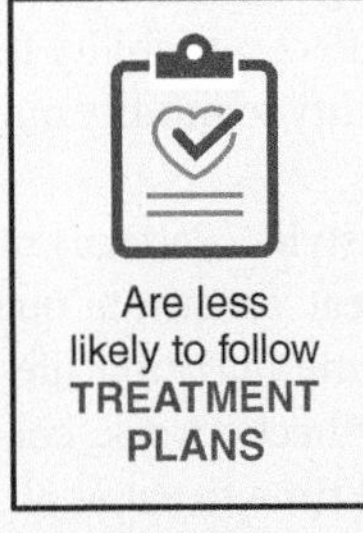
Are less
likely to follow
TREATMENT
PLANS

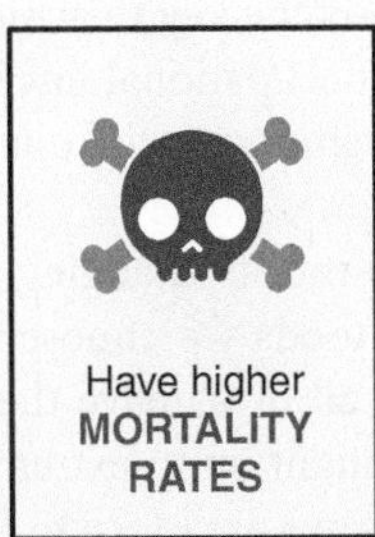
Have higher
MORTALITY
RATES

Fig. 1.3 Patients with low health literacy. (From Patients with low health literacy (cdc.gov)) www.cdc.gov/cpr/infographics/00_docs/healthliteracy.pdf

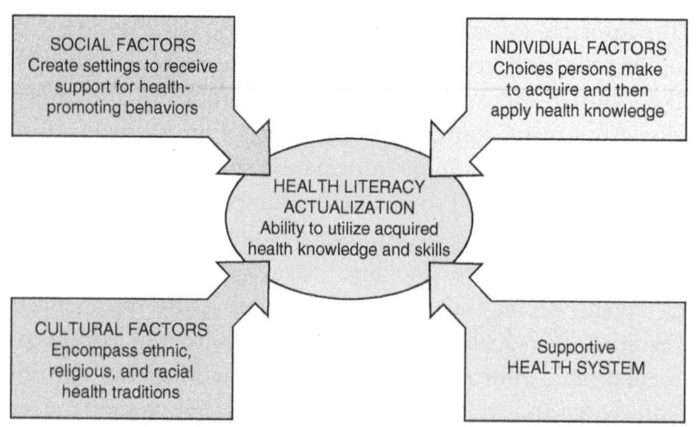

Fig. 1.4 Health literacy context.

health populations seeking greater involvement in their health care (Fig. 1.4).

Nurses are involved with the development of client health literacy (Box 1.2). Formal education may be conducted by school nurses who teach health courses; topics can be approached through the health and nutrition issues of the ethnic and cultural groups of the particular school's population. Nonformal education occurs when associations such as the American Heart Association or hospital wellness programs teach courses on risk-reducing lifestyle changes; these courses are usually open to the community. Informal education takes place when a nurse chats with a patient and his or her family, explaining the purpose of the dietary modifications recommended for the patient's particular disorder.

Researchers are advocating a multidimensional definition of health literacy as an ongoing process involving interactions between the individual and health professionals within the framework of health promotion, health treatment, health care services, and availability. Rather than health literacy defined as a skill level of an individual, this creates a dynamic relationship resulting in multiple levels of change. The variations of outcomes are dependent on the variety of factors composing the interactions. Box 1.2, Health Literacy: Clearly Stated sorts out the health literacy skills for those needing and those providing health information and services (Pleasant et al, 2016).

Modifying Nutrition Lifestyles

Never before have we had so much information about the effects of our personal behavior patterns on our level of health. Changing (or maintaining) our patterns of behaviors—and therefore our lifestyles—is the key to achieving wellness. Many social, community, and occupational forces affect our ability to change. Strategies and techniques ease our ability to modify our personal behaviors.

Modifying behaviors means changing lifestyles. Patterns of behaviors affecting the foods we choose to eat constitute our nutrition lifestyles. Not all of us have the same nutrition lifestyles. Some of us are caught up in extremely hectic work, college, or sports schedules; we are lucky to find time to eat at all. Others find our families of origin still at the center of our eating patterns; our families, however, may not have adopted recent recommendations to decrease the risks of diet-related diseases.

BOX 1.2 Health Literacy: Clearly Stated

What Is Health Literacy?

The Patient Protection and Affordable Care Act of 2010, Title V, defines health literacy as the degree to which an individual has the capacity to obtain, communicate, process, and understand basic health information and services to make appropriate health decisions.

Health Literacy Capacity and Skills

Capacity is the potential a person has to do or accomplish something. Health literacy skills are those people use to realize their potential in health situations. They apply these skills either to make sense of health information and services or provide health information and services to others.

Anyone who needs health information and services also needs health literacy skills to do the following:

- Find information and services
- Communicate their needs and preferences and respond to information and services
- Process the meaning and usefulness of the information and services
- Understand the choices, consequences, and context of the information and services
- Decide which information and services match their needs and preferences so they can act

Anyone who provides health information and services to others, such as a doctor, nurse, dentist, pharmacist, or public health worker, also needs health literacy skills to do the following:

- Help people find information and services
- Communicate about health and health care
- Process what people are explicitly and implicitly asking for
- Understand how to provide useful information and services
- Decide which information and services work best for different situations and people so they can act

(Modified from Centers for Disease Control and Prevention (CDC): *What is health literacy?* Revised September 1, 2020. Accessed January 9, 2021, from www.cdc.gov/healthliteracy/learn/index.html.)

Many of us are part of new social settings on campus and need to adjust to rigid schedules and school cafeteria menus. Yet, despite these variances, we have in common the ability to improve wellness through our nutrition lifestyles.

As health care professionals, we need to be concerned with our own nutritional patterns as well as those of our clients. To reflect a health-promotion perspective, individuals cared for by health professionals to maintain health or who are treated at ambulatory care centers are called clients. Those who are ill or recuperating from illness and are receiving care in hospitals or similar sites are called patients.

Enhancing personal health provides the stamina and well-being to fulfill the rigorous demands of the nursing practice. A fundamental responsibility of nursing is client education. When teaching clients about nutritional wellness, nurses also function as role models for the positive effects of enhanced nutrition lifestyles.

OVERVIEW OF NUTRIENTS WITHIN THE BODY

Which nutrients are the cornerstones of health and disease prevention? What do they do that makes them so important? Why can't we just take a nutrient pill?

TABLE 1.1 Known Essential Nutrients

Nutrient	Source
Carbohydrates	Glucose
Lipids (fats)	Linoleic acid, linolenic acid
Protein	Amino acids: histidine, isoleucine, leucine, lysine, methionine, phenylalanine, threonine, tryptophan, valine
Vitamins	Fat-soluble vitamins: A (retinol), D (cholecalciferol), E (tocopherol), K Water-soluble vitamins: thiamin, riboflavin, niacin, pantothenic acid, biotin, B_6 (pyridoxine), B_{12} (cobalamin), folate, C (ascorbic acid)
Minerals	Major minerals: calcium, phosphorus, sodium, potassium, sulfur, chlorine, magnesium Trace minerals: chromium, cobalt, copper, fluorine, iodine, iron, manganese, selenium, zinc
Water	Water

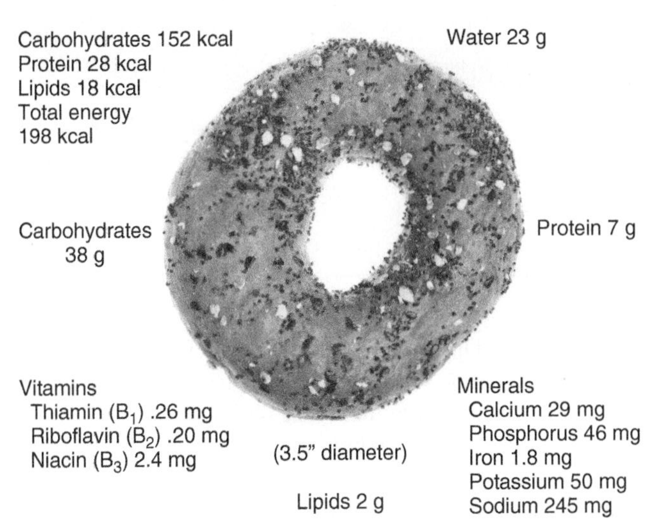

Fig. 1.5 Most foods contain a mixture of nutrients; a food's kilocalorie (kcal) content is based on the energy-yielding nutrients it contains. (Photo from http://www.thinkstockphotos.com; data from U.S. Department of Agriculture, Agricultural Research Service, Nutrient Data Laboratory: *USDA national nutrient database for standard reference* [Release 28], 2017. Accessed October 10, 2020 from https://www.ars.usda.gov/northeast-area/beltsville-md-bhnrc/beltsville-human-nutrition-research-center/methods-and-application-of-food-composition-laboratory/mafcl-site-pages/sr11-sr28/.)

Nutrient Categories

Nutrients can be divided into the following six categories:

1. Carbohydrates
2. Proteins
3. Lipids (fats)
4. Vitamins
5. Minerals
6. Water

Nutrients may be either essential or nonessential, depending on whether the body can manufacture them. When the body requires a nutrient for growth or maintenance but lacks the ability to manufacture amounts sufficient to meet the body's needs, the nutrient is essential and must be supplied by the foods in our diet. Table 1.1 lists the essential nutrients needed in our diet. Other nutrients, which the body can make, are called nonessential. Some nutrients have very specific functions, whereas others are diverse in their impact. Overall, the functions of essential nutrients in the body include the following:

1. ***Providing energy:***
   - Carbohydrates, proteins, and lipids provide energy.
   - Vitamins and minerals have indirect roles as catalysts for the body's use of energy nutrients.
2. ***Regulating body processes:***
   - Proteins, lipids, vitamins, minerals, and water are required.
   - Each vitamin serves a specific function related to regulation.
3. ***Aiding growth and repair of body tissues:***
   - Proteins, lipids, minerals, and water are essential for growth and repair.

FOOD, ENERGY, AND NUTRIENTS

Although the discussion to this point has focused on nutrients, we must remember that nutrients are found in foods. Because foods usually contain a mixture of nutrients, we often categorize a food on the basis of the predominant nutrient it contains. A bagel is a carbohydrate food and contains mostly complex carbohydrates, although it also contains protein, water, small amounts of vitamins and minerals, and an even smaller amount of lipids or fat (Fig. 1.5). The gold mine of nutrients found in whole foods (foods that are minimally processed) is one of the reasons why taking a nutrient-specific pill will not provide for all the necessities of the human body.

Energy

Let's consider the energy-containing nutrients of carbohydrates, protein, and lipids. These contain energy because they are organic. Being organic means they are composed of a structure that consists of hydrogen, oxygen, and carbon. Living or once-living things, including plants and animals, produce organic compounds. The carbon-containing structure identifies these nutrients as being organic. When these nutrients are oxidized (burned in the body), energy is released and available for use by the cells. Although vitamins are also organic, they do not provide energy for the human body. Only carbohydrates, proteins, and lipids are energy-yielding nutrients.

The energy released from food is measured in kilocalories (thousands of calories) or calories. Technically, a calorie is the amount of heat necessary to raise the temperature of a gram of water by 1° C (0.8° F). When someone asks how much energy is in an 8-ounce glass of skim milk, the correct response is 90,000 calories or 90 kilocalories. For numeric simplicity, we commonly refer to the calories in a food rather than using the correct term, kilocalories. To ensure accuracy, the term kilocalories (kcal) is used throughout this text.

Energy-yielding nutrients provide different amounts of energy (Table 1.2). Carbohydrates and proteins each provide

TABLE 1.2 Kilocalorie Values of Types of Foods

Nutrient	Kilocalorie Value per Gram
Carbohydrates	4
Protein	4
Lipids (fats)	9
Alcohol	7

4 kcal per gram. Lipids contain more than twice as much energy as carbohydrates or proteins, providing 9 kcal per gram. The kcal content of a specific food (e.g., a bagel) is based on the amount of carbohydrate, lipid, and protein energy contained in the food (see Fig. 1.5). When we consume energy-yielding foods, we usually ingest other nutrients as well, including vitamins, minerals, and water.

Another energy-yielding substance is alcohol. Alcohol provides 7 kcal per gram. Although alcohol provides energy, it is not considered a nutrient because the body does not need it. In fact, when alcohol is consumed in excess, the body treats it as a toxin. Breaking down or metabolizing alcohol is not only stressful to the body, but also uses essential nutrients that could be better used to nourish the body. Moderate consumption of alcohol, however, may be protective for heart disease. The beneficial components of alcohol-containing beverages such as red wine are phytochemicals—nonnutritive plant substances found in the ingredients (red grapes) used to produce the alcoholic beverages.

Moderate use of alcohol is defined as two servings or fewer per day for men and one serving for women. One serving of alcohol equals 12 ounces of beer, 5 ounces of wine, or 1.5 ounces of 80-proof spirits. Alcohol should be avoided if any of the following apply: driving a vehicle, being pregnant or breastfeeding, taking certain medications, and having certain medical conditions.

Although proteins, lipids, and carbohydrates provide energy, they—along with the other three nutrient categories, vitamins, minerals, and water—have other important functions. A brief introduction to each nutrient category follows.

Carbohydrates

Carbohydrates are a major source of fuel. They consist of simple carbohydrates, often called sugars, and complex carbohydrates, which include starch and most fiber. Simple carbohydrates are found in fruits, milk, and all sweeteners, including white and brown sugar, honey, and high-fructose corn syrup. Complex carbohydrates are found in cereals, grains, pastas, fruits, and vegetables. All, except fiber, are broken down to units of glucose, which is one of the simple carbohydrates. Glucose provides the most efficient form of energy for the body, particularly for muscles and the brain.

Most fiber cannot be broken down by the human digestive system; therefore, it provides little, if any, energy. However, consuming fiber is necessary for good health. Dietary fiber has several beneficial effects on the digestive and absorptive systems of the body. These effects range from preventing constipation to possibly reducing the risk of colon cancer and heart disease.

Proteins

Proteins, in addition to providing energy, perform an extensive range of functions in the body. Some of these functions are roles in the structure of bones, muscles, enzymes, hormones, blood, the immune system, and cell membranes. The linking of amino acids in various combinations forms proteins. Twenty amino acids are required to create all the necessary proteins to maintain life. Some amino acids are formed by the body, whereas others, called essential amino acids, must be consumed in foods. The nine essential amino acids are found in animal and plant sources. Animal sources include meat, fish, poultry, and some dairy products, such as milk and cheeses. Plant sources include grains, legumes (peas and beans that contain protein), seeds, nuts, and many vegetables (albeit in small amounts).

Although protein is important nutritionally, eating too much of it can be a problem. Eating substantially more than the recommended amounts of protein does not produce superhumans. Instead, our physical systems can become overworked. Excess protein is broken down to amino acids. The amino acids are then used for energy or broken down further in metabolic processes and are either stored as body fat or excreted through the kidneys in urine.

Lipids (Fats)

Fats are the densest form of energy available in foods and as stored energy in our bodies. Fats, or lipids, serve other purposes, such as functioning as components of all cell structures, having a role in the production of hormones, and providing padding to protect body organs. Essential fatty acids and the fat-soluble vitamins, A, D, E, and K, are found in food lipids. It is the fats in certain foods that make them taste so appealing.

Lipids are divided into three categories: triglycerides, phospholipids, and sterols. Triglycerides are called saturated, monounsaturated, or polyunsaturated fats according to the types of fatty acids they contain. Fatty acids are carbon chains of varying lengths and degrees of hydrogen saturation. The most common phospholipid is lecithin; among sterols, we hear most about cholesterol. Although we consume lecithin and cholesterol in food, our bodies manufacture them as well.

Fats and cholesterol are often in the news. Saturated fats or triglycerides found in some fat-containing foods, trans fats from processed fats, and dietary cholesterol are associated with increased blood lipid levels. Elevations of blood lipids, whether formed by our bodies or consumed in dietary sources, make up a risk factor for the development of coronary artery disease. Saturated fats, and to a certain extent polyunsaturated fats, also have been associated with increased risk for certain cancers. Coronary artery disease and cancer are serious public health diseases that affect millions of North Americans. Consequently, medical and health professionals emphasize the need to consume better types of fats and to moderate amounts of dietary cholesterol.

Vitamins

Vitamins are compounds that indirectly assist other nutrients through the complete processes of digestion, absorption, metabolism, and excretion. Thirteen vitamins are needed by the body, and each has a specific function. As noted earlier, vitamins provide no energy but assist in the release of energy from carbohydrates, lipids, and proteins.

Vitamins are divided into two classes on the basis of their solubility (i.e., ability to dissolve). The water-soluble vitamins include the B vitamins (thiamin, niacin, riboflavin, folate, cobalamin [B_{12}], pyridoxine [B_6], pantothenic acid, and biotin) and vitamin C. The fat-soluble vitamins, which dissolve in fats, are vitamins A, D, E, and K.

Vitamins are found in many foods; fruits and vegetables are particularly good sources. Because some foods are better sources of specific vitamins, eating a variety of foods is the best way to consume sufficient amounts.

Minerals

Minerals serve structural purposes (e.g., bones and teeth) in the body and are found in body fluids. Minerals in body fluids affect the nature of the fluids, which in turn influences muscle function and the central nervous system. The 16 essential minerals are divided into two categories: major minerals and trace minerals. Although this distinction is based on the quantity of minerals required by the body, all are equally important.

Minerals are plentiful in fruits, vegetables, dairy products, meats, and legumes. Although minerals are indestructible, some may be lost through food processing. For example, when whole-wheat flour is processed or refined to white flour, minerals such as phosphorus and potassium are lost and not replaced.

Water

Water is a major part of every tissue in the body. We can live only a few days without water. Water functions as a fluid in which substances can be broken down and reformed for use by the body. As a constituent of blood, water also provides a means of transportation for nutrients to and from cells.

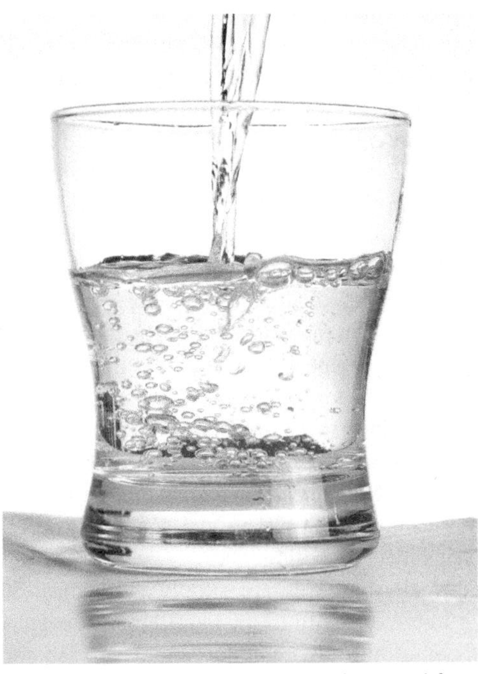

The need for water is more urgent than the need for any other nutrient. (From http://www.thinkstockphotos.com)

Many of us probably do not drink enough water or liquids to best meet the needs of our bodies. We should consume the equivalent of about 9 to 13 cups of water a day from foods and beverages (National Research Council [NRC], 2006). Awareness of the value of water consumption is growing as bottled water companies heavily advertise their products to the public. Bottled waters have become a fashionable alternative to other beverages. These products seem to offer convenience and status against which tap water cannot compete. Although more money may be spent on bottled water than is necessary, the health benefits are still achieved. Unflavored, plain water, whether purchased bottled or drunk from public water supplies, provides the best value; waters fortified with vitamins, minerals, and herbs are not necessary.

DIETARY STANDARDS

Simply knowing which nutrients are essential to life is not sufficient. We need to know how much of each nutrient to consume to be assured of basic good health. Similarly, eating foods without awareness of their nutrient value does not ensure an adequate intake of nutrients. Dietary standards provide a bridge between knowledge of essential nutrients and food consumption. They also provide a guide to adequate nutrient intake levels against which to compare the nutrient values of foods consumed.

Dietary Reference Intakes

In the United States, past dietary standards were based on providing nutrients in amounts that would prevent nutritional deficiency diseases. The current set of nutrient standards, Dietary Reference Intakes (DRIs), combines the classic concerns of deficiency diseases that were the original focus of nutrient recommendations with the contemporary interest of reducing the risk of chronic diet-related diseases, such as coronary artery disease, cancer, and osteoporosis. The DRIs also consider the availability of nutrients, food components, and the use of dietary supplements. They are designed to apply to various individuals and population groups.

Responsibility for dietary standards lies with the Standing Committee on the Scientific Evaluation of Dietary Reference Intakes of the Food and Nutrition Board, Institute of Medicine, and National Academy of Sciences, along with the participation of Health Canada. The DRIs are now the nutrient recommendations for the United States and Canada.

The DRIs are based on (1) reviewing the available scientific data about specific nutrient use, (2) assessing the function of these nutrients to reduce the risk of chronic and other diseases and conditions, such as coronary artery disease and cancer, and (3) evaluating current data on nutrient consumption levels among U.S. and Canadian populations.

Dietary Reference Intakes Lingo

The DRIs consist of the estimated average requirement, the recommended dietary allowance, adequate intake, the tolerable upper intake level, and acceptable macronutrient distribution ranges.

The estimated average requirement (EAR) is the amount of a nutrient needed to meet the basic requirements of half the individuals in a specific group that represents the needs of a population. The EAR considers issues of deficiency and physiologic functions. Public health nutrition researchers and policymakers primarily use the EARs to determine the basis for setting the RDAs.

The **recommended dietary allowance (RDA)** is the level of nutrient intake sufficient to meet the needs of almost all healthy individuals of a life-stage and gender group. The aim is to supply an adequate nutrient intake to decrease the risk of chronic disease. The RDA is based on EARs for that nutrient, plus an additional amount to provide for the particular need of each group. Some nutrients have an adequate intake, not an RDA.

Adequate intake (AI) is the approximate level of an average nutrient intake determined by observation of or experimentation with a particular group or population that appears to maintain good health. The AI is used when there are insufficient data to set an RDA.

The **tolerable upper intake level (UL)** is the level of nutrient intake that should not be exceeded to prevent adverse health risks. This amount includes total consumption from foods, fortified foods, and supplements. The UL is not a recommended level of intake but a safety boundary for total consumption. ULs exist only for nutrients for which adverse risks are known.

Acceptable macronutrient distribution ranges (AMDRs) are daily percentage energy intake values for the macronutrients fat, carbohydrate, and protein. For these energy-yielding nutrients, the following daily intake ranges are set to provide adequate energy and nutrients while offering reduced risk of chronic disorders:

- 45% to 65% of kcal intake from carbohydrate
- 20% to 35% of kcal intake from fat
- 10% to 35% of kcal intake from protein

The DRIs are designed to meet the needs of most healthy individuals. Individuals generally use the RDAs and AIs when assessing their nutrient intakes. People with special nutritional needs, such as those suffering from disease, injury, or other medical conditions, may have nutrient needs that are higher than the DRIs.

Use of Dietary Reference Intakes

The DRIs are widely used throughout the U.S. food systems, such as in the following activities:

- Planning meals for large groups, such as the military
- Creating dietary standards for governmental food assistance programs, such as the Special Supplemental Nutrition Program for Women, Infants and Children (WIC) and Supplemental Nutrition Assistance Program (SNAP)
- Interpreting food consumption information for individuals and populations

Although originally intended only for analysis of the diets of large groups of people, DRIs can be used for individuals if compared with an average intake over time. The intake of a single day does not have to meet the recommended levels. A comparison with the DRIs does not determine nutritional status but is only one of several measurements used to assess nutritional status, as follows:

- Meeting national nutrition goals such as those listed in *HP2030*
- Developing new food products, such as imitation products, that duplicate the nutrient values of the original

However, the DRI standards are not the basis of the nutrient information that appears on food and supplement products. The daily value (DV) is used for nutrition labeling and is based on dietary standards from 1968, when nutrition labeling was first implemented. When the current food labeling standards were revised in 1994, the U.S. Food and Drug Administration did not update the nutrient values. (See Chapter 2, Consumer Information and Wellness, for a detailed discussion of food labeling.)

Additional Standards

The **estimated energy requirement (EER)** is the DRI for dietary energy intake. The EER aims to maintain good health by providing energy intake levels to maintain individuals' body weights within specific age, gender, height, weight, and physical activity categories. These energy intake recommendations are an average of the need for each category. To avoid recommending potentially excessive intakes of energy, a margin of safety is not added; consuming too much energy may be a primary cause of obesity, a major public health issue that increases chronic disease risk.

Global Standards

Other countries have developed dietary standards on the basis of energy needs, food supply, or environmental factors that affect their populations. In addition, organizations such as the Food and Agriculture Organization of the United Nations, along with the WHO, have developed dietary standards that meet the practical needs of healthy adults worldwide.

Why are nutrient recommendations not the same for every country or population? After all, the needs of the human body must be the same around the world. The difference lies in the definitions and purposes of nutrient recommendations.

Standards may be designed to provide the basic amount of a nutrient to prevent deficiency symptoms or to supply sufficient amounts for basic good health. These amounts may differ substantially according to the nature of the nutrient, such as whether it is stored in the body. In addition, health professionals of a nation or organization may interpret the same scientific data differently, arriving at various recommended amounts.

Whether a standard is set to provide for only basic nutrient needs may depend on the availability of food. In the United States, where access to food is easy and the supply plentiful, the setting of nutrient recommendations higher than minimum levels is reasonable; most citizens have access to foods to meet those levels. In parts of the world where the food supply is more limited, the immediate goal is to supply as many individuals as possible with basic needs to prevent deficiencies.

Some values differ from the U.S. standards on the basis of the most common sources of nutrients worldwide. For example, most of the world relies heavily on plant protein sources, whereas North Americans use mainly animal sources. Recommended protein levels reflect this difference.

Ultimately all standards are simply guidelines. Standards represent a range of the nutrient requirements, even when set at a specific amount. Individual needs may vary, so consuming enough food to meet the basic amounts should be each person's nutritional goal.

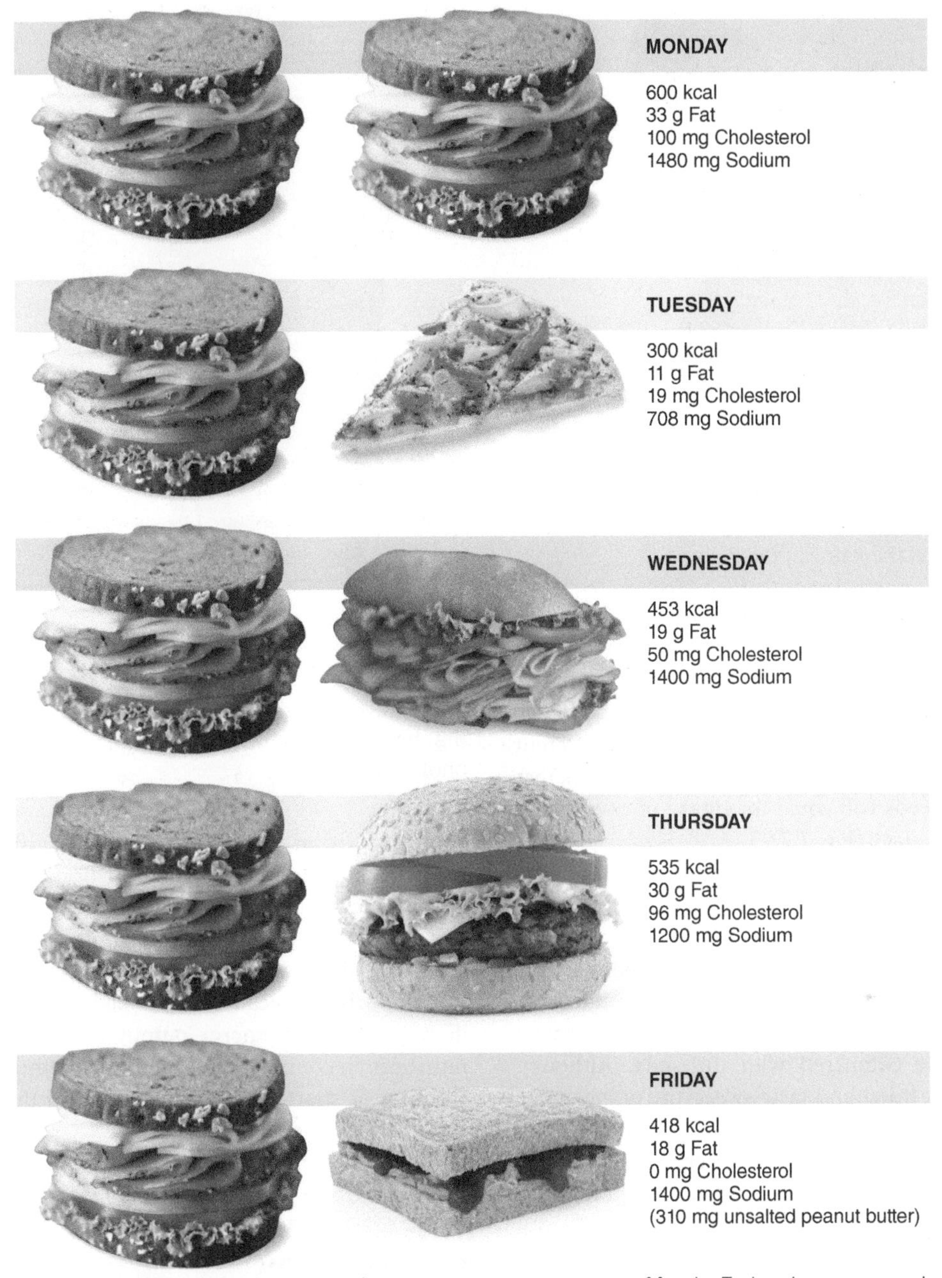

Fig. 1.6 An adequate eating pattern incorporates an assortment of foods. Eating the same sandwich every day may be convenient, but an assortment of foods over a 5-day period provides a daily average of fewer calories and a greater variety of nutrients. (Data from U.S. Department of Agriculture, Agricultural Research Service, Nutrient Data Laboratory: *USDA national nutrient database for standard reference* [Release 28], 2017. Accessed October 10, 2020, from https://www.ars.usda.gov/northeast-area/beltsville-md-bhnrc/beltsville-human-nutrition-research-center/methods-and-application-of-food-composition-laboratory/mafcl-site-pages/sr11-sr28/.)

ADEQUATE EATING PATTERNS

Knowing the DRIs makes nutrition seem simple. Just eat enough of the DRI nutrients, and good health seems ensured. However, we don't eat nutrients; we eat foods. For an eating pattern to be considered adequate, the foods we eat must provide all the essential nutrients plus fiber and energy. An adequate eating pattern takes into account assortment, balance, and nutrient density.

Assortment addresses the value of eating a variety of foods from every food group. Eating the same foods every day may be convenient but may not serve health and nutrient needs. The limited selection of foods may not contain sufficient amounts of essential nutrients and dietary fiber or may be high in some nutrients, such as fat, and low in others, such as vitamin A. As shown in Fig. 1.6, eating a ham and cheese sandwich every day may seem like a quick lunchtime solution, but an assortment of selections over a 5-day period provides a daily average of fewer calories, less fat, less cholesterol, and less sodium. A good strategy is to adopt a habit of selecting different foods for lunch or, at the least, rotating food choices throughout the week.

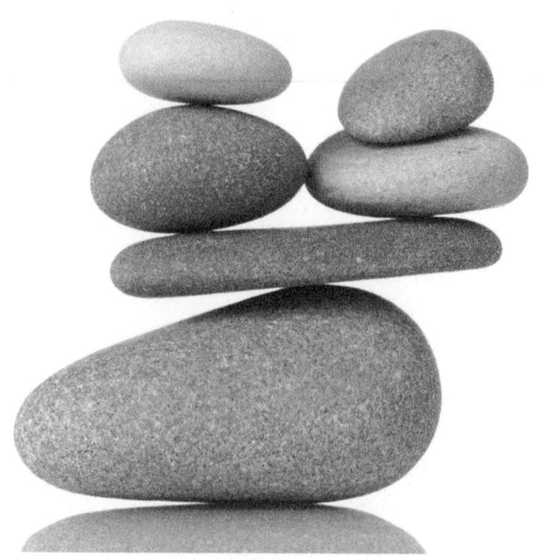

Fig. 1.7 A balance of nutrients in the diet helps ensure adequacy. (From http://www.thinkstockphotos.com)

An eating pattern exhibiting balance will provide foods from all the food groups in quantities so essential nutrients are consumed in proportion to one another, thus achieving a balance among the levels of nutrients eaten. The USDA's food guidance system MyPlate represents this concept by considering different food groups and numbers of servings. Balance also ensures that energy plus nutrient needs will equal the intake of energy and nutrients to satisfy adequacy (Fig. 1.7).

Nutrient density assigns value to a food on the basis of a comparison of its nutrient content with the kcal the food contains. The more nutrients and the fewer kcal a food provides, the higher its nutrient density. Fig. 1.8 demonstrates that a 12-ounce glass of orange juice contains many more nutrients than a 12-ounce soda, which contains "empty" kcal. The orange juice is nutrient dense compared with the soda. Although both may quench your thirst and taste sweet, the orange juice supplies so much more for similar kcal.

No single food contains all the nutrients essential for optimum health. An adequate eating pattern incorporates an assortment of foods.

Undernutrition, Overnutrition, and Malnutrition

Estimates of food consumption are often used to determine the nutritional status of individuals and populations. Sometimes, if the dietary intake is imbalanced, undernutrition, overnutrition, or malnutrition may be diagnosed.

Undernutrition is the consumption of not enough energy or nutrients compared with DRI values. This means either not eating enough food to take in all the essential nutrients or eating enough food for energy but choosing foods that lack certain nutrients. In the United States, some women do not consume enough of the vitamin folate, although the rest of their nutrient intake is adequate. Folate is very important during the childbearing years, as discussed in Chapter 7.

Overnutrition is consumption of too many nutrients and too much energy compared with DRI values. North Americans generally overconsume saturated fats, which is a risk factor for the development of heart disease.

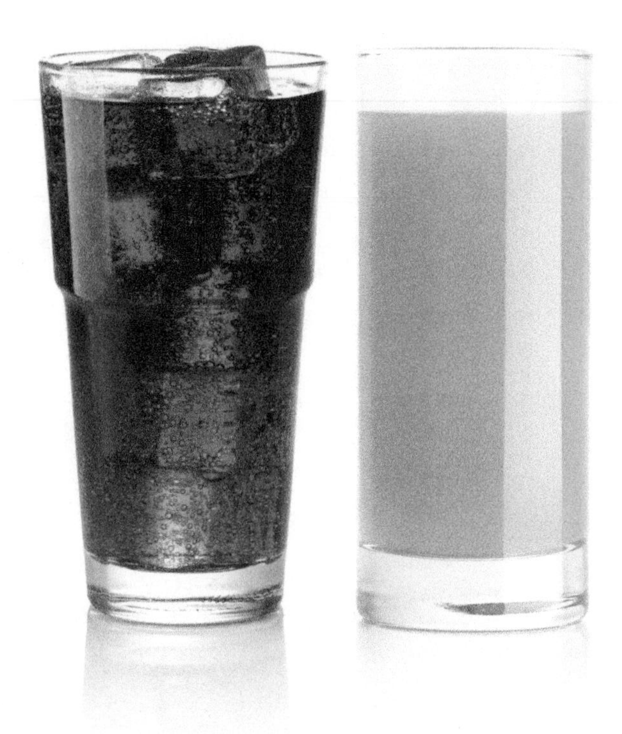

Fig. 1.8 The more nutrients and the fewer kcal a food provides, the higher its nutrient density. (From http://www.thinkstockphotos.com)

Malnutrition is a condition resulting from an imbalanced nutrient or energy intake. Malnutrition is both undernutrition and overnutrition—consumption of too few nutrients or too low an energy intake and excess nutrient or energy consumption. An obese man who consumes an excessive amount of kcal is malnourished because his intake is out of balance. His intake does not equal his energy output. A nutrient overdose is malnutrition. In contrast, a college student who constantly diets for slimness or sports, consuming less than the DRI for nutrients and energy, is also malnourished.

TOWARD A POSITIVE NUTRITION LIFESTYLE: SELF-EFFICACY

Achieving wellness is an ongoing process. We all experience times when meeting our personal dietary goals is easy and other times when it seems as if we will never regain a sense of control over our nutrition lifestyles. These ups and downs are all part of the process of achieving wellness.

To support our pathway toward achieving wellness, this section in each chapter will feature psychosocial strategies to enhance positive self-efficacy. Self-efficacy is our perception of our ability to have power over our lives and behaviors. Positive self-efficacy means believing that personal behaviors can be changed, and one has control over one's life. Negative self-efficacy refers to feeling as if one is powerless, with little control over circumstances. A sense of positive self-efficacy is essential to attaining and then maintaining nutrition lifestyles for optimum health. These strategies may be applicable in our own life situations and are useful for our clients as they, too, strive for enhanced self-efficacy.

SUMMARY

- Health is the merging and balancing of six physical and psychological dimensions: physical, intellectual, emotional, social, spiritual, and environmental. Wellness is a lifestyle that enhances our level of health, resulting in a sense of competency and achievement to modify behaviors to increase or maintain positive levels of health.
- Health promotion consists of strategies used to increase the level of the health of individuals, families, groups, and communities. Development of positive behaviors may depend on knowledge, techniques, and community supports.
- *Healthy People 2030 (HP2030)* is a set of national health goals and objectives for the United States that considers the overlapping of environmental and social determinants of health as affecting health outcomes.
- Health literacy is the ability to acquire and comprehend basic health concepts, such as nutrition, and apply them to one's own health decisions.
- Health context considers the influence of cultural, social, and individual factors on the acquisition of health literacy.
- Nutrition, the study of nutrients and the processes by which they are used by the body, uses six nutrient categories: carbohydrates, proteins, lipids (fats), vitamins, minerals, and water.
- The functions of essential nutrients are providing energy, regulating body processes, and aiding growth and repair of body tissues.
- Dietary Reference Intakes (DRIs) are a set of dietary standards intended to prevent nutrient deficiency diseases and to reduce the risk of chronic diet-related disorders.
- The DRIs include estimated average requirement (EAR), recommended dietary allowance (RDA), adequate intake (AI), tolerable upper intake level (UL), and acceptable macronutrient distribution range (AMDR).
- An adequate eating pattern considers assortment, balance, and nutrient density. If dietary intake is imbalanced, undernutrition, overnutrition, or malnutrition may occur.

THE NURSING APPROACH: CLINICAL JUDGMENT AND NEXT-GENERATION NCLEX® EXAMINATION-STYLE QUESTIONS

Nurses Assisting with Nutrition—Using the Nursing Process and the Clinical Judgment Measurement Model

The nursing process is a systematic method of thinking used widely by nurses to organize the care of individuals, groups, and communities. It is similar to the problem-solving method. The nursing process is cyclical, and is revised as patients' needs change. The steps of the nursing process can be remembered with the acronym ADPIE: assessment, diagnosis, planning, implementation, and evaluation. The nursing process components follow the sequence of assessing, diagnosing, planning, implementing, and evaluating. Legally, nurses are accountable by their licenses and scopes of practice to assess the patient's health care status, make a diagnosis about patient responses to actual or potential health problems, develop plans to meet identified needs, implement specific nursing interventions, and revaluate patient outcomes.

The Clinical Judgment Measurement Model

The Clinical Judgment Measurement Model (CJMM) and the item types were developed to effectively test clinical judgment, described as a necessary component to delivering effective and safe care and is the foundation of quality nursing care (Dickison et al, 2019; Manetti, 2019). There are six cognitive processes/skills measured in the CJMM (Dickison et al, 2019). These include:

- **Recognize cues:** Identifying significant data from many sources (assessment)
- **Analyze cues:** Connecting the data to the client's presentation—is this data expected? Unexpected? What are the concerns? (analysis)
- **Prioritize hypotheses:** Rank the hypotheses; concerns, client needs (analysis, diagnosis)
- **Generate solutions:** Use hypotheses to determine interventions for an expected outcome (planning)
- **Take actions:** Implement the generated solutions addressing the highest priorities or hypotheses (implementation)
- **Evaluate outcomes:** compare observed outcomes with expected ones (evaluation)

The Clinical Judgment Measurement Model and its relationship to the Nursing Process

The CJMM is a flexible model that presents the complex entities associated with decision making in a simplified manner (Dickison et al, 2019) and can guide nurse educators to measure the application of specific cognitive processes necessary for decision making and rendering clinical judgments. As an Action Model according to the NCSBN (Dickison et al, 2019), it closes the gap between what is taught in clinical nursing education and what is measured on the exam.

Steps of the Nursing Process/Clinical Judgment Measurement Model

Assessment/Recognize Cues

Definition: Collecting, organizing, and recording patient information obtained through interview, physical assessment, and reading patient charts and recognizing important data from many sources.

Example: The nurse asks a patient about his or her appetite and how the patient's culture may affect personal food choices and identifies significant data from many sources. The nurse also obtains the patient's height and weight, records fluid intake and urinary output, and monitors laboratory results.

Assessment may be comprehensive or focused, depending on the situation. The data recorded may be objective, sometimes referred to as signs (e.g., vomiting, grimacing, and moaning), or subjective sometimes referred to as symptoms (e.g., nausea and pain).

Diagnosis (Nursing)/Analyze Cues

Definition: A clinical judgment about patient responses to actual or potential health problems. After assessing the patient, the nurse selects cues for the specific individual patient. The nurse also connects the data or cues to the client's presentation.

The statement may have two or three parts. Examples of these statements are in the case studies. Example: Fluid overload related to decreased cardiac output and excess sodium intake as evidenced by blood pressure 170/90, pitting edema, jugular venous distention, and weight gain of 2 pounds in 1 week.

Prioritize hypotheses: Rank the hypotheses: concerns, client needs (analysis).

Definition: (1) Establishing priorities; (2) setting realistic, measurable patient outcomes; and (3) deciding which nursing interventions are best to use.

Continued

 THE NURSING APPROACH: CLINICAL JUDGMENT AND NEXT-GENERATION NCLEX® EXAMINATION-STYLE QUESTIONS—cont'd

Generating hypotheses is done to determine interventions for an expected outcome (planning). Example: The patient will gain 1 pound by August 31.

Planning/Generate Solutions

The plan of care should be developed by a team composed of health care professionals and in cooperation with the patient. The solutions generated may be prescribed by the physician or nurse practitioner, directed by the registered dietitian/nutritionist (RDN), or designed independently by the nurse.

Examples of solutions to support nutrition include the following:

- Provide snacks and supplements in between meals.
- Give medicine to counteract nausea, vomiting, or pain.
- Teach the patient guidelines for following the new diet.
- Assist the patient to choose appropriate selections from the hospital menu.
- Assist with eating because of weakness or other physical problems.

Independent nursing solutions generated are planned according to the analysis of cues related to the causes or contributing factors identified. When developing solutions, nurses must understand nutrition care for patients with a variety of health conditions. They must be able to support the solutions they select for individual patients with a scientific rationale. Examples of these rationales are in the case studies. Nurses are responsible for evidence-based practice, choosing solutions on the basis of proven nursing research results.

Implementation/Take Action

Definition: Carrying out the plan and taking action, as well as documenting the care provided. Implementing the generated solutions and addressing the highest priorities or hypotheses (implementation/take action).

Example: Provided 8 fluid ounces of a nutritional supplement twice a day between meals.

The RDN is the expert in food and nutrition. However, it is usually the nurse who interacts most often with the patient throughout the day and night and is therefore in a position to provide and coordinate the solutions developed by the interdisciplinary team.

Evaluation/Evaluate Outcomes

Definition: Assessing to what extent the patient outcomes were met and revising the solutions as needed. Also, comparing observed outcomes with expected ones (evaluation).

Example: The patient gained one-half pound within 5 days. Goal partially met.

The Next Generation NCLEX® (NGN) and the types of questions are based on The Clinical Judgment Measurement Model (CJMM) that will be included on the examination. Currently, the types of NGN test items that will be part of the new examination include enhanced hot spot/highlight, enhanced select all that apply (SATA), enhanced drag and drop, matrix/grid, and cloze (drop down). The new NCLEX® examination will be a combination of current NCLEX® item types and NGN items (Silvestri, 2020).

Current Test Question	Current Question Type	Current Cognitive Skill	Potential Cognitive Skill(s) That Can Be Measured	Additional Content Needed to Revise to NGN	Revised Question	NGN Item Type
The nurse is monitoring a client receiving a blood transfusion. The nurse would watch for which specific sign of a blood transfusion reaction? 1. Chills 2. Fatigue 3. Lack of appetite 4. Elevation in blood pressure	Multiple Choice	Recognize Cues	• Recognize cues • Analyze cues • Prioritize hypotheses • Generate solutions • Take actions	Add data to the question that indicates a transfusion reaction; data should not tell the student that the client is having a reaction. Add data to the question that would require differentiating between significant and insignificant data.	The nurse is administering a unit of blood and checks vital signs. The vital signs are: T 39.8° C, P 110 bpm, RR 20 bpm, BP 100/58 mm Hg, SpO_2 95% RA. The client complains of "feeling funny," lower back pain, chills, and feels flushed. Which prescribed measures would the nurse take to safely manage the care of this client? **Select all that apply**. 1. Stop the transfusion 2. Administer antibiotics 3. Administer furosemide 4. Administer acetaminophen 5. Administer diphenhydramine 6. Administer intravenous fluids	Enhanced hot spot/highlight, Enhanced SATA, Enhanced drag and drop, Cloze, Matrix/grid

NGN Test Item Types

1. ***Enhanced Hot Spot/Highlighting:*** requires the reader/test taker to highlight data that are relevant to answer the question.
2. ***Cloze:*** requires the reader/test taker to fill in two or more blanks to complete statements or tables, e.g., drug tables. Options that provide the missing information are listed for each blank.
3. ***Extended Multiple Response:*** (similar to the current Select All That Apply) requires the reader/test taker to select all of the choices that answer the question. Up to 10 choices may be provided.
4. ***Extended Drag and Drop:*** requires the reader/test taker to choose from a list of options to match them with selected complications, medications, client or nurse responses, etc.
5. ***Matrix/Grid:*** requires the reader/test taker to choose the status of multiple actions or assessments as part of a grid or table.

Case Study Types

Oermann and Gaberson (2017) differentiated three types of cases that focus on the patient experience:

1. ***Case Method:*** Short clinical scenario (1–2 sentences) that provides only the essential data; 1–2 related questions (usually do not require high-level thinking).
   a. What assessment information in this patient situation is the most important and of immediate concern for the nurse? (Identify the relevant information first to help you determine what is most important.) [Recognize Cues]
2. ***[Single-Episode] Case Study:*** Comprehensive clinical scenario that requires analysis and decision-making; multiple related high-level-thinking questions.
   a. What patient conditions are consistent with the most relevant information? (Think about priority collaborative problems that support and contradict the information presented in this situation.) [Analyze Cues]

Continued

THE NURSING APPROACH: CLINICAL JUDGMENT AND NEXT-GENERATION NCLEX® EXAMINATION-STYLE QUESTIONS—cont'd

3. ***Unfolding Case Study:*** Initial comprehensive clinical scenario that changes over time (several phases of care) as the patient's condition changes; requires analysis and decision-making; multiple related high-level-thinking questions for each phase of care.
   a. Which possibilities or explanations are most likely to be present in this patient situation? Which possibilities or explanations are the most serious or priority? (Consider all possibilities and determine their urgency and risk for this patient.) [Prioritize Hypotheses]
   b. What actions would most likely achieve the desired outcomes for this patient? Which actions should be avoided, are irrelevant, or are potentially harmful? (Determine the desired outcomes first to help you decide which actions are appropriate and those that should be avoided.) [Generate Solutions]
   c. Which actions are the most appropriate and how should they be implemented? In what priority order should they be implemented? (Consider health teaching, documentation, requested primary health care provider orders/prescriptions, nursing skills, collaboration with or referral to health team members, etc.) [Take Action]
   d. What patient assessment would indicate that your actions were effective? (Think about signs that would indicate an improvement, decline, or unchanged patient condition.) [Evaluate Outcomes]

Using the Nursing Approach Boxes

The Nursing Approach boxes describe experiences of nurses from a variety of settings and levels, including nurse practitioners and nurses from the hospital, the clinic, home health, occupational health, and schools. Regardless of the setting, the nurse is in a unique position to assess and help improve an individual's nutritional status. The nurse who has practical knowledge of basic nutrition will appreciate the importance of dietary intake in maintaining the patient's good health and in facilitating the patient's recovery from disease or injury. By ensuring that the patient receives adequate nutrition and hydration, the nurse acts as the patient's advocate for health, healing, and well-being.

While going through each The Nursing Approach box, answer the questions at the end of each case study by using clinical judgment strategies.

Case Study

The nurse is caring for a client who is on hemodialysis and fluid restrictions. The client is complaining of increased thirst. The nurse educates the client in actions to relieve thirst to promote adherence to the fluid restrictions. What are some of the actions the nurse suggests to help relieve the client of increased thirst?

Use an X to mark the undesirable assessment findings that require follow up by the nurse.

1. Warming fluids so that they are easier to swallow
2. Sucking on hard candy
3. Avoid adding lemon juice to the water to prevent a sour taste
4. Gargling with warmed mouthwash
5. Chewing gum
6. Put a mouthful of broken ice cubes in the mouth each hour

(Data from Dickison P, Haerling KA, Lasater K: Integrating the National Council of State Boards of Nursing Clinical Judgment Model into nursing educational frameworks. *Journal of Nursing Education* 58(2):72–78, 2019; Manetti W: Sound clinical judgment in nursing: A concept analysis, *Nursing Forum* 54:102–110, 2019; Oermann MH, Gaberson KB: *Evaluation and testing in nursing education* ed 5, New York, 2017, Springer Publishing; Silvestri L: *Higher-Cognitive-Level Test Questions: A Starting Point for Creating Next Generation NCLEX® (NGN) Test Items*, Elsevier, 2–3, 2020.)

APPLYING CONTENT KNOWLEDGE

Health promotion strategies often involve lifestyle changes. Bob needs to reduce his dietary fat intake because he is at risk for coronary vascular disease. He lives in a suburban community and takes a train into New York City, where he works. Although it is only a half mile to the train station, he usually drives his car there to save time. Breakfast is often coffee, with a midmorning break that consists of a Danish and more coffee. He obtains lunch from street vendors who sell hot dogs and sausage sandwiches. Bob usually eats dinner with his family, but it often features meat and potatoes, his favorites. Because he leaves early in the morning and returns tired in the evening, he says he doesn't know how to change his behavior.

Using the strategies of knowledge, techniques, and community supports, describe the education care plan that could be developed with Bob.

WEBSITES OF INTEREST

Academy of Nutrition and Dietetics
www.eatright.org
A resource about nutrition, health, wellness, and dietetic professionals.

Healthy People
www.healthypeople.gov
The official website of *Healthy People 2030.*

Nutrient Data Laboratory
www.ars.usda.gov/nutrientdata
A nutrient database of food items commonly consumed in the United States.

REFERENCES

Centers for Disease Control and Prevention (CDC): What is health literacy? 2016. From: www.cdc.gov/healthliteracy/learn/index.html. (Accessed 26 August, 2017).

Centers for Disease Control and Prevention/National Center for Health Statistics (CDC/NCHS): National Health and Nutrition Examination Survey. 2021 (last update). From: www.cdc.gov/nchs/nhanes/index.htm. (Accessed 13 September, 2021).

Centers for Disease Control and Prevention/National Center for Health Statistics (CDC/NCHS): What We Eat in America, DHHS-USDA Dietary Survey Integration. 2015. From: www.cdc.gov/nchs/nhanes/wweia.htm. (Accessed 22 August, 2017).

Dubos, R. (1968). *So Human the Animal*. New York: Scribner's.

National Center for Health Statistics (NCHS): *Healthy People 2020 Midcourse Review*, Hyattsville, MD, 2016. From: www.cdc.gov/nchs/data/hpdata2020/HP2020MCR-C29-NWS.pdf. (Accessed 18 August, 2017).

National Research Council (NRC). (2006). *Dietary Reference Intakes: The Essential Guide to Nutrient Requirements*. Washington, DC: The National Academies Press.

Pleasant, A., Rudd, R. E., O'Leary, C., et al. (2016). *Considerations for a new definition of health literacy*, Washington, DC, Discussion Paper, National Academy of Medicine. From: nam.edu/wp-content/uploads/2016/04/Considerations-for-a-New-Definition-of-Health-Literacy.pdf. (Accessed 28 August, 2017).

U.S. Department of Agriculture, Agricultural Research Service, Beltsville Human Nutrition Research Center, Food Surveys Research Group (Beltsville, MD) and U.S. Department of Health and Human Services, Centers for Disease Control and Prevention, National Center for Health Statistics (Hyattsville, MD) (USDA) et al: What we eat in America, National Health and Nutrition Examination Survey. From: www.ars.usda.gov/Services/docs.htm?docid=13793. (Accessed 18 August, 2017).

U.S. Department of Health and Human Services, Office of Disease Prevention and Health Promotion (USDHHS): Healthy People 2030: Framework, n.d. From: www.healthypeople.gov/2020/About-Healthy-People/Development-Healthy-People-2030/Framework. (Accessed 3 October, 2020).

World Health Organization: Preamble to the Constitution of the World Health Organization as adopted by the International Health Conference, New York, 19-22 June, 1946; signed on 22 July, 1946 by the representatives of 61 States (*Official Records of the World Health Organization*, no. 2, p. 100) and entered into force on 7 April, 1948. From: www.who.int/bulletin/archives/80(12)981.pdf. (Accessed 20 June, 2021).

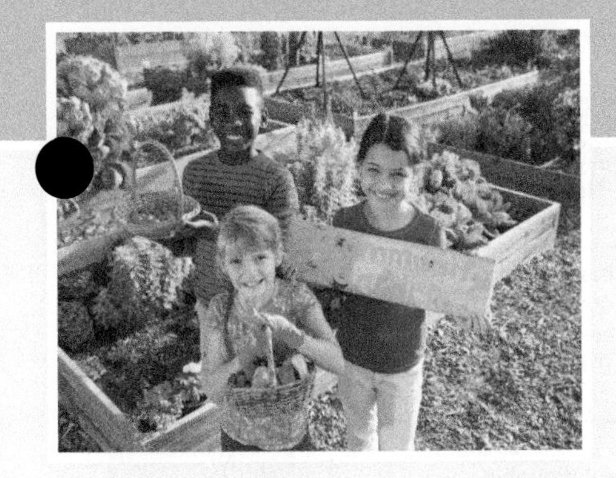

2

Personal and Community Nutrition

The nutritional status of our communities is a reflection of our individual nutritional health.

http://evolve.elsevier.com/GRODNER/FOUNDATIONS

LEARNING OBJECTIVES

- Identify factors that influence food selection.
- Describe the Dietary Guidelines for Americans, 2020–2025 (Dietary Guidelines).
- Discuss the relationship between *Dietary Guidelines*, MyPlate, and Daily Food Plan.
- List the information required on the Nutrition Facts panel.
- Explain the purpose of food label descriptors and health claims.

Have you ever thought about who is responsible for your health? Perhaps you thought of your parents, spouse, or significant other. Or possibly you have always taken your health for granted, not as something to actively work toward improving or maintaining. What influences your health behaviors? What about the health of the community in which you live or work? Have you ever considered the health status of the residents of your town or college community?

Factors affecting the main health indicators of HealthyPeople 2030 introduced in Chapter 1 occur on several levels of influence as presented in Fig. 2.1 NIMHD Research Framework. The levels of influence involve Individual, Interpersonal, Community, and Societal stages, which are intertwined within the domains of influence of Biological, Behavioral, Physical/Built Environment, Sociocultural Environment, and Health Care System through the lifespan. This research framework is envisioned to address and enhance factors supporting or impacting minority health goals, while mitigating and reducing health disparities. Therefore, specific factors within the levels and domains of influence will vary, depending on the individuals and larger populations for whom a similar framework could be applied.

Consequently, the health of the individual is tied to the overall health of the community and societal/institutional structures. Likewise, the health status of the community is influenced by the shared attitudes and actions of those who reside in it. To support promotion of good health, we must take responsibility for our personal health and the health of communities at large. This chapter considers strategies to improve our health by taking charge of our personal nutrition and becoming aware of the nutrition issues of our communities.

ROLE IN WELLNESS

As presented in Part 1, Chapter 1, wellness is a lifestyle through which we continually strive to enhance our level of health. Health is the merging and balancing of physical, intellectual, emotional, social, spiritual, and environmental dimensions. Considering these dimensions in relation to personal and community nutrition broadens our understanding. The physical health dimension is represented by the food guides presented in this chapter. By following the recommendations of the food guides, we may reduce the risk of diet-related diseases. Consumer decisions about food purchases and application of food safety recommendations depend on reasoning abilities that reflect the intellectual health dimension. The emotional health dimension may affect a person's ability to be flexible when adopting suggested guideline changes. If we (or our patients) have problems doing so, will we view ourselves as "failures"? The social health dimension is tested as we (and our patients) interact with family and friends while we attempt to follow the guidelines. Can we be role models for others without being perceived as threats? Many religions stress personal responsibility for caring for one's body, which embodies the spiritual health dimension. Part of that responsibility includes the foods we choose to eat. The environmental health dimension considers access to safe and conducive settings to support preparation and consumption of nutritious meals.

Levels of Influence*	Domains of Influence (Over the Lifecourse)					
	Biological	Behavioral	Physical/Built Environment	Sociocultural Environment	Health Care System	Health Outcomes
Individual	• Biological vulnerability and mechanisms	• Health behaviors • Coping strategies	• Personal environment	• Sociodemographics • Limited English • Cultural identity • Response to discrimination	• Insurance coverage • Health literacy • Treatment preferences	Individual Health
Interpersonal	• Caregiver–child interaction • Family microbiome	• Family functioning • School/work functioning	• Household environment • School/work environment	• Social networks • Family/peer norms • Interpersonal discrimination	• Patient-clinician relationship • Medical decision-making	Family/ Organizational Health
Community	• Community illness • Exposure • Herd immunity	• Community functioning	• Community environment • Community resources	• Community norms • Local structural discrimination	• Availability of services • Safety net services	Community Health
Societal	• Sanitation • Immunization • Pathogen exposure	• Policies and laws	• Societal structure	• Social norms • Societal structure discrimination	• Quality of care • Health care policies	Population Health

*Health Disparity Populations: Race/Ethnicity, Low SES, Rural, Sexual and Gender Minority
Other Fundamental Characteristics: Sex and Gender, Disability, Geographic Region

Fig. 2.1 NIMH Health Disparities Research Framework. (From National Institute on Minority Health and Health Disparities research framework. NIMHD, 2018. Adapted from https://nimhd.nih.gov/docs/research_framework/research-framework-slide.pdf. Accessed 17 October, 2020.)

The decisions individuals make about the food they eat determine their health and wellness. Health professionals often give advice about appropriate foods for patients to consume. Therefore, it is important for nurses in institutional and community settings to understand how personal factors and community issues that affect food availability, consumption and expenditure trends, consumer information, and food safety can influence a person's food behaviors. The effects of these personal and community factors on consumers' food decisions are some of the major topics of this chapter.

PERSONAL NUTRITION

As an adult, each of us is ultimately responsible for the quality of our dietary intake. Although external forces may affect our everyday food choices, we can decide to have the internal self-awareness to consciously modify those forces. Being accountable for our nutritional status and health may require adjustment of some personal goals to allow time to work on achieving a wellness lifestyle.

Food Selection

Our food preferences, food choice, and food liking affect the foods we select to eat. Although these terms reflect similar food-related behaviors, they are different (Logue, 2015). **Food preferences** are those foods we choose to eat when all foods are available at the same time and in the same quantity. Factors affecting preferences include genetic determinants and environmental effects. Genetic factors include inborn desires for sweet and salty flavors. Studies of taste receptors note that because of variations in genetic taste markers, some people are "super tasters." Super tasters may experience the taste of vegetables such as broccoli and Brussels sprouts as bitter and therefore avoid such foods, whereas other people find this flavor enjoyable (Moss, 2013). Cruciferous vegetables, such as broccoli and Brussels sprouts, contain a vast array of nutrients and substances that may be associated with a decreased risk for the development of certain cancers. If some people avoid them because of perceived bitter taste, will they be more at risk for cancers?

Environmental effects are learned preferences that are the result of cultural and socioeconomic influences. We often adjust our choices to match those around us. Because we are around our families the most, their influence is the most significant factor in the choices we make; therefore, the dietary patterns we experience as children affect us throughout our lives (Howard, Mallan, Byrne, Magarey, & Daniels, 2012). In fact, even the food a mother eats prenatally affects the preferences of her child in the future (Beauchamp & Mennella, 2011).

An indirect influence on food preferences is the media. Television, Internet, and digital media advertising are particularly potent forces that influence the foods we prefer and buy. Programs, websites, and social media spread messages about the food and lifestyle preferences of different socioeconomic groups. A TV show about a working-class family presents images of food intake associated with those of a lower socioeconomic status; dinner might be hot dogs and beans. In another TV show, an upper socioeconomic family might sit down to a meal of baked salmon and salad. Each unintentionally sends messages about appropriate and inappropriate food intake for individuals belonging to the perceived socioeconomic group.

Health promotion issues are tied to food preferences. If recommendations call for changes in foods for which preference is rooted in genetic determinants, the motivation for change needs to be different from when the food preference is environmentally learned. New preferences can be learned; genetic preferences are more difficult to change.

Food choice concerns the specific foods that are convenient to choose when we are actually ready to eat; rarely are all our preferred foods available at the same time to satisfy our preferences. Food choices are restricted by convenience. As a result of our hectic lifestyles, we tend to avoid foods that take a long time to prepare. Instead, we often repeatedly choose foods that are easy to prepare and eat, regardless of their nutritional value. Cost is also a factor. We sometimes weigh cost benefits against time benefits. If a food costs more but saves time, we may choose it. We may decide that a food item, even if nutrient dense, costs too much money for the benefits received. Again, nutritional value may not be a prime concern that affects food choice.

Entrepreneurs have developed a new niche in food preparation and choice. Packaged meal services, such as Blue Apron and Hello Fresh, deliver all the ingredients for a complete meal to a person's or family's home but not the actual cooked meal. Instead, simple cooking instructions using the foods provided allow for preparation of interesting complete meals without the need of grocery shopping. The benefits include saving time by not shopping, less food waste as the package contains just the right amounts of ingredients, and the satisfaction of actually cooking a meal. The added cost is worth these benefits to those who may subscribe to the meal delivery services.

Food liking considers which foods we really like to eat. We may want to eat foods that enhance our health, but we like to eat chocolate cake, for example. We constantly weigh all the factors of preference, choice, and liking when we select the foods we eat. Ultimately, these three types of food behaviors greatly affect individual nutritional status (Logue, 2015).

These three food behaviors may be covertly manipulated when the food industry develops and markets foods that appeal to our biological preferences for sugar, salt, and fat. We may become "hooked" into craving processed food products that contain high levels of added sugar, salt, and fat. Physiologic changes that occur create an addiction-like response. These preferences are reinforced by repeated consumption and through advertising promoting the taste of and "having the fun" of consuming these processed products. Marketing strategies of major food corporations have powerful means to mold our food taste preferences (Moss, 2013). Media promotions and product availability may influence selection by consumers because of convenience, including accessibility, cost, and time saving, often with no consideration of nutritional value. Food liking evolves from, and may be the result of, repeated exposures. Although some people are able to moderate their consumption of less nutrient-dense food products, others cannot, thereby affecting their nutritional status and health determinants.

It is the small steps we take that eventually lead to cumulative change. As we study different aspects of food and nutrition, suggestions will be presented that move us and our patients toward significant change. These suggestions will lead to the formation of new personal food habits.

COMMUNITY NUTRITION

The nutritional status of our communities reflects our individual nutritional health. Perhaps the most significant factor affecting the nutritional status of communities is economics. Having sufficient funds to purchase adequate food supplies is a necessity. Public health nutrition efforts to prevent nutrient deficiencies include two federal government programs. The Supplemental Nutrition Assistance Program (SNAP), formerly known as the Food Stamp Program, provides individuals and families whose income is below certain levels with nutrition assistance. Another program is the Special Supplemental Nutrition Program for Women, Infants, and Children (WIC). The WIC program provides nutrition counseling and supplemental foods, as well as referrals to other health care and social services, to women who are pregnant or breastfeeding and to infants and children up to the age of 5 who are at nutritional risk. Both programs are provided through the Food and Nutrition Service of the U.S. Department of Agriculture (USDA) and have a significant impact on improving the nutritional status of those who participate. Additional government programs are discussed in Chapter 10.

Another level of public health nutrition is aimed at the nutrient excesses of our dietary intake. In the late 1970s a new era in nutrition recommendations began in the United States. Rather than focusing on nutrient deficiencies as a cause of poor health, health professionals began to notice that the cause of an increasing amount of chronic illness was possibly tied to excessive intake of certain nutrients, such as saturated fats, cholesterol, sodium, and sugars. As knowledge of diet-related diseases (e.g., heart disease, hypertension, cancer, diabetes, osteoporosis, and obesity) has improved, sets of dietary recommendations from different government agencies and voluntary health and scientific associations have evolved to address this issue.

Each set of recommendations serves a different purpose. For example, recommendations from the American Heart Association focus on lifestyle and dietary factors that affect risk factors of coronary artery disease, whereas those of the American Cancer Society center on issues related to cancer development. Despite differences in the focus of the recommendations, consensus exists on the guidelines for maintaining general good health. These recommendations are incorporated into our national goals. All recommendations tend to suggest reducing intake of saturated fat, *trans* fat, total fat, cholesterol, sodium, sugar, and excessive kilocalories and increasing our intake of healthier fats, fiber, complex carbohydrates, fruits, and vegetables. These goals form the basis of health promotion efforts to implement primary, secondary, and tertiary prevention strategies. Education at the community level that reaches as many individuals and families as possible continues to be a challenge for health professionals.

The recommendations are still needed because four of the ten most common leading causes of death in the United States

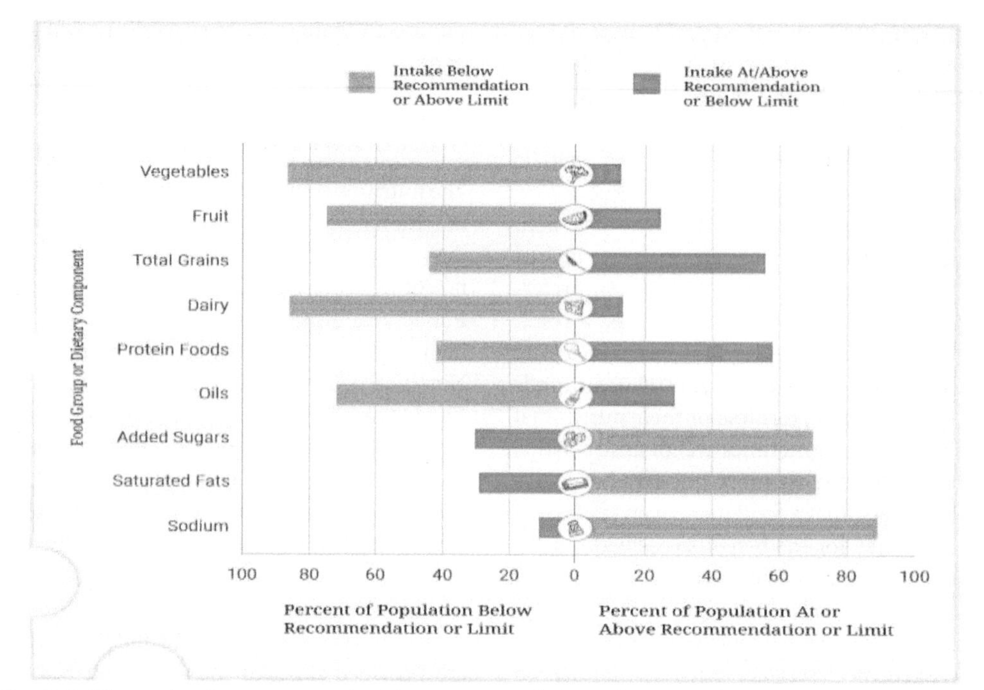

Fig. 2.2 Dietary intakes compared with recommendations. Percent of the U.S. population aged 1 year and older who are below, at, or above each dietary goal or limit. (Data from What We Eat in America, NHANES 2007–2010 for average intakes by age-sex group. Healthy U.S.-Style Food Patterns, which vary based on age, sex, and activity level, for recommended intakes and limits; U.S. Department of Health Human Services (USDHHS), U.S. Department of Agriculture (USDA). *2015–2020 Dietary Guidelines for Americans*, ed 8. December 2015. Available at http://health.gov/dietaryguidelines/2015/guidelines/ Accessed 1 November, 2020.)

are diet-related disorders—heart disease, cancers, stroke (cerebrovascular disease), and diabetes mellitus (a disorder of carbohydrate metabolism) (National Vital Statistics Reports, 2019).

Dietary Guidelines for Americans

In response to the dietary recommendations, the USDA and the USDHHS developed the *Dietary Guidelines for Americans*, which were first released in 1980. These guidelines are updated every 5 years and are intended for healthy Americans older than 2 years of age. The *2020–2025 Dietary Guidelines for Americans* are based on the latest scientific knowledge about diet, physical activity, and other health issues. This knowledge is used to formulate lifestyle and dietary pattern recommendations that will contain adequate nutrients, promote health, maintain active lifestyles, and decrease the risk of chronic diseases. As such, the *Dietary Guidelines* serve as the foundation of federal nutrition policy and education (USDA & USDHHS, 2020).

The American public consumes insufficient amounts of certain nutrients, such as vitamin D, calcium, potassium, and dietary fiber but an excess of solid fats and added sugars (SoFAS), refined grains, sodium, and saturated fat. This combination has resulted in an excessive energy intake that has led to a majority of Americans' being overweight or obese (Fig. 2.2).

The current *2020–2025 Dietary Guidelines for Americans* (hereafter referred to simply as *Dietary Guidelines*) focuses on the goals of "good health and optimal functionality across the life span" with consideration of the malnutrition (deficiency of nutrient intake) and weight issues of the population at large (USDA & USDHHS, 2020). Consequently, to attain these goals a lifestyle (behavioral) and lifespan approach is suggested. This approach centers on a total diet concept low in processed foods. To implement a total diet concept that is balanced in energy and nutrient content, dietary patterns are the focus to emphasize portion size and greater consumption of plant foods, such as vegetables, beans, fruits, whole grains, and nuts and seeds; increased intake of low-fat dairy products; and moderate amounts of poultry, lean meats, and eggs. In addition, lower intake of foods with added sugars and solid fats supports energy balance goals.

To sustain this endeavor, community support continues to be critical, so that on a population level, individuals and families can adopt these guidelines whether eating at home, at school or work, or in restaurants. Local food availability is a concern to ensure that more nutrient-dense foods are affordable and accessible in all settings from the neighborhood supermarket to fast-food restaurants. The techniques to prepare simple homecooked meals and strategies of food safety are prerequisites for achieving the goals of the *Dietary Guidelines*. These techniques and strategies can be taught in nonformal and formal educational settings, including health care clinics, public health departments, faith-based organizations, and print and electronic media.

BOX 2.1 The Guidelines: Make Every Bite Count With *Dietary Guidelines for Americans*

The following four major guidelines, if implemented, would assist everyone to practice health-promoting dietary patterns.

1. **Follow a healthy dietary pattern at every life stage.**
   At every life stage—infancy, toddlerhood, childhood, adolescence, adulthood, pregnancy, lactation, and older adulthood—it is never too early or too late to eat healthfully.
2. **Customize and enjoy nutrient-dense food and beverage choices to reflect personal preferences, cultural tradition, and budgetary considerations.**
   A healthy dietary pattern can benefit all individuals, regardless of age, race, or ethnicity, or current health status. The *Dietary Guidelines* provides a framework intended to be customized to individual needs and preferences, as well as the foodways of the diverse cultures in the United States.
3. **Focus on meeting food group needs with nutrient-dense foods and beverages, and stay within calorie limits.**
   An underlying premise of the *Dietary Guidelines* is that nutritional needs should be met primarily from foods and beverages—specifically, nutrient-dense foods and beverages. Nutrient-dense foods provide vitamins, minerals, and other health-promoting components and have no or little added sugar, saturated fat, and sodium. A healthy dietary pattern consists of nutrient-dense forms of foods and beverages across all food groups, in recommended amounts, and within calories limits.
   The core elements that make up a healthy dietary pattern include:
   - **Vegetables of all types**: dark green; red and orange; beans, peas, and lentils; starchy; and other vegetables
   - **Fruits**, especially whole fruit
   - **Grains**, at least half of which are whole grain
   - **Dairy**, including fat-free or low-fat milk, yogurt, and cheese, and/or lactose-free versions and fortified soy beverages and yogurt as alternatives
   - **Protein foods**, including lean meats, poultry, and eggs; seafood; beans, peas, and lentils, and nuts, seeds, and soy products
   - **Oils**, including vegetable oils and oils in food, such as seafood and nuts
4. **Limit foods and beverages higher in added sugars, saturated fat, and sodium, and limit alcoholic beverages.**
   At every stage, meeting food group recommendations—even with nutrient-dense choices—requires most of a person's daily calories needs and sodium limits. A healthy dietary pattern doesn't have much room for extra added sugars, saturated fat, or sodium—or for alcoholic beverages. A small amount of added sugars, saturated fat, or sodium can be added to nutrient-dense foods and beverages to help meet food group recommendations, but foods and beverages high in these components should be limited. Limits are:
   - **Added sugars:** Less than 10% per day starting at age 2. Avoid foods and beverages with added sugars for those younger than age 2.
   - **Saturated fat:** Less than 10% of calories per day starting at age 2.
   - **Sodium:** Less than 2,300 mg per day—and even less for children younger than age 14.
   - **Alcoholic beverages:** Adults of legal drinking age can choose not to drink, or to drink in moderation by limiting intake to 2 drinks or less in a day for men and 1 drink for women. Drinking less is better for health than drinking more. There are some adults who should not drink alcohol, such as women who are pregnant.

(From U.S. Department of Agriculture and U.S. Department of Health and Human Services. *Dietary Guidelines for Americans*, 2020–2025, ed 8. Pages ix–x, December 2020, from DietaryGuidelines.gov. Accessed 7 January, 2020.)

Box 2.1 lists the four major guidelines that if implemented would assist everyone to practice consumption of dietary patterns that are health-promoting.

Additional details regarding the *Dietary Guidelines* are available at https://www.dietaryguidelines.gov.

As nurses work within communities and hospital settings, the *Dietary Guidelines* provide nutrient and health recommendations on which community programming and patient education can be based.

Lifestyle Applications

Your patients and patients would certainly like to follow the *Dietary Guidelines*, but how should they do this? Their busy schedules barely allow time to eat much of anything. Ask them to consider the following nutrition-related suggestions:

- In the morning, choose dry cereals and bread products (e.g., English muffins) that contain whole grains, and alternate or mix these with lower fiber favorites. If no time can be found for breakfast, stock up on portable juices and portable fruit, such as apples, bananas, dried fruits, or a handful of nuts, which can be eaten on the way to class or work. Bring fruit and nuts in backpacks or briefcases for a quick snack.
- Be creative with vending machine selections. Choose healthier fat and lower sugar selections such as raisins, bagel chips, pretzels (rub off the excess salt), popcorn, and nuts or trail mix. Some vending machines stock small cans of tuna, yogurt, and fruit. Contact the staff responsible for filling the vending machines to request healthier selections.
- If lunch and dinner are on the run and fast-food drive-throughs are the only option, select lower fat items such as grilled chicken sandwiches or plain hamburgers without the sauce. Don't order French fries or milkshakes every time, but instead alternate them with salads and low-fat milk, juice, or water. Major restaurant chains list nutrition information on their company websites.
- Perhaps lunch and dinner are in a college or employee cafeteria. Try to select turkey, chicken (without the skin), fish, and lean beef dishes. Include whole-grain bread, a grain (rice or pasta), several vegetables, and salad. Try fruit for dessert; it is good with frozen low-fat yogurt, if available.
- Maybe your patients don't really eat "meals" but eat snacks throughout the day. This is called grazing. It is possible to graze and follow the *Dietary Guidelines* by choosing wholesome foods instead of candy bars and soda. High-quality grazing foods often available include bagels (with a little cream cheese), yogurt, fruit, pretzels, pizza (but not daily because of the high-fat content of the cheese), and dry cereals with milk. Care must be taken to control for overall calorie intake. Others may plan 5 to 6 mini-meals to be consumed through the day to maintain energy levels.

Encourage your patients, the next time they are food shopping or grabbing a snack or meal, to stop a moment to consider the best choices available (Box 2.2).

BOX 2.2 Implementing Dietary Guidelines: Easier Said Than Done

As most of us become familiar with the *Dietary Guidelines for Americans* recommendations and MyPlate, we probably reflect on the different food choices available to us and what changes we could most easily implement. But many low-income and unemployed individuals and families don't have the luxury of deciding among a variety of available foods. Instead, their problem is one of food insecurity.

Food insecurity is the limited access to safe, nutritious food, and it may be measured as a marker of undernutrition among people who are also poor and isolated from mainstream society. Retarded growth and iron deficiency, along with food insecurity, may lead to health disparities because of income, race, and ethnicity. The available financial resources of the households of such individuals and families may not stretch far enough to provide sufficient quantities of high-quality foods. A recurring strain for these families is to provide enough food for their children and themselves; sometimes they may all experience hunger.

In this context the definition of hunger is not just the physiologic need for food. Instead a social definition of hunger is the inability to access enough food to feel nourished and satisfied.

Although government programs like Supplemental Nutrition Assistance Program (SNAP) and the Women, Infants, and Children's Program (WIC) and private nonprofit food banks do fill hunger gaps, they are often insufficient to provide enough food for all of those in need. During the COVID-19 pandemic, the effects of unemployment, underemployment, and lack of paid sick time economically impacted Americans to an extent that not only was food insecurity occurring, but also a more severe measure of "sometimes or often not enough to eat" was happening. Groups found to be most affected were those experiencing poverty; Latinx and Black families; individuals without a college degree; and children. About 1 in 5 Black and Latinx people reported not having sufficient food to consume as compared with 1 in 14 White and Asian adults. One in 4 of the families experiencing these levels of hunger had usual incomes above $50,000 per year. The repercussions of this impact are not only felt on our economic status, but also on our everyday physical and mental health status.

When patients struggle to adopt new dietary guidelines, consider and be curious about the potential range of food choices easily available to them.

(Data from Schanzenbach DW: *Not Enough to Eat: COVID-19 Deepens America's Hunger Crisis*, September 2020. Food Research & Action Center (FRAC). From: https://frac.org/wp-content/uploads/Not-Enough-to-Eat_Hunger-and-COVID.pdf. Accessed 4 January, 2021.)

FOOD GUIDES

When we are armed with the latest nutrient recommendations, we can easily apply this knowledge to the way we eat every day. Because we think about what food to eat rather than what nutrients we need, these nutrient recommendations are most useful when translated into real food. To help us do this, food guides have been developed.

MyPlate

How do we and our patients implement the recommendations of the *Dietary Guidelines* on an everyday basis? The MyPlate food guidance system is designed to guide us through our food selections to meet the goals of the *Dietary Guidelines* (USDA, n.d.). The creation of MyPlate considers the current patterns of consumption of Americans plus the recommendations of the *Dietary Guidelines* and the Dietary Reference Intakes (DRIs). The result is a total diet that meets the nutrient needs from foods while limiting dietary components that are often eaten in excess. A tool to use in conjunction with MyPlate is the Nutrition Facts label on food products.

MyPlate is an Internet-based interactive tool providing recommendations based on a person's age, sex, and activity level. Individuals can go directly to the website (www.choosemyplate.gov) and enter their own data to receive personalized guides to the food group servings to meet their needs. The food groups on the MyPlate visual are grains, vegetables, fruits, and protein plus dairy (Fig. 2.3). MyPlate is intended for adults. Resources can be found at www.choosemyplate.gov that focus on other specific target groups, such as preschoolers, children, college students, dieters, and pregnant and breastfeeding women, as well as educators/teachers and health care professionals. MyPlate also provides guidance for various types of food consumption, such as Hacking Your Snacks (Fig. 2.4). For individuals who do not have a computer or access to one or who don't have computer skills, hard-copy print materials are available.

By following the interrelated recommendations of MyPlate, the following results can be expected:

- Increasing intake of vitamins, minerals, dietary fiber, and other essential nutrients, especially those often consumed at low levels in typical diets
- Lowering intake of saturated fats, *trans* fats, and cholesterol and raising intake of fruits, vegetables, and whole grains, thereby decreasing risk for some chronic diseases
- Balancing intake with energy needs, thereby preventing weight gain and/or promoting a healthy weight

The recommendations represent the following four themes:

Variety: Eat foods from all food groups and subgroups.

Proportionality: Eat more of some foods (fruits, vegetables, whole grains, and fat-free or low-fat milk products) and less of others (foods high in saturated or *trans* fats, added sugars, cholesterol, salt, and alcohol).

Moderation: Choose types of foods that limit intake of saturated or *trans* fats, added sugars, cholesterol, salt, and alcohol.

Activity: Be physically active every day.

The simple MyPlate symbol reminds us and our patients to make healthy food choices and to be physically active. The significant concepts of the symbol are highlighted in Fig. 2.3.

Other Food Guides

Not all health professionals view the recommendations of MyPlate as the soundest to improve and maintain health. Some cite the rising incidence of diet-related disorders as evidence that MyPlate recommendations do not meet our health goals. These disorders include T2D, obesity, and metabolic syndrome (MetS or syndrome X), a group of heart disease risk factors including abdominal obesity, insulin resistance, high blood pressure, and abnormal blood lipid levels. It is also possible that MyPlate is not being followed correctly, resulting in continuing diet-related disorders. As noted earlier, the dietary intake of most Americans is unbalanced compared with the recommendations of MyPlate. Intake of meats and grains is higher than recommendations, and consumption of dairy, fruits, and vegetables is lower (Centers for Disease Control and Prevention [CDC], 2018).

One of the first alternative plates to address these concerns was developed by the Nutrition Source of the Department of Nutrition, Harvard School of Public Health (HSPH). Compared with MyPlate, the Healthy Eating Plate provides more guidance as to which types of foods in each category to choose on a daily basis. Based on accumulated scientific research, the Healthy Eating Plate includes only whole-grain sources, with limited intake of refined grains, and also highlights plant sources of protein, such as nuts and legumes, and identifies sources of healthful plant oils. Fish, poultry, beans, and nuts are listed as protein sources that are lower in saturated fat and dietary cholesterol. Red meat is to be used sparingly or infrequently. Rather than suggesting, as MyPlate does, dairy as a beverage or food to be consumed at every meal, the Healthy Eating Plate recommends water or nonsugary beverages. In addition, the Healthy Eating Plate includes recommendations for daily exercise and weight control. The Healthy Eating Plate can be accessed at www.hsph.harvard.edu/nutritionsource/healthy-eating-plate.

Alternative and ethnic food guides are also available, providing specific food selections that conform to the general MyPlate categories. These guides recognize that dietary patterns other than the standard American diet offer opportunities to decrease the risk of diet-related disorders. An alternative food guide is represented by the Power Plate, created by the Physicians Committee for Responsible Medicine. The Power Plate consists of whole grains, legumes, and abundant amounts of fruits and vegetables and may be accessed at www.pcrm.org/health/diets/pplate/power-plate. The Power Plate is a vegan dietary pattern centered on a plant-based dietary intake that eliminates animal-derived foods and nutrients, thereby significantly reducing saturated fat and dietary cholesterol (discussed further in Chapter 6).

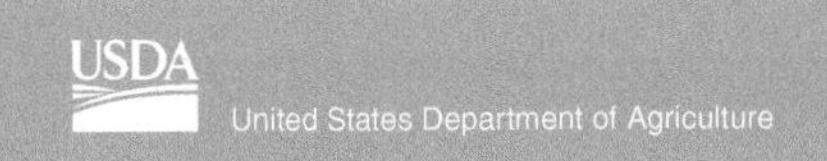
USDA
United States Department of Agriculture

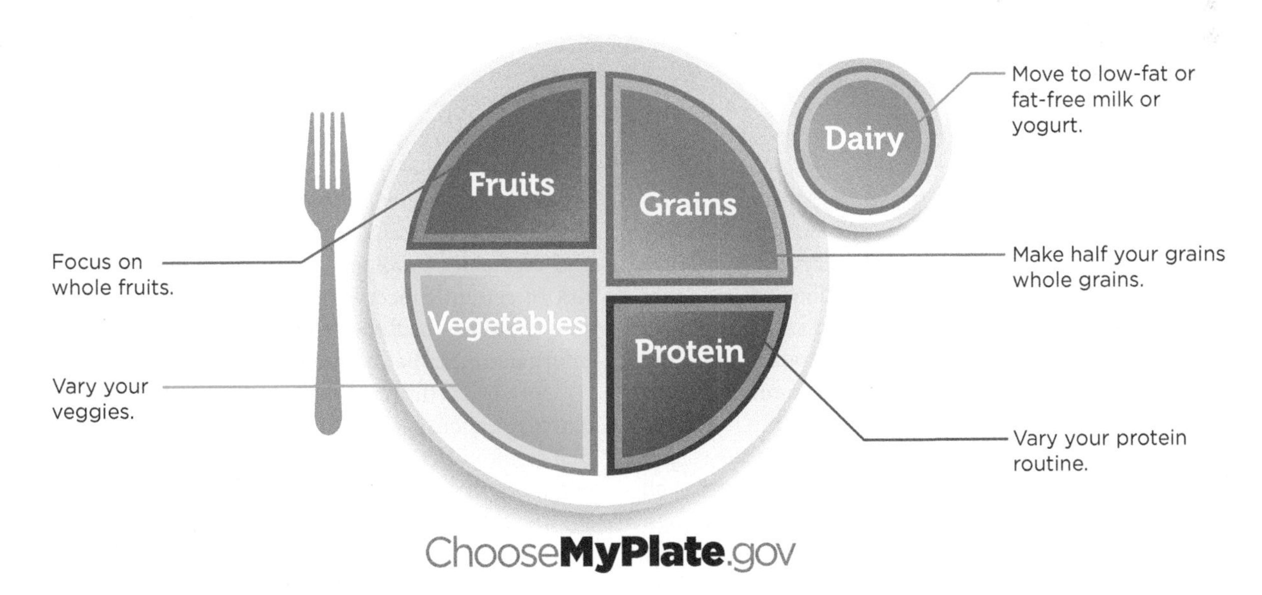

Find your healthy eating style. Everything you eat and drink over time matters and can help you be healthier now and in the future.

Vary your veggies.
Move to low-fat or fat-free milk or yogurt.
Make half your grains whole grains.
Vary your protein routine.

Limit
Limit the extras.
Drink and eat beverages and food with less sodium, saturated fat, and added sugars.

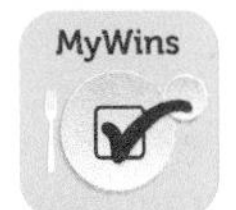
MyWins
Create 'MyWins' that fit your healthy eating style.
Start with small changes that you can enjoy, like having an extra piece of fruit today.

Fig. 2.3 MyPlate, MyWins: Make it yours. (Available at https://www.myplate.gov/. Accessed 1 November, 2020.)

Continued

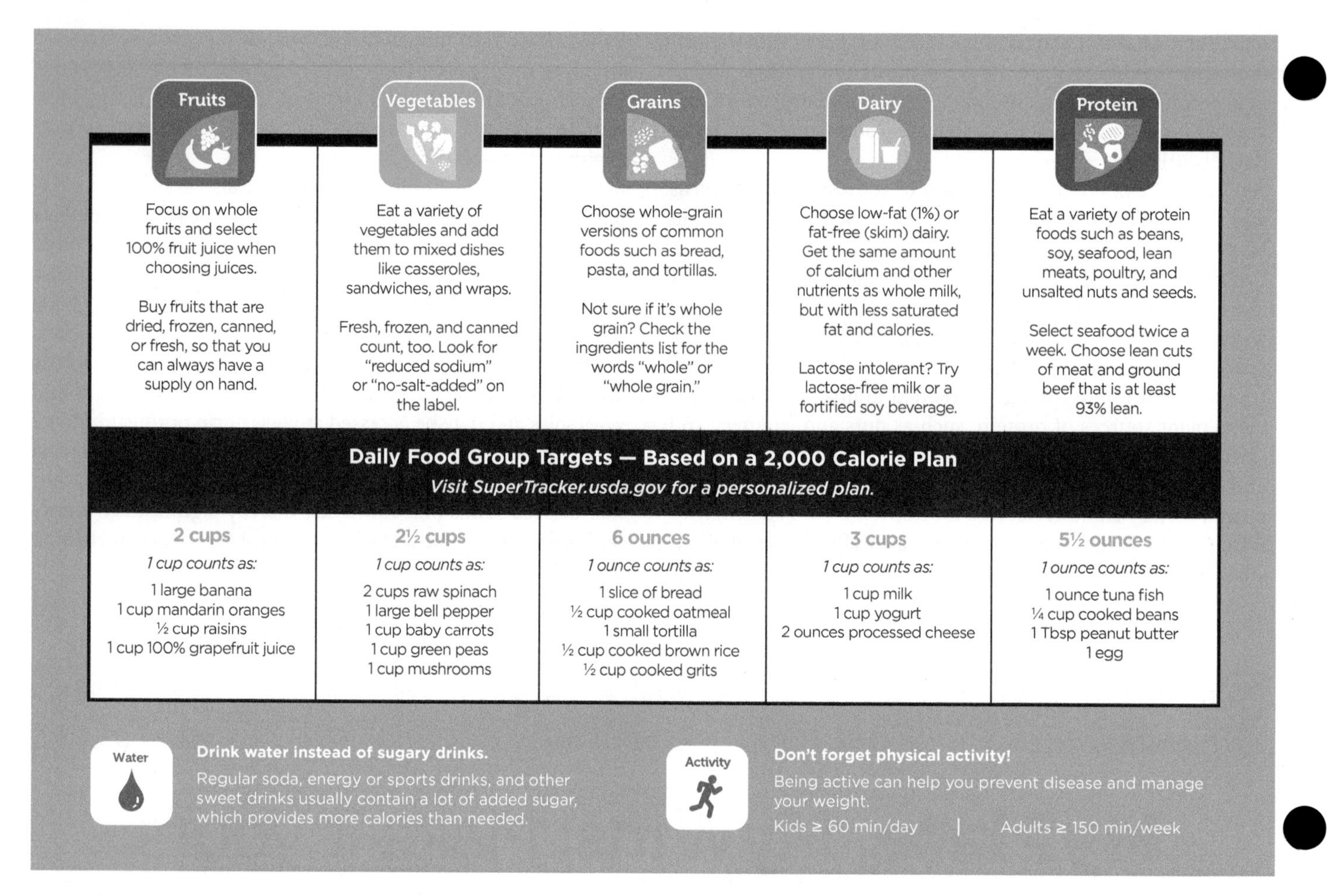

Fig. 2.3—cont'd

Ethnic food guides applicable to North America, including the Mediterranean, Asian, Latino, and African Heritage Diet Pyramids, developed by the Oldways Preservation Trust, are accessible at https://oldwayspt.org/traditional-diets. These guides differ from MyPlate in the number of servings of animal foods, legumes, varieties of fruits and vegetables, nuts, and seeds recommended. Other countries and commonwealths have food guides reflecting their national food supply, food consumption patterns, and nutritional status. Although the shapes of the guides may differ from MyPlate of the United States, all recommend similar distributions of food category servings. Ethnic and national food guides may be useful to nurses caring for patients from various cultures and countries.

"HAVE A PLANT"

Perhaps you have noticed banners and brochures in your local supermarket that proclaim, "Have a Plant" and other posters advising increased consumption of fruits and vegetables. This program represents the first partnership of government, not-for-profit agencies, and private industry to improve the health of Americans. By increasing consumption of fruits and vegetables by all age groups, the program may reduce the risk of certain cancers, diabetes, stroke, and high blood pressure (Produce for Better Health Foundation, 2020). Additional information can be accessed at https://fruitsandveggies.org/.

The CDC is the federal agency leading this public health initiative to encourage and motivate consumers to adopt strategies that result in the consumption of 2 to 6½ cups (4–13 servings) of fruits and vegetables as recommended daily. If consumers do so, the goals of the *Dietary Guidelines for Americans, Healthy People*, and other dietary recommendations may be achieved.

Research shows that for American adults the median intake of fruits a day is about 1.1 times a day, compared with the recommended four servings (2 cups); for vegetables, the median intake is about 1.6 times a day, compared with the recommended five servings (2½ cups) (Fig. 2.5). Overall, about 50% of American adults report consuming less than one fruit or vegetable daily (Bentley, 2017; CDC, 2018). Therefore, most Americans do not meet the recommended five servings (~2 to 2½ cups each) of

Hacking your snacks

Planning for healthy snacks can help satisfy hunger in between meals and keep you moving towards your food group goals.

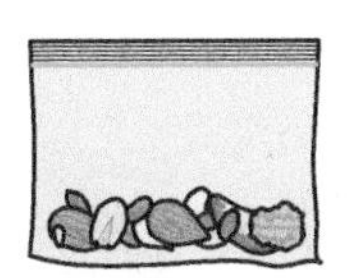

Build your own

Make your own trail mix with unsalted nuts and add-ins such as seeds, dried fruit, popcorn, or a sprinkle of chocolate chips.

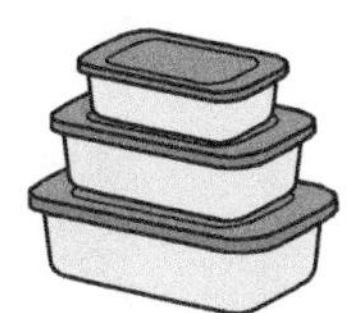

Prep ahead

Portion snack foods into baggies or containers when you get home from the store so they're ready to grab-n-go when you need them.

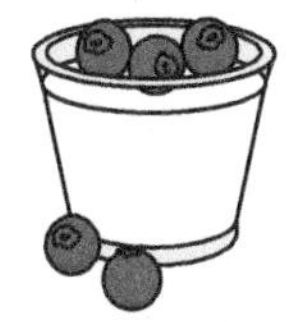

Make it a combo

Combine food groups for a satisfying snack—yogurt and berries, apple with peanut butter, whole-grain crackers with turkey and avocado.

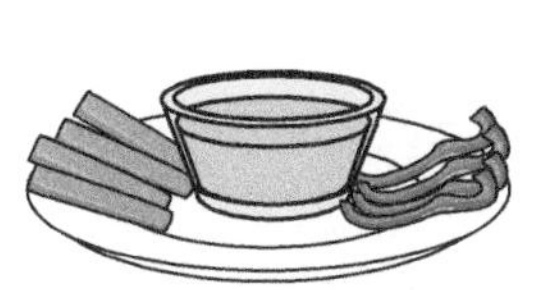

Eat vibrant veggies

Spice up raw vegetables with dips. Try dipping bell peppers, carrots, or cucumbers in hummus, tzatziki, guacamole, or baba ganoush.

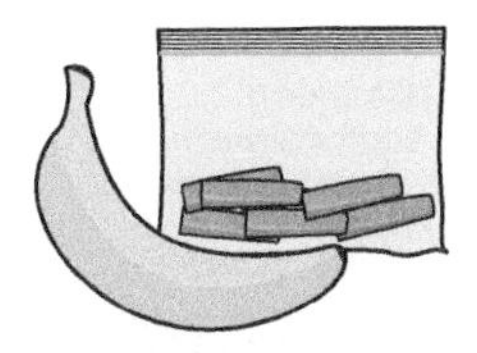

Snack on the go

Bring ready-to-eat snacks when you're out. A banana, yogurt (in a cooler), or baby carrots are easy to bring along and healthy options.

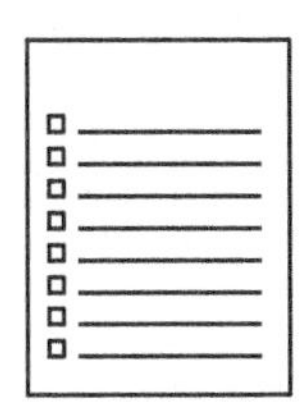

List more tips

Fig. 2.4 MyPlate, MyWins Tips: Hacking Your Snacks. (Modified from https://www.myplate.gov/. Accessed 1 November, 2020.)

fruits and vegetables a day, even though this amount is the minimum amount recommended by MyPlate.

By focusing on only fruits and vegetables, the "Have a Plant" campaign becomes an easy way to decrease intake of fats because fruits and vegetables are naturally low in fat. Consumption of fiber, vitamin C, and beta carotene will increase. These nutrients, in addition to their functions as essential nutrients, are recognized as having the potential to reduce the risk for the development of heart disease and certain cancers. Fruits and vegetables are also excellent sources of antioxidants and phytochemicals, for which potential health benefits are continually being uncovered.

Although it may be difficult to determine the percentage of daily dietary fat consumed, it is easy to count the number of servings of fruits and vegetables. If more fruits and vegetables are eaten every day, cravings for high-fat foods will tend to decrease.

Criteria for Future Recommendations

Although the current recommendations are expected to provide sound advice for the time being, other organizations may issue their own guidelines in the future. Which guidelines should we follow? Should we change our eating habits and revise patient dietary recommendations for each new study? Or, to avoid confusion, should new recommendations just be ignored?

Following are criteria to use to evaluate future dietary guidelines and recommendations:

1. Consider the source of the nutrition advice. Are the recommendations from a federal government agency? If so, the work of these agencies is usually reviewed by health and nutrition professionals before release to the public. If the advice is from a private nonprofit group, is the group nationally recognized? A number of well-respected organizations are devoted to the prevention and treatment of specific diseases, such as the American Heart Association, American Cancer Society, and American Diabetes Association. In addition, there are professional associations, including the Academy of Nutrition and Dietetics and the Society for Nutrition Education and Behavior, that specialize in the relationship between nutrition and health.
2. Assess the comprehensiveness of the recommendations. Do the recommendations address only one health problem? If so, is that a health problem that affects your patients? Would following these recommendations have any negative effects? If they were followed, would a category of nutrients be under consumed? Recommendations addressing several health issues are usually more complete and provide a higher level of prevention and health promotion.
3. Evaluate the basis of the recommendations. How were the recommendations determined? The current recommendations

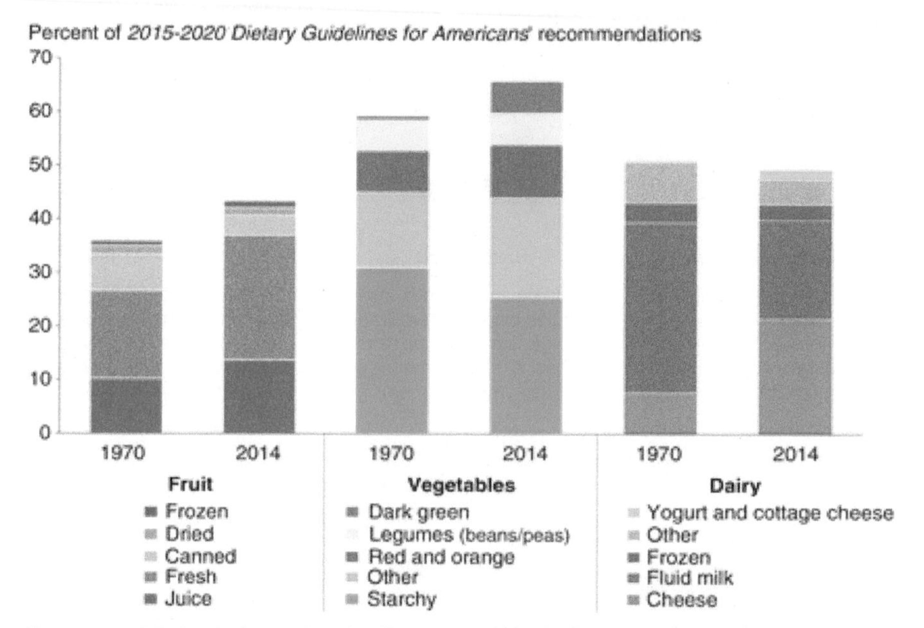

Based on a 2,000-calorie-per-day diet. Segments within the food group bars reflect the subgroups' relative consumption amounts.
Loss-adjusted food availability data serve as a proxy for consumption.
Dark green vegetables—broccoli, romaine lettuce, spinach, and others. Legumes—black beans, red kidney beans, peas, lentils, and others. Red and orange vegetables—carrots, tomatoes, pumpkin, and others. Other vegetables—cabbage, celery, cucumbers, head lettuce, onions, and others. Starchy vegetables—potatoes, green peas, corn, and others. Other dairy includes evaporated milk, condensed milk, dry milk products, half and half, and eggnog.
Source: USDA, Economic Research Service, Loss-Adjusted Food Availability Data and *2015-2020 Dietary Guidelines for Americans*.

Fig. 2.5 Americans have increased consumption of fruits and vegetables but still do not meet dietary recommendations. (From Bentley J: U.S. still out of balance with dietary recommendations, *Amber Waves*, 2017. From https://www.ers.usda.gov/amber-waves/2017/july/us-diets-still-out-of-balance-with-dietary-recommendations. Accessed 21 September, 2017.)

BOX 2.3 Types of Research

Experimental Study
Consists of an experimental group receiving treatment (or dietary change) and a control group receiving no treatment (or dietary change); differences, if any, are then noted; called a clinical or laboratory study.

Case Study
Analyzes an individual case of a disease or health difference to determine how factors may influence health; a naturalistic study because no manipulation of dietary intake or behaviors occurs.

Epidemiologic Study
Studies populations; tracks the occurrence of health or disease processes among populations; may use historical data, surveys, and/or medical records to determine possible factors influencing the health of a group of people.

are based on many research studies on the relationships between diet and disease. If new recommendations are issued, are they based on the results of new studies? If so, how many and what kinds of studies (Box 2.3)? Collecting this type of information means doing more than just listening to a 2-minute radio announcement or a 5-minute television report. Some newspaper articles contain in-depth evaluations of research; others just skim the surface. It may be necessary to read the original study in the library or on the Internet or to discuss the recommendations with other health professionals.

4. Estimate the ease of application. Can the recommendations be easily adopted? Are they presented in terms of foods (easier to apply) or nutrients (harder to apply)? Is a degree in nutrition needed to understand them?

CONSUMER FOOD DECISION MAKING

Community supports can have an impact on the quality of personal nutrition. Most important are the consumer decisions a person makes daily when buying food to be prepared in the home or when eating out.

Food Selection Patterns

Food selection patterns may be estimated by assessing government data gathered through national surveys and programs. One approach is to compare a patient's choices with the national recommendations of the online site ChooseMyPlate, (available at www.choosemyplate.gov).

According to research, the public's attention has changed to appealing to health and wellness as a way to "feel good." This approach is less intimidating than "looking good." Consequently, the goal of "feeling good" is easier to achieve. Improving preparation skills and food choices is an option by which individuals and families can accomplish "feeling good" by implementing some strategic planning and use of selected resources (Hartman Group, 2017).

Application to Nursing

When working with clients and patients, we can be aware of their attitudes toward nutrition and dietary change. Although changing dietary intake is a prime strategy to reduce the risk of diet-related chronic disorders, many Americans are not interested in changing their eating behaviors. In addition, the belief that snacking is unhealthy is unfortunate. Snacks do not have to be high fat, high sodium, or calorie laden. Consuming additional fruits, vegetables, and whole-grain foods is often best accomplished through wisely selected additional "mini-meals" or snacks (see Fig. 2.4). We may need to educate or remind patients about the nutritional benefits of dietary change as a disease-prevention strategy, and we should definitely emphasize the positive value of snacking on wholesome foods. Providing patients with simple techniques for changing food selection habits is crucial.

Food Consumption Trends

Food consumption trends reflect the food decisions Americans made in the past. Tracking these trends is the responsibility of the USDA. Following changes in consumption trends across the years for specific foods reveals information about food substitutions, including food prices or technologic changes that bring new types of food products to the marketplace (see Fig. 2.5). Food consumption trends now show that generally Americans spend more on food-away-from-home sales compared with purchases for food at home (Morrison, 2017; Bentley, 2020) (see Fig. 2.6).

Implications of food consumption trends. Food consumption trends affect the nutritional status of the U.S. population. Consumption can be gauged from grocery purchase data, which show that Americans underspend on fruits, vegetables, and whole grains and overspend on fats, refined grains, sweets, and convenience foods (Guthrie, Lin, Okrent, & Volpe, 2013). Grocery purchase data cover just food purchased for home consumption. They do not show the impact of away-from-home food consumption, which now constitutes more than one third of daily caloric intake for the average American. Away-from-home foods tend not be as wholesome as at-home foods (Guthrie et al., 2013). Therefore, guidance is needed regarding strategies to make more health-promoting food choices even if eating away-from-home foods.

Factors affecting these trends may include cost, availability, knowledge, and time. Income differences may account for the varying consumption levels. Lower income households report consuming fewer fruits and vegetables than other households.

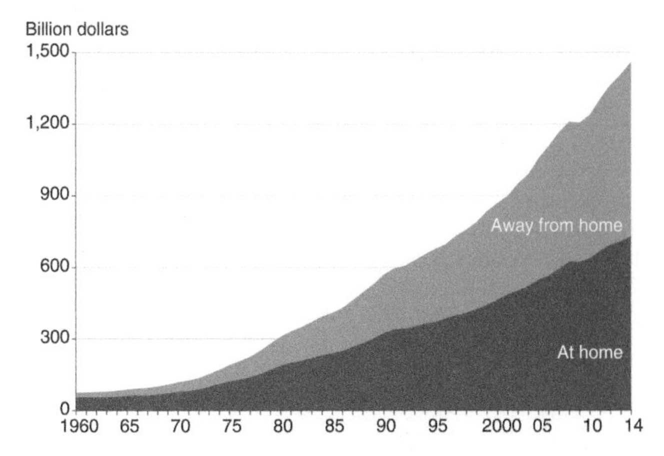

Fig. 2.6 U.S. food-away-from home sales topped food-at-home sales. As of 2019, spending for U.S. food away-from-home continues to surpass food-at-home spending. (From Morrison RM: *Food prices and spending.* Accessed 21 September, 2017, from www.ers.usda.gov/data-products/ag-and-food-statistics-charting-the-essentials/food-prices-and-spending.)

Costs of fruits and vegetables have been rising because of increased energy and production costs. Because consumers expect seasonal produce to be available year round, transportation costs rise as produce travels halfway around the world to arrive on our grocers' stands. Although all households are affected, price increases for produce in any form (fresh, frozen, or canned) limits the food-buying power of lower income households more.

Cost may be tied to availability. If under-consumed foods are in limited supply to be purchased, the price may be higher than if they are easily available. If communities have access to reasonably priced nourishing foods, residents will purchase and eat healthier foods. Improving such access may mean increasing the number of food outlets in both rural and urban areas (Dutko, Ver Ploeg, & Farrigan, 2012). Food deserts are areas where residents do not have adequate access to affordable and quality sources from which to purchase food. There simply are not enough supermarkets or grocery stores to meet the needs of the population. Although poverty is a common factor in both rural and urban communities, other determinants, such as inadequate public or personal transportation and communities of color, may increase the likelihood of food deserts (ERS-USDA, 2020). Elimination of food deserts will provide access to wholesome foods for residents while strengthening the economic viability of communities through increased food retail employment opportunities. See the *Personal Perspectives* box From Food Desert to Food Oasis, One Casserole at a Time to consider unique community-driven solutions.

Does knowledge affect food consumption trends? Everyone knows that fruits and vegetables are healthier options than

PERSONAL PERSPECTIVES

From Food Desert to Food Oasis, One Casserole at a Time

The Arthur M. Blank Family Foundation (www.blankfoundation.org), founded in 1995, seeks to sponsor creative positive approaches to improve and enrich the lives of individuals, as well as the community at large. The following excerpt, written by John Bare, Vice President for Programs of the Foundation, describes how innovative solutions evolved in response to concerns about food deserts in a Georgia community.

When a leader of a local Baptist church made a plea to teach young people the value of casseroles, I knew we were on to something.

It turns out the casserole, long a staple of church suppers, may be the ultimate example of a do-it-yourself family food experience. The casserole is about efficiency, relying on the know-how to organize multiple seasonal ingredients into a dish that will stretch the family food dollar. Every casserole is a teaching moment, pulling the kids into the kitchen to learn alternatives to drive-through fast food. The casserole is about friends and family, as parents traditionally kept a couple in the freezer to give to a neighbor suffering a hardship. All roads to a new food system run through the casserole.

In our food initiative, led by the Atlanta Falcons Youth Foundation, we had initially used vocabulary from public health—lots of talk about food deserts and food insecurity, all supported by maps. Not a mention of casseroles.

The residents we aimed to serve, however, talked about food in different ways. And what we learned from residents helped us reimagine our strategy. What emerged—the Georgia Food Oasis campaign—is now helping families across the state pursue their own ideas of how to eat, cook, and grow more fruits and vegetables.

Launched in Atlanta, Augusta, Columbus, and rural north Georgia, the Georgia Food Oasis campaign is bringing together community residents so they can raise the profile of existing local programs that help families eat, cook, and grow fruits and vegetables. Through this convening, residents also set priorities for local innovation. Thanks to this two-pronged approach, Georgia Food Oasis helps communities maximize the benefits of existing farmers' markets, community gardens, and food pantries while at the same time rallying support for new programs that fill gaps.

By listening and responding to residents, here's what we learned:

Changing the food profile of a neighborhood is doable. In two of the toughest neighborhoods in Atlanta, we've seen a pop-up retail market and a nonprofit neighborhood grocery change retail shopping behavior in one growing season. Leaders should take on the food issue with excitement, not fearful rhetoric. There are wins to be had through increased resident purchasing of fruits and vegetables.

- Language matters. Residents want more choices in their neighborhood—more choices with schools, parks, and, yes, food. They want to cook up their own food future. They don't want nags, finger-pointers, or lectures from the food police.
- Food access is not a binary problem. That is, by technical definition, a neighborhood is either a "food desert" or not. But the presence or absence of a grocery store hardly tells the full story. We heard more about other barriers—transportation, price, quality of produce, and not being welcome in local stores. Turning a neighborhood into a food oasis is about addressing whatever is limiting choice. It's often not just the presence or absence of a store.
- Food access changes through relationships, not transactions. For well-intended foundations and nonprofits ready to launch work in new communities, it's easy to slip up and focus on the latter instead of the former. It's more important to start by developing authentic relationships with residents. Do that, and you'll be surprised at how many barriers to change begin to melt away.
- When you hear about the need for more research in a neighborhood, be skeptical. Remember your research turns residents into human subjects. Start with the assumption that you have enough information—however imperfect—to support action, not research.
- It's critical to know enough about existing local programs. These programs can let residents know what they can do today to eat, cook, and grow fruits and vegetables. Residents are more engaged when, for the first time, they see all the services available. Hint: Compile this directory through resident-led organizing, not research from outsiders.

In the end, Georgia Food Oasis understands that food is central to community building. By focusing on residents' demand for fruits and vegetables, Food Oasis leads with irrefutable evidence that it is, in fact, worth the effort to remove barriers to access. From participation in cooking lessons to the rise in SNAP transactions at farmers markets to the pursuit of more community gardens, we're overwhelmed—and overjoyed—by the demand. If you don't have evidence of demand, see earlier: Focus on relationships. Residents want choices, and you've got to lift up the voices of residents to succeed.

(From Bare J: *From food desert to food oasis, one casserole at a time*, February 17, 2016. Accessed September 26, 2017, from https://www.healthyfoodaccess.org/resources-tools-perspectives-from-food-oasis-one-casserole-at-a-time.)

processed food and snacks, yet highly processed foods and snacks are too often chosen. So what knowledge is needed? Generally, many consumers could learn how to prepare a wider variety of vegetables, so they taste and look good and are safe to eat. Consumers need to know that frozen fruits and vegetables can be as nutritious as fresh and are available year-round. Teaching how to buy and prepare foods is an adjunct goal of nutrition education. In addition, efforts by the government and private industry to make food labels and point-of-purchase information easier to understand and apply may increase preference for nourishing foodstuffs (Guthrie et al., 2013).

Time as a factor in consumption trends encompasses the limiting of time to shop and prepare meals by work, school, and family responsibilities, as well as other distractions of contemporary lifestyles (such as increasing use of digital technology). As Michael Pollan, author of *Cooked: A Natural History of Transformation* (2013), remarks:

"Survey research confirms we're cooking less and buying more prepared meals every year. The amount of time spent preparing meals in American households has fallen by half since the mid-sixties, when I was watching my mom fix dinner, to a scant twenty-seven minutes a day. (Americans spend less time cooking than people in any other nation, but the general downward trend is global.) And yet at the same time we're talking about cooking more—and watching cooking, and reading about cooking, and going to restaurants designed so that we can watch the work performed live. We live in an age when professional cooks are household names, some of them as famous as athletes or movie stars. The very same activity that many people regard as a form of drudgery has somehow been elevated to a popular spectator sport."

Although these trends reflect per capita consumption patterns based on the total population, it is our individual consumer food decisions that have the greatest influence on our personal level of wellness.

Effective Food-Buying Styles

This chapter is full of information about consumer decisions, but how is it to be applied? How do you and your clients become better shoppers? The first step is to tailor a shopping style to one's particular situation.

Consider the following issues to formulate the most effective approach to food shopping:

1. Food budget: A food budget should consider the funds needed to keep a moderate amount of food in the home and the money spent on meals away from home.
2. Consumer diversity: Buying food for a single young adult is different from buying for a family. Lifestyles of household members affect the numbers and types of meals served and the kinds and amounts of food served.
3. Dietary preferences: We all have food preferences based on ethnicity, habits, chronic illness, or ethical views such as vegetarianism. Each preference affects food-buying selections.
4. Shopping frequency: Each household works best with a shopping plan—perhaps weekly, every 2 weeks, or on the way home from school or work when things are needed.
5. Location and types of food stores: Different types of food stores provide a range of services and products. Conventional supermarkets, superstores, supercenters, and super warehouse stores are valuable for fresh produce, perishables, and basic grocery items; wholesale clubs and limited assortment warehouse stores are good for bulk foods at low prices; specialty stores offer unique foods at high prices; and convenience stores "save the day."

CONSUMER INFORMATION AND WELLNESS

The more information consumers have about the food they eat, the better they can choose foods that contribute to wellness. Nutrition education is necessary for consumers to use the additional information appropriately.

Food Labeling

Food labels are the best way for consumers to see how individual foods fit their nutritional needs. The function of food labels is twofold. The first is to help consumers select foods with the most health-providing qualities. The second is to motivate food companies to enhance the nutritional value of food products because labels reveal ingredient and nutrient content.

Food labeling for processed foods in the United States is based on standards established under authority of the 1990 Nutrition Labeling and Education Act. Although nutrition labeling is mandatory for most processed products, it is voluntary for fresh meat, poultry, fish, milk, eggs, and produce. It is expected that by 2022, the revised format for Nutrition Facts label will be universally used on all processed food products. A side-by-side comparison of the original label to the revised label for processed foods is available at Original versus New Label—Side-by-Side Comparison (https://www.fda.gov/downloads/Food/GuidanceRegulation/GuidanceDocumentsRegulatoryInformation/LabelingNutrition/UCM501646.pdf).

The revision updates the original label that was implemented more than 20 years ago. Updates are based on current scientific data, recent nutrition and public health research, improved dietary recommendations from health promotion/disease prevention organizations, and concerns from interested citizens (U.S. Food and Drug Administration [FDA], 2017) (Fig. 2.7).

Changes include reassessing serving sizes to reflect the amount of a product that is most commonly consumed (Fig. 2.8). A new addition is the listing of "added sugars" in grams, which provides information needed for consumers to assess their intake from added sugar. Recommendations suggest that no more than 10% of total daily calories should come from added sugar. Another modification is that, in the list of required vitamins and minerals (in addition to sodium), vitamin D and potassium have been added to calcium and iron, whereas vitamin C and vitamin A are no longer required but may be listed.

The Nutrition Facts panel on the food packaging must list the quantities of energy (kcal), fat, and the following other specific nutrients in a serving:

- Total food energy
- Food energy from fat
- Total fat
- Saturated fat
- *Trans* fat
- Cholesterol
- Sodium
- Total carbohydrates
- Dietary fiber
- Sugars
  - Added sugars
- Protein
- Vitamin D
- Calcium
- Iron
- Potassium

The **daily values (DVs)**, a system created for food labeling, reflects the amount of a nutrient needed as general nutrition guidance, based on a 2000-kcal diet. For each serving, the percent of daily value (%DV) for the nutrients that are required must be listed on the label. This shows consumers how much of a day's ideal intake of a particular nutrient they are eating. DVs for selected nutrients and food components based on a 2000-calorie diet also reveal the percent present in a single serving of the product. In addition, the actual amount contained must be listed, addition to the %DV. This includes vitamin D, calcium, iron, and potassium. Amounts of other vitamins and minerals can be voluntarily listed. The DVs of sodium, dietary fiber, and vitamin D are updated to reflect recommendations from the Institute of Medicine of the National Institutes of Health and the *Dietary Guidelines*.

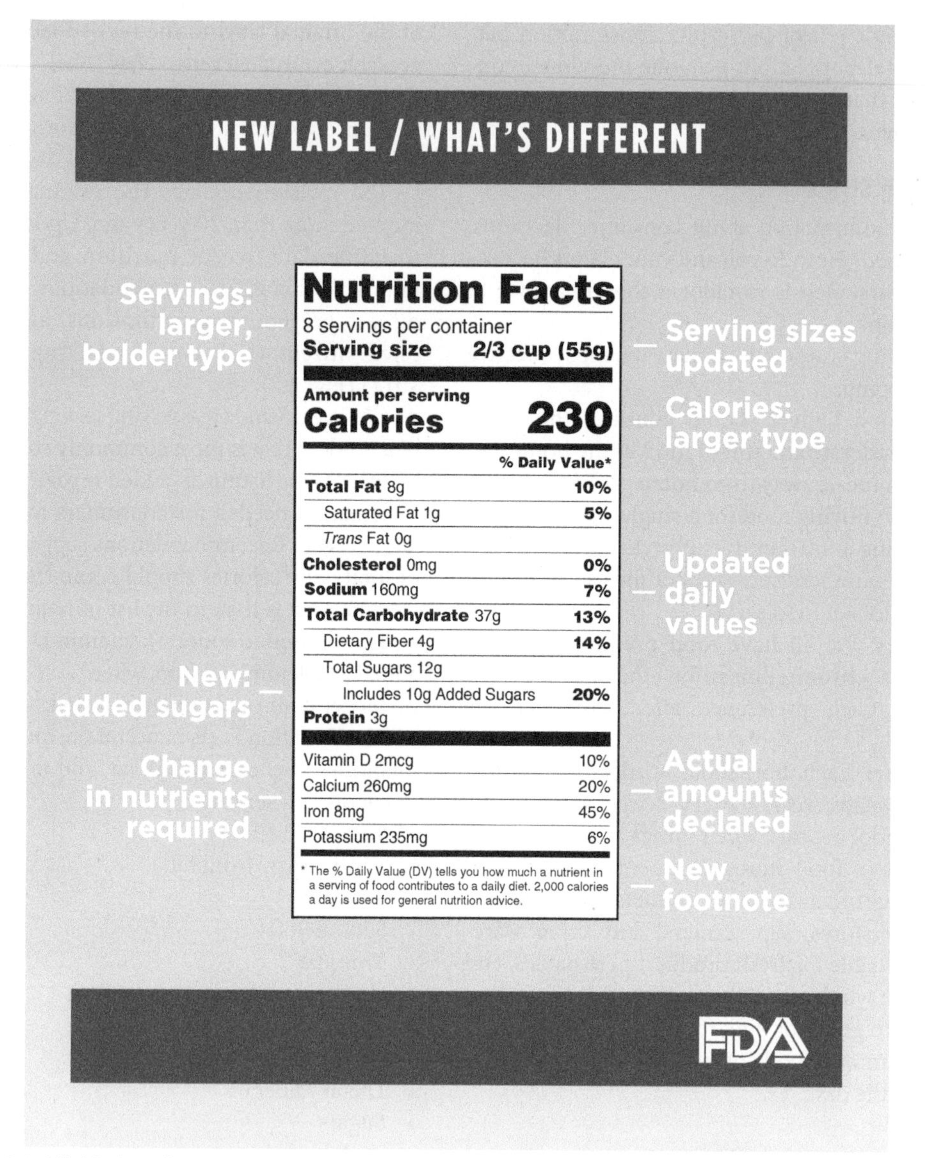

Fig. 2.7 Highlights of what's different on the new label. (From U.S. Food and Drug Administration FDA, Center for Food Safety and Applied Nutrition: Changes to the Nutrition Facts Label, Silver Spring, MD, Author. From: www.fda.gov/Food/GuidanceRegulation/GuidanceDocumentsRegulatoryInformation/LabelingNutrition/ucm385663.htm Accessed 31 October, 2020.)

Uses of Percent of Daily Values Information

The %DV is useful to make comparisons between products, to assess nutrient content claims, and to choose a mix of foods to balance nutrient intake as part of a total daily dietary intake. Making comparisons among %DVs of similar products is possible if the serving sizes are the same. Which brand has the lowest fat content? Which has the highest fiber content? Assessing nutrient content claims is simple when using %DV. By considering the %DVs of fiber in two food products, the consumer can quickly determine the better source of fiber. This can be used for any nutrient content claim. Using %DV to balance nutrient intake is accomplished by combining foods high in %DV of a particular nutrient, such as fat, with foods low in %DV of that nutrient. A person's daily intake of fat can still be less than 100%DV.

Uniform Definitions for Food Descriptors

Uniform definitions for food descriptors, such as light and low fat, for nutrient content claims are now clearly established and must be consistently used for all foods (FDA, 2013) (Box 2.4). This information helps consumers who try to control their intakes of specific nutrients and food components.

Manufacturers have increased the proportion of whole-grain ingredients in many products so consumers can more easily achieve the *Dietary Guidelines*' recommendation to consume at least 3 ounces of whole grains daily—and to remain competitive with other products. The Whole Grains Council, an Oldways Program that includes scientists, manufacturers, and chefs, developed two stamps to appear on packaging that identify the whole-grain content of a product. The "100% Whole Grain Stamp" on a product signifies that all of the grain ingredients

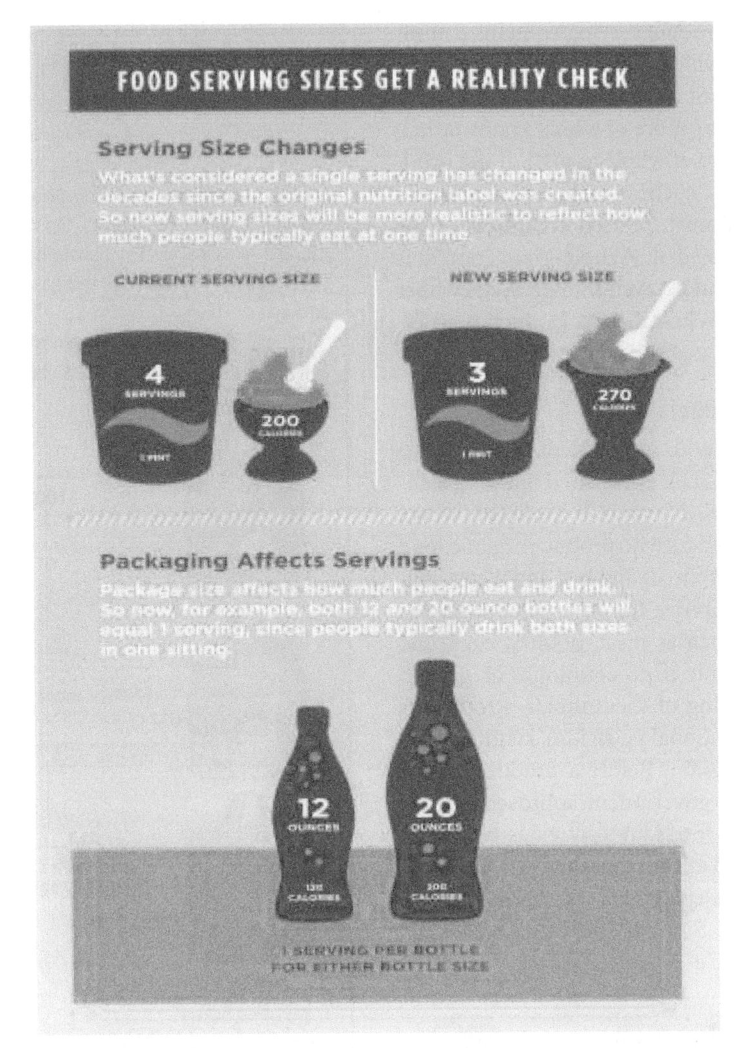

Fig. 2.8 Food serving sizes get a reality check. (From U.S. Food and Drug Administration, Center for Food Safety and Applied Nutrition: *Changes to the nutrition facts label*, Silver Spring, MD, 2017, Author. From: www.fda.gov/consumers/consumer-updates/food-serving-sizes-get-reality-check Accessed 31 October, 2020.)

BOX 2.4 Food Descriptors

Free
Contains only a tiny or insignificant amount of fat, cholesterol, sodium, sugar, and/or calories. For example, a "fat-free" product contains less than 0.5 g of fat per serving.

Low
"Low" in fat, saturated fat, cholesterol, sodium, and/or calories; can be eaten fairly often without exceeding dietary guidelines. So, "low in fat" means no more than 3 g of fat per serving.

Lean
Contains less than 10 g of fat, 4 g of saturated fat, and 95 mg of cholesterol per serving. "Lean" is not as lean as "low." "Lean" and "extra lean" are U.S. Department of Agriculture terms for use on meat and poultry products.

Extra Lean
Contains less than 5 g of fat, 2 g of saturated fat, and 95 mg of cholesterol per serving. Although "extra lean" is leaner than "lean," it is still not as lean as "low."

Reduced, Less, Fewer
Contains 25% less of a nutrient or calories. For example, hot dogs might be labeled "25% less fat than our regular hot dogs."

Light/Lite
Contains one third fewer calories or one half the fat of the original. "Light in sodium" means a product with one half the usual sodium.

More
Contains at least 10% more of the daily value of a vitamin, mineral, or fiber than the usual single serving.

Good Source of ...
Contains 10% to 19% of the daily value for a particular vitamin, mineral, or fiber in a single serving.

(From U.S. Food and Drug Administration, Center for Food Safety and Applied Nutrition: Guidance for industry: A food labeling guide, College Park, MD, 2013, Author. From https://www.fda.gov/media/81606/download. Accessed 31 October, 2020.)

are whole grains and that each product serving contains a minimum of 16 g of whole grains, which equals 1 ounce of whole grains. The "Basic Whole Grain Stamp" means that each product serving contains at least 8 g or more of whole grains or half a full serving (equaling 0.5 ounce of whole grains). If the product also contains refined grains, such as extra bran, germ, or refined flour, the Basic Stamp must be used regardless of the total amount of whole grains provided. (Whole-grain content is not the same as dietary fiber content, even though dietary fiber is part of the whole grain.) The Whole Grains Council is accessible at wholegrainscouncil.org.

Organic Food Standards and Labels

Fresh produce and a variety of foods are labeled "organic." Just what does organic mean? The USDA established national standards for food products to be labeled organic, regardless of where they are grown or processed. Farmers who produce organic food focus on the use of renewable resources and soil and water conservation to maintain and/or improve the environment for the future. Animal-derived foods such as meat, poultry, eggs, and dairy products are labeled organic if no antibiotics or growth hormones are used in the rearing of the animals. Produce is grown without the use of conventional pesticides, synthetic fertilizers, bioengineering, or radiation. Before a product can be labeled organic, certification by government-approved inspectors is required of farms where foods are grown, as well as of companies that process foods, to ensure that the USDA organic standards are followed (U.S. Department of Agriculture & Agricultural Marketing Service USDA, AMS, 2016).

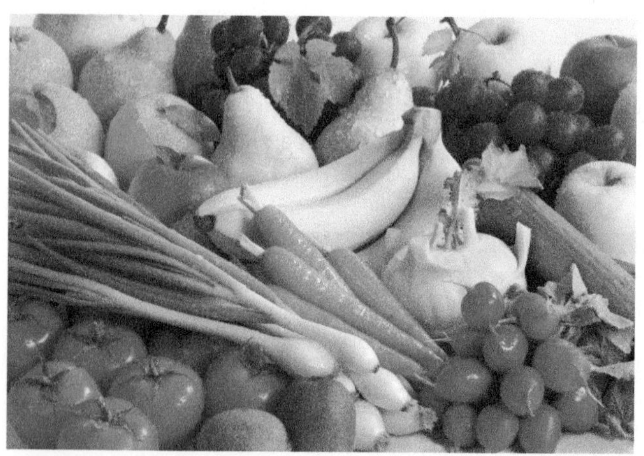

Consumption of fruits and vegetables may reduce the risk of diet-related disorders. (From http://www.thinkstockphotos.com)

Specific labeling rules exist for foods containing organic ingredients (U.S. Department of Agriculture & Agricultural Marketing Service USDA, AMS, 2016). Single-ingredient foods may use the organic seal and the word organic on labeling or on display posters. These foods may include fresh fruits, vegetables, cheese, cartons of eggs or milk, meat packages, and other single-ingredient foods. When foods contain more than one ingredient, specific labeling categories are followed (Box 2.5).

The term natural may also be used, but it is not the same as organic. Natural often signifies that the ingredients of a product are less processed and more wholesome but does not address how the ingredients were grown or the animals reared. Organic means that the food is certified as fulfilling the USDA organic standards for farming and/or rearing of animals, not how the ingredients have been processed during the manufacturing procedures. Organic soda prepared from organically grown sugar and/or high-fructose corn syrup and flavorings is not more nutrient dense or natural than a soda from a national beverage company containing similar ingredients grown under conventional means. Consumers need to be savvy about the nutrient density of the foods chosen regardless of whether the product meets USDA organic standards (see Box 2.5).

Application to nursing. Check the Nutrition Facts panels for products purchased regularly. Ingredients may be changed by manufacturers, and similar products may be created from

BOX 2.5 Labeling Definitions for Organic Foods

Look for the U.S. Department of Agriculture (USDA) organic seal on raw, fresh products, and processed products that contain organic agricultural ingredients. Or the seal may appear on a sign above an organic produce display.

On multi-ingredient products, the seal is usually placed on the front of the package (principal display panel); however, it may be placed anywhere on the package. When you see this seal, you know the product is at least 95% organic.

The seal may be printed in green and brown (as shown), in black and white, or outlined in black on a transparent background.

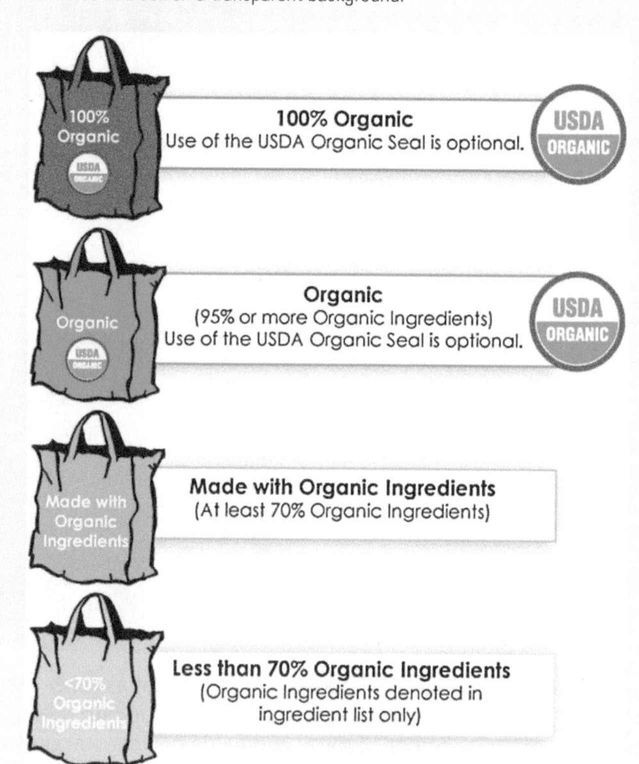

100% Organic
100% Organic
Use of the USDA Organic Seal is optional.
USDA ORGANIC
Organic
Organic
(95% or more Organic Ingredients)
Use of the USDA Organic Seal is optional.
USDA ORGANIC
Made with Organic Ingredients
Made with Organic Ingredients
(At least 70% Organic Ingredients)
<70% Organic Ingredients
Less than 70% Organic Ingredients
(Organic Ingredients denoted in ingredient list only)

(From U.S. Department of Agriculture, National Organic Program, Agricultural Marketing Service: *Understanding organic labeling*, Washington, DC, 2016. Author. From https://www.ams.usda.gov/sites/default/files/media/Labeling%20Organic%20Products.pdf. Accessed 31 October, 2020.)

 TEACHING TOOL

Just the Facts: Using Labels to Teach Nutrition Literacy

Health care providers view nutrition as a basic component of health education and refer patients to nutritionists for nutrition education. Nurses are in the position to reinforce nutrition concepts first presented by dietitian/nutritionists. Although physicians may be viewed as the experts on health, patients who have low literacy skills tend to use their social network of family and friends for health and nutrition information. Consequently, for interventions to be successful, members of social networks should be included. The approach should be visual, interactive, and culturally appropriate. This lesson on label comprehension fits these three criteria.

Patients should be presented with three boxes of cereal or Nutrition Facts labels from three cereal products. Choose three different products. For example, include a heavily presweetened cereal, a lightly sweetened cereal, and one with no added sweeteners. Ask the following questions:

Which has the most kcal per serving? This may be affected by weight, volume of the cereal (popped with air), and the density of added ingredients like raisins.

Which has the largest serving size? Serving sizes are the same by weight for all products in a food category.

Which contains the most dietary fat? Fat is not an issue with cereals, except for granola.

Which contains the most sodium? Some cereals contain about 300 mg, which is high for sodium-sensitive patients.

Which contains the most added sugars? Added sugars can range from none to 13 g per serving.

How many calories come from added sugars? Multiply the number of grams of sugars by 4 kcal. By dividing this number by the total kcal per serving and multiplying the decimal by 100, you can determine the percentage of sugar content.

Which contains the most fiber? Fiber content can range from none to about 5 g per serving.

As your study of nutrition continues, you may add other questions and be able to relate patient responses to preventive health issues of diet-related diseases or to address specific dietary needs of a patient's nutrition recommendations.

(Data from Lee SY, Arozullah AM, Cho YI: Health literacy, social support, and health: a research agenda, *Soc Sci Med* 58(7):1309–1321, 2004.)

different formulations. This may result in modifications of ingredients and serving sizes that affect calories and nutrient content. See the *Teaching Tool* box Just the Facts: Using Labels to Teach Nutrition Literacy for information on how to help patients evaluate food labels.

Health Claims

Health claims relating a nutrient or food component to the risk of a disease or health-related condition now appear on food labels. Only health claims approved by the FDA may be on the label. This information helps consumers select those foods that can keep them healthy and well.

So far, the health claims allowed include relationships between the following:

- Potassium and reduced risk of high blood pressure (hypertension)
- Plant sterol and plant stanol esters and heart disease (Plant sterols and stanols are substances found naturally in certain plant foods that provide health benefits.)
- Whole grains and reduced risk of heart disease and certain cancers
- Soy protein and reduced risk of heart disease
- A diet with enough calcium and a lower risk of osteoporosis
- A diet low in total fat and a reduced risk of some cancers
- A diet low in saturated fat, cholesterol, and *trans*-fat and a reduced risk of coronary heart disease
- A diet rich in fiber-containing grain products, fruits, and vegetables and a reduced risk of some cancers
- A diet rich in fiber-containing grain products, fruits, and vegetables and a reduced risk of coronary heart disease
- A diet low in sodium and a reduced risk of high blood pressure
- A diet rich in fruits and vegetables and a reduced risk of some cancers
- Folic acid and a decreased risk of neural tube defect–affected pregnancy
- Dietary sugar alcohols and a reduced risk of dental caries (decay)
- Fluoridated water and reduced risk of dental caries (decay)
- Soluble fiber from certain foods, such as whole oats and psyllium seed husk, as part of a diet low in saturated fat and cholesterol and a reduced risk of heart disease

Food labeling legislation also covers dietary supplements. The Dietary Supplement Health and Education Act of 1994 (DSHEA) requires the FDA to prove that a dietary supplement is unsafe or adulterated or has false or misleading labeling. The act does not allow claims about diagnosis, treatment, or prevention of disease but does allow that claims of certain benefits must be truthful. A standard statement is required on the label by the FDA (FDA, Office of Dietary Supplement Programs [ODSP], 2019).

TOWARD A POSITIVE NUTRITION LIFESTYLE: LOCUS OF CONTROL

Do things just happen to you? Does it seem as if school, family, or society affect what you do without your input? Or do you feel that you have control over what takes place? Do you have a life plan (or weekly plan) that you follow? **Locus of control** is the perception of one's ability to control life events and experiences. Having an internal locus of control means feeling as if you can influence the forces with which you come into contact. You have an inner sense of your ability to guide life events. An external locus of control is defined as the perception that you are not able to control what happens to you and that outside forces have power over what you experience.

Let's apply these concepts to your style of making food choices when shopping. In particular, consider the nutritional implications of locus of control. If you have an internal locus of control, you may develop a basic plan of the types of nutritious foods to be purchased during a shopping trip. You may make a few unplanned purchases, but they would be limited. You feel in control of your choices. Having an external locus of control means you might start out with a shopping list, but you are probably easily swayed by in-store promotions, coupons, and even colorful packaging to select products not on your list. You often buy more than needed because so much "looked good."

Awareness of our type of locus of control allows us to develop strategies to improve our food decisions. Individuals with an internal locus of control tend to develop their own approaches for changing food-related behaviors; those with an external locus of control may need a structured program or group support to provide guidance to modify their food behaviors.

SUMMARY

- Personal nutrition is composed of the dietary choices an individual makes that affect health and nutritional status.
- Food preferences, food choice, and food liking influence selection. These may be altered by biological tendency, availability, media, and marketing.
- Community nutrition reflects the nutritional health of the individuals within the community.
  - Public health programs such as SNAP and WIC focus on the prevention of nutrient deficiencies on the individual and community levels. Other government and private organizations representing specific diet-related disorders such as the American Heart Association and American Diabetes Association develop recommendations to reduce excessive intake of energy and nutrients.
- *Dietary Guidelines* provides lifestyle and dietary pattern recommendations that ensure nutrient adequacy and primary disease prevention.
- MyPlate is an interactive food guide to implement the *Dietary Guidelines* recommendations.
- The requirement for consumer information on food product packaging increases the probability that decisions about food choice are based on nutritional value as well as on taste, cost, and availability.
- FDA food labeling regulations require the following:
  - The Nutrition Facts panel must list the quantity of energy (fat), fat, and other specified nutrients per serving listed as percentage of daily values.
  - Food descriptors are defined to ensure uniformity of meaning.
  - Health claims approved by the FDA may appear on food labels.
- Organic food standards established by the USDA determine labeling of products containing multiple ingredients.

THE NURSING APPROACH

Clinical Judgment and Next-Generation NCLEX® Examination-Style Questions

The Clinical Judgment Measurement Model (CJMM) includes six measured cognitive processes/skills including their descriptions (Dickison et al, 2019).

1. **Recognize Cues/Assessment:** Identifying specific data from many sources (assessment). Each learning session should begin with an assessment of the patient's learning needs and goals identified by the nurse and patient.
2. **Analyze Cues/Analysis:** Linking the data to the patient's presentation—is this data expected? Unexpected? What are the concerns?
3. **Prioritize hypotheses/Analysis:** Analyze the hypotheses; concerns, patient needs (analysis, diagnosis). What priority methods will facilitate change?
4. **Generate solutions/Planning:** Use hypotheses to determine interventions and plans for an expected outcome.
5. **Implementation/Take Action:** Implement the generated solutions related to the highest priorities or hypotheses.
6. **Evaluate outcomes/Evaluation:** Compare observed outcomes with expected ones (evaluation) and the item types that effectively test clinical judgment.

Case Study

A 24-year-old slightly overweight female wants to lose weight. She states that this is difficult because she mostly eats takeout food for the majority of her meals. Several of her friends are on fad diets, and she is interested in trying one. She lives with her mother, who is obese, and wants to help herself and her mother make healthier choices. She asks a friend, who is a nurse, about information on healthier eating. The nurse tells her that good food guidelines are available. She could consider following these strategies if she decides to change her eating habits.

Put an X to mark the five strategies that encourage healthier eating patterns.

1. Follow a healthy eating pattern across the life span
2. Choose a variety, nutrient-poor, with excess amount of food
3. Limit calories from added sugars and saturated fats, and reduce sodium intake
4. Do not use sugar substitutes
5. Support healthy eating patterns for all
6. Shift to healthier food and unsweetened beverage choices.
7. Avoid cultural and personal preferences to make shifts easier to accomplish and maintain.
8. Focus on variety, nutrient density, and portion size

(Data from Dickison P, Haerling KA, Lasater K: Integrating the National Council of State Boards of Nursing Clinical Judgment Model into nursing educational frameworks. *Journal of Nursing Education* 58(2): 72–78, 2019.)

APPLYING CONTENT KNOWLEDGE

Jennifer and Peter are in their late 40s. Recently Peter was diagnosed with high blood cholesterol levels. His doctor told him to cut down on fats and cholesterol, but he is confused about what to order at the daily business lunches he must attend. Jennifer has noticed that she is starting to put on weight and wonders whether the change has to do with perimenopause or whether she is just eating more than usual. In addition, Jennifer's mother has just moved in with them because she could no longer afford her own home. Jennifer is concerned because her mother seems to eat little during the day. Her mother is alone all day because Jennifer and Peter work. What advice might you give to this family?

WEBSITES OF INTEREST

ChooseMyPlate Food Guidance System
www.ChooseMyPlate.gov
The official "home" of MyPlate, the interactive food guidance system.

Oldways Preservation Trust
oldwayspt.org
A nonprofit organization promoting good health through heritage.

U.S. Food and Drug Administration (FDA)
www.fda.gov
Gateway website connecting areas serviced and supervised by the FDA.

REFERENCES

Beauchamp, G. K., & Mennella, J. A. (2011). Flavor perception in human infants: development and functional significance. *Digestion*, *83*(Suppl 1), 1–6.

Bentley J.: July, 2017. U.S. Still Out of Balance with Dietary Recommendations. *Amber Waves*. From: <https://www.ers.usda.gov/amber-waves/2017/july/us-diets-still-out-of-balance-with-dietary-recommendations/>. (Accessed 18 October, 2020).

Centers for Disease Control and Prevention (CDC). (2018). *State indicator report on fruits and vegetables*. Atlanta, GA: Author. From: <https://www.cdc.gov/nutrition/data-statistics/2018-state-indicator-report-fruits-vegetables.html>. (Accessed 18 October, 2020).

Dutko, P., Ver Ploeg, M., & Farrigan, T. (2012). *Characteristics and influential factors of food deserts (ERR-140)*. Washington, DC: U.S. Department of Agriculture, Economic Research Service.

Guthrie J., Lin B.-H., Okrent A., Volpe R.: 2013. Americans' food choices at home and away: How do they compare with recommendations? *Amber Waves*. From: <www.ers.usda.gov/amber-waves/2013-february/americans-food-choices-at-home-and-away.aspx#.UdN7InDD8iQ/>. (Accessed 5 July, 2013).

Hartman Group. (2017). *Health + wellness 2017, executive summary*. Bellevue, WA: The Hartman Group, Inc.

Howard, A. J., Mallan, K., Byrne, R., Magarey, A., & Daniels, L. (2012). Toddlers' food preferences: the impact of novel food exposure, maternal preferences and food neophobia. *Appetite*, *59*, 818–825.

Logue. A. W. (2015). *The psychology of eating and drinking: An introduction* (4th ed.). New York: Taylor & Francis Books Inc.

Morrison R.M.: (2017). Food prices and spending. *Amber Waves*. From: <www.ers.usda.gov/data-products/ag-and-food-statistics-charting-the-essentials/food-prices-and-spending/>. (Accessed 21 September, 2017).

Moss. M. (2013). *Salt, sugar, fat: How the food giants hooked us*. New York: Random House.

National Vital Statistics Reports Deaths: 24 June, 2019. Leading Causes for 2017, 68(6). From: <https://www.cdc.gov/nchs/data/nvsr/nvsr68/nvsr68_06-508.pdf>. (Accessed 18 October, 2020).

Pollan. M. (2013). *Cooked: A natural history of transformation*. New York: The Penguin Press.

Produce for Better Health Foundation (PBHF): *Research and Consumer Insights*. From: <https://fruitsandveggies.org>. (Accessed 18 October, 2020).

U.S. Department of Agriculture (USDA): n.d. ChooseMyPlate.gov. From: <www.choosemyplate.gov>. (Accessed 18 October, 2020).

U.S. Department of Agriculture, Agricultural Marketing Service (USDA, AMS): 2016. Organic Certification and Accreditation; Organic Labeling. From: <www.ams.usda.gov/services/organic-certification> and <www.ams.usda.gov/rules-regulations/organic/labeling>. (Accessed 31 October, 2020).

U.S. Department of Agriculture, Economic Research Service (ERS-USDA): Food Access Research Atlas (Updated 31 October, 2019). From: <www.ers.usda.gov/data-products/food-access-research-atlas/download-the-data/#Current%20Version>. (Accessed 31 October, 2020).

U.S. Department of Agriculture and U.S. Department of Health and Human Services. December 2020. *Dietary Guidelines for Americans, 2020–2025*, ed 9. Available at DietaryGuidelines.gov. (Accessed 7 January, 2020).

U.S. Food and Drug Administration (FDA), *Center for food safety and applied nutrition: Changes to the nutrition facts label*, Silver Spring, MD, Author. (Updated: 16 August 2019) From: <www.fda.gov/Food/GuidanceRegulation/GuidanceDocumentsRegulatoryInformation/LabelingNutrition/ucm385663.htm>. (Accessed 1 November, 2020).

U.S. Food and Drug Administration, Office of Dietary Supplement Programs (FDA, ODSP): *Dietary supplements*, College Park, MD, Author. Updated: 8/16/2019. From: <www.fda.gov/Food/DietarySupplements/default.htm>. (Accessed 1 November, 2020).

3

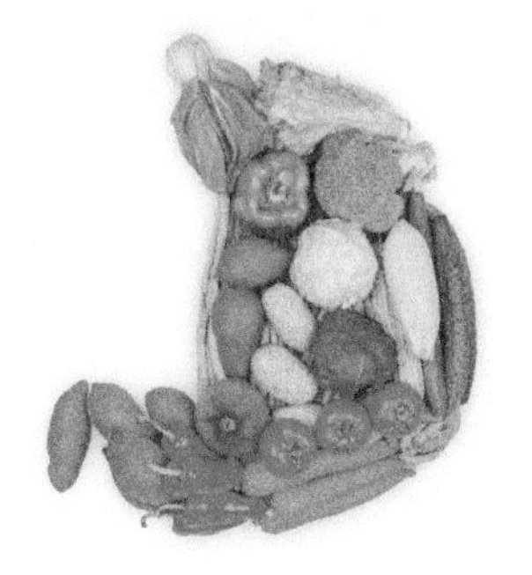

Digestion, Absorption, and Metabolism

The digestive system, which is responsible for processing foods, is itself dependent on the body's nutrient intake for its maintenance.

http://evolve.elsevier.com/GRODNER/FOUNDATIONS

LEARNING OBJECTIVES

- List the organs of the gastrointestinal (GI) tract and their functions.
- Identify other structures and organs supportive of digestion and absorption.
- Describe the three types of muscular actions of the GI tract.
- Discuss the digestive and absorption roles of the small intestine.
- Explain the function of metabolism.

ROLE IN WELLNESS

Gulping down breakfast on the way to class or work, skipping lunch, and then eating dinner late may not seem to affect the health status of adults. However, if this kind of eating becomes routine, it characterizes an individual's lifestyle and may negatively influence health status.

The body's health is based on the nutrients available to support growth, maintenance, and energy needs. Inadequate nutritional intake can affect the body's ability to use the foods consumed. The digestive system, which is responsible for processing foods, depends on nutrient intake for its maintenance. Although the body is resilient, we stress our physical limits when we adopt habits that do not support optimal health. A primary way to decrease the risk of future disease and achieve wellness is to use lifestyle choices that support positive health behaviors.

Physical health begins with the gastrointestinal (GI) tract as the first step to maintain body functioning; unless nutrients in foods are digested and absorbed, life cannot continue. The decision and follow-through to change lifestyle behaviors to positively improve health in relation to digestive disorders is an aspect of intellectual health. An individual's emotional state and ability to handle stress may increase the risk of several disorders of the GI tract. Consequently, the emotional health effects of lifestyle behaviors may be related to constipation, diarrhea, and heartburn. Reducing the causes of intestinal gas helps guard against socially embarrassing moments. Our food choices and styles of eating may affect the level of flatus experienced. Negativity associated with body smells is defined by society and thus affects our social health dimension. Respecting the sanctity of the human body, thereby acknowledging our spiritual health dimension, may include one's willingness to follow dietary and lifestyle changes to enhance the functioning of the GI tract (see the *Cultural Diversity and Nutrition* box Wholeness of Body, Mind, and Self). The environmental health dimension considers how we organize our lifestyles to allow adequate time for preparation and consumption of meals.

This chapter presents a brief orientation to the processes of digestion, absorption, and metabolism. These processes work together to provide all body cells with energy and nutrients.

DIGESTION

The main organs of the digestive system form the gastrointestinal (GI) tract, or alimentary canal, which creates an open tube that runs from the mouth to the anus (Fig. 3.1 and Box 3.1). Everything we eat is processed through the GI tract. The digestive system consists of a series of organs that prepare ingested nutrients for digestion and absorption and protect against

CULTURAL DIVERSITY AND NUTRITION

Wholeness of Body, Mind, and Self

This text's presentation of digestion and absorption is based on Western perspectives. To most Westerners, body organs tend to be viewed separately from mind and spiritual influences. In contrast, *Ayurveda*, the name given by traditional Indian medicine that means "the science of life," is based on living a balanced life. Consequently, Ayurveda regards physical disorders as imbalance of the body (organs) or life. Treatment works to bring balance or harmony back to the individual's life. The wholeness of life is represented by body (*shira*), mind (*manas*), and self (*atman*). All three require attention to achieve and maintain health. Because each component is important, Ayurveda is a holistic approach recognizing the interdependent roles of body, mind, and self. A person is viewed as a combination of three forces or humors called *doshas*. Each person is a different combination of these forces, which are *vata*, *pitta*, and *kapha*. *Vata* is a force similar to air; *pitta*, a force similar to fire; and *kapha*, a force like mucus and water. Health occurs when these *doshas* are in balance; otherwise disease occurs. If *pitta* is too strong, fever, ulcers, and liver disorders may occur. An individual would need to strengthen the other *doshas* through (1) changes in behaviors and food choices, (2) use of natural medicines, and (3) yoga and meditation to decrease *pitta* and regain balance.

Application to Nursing

This concept may assist clients to understand that their health may be affected by other components of their lives. Sometimes health concerns force us to confront factors that may influence our ability to maintain health or to achieve balance in our lives.

(Data from Ninivaggi, FJ: Ayurveda: A comprehensive guide to traditional Indian medicine for the West, Westport, CT, 2008, Praeger Press.)

BOX 3.1 Digestive System Organs

Segments of the Digestive Tract

Mouth
Oropharynx
Esophagus
Stomach
Small intestine
Duodenum
Jejunum
Ileum
Large intestine
Cecum
Colon:
 Ascending colon
 Transverse colon
 Descending colon
 Sigmoid colon
Rectum
Anal canal

Accessory Organs

Salivary glands
Parotid gland
Submandibular gland
Sublingual gland
Tongue
Teeth
Liver
Gallbladder
Pancreas
Vermiform appendix

consumed microorganisms and toxic substances. To accomplish these actions, several processes take place. These processes—ingestion, digestion, absorption, and elimination—depend on the motility or movement of the GI wall and the secretions of digestive juices and enzymes.

The Mouth

Are you hungry? Are you thinking about your favorite food? Is your mouth watering? Our mouths really do "water" when we think about or begin to eat foods. However, it is not actually water we sense but a thin mucus-like fluid called saliva. Saliva is the term for the secretions of the three sets of salivary glands of the mouth. As exocrine glands, each set of salivary glands produces a different type of secretion that is released into the mouth. The parotid glands create watery saliva that supplies enzymes; the submandibular glands produce mucus and enzyme components; and the sublingual glands, the smallest, create a mucous type of saliva. A reflex mechanism controls these secretions.

Food in the mouth stimulates chemical and mechanical digestion. Chemical digestion occurs through the action of saliva that not only moistens the foods we chew but also contains amylase, an enzyme that begins the digestive process of starches.

Another digestive process that occurs in the mouth is mechanical digestion, which depends on teeth. Teeth rhythmically tear and pulverize food. The enamel covering teeth is the hardest substance in the body and therefore protects teeth from the harsh effects of chewing. (See the *Personal Perspectives* box Which Came First, the Fork and Knife or the Overbite?) The tongue assists with mechanical digestion by guiding food into chewing positions and then leading the pulverized food into the esophagus. Another function of the tongue is that of taste. More than 2000 taste buds are responsible for our sensations of sweet, bitter, sour, and salty when we taste foods (Fig. 3.2).

As toddlers, we have the highest number of taste buds and a higher degree of taste sensitivity, so bland foods are more appealing. The number of taste buds declines as we grow older, explaining why older adults have diminished taste sensitivity. Older adults may need to be encouraged to avoid the use of too much salt, particularly if they have hypertension or cardiac disorders.

Our sense of smell works along with our taste bud sensations. These two combined senses actually account for the perception (and enjoyment) of the flavors of different foods. Our positive or negative response to specific foods based on our sensory perception affects our food choices (Mahan et al, 2017).

Portions of the pulverized or masticated food are formed into the shape of a ball called a bolus. The tongue effortlessly forms the bolus, which is then swallowed and passed by the epiglottis into the esophagus within about 5 to 7 seconds. The epiglottis is a flap of tissue that closes over the trachea to prevent the bolus from entering the lungs.

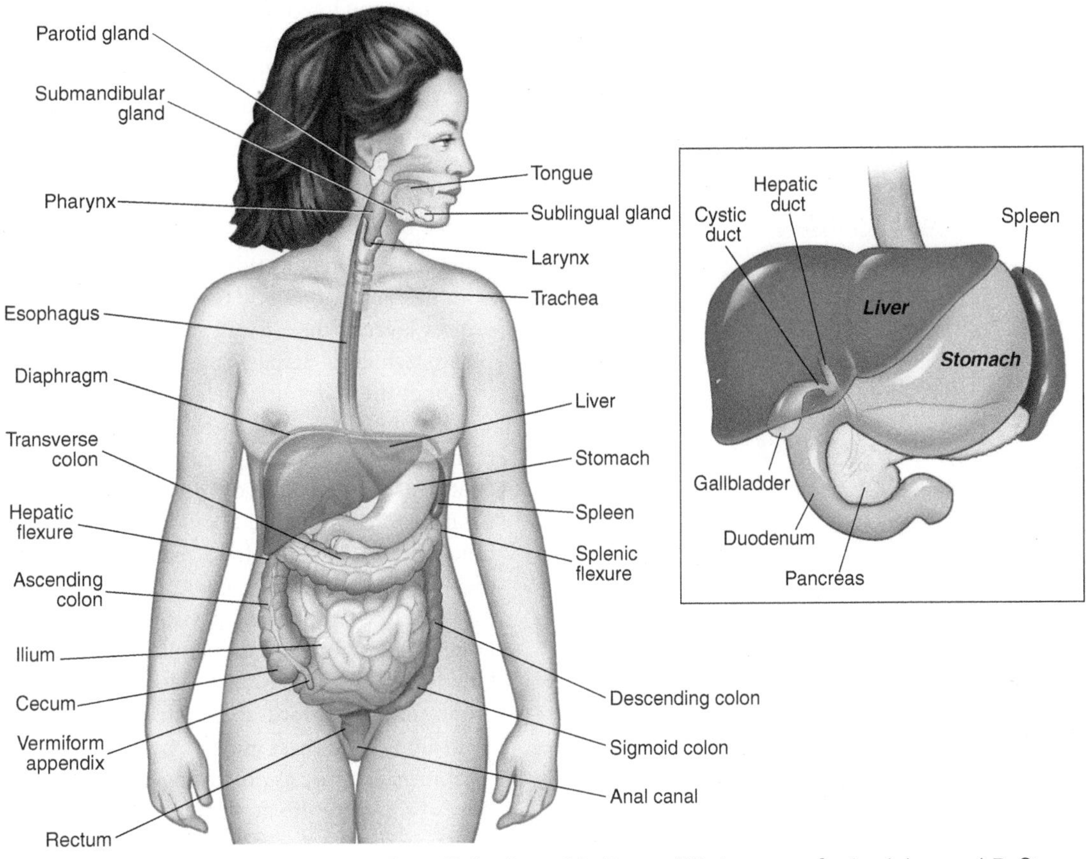

Fig. 3.1 The digestive system. (From Thibodeau GA, Patton KT: *Anatomy & physiology*, ed 5, St Louis, 2003, Mosby.)

PERSONAL PERSPECTIVES

Which Came First, the Fork and Knife or the Overbite?

Bee Wilson has written a fascinating account about how we cook around the world and through the centuries in *Consider the Fork: A History of How We Cook and Eat*. Her research reveals the past dangers of cooking throughout history, from young children wandering into the flames of families' cooking hearths to the use of young boys or dogs to spin roasting meats to prevent charring and uneven cooking while being exposed to searing heat from open flames. Here we consider an example of human physiologic change.

We tend to forget that human physiology changes very slowly over the passage of time. Of course, we consider ourselves different than the Neanderthals in our choice of food preparation methods, such as cooked rather than raw, and how we consume foods based on our cultural customs, ranging from using fingers, knives, or forks to chopsticks. According to the historical research of Charles Loring Brace, an anthropology professor, one of the substantial physical changes to human anatomy occurred as recently as the late eighteenth century: the overbite of the jaw. Previously, an "edge-to-edge" bite of the top jaw meeting the edge of the lower jaw prevailed and an overbite was not to be found.

The potential cause appears to be not a change in what we eat but how we eat our food. In the past a large quantity of food was put into one's mouth. What could not be contained in the oral cavity was then ripped off by clenching one's teeth. In this circumstance, an edge-to-edge bite was the efficient way to "cut" the food away from one's mouth. A knife could, carefully, be used to achieve the same purpose, but teeth were safer.

This significant change in physiology may have come about because of how knives, with the assistance of forks to hold the food still, allowed foods to be cut into bite-sized pieces to more easily be chewed. As customs around food evolved, cultures prized the genteel nature of cutting food into smaller and smaller pieces that barely required chewing. Therefore, the overbite—of the top jaw hanging over the lower jaw—emerged as the tearing role of the teeth became obsolete.

Although the knife had been around a very long time, the newer use of the fork to ease the cutting of bite-sized pieces of food allowed the overbite to evolve. We can just wonder what the next physiologic change may be!

(Data from Wilson B: *Consider the fork: A history of how we cook and eat*, New York, 2012, Basic Books.)

The Esophagus

The esophagus is a muscular tube through which the bolus travels from the mouth to the stomach. The process begins at the top of the esophagus when peristalsis, the involuntary movements of circular and longitudinal muscles, begins and draws the bolus farther into the GI tract. This mechanical action further breaks down the size of foodstuff and increases its exposure to digestive secretions. Muscular actions depend on the four layers of tissues that form the tube of the GI tract (Fig. 3.3). The mucosa is composed of mucous membrane and forms the inside layer. Under the mucosa is the submucosa, a layer of connective tissue. Digestion depends on the blood vessels and nerves of the submucosa to regulate digestion. Surrounding the submucosa is a thick layer of muscle tissue called the muscularis. The outermost layer of the GI wall is made of serous membrane called serosa, which is actually the visceral layer of the peritoneum that lines the abdominal pelvic cavity and covers organs.

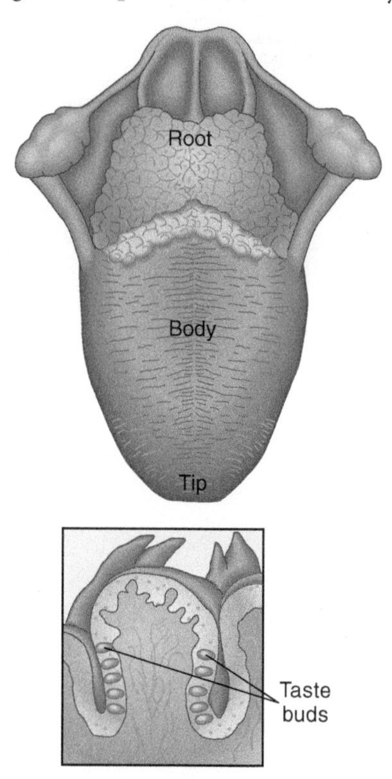

Fig. 3.2 (A) Parts of the tongue. (B) A detailed site of taste buds. (From Thibodeau GA, Patton KT: *Anatomy & physiology*, ed 5, St Louis, 2003, Mosby.)

The coordination of these layers provides the varied movements required for digestion. Essentially, muscular action controls the movement of the food mass through the GI tract. Churning action within a segment of the GI tract allows secretions to mix with the food mass. Circular muscles surround the GI tube. Rhythmic contractions of these muscles cause the wavelike motions of peristalsis, moving food downward. Longitudinal muscles run parallel along the GI tube. The combined effect of the circular and longitudinal muscles causes segmentation, a forward-and-backward movement that assists in controlling food mass movement through the GI tract.

Sphincter muscles are stronger, circular muscles that act as valves to control the movement of the food mass in a forward direction. In effect, sphincter muscles prevent reflux by forming an opening when relaxed and closing completely when contracted. At the bottom of the esophagus, the cardiac sphincter controls the movement of the bolus from the esophagus into the stomach. It also prevents the acidic contents of the stomach from moving upward back through the esophagus.

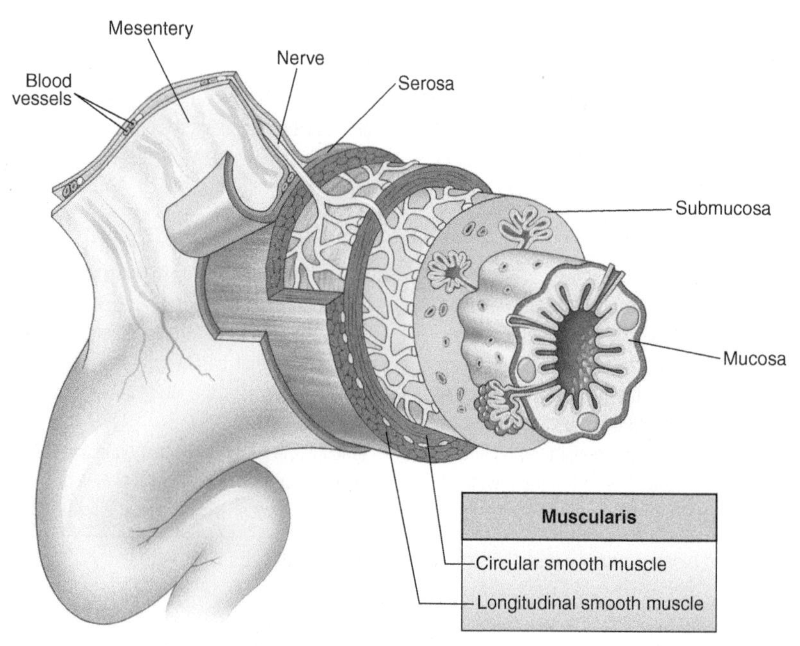

Fig. 3.3 Muscle layers of the gastrointestinal tract. (From Thibodeau GA, Patton KT: *Anatomy & physiology*, ed 5, St Louis, 2003, Mosby.)

The Stomach

Functions of the stomach include the following:

- Holding food for partial digestion
- Producing gastric juice
- Providing muscular action that, combined with gastric juice, mixes and tears food into smaller pieces
- Secreting the intrinsic factor for vitamin B_{12} absorption
- Releasing gastrin
- Assisting in the destruction, through its acidity of secretions, of pathogenic bacteria that may have inadvertently been consumed

When the bolus passes through the cardiac sphincter, it enters the fundus, the upper portion of the stomach that connects with the esophagus. The other divisions of the stomach include the body, or center portion, and the pylorus, the lower portion. The stomach wall contains gastric mucosa with gastric pits. At the base of the pits are the gastric glands whose chief cells create gastric juice, a mucous fluid containing digestive enzymes, and parietal cells, which secrete stomach acid called hydrochloric acid.

Gastric secretions occur in three phases: cephalic, gastric, and intestinal (Sullivan et al, 2014). The cephalic phase is called the psychic phase because mental factors can stimulate gastrin, a hormone secreted by stomach mucosa. In the gastric phase, gastrin increases the release of gastric juices when the stomach is distended by food. The third phase is the intestinal phase, in which the gastric secretions change as chyme, a semiliquid mixture of food mass, passes through to the duodenum. Gastric secretions are inhibited by exocrine and nervous reflexes of gastric inhibitory peptides, secretin, and cholecystokinin (CCK) (also called pancreozymin), a hormone secreted by intestinal mucosa.

Some gastric juices provide acidity in the stomach to assist the effective function of certain enzymes. As agents of chemical digestion, enzymes are specific in action, working only on individual classes of nutrients and changing substances from one form to a simpler form. Enzymes are "organic catalysts" formed from protein structures. They function at specific pH levels and are continually created and destroyed. Specific enzymes are required for energy release and digestion.

Hormones regulate the release of gastric juices and enzymes, acting as messengers between organs to cause the release of needed secretions. In digestion, hormones affect the secretions from the stomach, intestines, and gallbladder. These secretions may slow or speed digestion and may affect the pH levels of gastric juice. Overall, the mechanical and chemical actions work together to complete the process of digestion.

Gastric motility, or movement of the food mass through the stomach, requires 2 to 6 hours. The churning and mixing of the food mass with gastric juices create a semiliquid mixture called chyme. When chyme enters the pylorus section of the stomach, it causes distention and the release of the hormone gastrin. Gastrin sends a message that hydrochloric acid (HCl) is needed to continue the breakdown of chyme. As HCl is released from the stomach lining, thick mucus is also secreted to protect the stomach walls from the harsh HCl.

Every 20 seconds chyme is released into the duodenum, the upper portion of the small intestine; this action is controlled by the hormonal and nervous system mechanism of enterogastric reflex. This consists of duodenal receptors in the mucosa that are sensitive to the presence of acid and distention. The impulses over sensory and motor fibers in the vagus nerve cause a reflex restriction of gastric peristalsis. For example, the gastric inhibitory peptide released in response to fats in the duodenum decreases peristalsis of stomach muscles and slows chyme passage. The result is decreased motility, which is why the stomach empties more slowly when a person eats a high-fat diet.

The combined action of mechanical digestion (the strong muscular movements of peristalsis) and chemical digestion (the effects of the gastric juices) works to prepare nutrients for the process of absorption. Chyme is kept in the stomach by the actions of the pyloric sphincter, which slowly releases it into the duodenum.

The Small Intestine

The chyme entering the duodenum soon moves through to the jejunum and ileum of the small intestine. It takes about 5 hours for chyme to pass through the small intestine because of the action of segmentation and peristalsis. Segmentation in the duodenum and upper jejunum mixes chyme with digestive juices from the pancreas, liver, and intestinal mucosa. Peristalsis is controlled by intrinsic stretch reflexes and is initiated by CCK, the hormone secreted by intestinal mucosa.

In the small intestine the nutrients in chyme are prepared for absorption. The small intestine is the major organ of digestion, and the final stages of the digestive process occur here. Because it is also the site of almost all the absorption of nutrients, the intestinal lining must be able to accommodate the actions of both digestion and absorption. The intestinal walls are covered with a thin layer of mucus, which protects the walls from digestive juices. The walls are also adapted to enhance the absorption process. Finger-like projections called villi greatly increase the amount of mucosal layer available for the absorption of nutrients (Fig. 3.4). On the villi are hair-like projections called microvilli that also enhance absorption by their structure and movements.

As chyme enters the small intestine, hormones begin sending messages that regulate the release of digestive juices to continue the process of chyme digestion. Some hormones are provided by the small intestine; several are released by other organs into the small intestine. These secretions include enzymes from the small intestines, bile produced in the liver, and digestive juices from the pancreas.

One of the first hormones released by the small intestine is secretin. This hormone causes the pancreas to send bicarbonate to the small intestine to reduce the acidic content of the chyme. As the acidic level decreases, other pancreatic juices enter and begin their work. Another hormone secreted by the small intestine is CCK, which initiates pancreatic exocrine secretions, acts against gastrin by inhibiting gastric HCl secretion, and activates the gallbladder to contract, causing bile to be released into the duodenum.

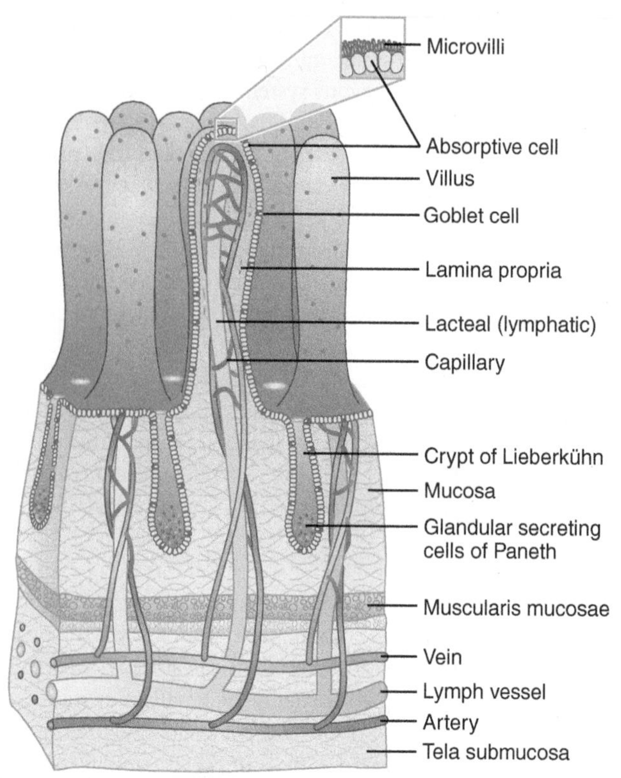

Fig. 3.4 Structure of the intestinal wall. The circular folds, villi, and microvilli multiply the surface area and enhance absorption. (From Mahan LK, et al, editors: *Krause's food & the nutrition care process*, ed 13, Philadelphia, 2012, Saunders.)

TABLE 3.1 Digestive Processes

Mechanism	Description
Ingestion	Process of taking food into the mouth, starting it on its journey through the digestive tract
Digestion	A group of processes that break complex nutrients into simpler ones, thus facilitating their absorption; mechanical digestion physically breaks large chunks into small bits; chemical digestion breaks molecules apart
Motility	Movement by the muscular components of the digestive tube, including processes of mechanical digestion; examples are peristalsis and segmentation
Secretion	Release of digestive juices (containing enzymes, acids, bases, mucus, bile, or other products that facilitate digestion); some digestive organs secrete endocrine hormones that regulate digestion or metabolism of nutrients
Absorption	Movement of digested nutrients through the gastrointestinal mucosa and into the internal environment
Elimination	Excretion of the residues of the digestive process (feces) from the rectum, through the anus; defecation

(Data from Thibodeau GA, Patton KT: *Anatomy & physiology*, ed 5, St Louis, 2003, Mosby.)

Bile, which is secreted by the liver and stored in the gallbladder, is released to emulsify fats, aiding in the digestion of lipids. The emulsification creates more surface area, allowing lipid enzymes to digest fats to their component parts. The liver continuously secretes bile, and CCK and secretin spur the gallbladder to release bile for the digestion of fats. In addition, the small intestine produces enzymes to assist in the digestive process. Although much of the chyme is absorbed, the rest—which usually consists of fiber, minerals, and water—passes through the next sphincter (ileocecal valve) and into the large intestine (ascending colon).

The Large Intestine

The large intestine consists of the cecum, colon, and rectum. The cecum is a blind pocket; therefore, the mass bypasses it and enters the ascending colon, which leads into the transverse colon running across the abdomen over the small intestine to the descending colon. The descending colon extends down the left of the abdomen into the sigmoid colon and leads into the descending colon, on to the rectum, and into the anal canal. Finally, any remaining mass passes out through the anus. The journey through the large intestine takes about 9 to 16 hours.

In the large intestine or colon, final absorption of any available nutrients, usually water and some minerals, occurs. Bacteria residing in the large intestine produce several vitamins, which are then absorbed. Water is withdrawn from the fibrous mass, forming solidified feces. Mucous glands in the intestinal wall create mucus that lubricates and covers feces as it forms. Again, peristalsis continues to move substances through the GI tract, resulting in the excretion of feces from the colon through the anus, the last sphincter muscle of the GI tract.

The movement of the food mass through the GI tract is controlled to enhance digestion and absorption. During passage through the GI tract, more than 95% of the carbohydrates, fats, and proteins ingested are absorbed. Some minerals, vitamins, and trace elements may be less absorbed (Sullivan et al, 2014). Table 3.1 summarizes the primary mechanisms of the digestive system. Details of carbohydrate, protein, and lipid digestion follow in specific chapters.

ABSORPTION

Although the food mass has possibly spent several hours in the tube of the GI tract, it is not yet actually inside the body until its nutrient components are absorbed. Absorption is the process by which substances pass through the intestinal mucosa into the blood or lymph. Transport processes provide the means for nutrients to actually pass through the wall of the small intestine. These include passive diffusion and osmosis, facilitated diffusion, energy-dependent active transport, and engulfing pinocytosis (Fig. 3.5).

Passive diffusion occurs when pressure is greater on one side of the membrane and the substance then moves from the area of greater pressure to less pressure, allowing molecules to travel through capillaries. Facilitated diffusion takes place when, despite positive pressure flow, molecules may be unable to pass through membrane pores unless aided. Specific integral membrane proteins support the movement

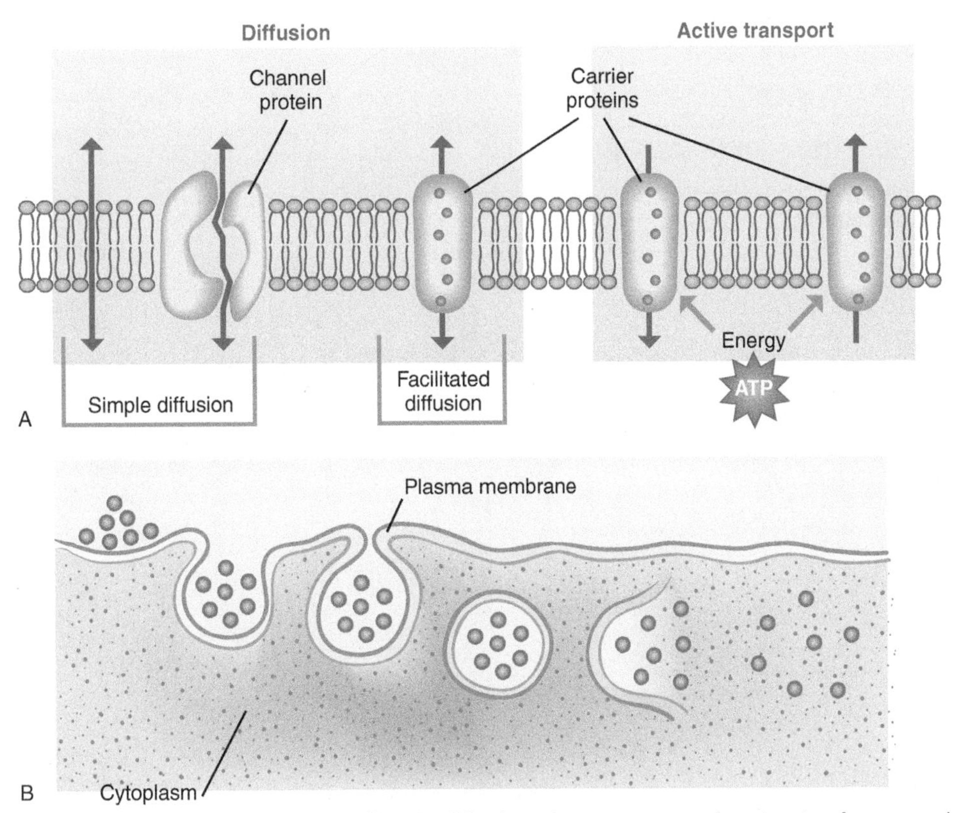

Fig. 3.5 (A) Methods of absorption. Simple diffusion, the movement of molecules from a region of high concentration to low concentration; facilitated diffusion, the movement of molecules by a carrier protein across the cell membrane from a region of high to low concentration; *active transport*, the movement of molecules and ions by means of a carrier protein against fluid pressures that require expenditure of cellular energy. *ATP*, Adenosine triphosphate. (B) Pinocytosis. (**A** from Mahan LK, Raymond JL, eds: *Krause's food & the nutrition care process*, ed 13, Philadelphia, 2012, Saunders; **B** from Nix S: *Williams' basic nutrition & diet therapy*, ed 12, St Louis, 2005, Mosby.)

by bringing the larger nutrient molecules through the capillary membrane.

Energy-dependent active transport happens when fluid pressures work against the passage of nutrients. As an active process, it requires energy. This energy is supplied by the cell and a "pumping" mechanism, which are assisted by a special membrane protein carrier. Engulfing pinocytosis takes place when a substance, either a fluid or a nutrient, contacts the villi membrane, which then surrounds the substance and creates a vacuole that encompasses the substance. Passing through the cell cytoplasm, the substance is then released into the circulatory system. The amounts of vitamins and minerals absorbed depend on the body's storage levels and immediate need for these nutrients. Nutrients such as fats, carbohydrates, and protein are easily absorbed regardless of the level of need. The structure of the small intestine, the site of almost all nutrient absorption, allows for efficient absorption to occur. The microvilli are sensitive to the exact nutrient needs of the body. Their wavelike motions, caused by peristalsis, result in the most exposure of the nutrient-laden chyme to the absorbing cells. This exposure allows needed nutrients to leave the GI tract and pass through the microvilli cells. At this point the nutrients are truly "inside" the body.

Various factors may affect absorption of nutrients. Combinations of naturally occurring substances, such as fiber or binders, may move nutrients through the GI tract too quickly for optimum absorption to occur. Individual nutrient absorption and other issues of bioavailability are addressed in other chapters. The relationship between food and drug absorption is also an important issue of medical treatment. Ingesting a medication with food may decrease the absorption rate of the medication and may interfere with the absorption of other nutrients contained in the food consumed. This issue is explored in depth in Chapter 11.

Once "inside" the body, the nutrients enter the circulatory systems of the bloodstream or lymphatic system. The general circulatory or blood system receives absorbed protein, carbohydrates, small parts of broken-down fats, and most vitamins and minerals. This system transports these nutrients throughout the body. The lymphatic system, a secondary circulatory system, receives large lipids and fat-soluble vitamins. The nutrients traveling in the lymphatic system are deposited into the bloodstream near the heart. All nutrients then circulate throughout the body in the blood, providing for the nutrient requirements of cells.

Soon after entering the bloodstream, nutrients pass by the liver. This arrangement allows the liver to have "first choice" of

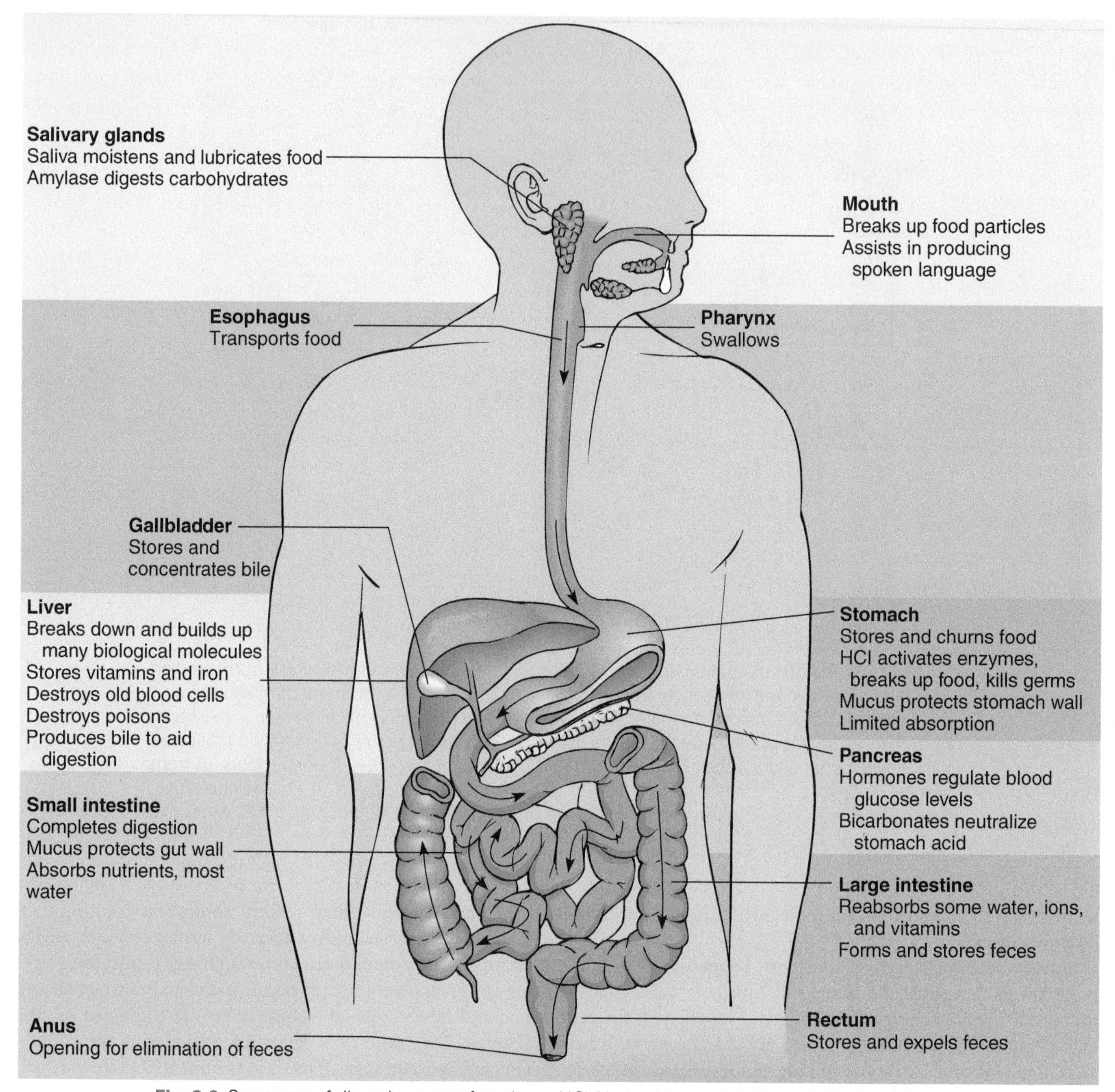
Salivary glands
Saliva moistens and lubricates food
Amylase digests carbohydrates
Mouth
Breaks up food particles
Assists in producing spoken language
Esophagus
Transports food
Pharynx
Swallows
Gallbladder
Stores and concentrates bile
Liver
Breaks down and builds up many biological molecules
Stores vitamins and iron
Destroys old blood cells
Destroys poisons
Produces bile to aid digestion
Stomach
Stores and churns food
HCl activates enzymes, breaks up food, kills germs
Mucus protects stomach wall
Limited absorption
Pancreas
Hormones regulate blood glucose levels
Bicarbonates neutralize stomach acid
Small intestine
Completes digestion
Mucus protects gut wall
Absorbs nutrients, most water
Large intestine
Reabsorbs some water, ions, and vitamins
Forms and stores feces
Anus
Opening for elimination of feces
Rectum
Stores and expels feces

Fig. 3.6 Summary of digestive organ functions. *HCl*, Hydrochloric acid. (From Rolin Graphics.)

the available nutrients. The liver is a powerhouse organ that provides a wide variety of services and substances; thus, its nutrient needs are a priority. From there, the bloodstream's journey of nutrients continues to the heart to also give it a prime nutrient selection. The journey then continues through the circulatory system to all cells. Some nutrients end up in nutrient storage sites of the body. These sites include the bones, liver, and kidneys. Other nutrients, if not discarded or used by cells, are filtered out of the blood by the kidneys to be reabsorbed or excreted in urine.

Elimination

The expulsion of feces or body waste products is called defecation. When the rectum is distended because of waste accumulation, the reflex to defecate occurs. The residue may include substances such as cellulose and other dietary fibers and connective tissue from meat collagen that are unable to be digested by human enzymes. Undigested fats may combine with dietary minerals, such as calcium and magnesium, and form residue. Additional residue may include water, bacteria, pigments, and mucus. Fig. 3.6 summarizes the functions of the digestive

TEACHING TOOL

Digesting Food: A Primer for Clients and Patients

As health care professionals, we may assume our clients understand the way the body works as easily as we do. More than likely, however, their knowledge is limited, and even if they studied digestion years ago in a health education class, they may have forgotten or replaced facts with misinformation.

When working with clients for health promotion or with patients recovering from GI disorders, the nurse should consider using the summary of digestive organ functions (see Fig. 3.6) as a teaching tool. A visual review of the digestive organs and processes can give clients and patients a clearer concept of the purposes of dietary recommendations, and they may therefore find compliance easier.

system, and the *Teaching Tool* box Digesting Food: A Primer for Clients and Patients provides suggestions for client and patient teaching.

Overall food transit times for nutrients to move from our plate to our cells are as follows:

Chewing and swallowing	Depends on texture and quantity
Esophagus	5–7 seconds
Stomach	2–6 hours
Small intestine	Approximately 5 hours
Large intestine	9–16 hours
Total	16–27 hours ingestion to elimination

Digestive Process Throughout the Life Span

Over the course of the life span, the main and accessory organs of digestion develop and change. The immature GI tract, particularly the intestinal mucosa of a young infant, may allow intact proteins to be absorbed without complete digestion occurring. This incomplete digestion may result in an allergic response by the immune system and is part of the reason to delay the introduction of solid foods (e.g., cereals) until the GI tract has matured sufficiently. Another age-related condition is lactose intolerance, in which the body ceases to produce lactase, the enzyme that breaks down the milk carbohydrate of lactose. For some people, this occurs once the primary growth needs for nutrients contained in milk is met. For others, it may not occur until adulthood or not at all. Older adults sometimes experience lactose intolerance when the secretion of enzymes, including lactase, decreases as part of the aging process. Conditions of the middle years include gallbladder disease and peptic ulcers (sores that may occur on the epithelial surfaces of the stomach or small intestine). Older years may be marked by problems of constipation and diverticulosis. These conditions may be associated with age-related reductions in peristalsis and physical activity and may be worsened by a lifelong history of chronic low dietary fiber consumption. GI disorders are discussed in Chapter 13. Other issues related to aging are discussed in other chapters, particularly Chapter 10.

METABOLISM

It is hard to imagine that a lunch consisting of tuna on rye bread will actually end up being part of the cells of the body. Fortunately, the human body is able to transform the nutrients of the sandwich into substances usable by cells. **Metabolism** is a set of processes through which absorbed nutrients are used by the body for energy and to form and maintain body structures and functions. The two main processes of metabolism involve catabolism and anabolism. Catabolism is the breakdown of food components into smaller molecular particles, which causes the release of energy as heat and chemical energy. Anabolism is the process of synthesis from which substances are formed, such as new bone or muscle tissue. Both processes happen within cells at the same time.

When nutrients finally reach individual cells, they may be chemically changed through anabolism to help form new cell structures or to create new substances such as hormones and enzymes. Some vitamins and minerals assist in the use of other nutrients within the cell. They act as catalysts or coenzymes to initiate and support the transformation and use of carbohydrates, proteins, and lipids. Other nutrients may be used as energy to continue life-supporting processes. These processes include the energy needed to support deoxyribonucleic acid (DNA) reproduction and create proteins and other molecules, nerve impulses, and muscle contractions. Some energy is stored in a ready-to-use state. Specific metabolic functions of individual nutrients are discussed in Chapters 4 to 8.

Waste products from metabolism are discarded by the cells and wind up circulating in the blood. They are then excreted through the lungs, kidneys, or large intestine. The lungs release excess water and carbon dioxide. The kidneys filter and excrete metabolic waste and excess vitamins and minerals but reabsorb nutrients that the body needs to retain. Waste products may also be discarded through the large intestine in feces. Fortunately, we do not have to consciously control these processes. Our responsibility is to provide an adequate selection of nutrients through the foods we choose to eat and to eat those foods in a way that enhances the functioning of the GI tract.

Metabolism Throughout the Life Span

Metabolic changes are most noticeable later in life as the amount of food energy required decreases in relation to lowered metabolic rates. Nutrient needs, however, remain constant. As we (and our clients) enter the middle years and beyond, our challenge is to meet nutrient needs while maintaining or reducing our kcal needs to equal actual metabolic use. Recognition of this change can forestall the unexpected weight gain that appears to accompany aging in the United States.

Some of our lifestyle behaviors affect the functioning and health of our GI tracts and therefore influence our nutritional status (see the *Social Issues* box Hunger Versus Appetite Versus Time). Some common GI tract health problems are caused by the everyday decisions that we make, but that can be changed. Some common GI tract health problems are caused by lifestyle behaviors that can be changed. Prevention suggestions and treatment strategies for heartburn, intestinal gas, and constipation consider the effect of lifestyle behaviors. Although vomiting and diarrhea are not usually related to lifestyle, each has an impact on the functioning of the GI tract. Prevention suggestions and treatment strategies for some common GI tract health problems are considered in Chapter 13. (See the *Health Debate* box Are Specialty Yogurts the Key to "Regularity"?)

HEALTH DEBATE

Are Specialty Yogurts the Key to "Regularity"?

Yogurts, which contain at least the starter probiotic cultures *Lactobacillus bulgaricus* and *Streptococcus thermophilus*, are recognized for their health-promoting value, particularly for the digestive tract. Probiotics can replace or push out problematic bacteria, thereby possibly decreasing gas, bloating, and constipation. Some sustain the immune system and may be preventive against antibiotic-related diarrhea.

Many yogurt brands contain additional probiotics such as *Lactobacillus rhamnosus*, *Lactobacillus casei*, and *Bifidobacterium animalis DN-173 010* (trademarked by Dannon as *Bifidus regularis* in the United States). These cultures, when listed as "live and active" ingredients of products, are probiotics—beneficial bacteria microorganisms that reside in the small intestine. In addition to yogurt, foods such as kefir, aged cheese, sauerkraut, kimchi, tempeh, and miso soup also contain the live probiotic bacteria.

But probiotics are not the only beneficial microorganisms found in the ecosystem or microbiome of our GI-tract, nor do we have to directly consume probiotics. As prebiotics, types of dietary fiber that when consumed feed healthy gut bacteria (discussed further in Chapter 13).

Marketing campaigns present certain yogurt products, such as *Activia* by Dannon, as able to "naturally regulate your digestive system," because of the added probiotics. Other yogurt brands contain even more probiotics than *Activia*, which also influence the digestive and immune systems, as well as foods that contain prebiotics.

Should we consume probiotics from heavily marketed (expensive and quite sweet) designer food products or from more traditional yogurt products containing similar probiotics? Should probiotics even be a concern, or should they be viewed as a dietary supplement? Do we really need to buy special (and sweetened) products to be "regular"?

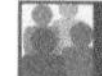

SOCIAL ISSUES

Hunger Versus Appetite Versus Time

Our daily schedules often determine our responses to hunger. Ever notice how differently you eat during the week compared with the weekend? The weekday mosaic of classes, studying, work, and possibly sports training often makes fitting in time to get to the campus cafeteria a Herculean feat. Or, if you prepare your own meals, time must be set aside for buying and cooking foods. Weekends may be more leisurely without classes or work, or perhaps we find time for socializing.

Yet, somehow, we manage. Although fewer meals may be eaten during the week, we are not any less hungry, nor are our energy needs lower. Sometimes, chaotic schedules may be accommodated by telling ourselves we are not really hungry, or we just do not have time to eat.

How can we do that? Isn't hunger a physiologic need for energy and nutrients? Can we just think ourselves through the hunger sensation? To understand this process, we need to explore the feeding regulating mechanism of the body.

Our sense of hunger and satiety is governed by the *hypothalamus*, a small portion of the brain. Its purpose is to maintain homeostasis (a state of balance) by regulating food intake through a feeding (hunger) center and a satiety center. The response of the hypothalamus, which initiates the hunger sensation, is thought to be related to either low blood glucose levels or to the lack of chyme in the stomach.

When we eat, blood glucose levels rise, and chyme is once again in the stomach. The hypothalamus responds by providing a feeling of satiety or satisfaction, and we stop eating.

When we "feel" hungry, we are recognizing the internal stimuli of hunger. Perhaps our stomach seems to be rumbling or "empty" or we are "starving." These sensations are tied to physical events in our bodies. When we act on these signals, we eat. However, we can also choose to ignore them. This means that we cognitively override the sensation and do not respond. There are physical mechanisms to cope with the lack of new energy sources, but it is still stressful to our bodies.

External stimuli also affect our desire or appetite for eating. Referred to as environmental cues, these stimuli include the smell and sight of food, which may artificially increase our hunger. Simply seeing a food commercial on television or talking about food can excite the feeding center, even if the stomach is not actually "empty." We also associate eating with specific social settings and time of day, regardless of our physical need for food. How can a birthday be celebrated without a cake? Religious holidays are often associated with special foods or meals. Throughout our elementary school experience, we ate lunch when we were scheduled, not necessarily when we were hungry.

All those years of eating by schedules and events have led us to adapt by overriding our cognitive cues about our real sense of hunger. Now, when personal schedules are more individualized, we may find that the external stimuli supporting our appropriate intake of food are gone; we must develop our own cues to ensure optimal nutritional intakes.

(Data from Logue AW: *The psychology of eating and drinking: An introduction*, ed 4, New York, 2015, Freeman; and Mahan LK, Raymond JL, editors: *Krause's food & the nutrition care process*, ed 14, Philadelphia, 2017, Saunders.)

TOWARD A POSITIVE NUTRITION LIFESTYLE: CONTRACTING

Have you ever made a bet? Contracting is similar to making a bet with a friend, except the object of the bet is a health behavior. A contract is a specific agreement with oneself or between you and a friend, spouse, or other relative. The agreement represents your willingness to attempt to change a health-related behavior. The advantage to contracting is that the goal or behavior change is clearly defined and observable. You also decide on a specific period within which to achieve the goal. As with a bet, you determine a reward or penalty for not completing the contract. (Yes, contracts with oneself are much easier to break.) The expectation is that practicing a new health-related behavior for a specific period makes the change permanent.

A contract with oneself might be to drink eight glasses of water a day for a week to relieve constipation. The change to increase fluid intake is a behavior you can directly control and observe. Although the aim is to alleviate constipation, which may not be a behavior you can consciously change, you can reduce its risk factors. At the end of the week, your reward could be to see a movie with a friend, whereas the penalty might be to clean out your messy bedroom closet.

Perhaps you have noticed that you regularly work through lunch and eat at your desk. The result is that heartburn has become a regular discomfort, and a discussion of remedies is often the topic of work breaks. A co-worker complains that she seems unable to break her habit of buying a high-calorie Danish pastry with her coffee each morning. You could contract with her that for the next 2 weeks you will eat lunch away from your desk, either in the employee cafeteria or at a local restaurant. She contracts with you that she will buy fruit instead of a Danish pastry for her morning snack. If you both complete the contracts, a reward could be to lunch together at a special restaurant. If only one person completes a contract, the penalty could be for the "loser" to pack a brown bag lunch for a week for the "winner." Contracting is applicable to many aspects of contemporary lifestyles and is limited only by our imagination.

SUMMARY

- GI tract organs include the mouth, esophagus, stomach, small intestine, and large intestine.
- Other supportive structures and organs are the teeth, tongue, salivary glands, liver, gallbladder, and pancreas.
- The small intestine is the main site of nutrient digestion and absorption.
- Digestion and absorption are achieved through mechanical and chemical digestion.
- Mechanical digestion consists of chewing, peristalsis, segmentation, and the actions of sphincter muscles, which regulate the movement of foodstuff through one organ to the next.
- Chemical digestion is the actual breakdown of substances resulting from the production and storage of gastric and digestive secretions.
- Nutrients, once absorbed, are transported through the blood circulatory system or the lymphatic system, becoming available to all cells.
- Once nutrients reach the cells, metabolism may occur at once. Metabolic changes allow the nutrients to fulfill many cell functions.
- Digestion, absorption, and metabolism work together to provide all body cells with energy and nutrients.

THE NURSING APPROACH: CLINICAL JUDGMENT AND NEXT-GENERATION NCLEX® EXAMINATION-STYLE QUESTIONS

Case Study

A client comes to the clinic complaining of digestive problems. The nurse explains that, "Everything we eat is processed through the gastrointestinal (GI) tract. The **digestive system** consists of a series of organs that prepare ingested nutrients for **digestion** and absorption and protect against consumed harmful microorganisms and toxic substances." To accomplish these actions, several processes take place.

Use an X to mark each of the processes of the digestive system.

Number	Process
1.	Metabolism
2.	Ingestion
3.	Elimination
4.	Digestion
5.	Secretion
6.	Absorption

APPLYING CONTENT KNOWLEDGE

James, a senior at the local university, is completing his internship at the rock radio station while continuing to work at his part-time job. Without any time to spare, he has been eating meals whenever he can, often from fast-food restaurants. These meals are usually gobbled quickly in his car. Lately, though, he is feeling stressed and is experiencing heartburn. List three lifestyle behaviors that James could change to possibly reduce heartburn.

WEBSITES OF INTEREST

Healthfinder.gov

health.gov/myhealthfinder

Provides a wealth of information and tools on health, coordinated by the National Health Information Center, U.S. Department of Health and Human Services.

American Dental Association

www.ada.org

Source of up-to-date news items and search tools related to oral health.

National Digestive Disease Information Clearinghouse (NDDIC)

www.niddk.nih.gov/health-information/digestive-diseases/digestive-system-how-it-works

Sponsored by the National Institute of Diabetes and Digestive and Kidney Diseases, the Health Information Center provides health and education materials such as *Your Digestive System & How It Works*

REFERENCES

Mahan, L. K., & Raymond, J. L. (Eds.). (2017). *Krause's food and the nutrition care process* (14th ed.). Philadelphia: Saunders.

Sullivan, S., Alpers, D., & Klein, S. (2014). Nutritional physiology of the alimentary tract. In A. C. Ross, B. Caballero, R. J. Cousins, C. L. Tucker, & T. R. Ziegler (Eds.), *Modern nutrition in health and disease* (11th ed.). Philadelphia: Wolters Kluwer/Lippincott Williams & Wilkins.

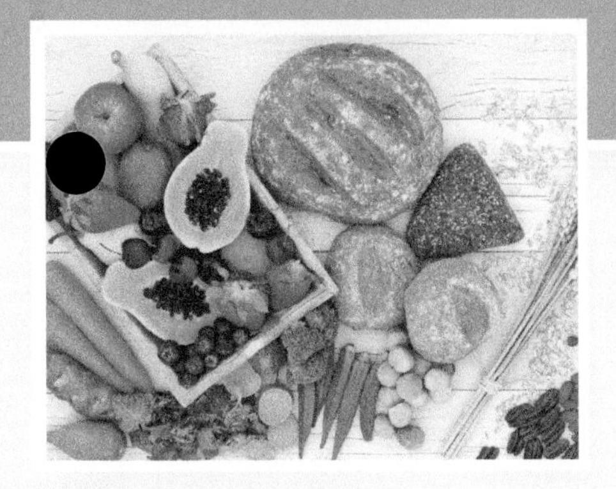

4

Carbohydrates

Nature has provided us with an excellent source of energy: carbohydrates. Found primarily in plants, carbohydrates are a convenient and economical source of calories for people throughout the world.

http://evolve.elsevier.com/GRODNER/FOUNDATIONS

LEARNING OBJECTIVES

- Identify the simple carbohydrates and their components.
- Explain the different types of complex carbohydrates.
- List the dietary recommendations (Dietary Reference Intake and Acceptable Macronutrient Distribution Range) for carbohydrates.
- Discuss the functions of carbohydrates as a source of energy and dietary fiber.
- Describe the differences and health benefits of soluble and insoluble fiber.
- Compare the nutrient content of refined versus unrefined grains.

ROLE IN WELLNESS

Nature has provided us with an excellent source of energy: carbohydrates. Found primarily in plants, carbohydrates are a convenient and economical source of calories for people throughout the world. Carbohydrates are organic compounds composed of carbon, hydrogen, and oxygen. These compounds consist of simple carbohydrates, such as glucose and sucrose, and complex carbohydrates, which include starch and dietary fiber. Each type of carbohydrate serves a distinct role in nourishing the body.

In addition to serving as an energy source, some carbohydrates are also used as sweetening agents. When carbohydrate sweeteners are found naturally in foods, such as in fruits, they are accompanied by essential nutrients. The sweetness makes eating nutrient-dense foods even more enjoyable. Some carbohydrates also supply dietary fiber.

The energy value of carbohydrates was discovered in 1844 (Dolan & Adams-Smith, 1978). Recognition that increasing our consumption of carbohydrates from grains, vegetables, and fruits provides preventive health benefits is more recent. Increased levels of complex carbohydrates, particularly dietary fiber, appear to reduce the risk factors associated with chronic diet-related disorders such as heart disease, diabetes, and some cancers.

The Dietary Reference Intake (DRI) for carbohydrates is 130 g/day for adults between 19 and 30 years of age. The acceptable macronutrient distribution range (AMDR) for carbohydrates is 45% to 65% of kcal intake per day as primarily complex carbohydrates (National Research Council [NRC], 2006). The U.S. Department of Agriculture (USDA) and U.S. Department of Health and Human Services (USDHHS) *Dietary Guidelines for Americans, 2020–2025*, concurs, recommending that we emphasize a plant-based diet consisting of fruits, vegetables, cooked dried beans and peas, whole grains, and seeds (USDA/USDHHS, 2020).

This advice is reflected in the nutrition guide MyPlate. More than threeq-uarters of MyPlate consists of food groups that are excellent sources of carbohydrates: fruits, vegetables, and grains. Although recommendations vary according to individual needs, average suggestions of 2 cups of fruits, 2½ cups of vegetables, and 6 ounces of grains (bread, cereal, rice, and pasta), with at least half being whole grains, provide adequate amounts of complex carbohydrates (Box 4.1).

Considering carbohydrates through the health dimensions provides perspective on their role in wellness. The physical health dimension depends on our ability to provide our bodies with enough carbohydrate kcal for energy and enough complex carbohydrates and fiber consumption for optimum body functioning. Issues related to the role of carbohydrates are often in the headlines. Our ability to process research findings and make decisions about our food choices reflects our level of intellectual, or reasoning, health dimension. For some of us, emotional health may depend on the ability to distinguish hypoglycemic

BOX 4.1 MyPlate: Grains

MyPlate provides a wealth of resources about nutrients, foods, portion sizes, and activity levels related to caloric needs. Highlights of grain food sources are listed here, but the reader should explore the MyPlate site, at ChooseMyPlate.gov, to customize the information to individual needs.

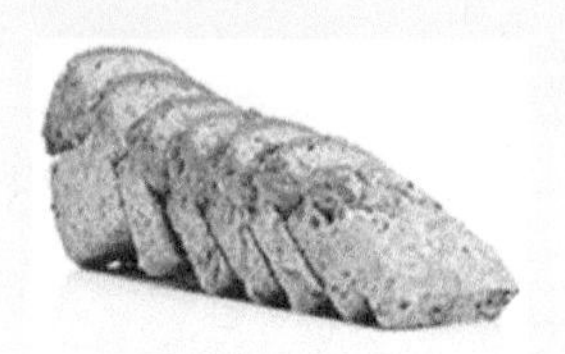

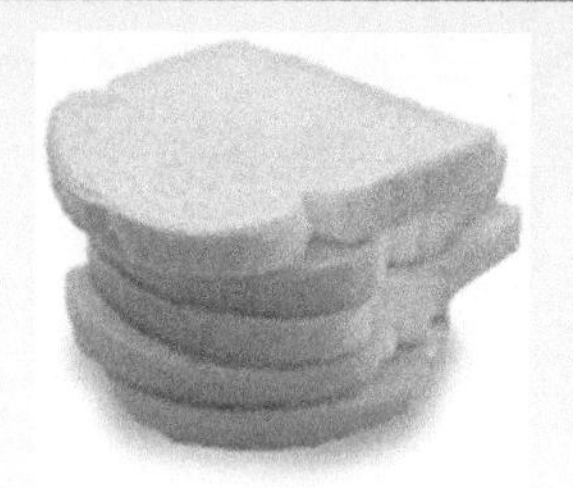

What Foods Are in the Grains Group?

Any food made from wheat, rice, oats, cornmeal, barley, or another cereal grain is a grain product. Bread, pasta, oatmeal, breakfast cereals, tortillas, and grits are examples of grain products.

Grains are divided into two subgroups, whole grains and refined grains. Whole grains contain the entire grain kernel—the bran, germ, and endosperm. Examples of whole grains include whole-wheat flour, bulgur (cracked wheat), oatmeal, whole cornmeal, and brown rice. Refined grains have been milled, a process that removes the bran and germ. This is done to give grains a finer texture and improve their shelf life, but it also removes dietary fiber, iron, and many B vitamins. Some examples of refined grain products are white flour, degermed cornmeal, white bread, and white rice.

Most refined grains are enriched. This means certain B vitamins (thiamin, riboflavin, niacin, folic acid) and iron are added back after processing. Fiber is not added back to enriched grains. Check the ingredient list on refined grain products to make sure that the word enriched is included in the grain name. Some food products are made from mixtures of whole grains and refined grains.

What Counts as an Ounce-Equivalent of Grains?

In general, 1 slice of bread, 1 cup of ready-to-eat cereal, or ½ cup of cooked rice, cooked pasta, or cooked cereal can be considered as 1 ounce-equivalent from the Grains Group. The following table lists specific amounts that count as 1 ounce-equivalent of grains toward your daily recommended intake. In some cases the number of ounce-equivalents for common portions is also shown.

OUNCE-EQUIVALENT OF GRAINS TABLE

		Amount That Counts as 1 Ounce-Equivalent of Grains	Common Portions and Ounce-Equivalents
Bagels	WG[a]: whole wheat RG[a]: plain, egg	1-inch mini bagel	1 large bagel = 4 ounce-equivalents
Biscuits	RG[a]: baking powder/buttermilk	1 small (2-inch diameter)	1 large (3-inch diameter) = 2 ounce-equivalents
Breads	WG[a]: 100% whole wheat RG[a]: white, wheat, French, sourdough	1 regular slice 1 small slice, French 4 snack-size slices rye bread	2 regular slices = 2 ounce-equivalents
Bulgur	WG[a]: cracked wheat	½ cup, cooked	
Cornbread	RG[a]	1 small piece (2½ inches × 1¼ inches × 1¼ inches)	1 medium piece (2½ inches × 2½ inches × 1¼ inches) = 2 ounce-equivalents
Crackers	WG[a]: 100% whole wheat, rye RG[a]: saltines, snack crackers	5 whole-wheat crackers 2 rye crisp breads 7 square or round crackers	
English muffins	WG[a]: whole wheat RG[a]: plain, raisin	½ muffin	1 muffin = 2 ounce-equivalents
Muffins	WG[a]: whole wheat RG[a]: bran, corn, plain	1 small (2½-inch diameter)	1 large (3½-inch diameter) = 3 ounce-equivalents
Oatmeal	WG[a]	½ cup, cooked 1 packet instant 1 ounce (⅓ cup), dry (regular or quick)	
Pancakes	WG[a]: whole wheat, buckwheat RG[a]: buttermilk, plain	1 pancake (4½-inch diameter) 2 small pancakes (3-inch diameter)	3 pancakes (4½-inch diameter) = 3 ounce-equivalents
Popcorn	WG[a]	3 cups, popped	1 mini microwave bag or 100-calorie bag, popped = 2 ounce-equivalents
Ready-to eat breakfast cereal	WG[a]: toasted oat, whole wheat flakes RG[a]: corn flakes, puffed rice	1 cup, flakes or rounds 1¼ cup, puffed	
Rice	WG[a]: brown, wild RG[a]: enriched, white, polished	½ cup cooked 1 ounce, dry	1 cup, cooked = 2 ounce-equivalents
Pasta: spaghetti, macaroni, noodles	WG[a]: whole wheat RG[a]: enriched, durum	½ cup, cooked 1 ounce, dry	1 cup, cooked = 2 ounce-equivalents
Tortillas	WG[a]: whole wheat, whole grain corn RG[a]: flour, corn	1 small flour tortilla (6-inch diameter) 1 corn tortilla (6-inch diameter)	1 large tortilla (12-inch diameter) = 4 ounce-equivalents

[a]Products are available both in whole-grain and refined-grain forms.
RG, Refined grains; *WG*, whole grains.
(Modified from U.S. Department of Agriculture, Center for Nutrition Policy and Promotion: *Choose My Plate*, Alexandria, VA, updated November 2017, Author. Accessed 26 January, 2018, from https://www.choosemyplate.gov/grains.)

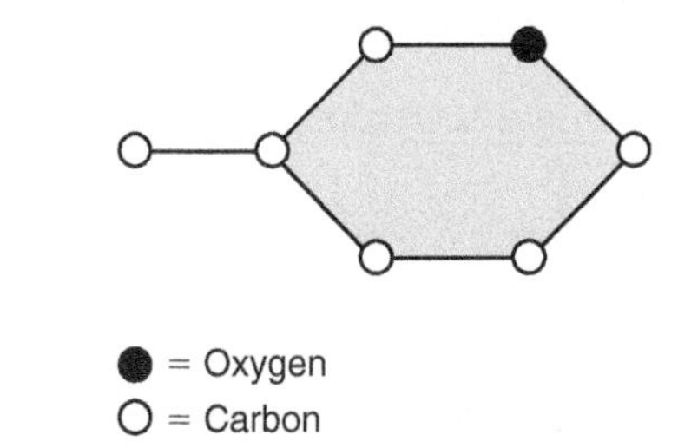

Fig. 4.1 Structure of a molecule of carbohydrate.

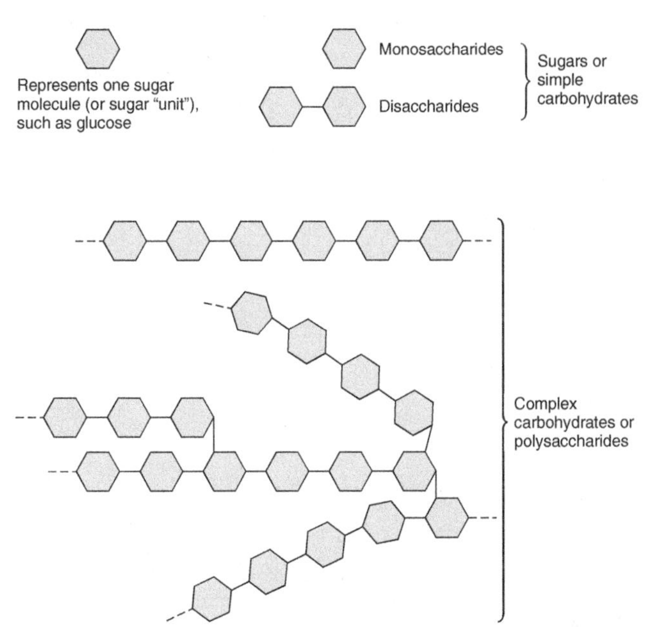

Fig. 4.2 Structure of monosaccharides, disaccharides, and polysaccharides.

(low blood glucose) symptoms. If we are aware of our personal response to normal hypoglycemia, can we then distinguish real emotional issues from those caused by hypoglycemia? The social health dimension also may be tested. Social groups can support change or make changes more difficult to achieve. Will you or your client feel comfortable snacking on a banana (a good fiber source) while other people are unwrapping chocolate bars? The spiritual health dimension has ties to carbohydrates because several religions view bread, a carbohydrate, as the "staff of life." The environmental health dimension may affect our available sources of carbohydrates. Are whole-grain products and snacks accessible and affordable, or are overly refined or excessively sweet carbohydrate foods the only options?

FOOD SOURCES

The carbohydrates we consume are primarily from plant sources. As plants grow, they capture energy from the sun and chemically store it as carbohydrates. This process, called photosynthesis, depends on water from the earth, carbon dioxide from the atmosphere, and chlorophyll in the plant leaves to form carbohydrates.

All carbohydrates are organic compounds composed of carbon, hydrogen, and oxygen in the form of simple carbohydrates or sugars (Fig. 4.1). When linked together, these simple sugars form three sizes of carbohydrates: monosaccharides, disaccharides, and polysaccharides (Fig. 4.2).

Monosaccharides are composed of single carbohydrate units. Glucose, fructose, and galactose are monosaccharides. Disaccharides consist of two single carbohydrates bound together. Sucrose, maltose, and lactose are disaccharides.

Polysaccharides consist of many units of monosaccharides joined together. Starch and fiber are food sources of polysaccharides, whereas glycogen is a polysaccharide stored in the liver and muscles.

The three sizes of carbohydrates are divided into two classifications: simple carbohydrates (monosaccharides and disaccharides) and complex carbohydrates (polysaccharides) (Table 4.1). Both are valuable sources of carbohydrate energy. There are differences, however, between the health values of simple and complex carbohydrates found in the foods we consume. Although simple carbohydrates primarily provide energy in the form of glucose, fructose, and galactose, complex carbohydrates may provide fiber in addition to glucose.

CARBOHYDRATE AS A NUTRIENT WITHIN THE BODY

Function

Carbohydrates provide energy, fiber, and naturally occurring sweeteners (sucrose and fructose). Energy is the only real nutrient function of carbohydrates; the roles of fiber and carbohydrate sweeteners are discussed later in this chapter. Carbohydrates supply energy in the most efficient form for use by our bodies. If enough carbohydrate is provided to meet the energy needs of the body, protein can be spared or saved to use for specific protein functions. This service of carbohydrates is called the protein-sparing effect.

When adequate amounts of carbohydrates are available, both carbohydrates and small amounts of fats are used for energy. When there are not enough carbohydrates available, fat is metabolized, resulting in the formation of ketones, intermediate products of fat metabolism. The body without distress easily disposes of low levels of ketones. If carbohydrate levels continue to be insufficient to meet energy demands, increased levels of ketones overwhelm the physiologic system and ketoacidosis develops; ketoacidosis affects the pH balance of the body, which can be lethal if uncontrolled. Although lipids and proteins can, if necessary, provide energy for most bodily needs, the brain and nerve tissues function best on glucose from carbohydrates.

Digestion and Absorption

Our food sources of carbohydrates tend to be disaccharides (sugars) and polysaccharides (starches). The gastrointestinal (GI) tract has the role of digesting carbohydrates into monosaccharides for easy absorption. The digestive process begins in the mouth. Mechanical digestion breaks food into smaller pieces

TABLE 4.1 Dietary Carbohydrates

Carbohydrate Type	Common Name	Naturally Occurring Food Sources
Simple		
Monosaccharides		
Glucose	Blood sugar	Fruits, sweeteners
Fructose	Fruit sugar	Fruits, honey, syrups, vegetables
Galactose	—	Part of lactose, found in milk
Disaccharides		
Sucrose (glucose + fructose)	Table sugar	Sugarcane, sugar beets, fruits, vegetables
Lactose (glucose + galactose)	Milk sugar	Milk and milk products
Maltose (glucose + glucose)	Malt sugar	Germinating grains
Complex		
Polysaccharides		
Starches (strings of glucose)	Complex carbohydrates	Grains, legumes, potatoes
Fiber (strings of monosaccharides, usually glucose)	Roughage	Legumes, whole grains, fruits, vegetables

TEACHING TOOL

Lacking Lactose? No Problem!

Lactose intolerance is not an illness and should not undermine a person's sense of wellness. To ensure that clients receive an adequate supply of nutrients usually consumed in lactose-containing dairy products—especially calcium, riboflavin, and vitamin D—without the use of supplements, consider making the following suggestions:

- Experiment with different portion sizes of lactose-containing foods to determine individual levels of tolerance; small amounts up to ½ cup consumed throughout the day can often be tolerated.
- Use over-the-counter lactase-enzyme tablets when consuming dairy products (currently available as Lactaid, Lactase, Dairy Ease, and others).
- If available, purchase lactose-reduced dairy products such as milk, ice cream, and soft cheeses.
- Try out different milk alternatives such as soy milk and other nondairy beverages. However. choose only products fortified with calcium, vitamin D, and B_{12} to obtain nutrients similar to those from dairy products.
- Consume foods high in nutrients found in lactose-containing foods; high-calcium foods include broccoli, eggs, kale, spinach, tofu, shrimp, canned salmon, sardines with bones, and calcium-fortified orange juice.
- Consume hard cheeses (in moderate amounts because of fat content) that contain lower lactose levels, such as Swiss, Cheddar, Muenster, Parmesan, Monterey, and provolone.
- Avoid softer cheeses (or experiment to learn level of tolerance), such as ricotta, cottage, mozzarella, Neufchatel, and cream.
- Test tolerance of different brands of yogurt; lactose levels may vary according to variations in processing. Generally, lactase bacteria in yogurt culture hydrolyzes some of the lactose.
- Consider supplementation if these dietary modifications are not achieved; consult with a dietitian/nutritionist for an appropriate supplement.

and mixes the carbohydrate-containing food with saliva, which contains an amylase called ptyalin. This begins the hydrolysis of starch into the simpler carbohydrate intermediary forms of dextrin and maltose. In the small intestine, intestinal enzymes and specific pancreatic amylase work on starch intermediary products to continue the breakdown to monosaccharides.

Enzymes specific for disaccharides (lactase for lactose, sucrase for sucrose, maltase for maltose) are secreted by the small intestine's brush-border cells, which then hydrolyze disaccharides into monosaccharides. (For more information, see the *Cultural Diversity and Nutrition* box The Missing Enzyme and the *Teaching Tool* box Lacking Lactose? No Problem!) After an active absorption process (i.e., one that requires energy input), absorptive cells in the small intestine take up these monosaccharides. Once glucose, fructose, and galactose enter the villi, the portal blood circulatory system transports them to the liver. The liver removes fructose and galactose and converts them to glucose. This glucose may be used immediately for energy or for glycogen formation, a storage form of carbohydrate providing an always-ready source of energy. Fig. 4.3 summarizes carbohydrate digestion.

Glycogen: Storing Carbohydrates

Glycogen is carbohydrate energy stored in the liver and in muscles. The amount held in the muscles of an adult is 150 g (600 kcal); 90 g (360 kcal) are stored in the liver. Retrieved as needed for energy, glycogen is quickly broken down by enzymes to produce a surge of energy. The process of converting glucose to glycogen is glycogenesis.

Glycogen levels can be significantly increased through physical training and dietary manipulations (see Chapter 9). It is still considered a relatively limited source of energy compared with the amounts of energy stored in body fat.

Metabolism

A primary aspect of carbohydrate metabolism is the maintenance of blood glucose homeostasis between 70 and 100 mg/dL. Sources of blood glucose, the most common sugar in the blood, may be carbohydrate and noncarbohydrate. Dietary starches and simple carbohydrates provide blood glucose after digestion and absorption; glycogen stored in the liver and muscle tissue

CULTURAL DIVERSITY AND NUTRITION

The Missing Enzyme

Approximately 70% of the adult world population is unable to easily digest the lactose found in milk. Among White North Americans, Europeans, and Australians, about 5% to 17% have lactose maldigestion. Those of mixed ethnicity tend to experience a lower prevalence (Lomer, 2008). This condition, lactose intolerance, occurs when the body does not produce enough lactase, a digestive enzyme that breaks lactose into glucose and galactose. When the lactose sits in the large intestine, bacteria begin to ferment the undigested lactose, causing diarrhea, bloating, and increased gas formation.

Lactase deficiency may have a primary or secondary cause. Primary lactose intolerance is caused by a genetic factor that limits the ability to produce lactase. Although small amounts of lactose can often be tolerated, the level of lactase produced cannot be enhanced. The condition is common among Asian, Pacific Islander, Black, Hispanic, Latino, and Native Americans. In the United States the prevalence of lactose intolerance caused by maldigestion or low lactose levels is approximately 75% in Black and Native Americans, 90% in Asian/ Pacific Islanders, 50% in Hispanic Americans, and lowest among White people.

One explanation for primary lactose intolerance is that the ability to digest milk is age related. Consider that the milk of mammals, including humans, was intended for the young to consume during periods of major growth. The ability to digest milk may diminish because the biological need is lessened as maturity is reached. Older adults may also experience lactose intolerance when the aging process diminishes the production of some digestive enzymes, such as lactase. The recent identification of a genetic variation is valuable for future diagnostic testing to determine risk for and severity of lactose intolerance earlier in life.

Sometimes, secondary lactose intolerance occurs when a chronic GI illness affects the intestinal tract, reducing the amount of lactase produced (see Chapter 13). Even a bout of an intestinal virus or flu can cause temporary lactose intolerance. Most individuals in whom this occurs recover and are again able to digest lactose.

Application to nursing: Health professionals can guide clients to determine what amounts of lactose-containing foods can be tolerated despite low lactase levels. Fine-tuning eating styles may require the assistance of a registered dietitian/nutritionist (RDN) to ensure adequate consumption of calcium-containing foods. Depending on the severity of the sensitivity, advice to clients may include additional label reading for lactose-containing foods and medications, especially for clients dealing with conditions such as irritable bowel syndrome.

(Data from Lomer MC, Parkes GC, Sanderson JD: Lactose intolerance in clinical practice—myths and realities, *Aliment Pharmacol Ther*, 27:93–103, 2008; National Institutes of Health: *Definition & Facts for Lactose Intolerance*, Washington, DC, 2018, National Institute of Diabetes and Digestive and Kidney Diseases Health Information Center. Accessed 3 December, 2020, from, https://www.niddk.nih.gov/health-information/digestive-diseases/lactose-intolerance/definition-facts#morelikely)

is converted back to glucose in a process called glycogenolysis. Intermediate carbohydrate metabolites are also a source of blood glucose. The metabolites include lactic acid and pyruvic acid, which occur when muscle glycogen is used for energy.

Noncarbohydrates can also provide blood glucose. Gluconeogenesis is the process of producing glucose from fat. It is not as efficient as using carbohydrate directly for glucose. As fat is metabolized into fatty acids and glycerol (see Chapter 5), the smaller glycerol portion can be converted by the liver into glycogen, which is then available for glucose needs through glycogenolysis. Protein, which is composed of numerous combinations of amino acids, also may be a source of glucose. Some of these amino acids are glucogenic; if they are not used for protein structures, they can be metabolized to form glucose. Carbohydrate as an energy source is also discussed in Fig. 9.2.

Blood glucose is a source of energy to all cells. Glucose may be used immediately as energy or converted to glycogen or fat; both conversions provide energy for the future. Although glycogen can be converted back to glucose, the conversion of glucose to fat is irreversible. Glucose cannot be formed again but is stored as fat and, if needed, is metabolized later as fat, although its original source was carbohydrate.

Glucose is essential for brain function and cell formation, particularly during pregnancy and growth. Because the body can form glucose through gluconeogenesis from protein and fat, glucose technically is not an essential nutrient. Gluconeogenesis can provide some glucose but not enough to meet essential needs if dietary carbohydrate is insufficient. To compensate (as previously discussed), ketone bodies can be used for energy. Ketone bodies are created when fatty acids are broken down for energy when sufficient carbohydrates are unavailable; this process of fat metabolism, however, is incomplete. If dietary carbohydrate continues to be insufficient, a buildup of ketones results, which causes ketosis, possibly leading to acid–base imbalances in the body.

Blood Glucose Regulation

Metabolism of glucose and regulation of blood glucose levels are controlled by a sophisticated hormonal system. Insulin, a hormone produced by the beta cells of the islets of Langerhans, lowers blood glucose levels by enhancing the conversion of excess glucose to glycogen through glycogenesis or to fat stored in adipose tissue. Insulin also eases the absorption of glucose into the cells so the use of glucose as energy is increased.

Whereas insulin lowers blood glucose levels, other hormones raise glucose levels. The pancreas produces two hormones with this function: glucagon and somatostatin. Glucagon stimulates conversion of liver glycogen to glucose, assisting the regulation of glucose levels during the night; somatostatin, secreted from the hypothalamus and pancreas, inhibits the functions of insulin and glucagon. Several adrenal gland hormones also have a role in raising blood glucose levels. Epinephrine enhances the fast conversion of liver glycogen to glucose. Steroid hormones function against insulin and promote glucose formation from protein. Produced by the pituitary gland, growth hormone and adrenocorticotropic hormone (ACTH) function as insulin inhibitors. The thyroid hormone thyroxine affects blood glucose levels by enhancing intestinal absorption of glucose and releasing epinephrine. Hypoglycemia (abnormally low blood glucose level) and diabetes mellitus (DM) (abnormally high blood

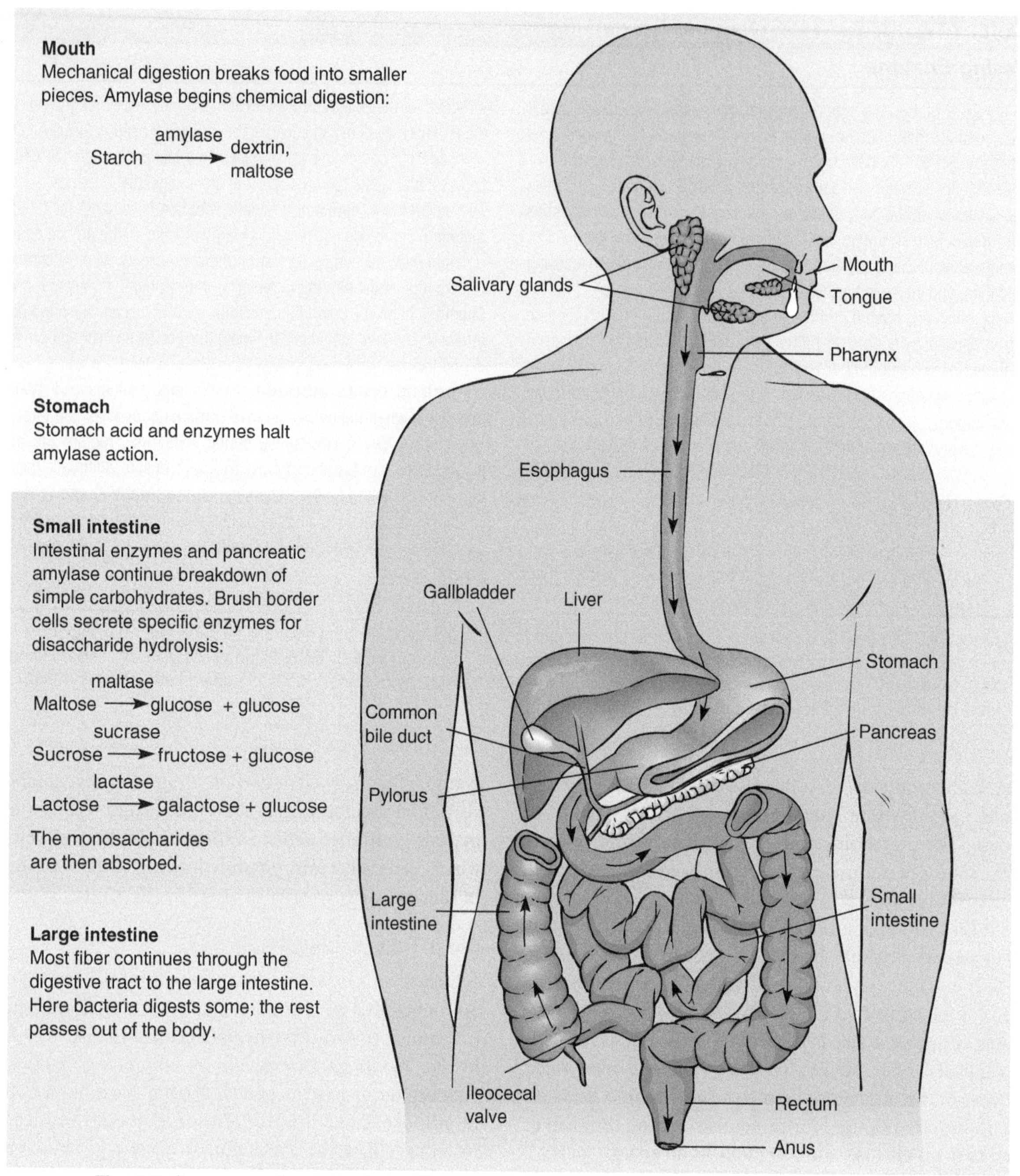

Mouth
Mechanical digestion breaks food into smaller pieces. Amylase begins chemical digestion:
amylase
Starch → dextrin, maltose
Stomach
Stomach acid and enzymes halt amylase action.
Small intestine
Intestinal enzymes and pancreatic amylase continue breakdown of simple carbohydrates. Brush border cells secrete specific enzymes for disaccharide hydrolysis:
maltase
Maltose → glucose + glucose
sucrase
Sucrose → fructose + glucose
lactase
Lactose → galactose + glucose
The monosaccharides are then absorbed.
Large intestine
Most fiber continues through the digestive tract to the large intestine. Here bacteria digests some; the rest passes out of the body.
Salivary glands
Mouth
Tongue
Pharynx
Esophagus
Gallbladder
Liver
Stomach
Common bile duct
Pancreas
Pylorus
Large intestine
Small intestine
Ileocecal valve
Rectum
Anus

Fig. 4.3 Summary of carbohydrate digestion and absorption. (From Rolin Graphics.)

glucose level) may occur when these systems cannot regulate glucose within normal levels. These conditions are discussed in Chapter 15.

Glycemic Index and Glycemic Load

Although the sophisticated hormonal system controls the metabolism and regulation of blood glucose levels, it is most likely that the composition of foods we consume differ significantly in their effects on blood glucose levels. To account for this, the concepts of glycemic index and glycemic load are used. Glycemic index is the ranking of foods according to the level to which a food raises blood glucose levels compared with a reference food such as a 50-g glucose load or white bread containing 50 g carbohydrate (Keim et al, 2014). A ranking of 100 is the highest glycemic index level—that is, it raises blood glucose levels the highest. Note the glycemic index rankings of commonly consumed foods listed in Table 4.2.

The glycemic index of a food is affected by the following factors:

- The physical form, such as a baked potato compared with a mashed potato
- The fat and protein content in addition to carbohydrate, which slows digestion

TABLE 4.2 Glycemic Index Comparisons of Commonly Consumed Foods

Glycemic Index	Food
60	Mini-wheat cereal (WG)
60	Raisin bran cereal (WG)
92	Cornflake cereal (RG)
60	Whole-grain bread (WG)
72	White bread (RG)
72	Bagel (RG)
30	Spaghetti/whole wheat (WG)
60	Spaghetti (RG)
50	Brown rice (WG)
60	White rice (RG)
30	Skim milk
40	Apple juice
50	Orange juice
63	Cola
70	Sports drinks
33	Pear
40	Apple
48	Orange
50	Banana
50	Sweet potato
90	Potato (baked, no fat)
14	Peanuts
22	Cashews
30	Legumes (lentils, chickpeas)

GI, Glycemic index; *RG*, refined grains; *WG*, whole grains.
(Data from Atkinson FS, Foster-Powell K, Brand-Miller JC: International table of glycemic index and glycemic load values: 2008, *Diabetes Care* 31(12):2281–2283, 2008.)

- The ripeness, such as in fruits and vegetables, which increases glucose content
- The fiber content, which slows digestion
- The botanic variety of a food, such as the different glycemic indexes of rice species

Because the glycemic index assesses only one food item, another measurement tool is needed because we usually eat several foods at the same time. This is accounted for by the glycemic load, which considers the total glycemic index effect of a mixed meal or dietary plan. It is calculated as the sum of the products of the glycemic index for each of the foods multiplied by the amount of carbohydrate in each food (Keim et al, 2014). Given that glycemic load accounts for the mixed consumption of foods, it measures the quantity and quality of the effect of carbohydrate on blood glucose and the resulting effect on insulin release (Gallagher, 2012).

Recent epidemiologic work notes associations between glycemic index and glycemic load and the risk of chronic diseases such as T2D mellitus (T2DM), cardiovascular disease, and diet-related cancers of the colon and breast. Seemingly, limiting consumption of foods that produce a high glycemic index and overall high glycemic load may reduce risk. Public health recommendations, however, will most likely not be forthcoming until long-term clinical trials demonstrate a clear role for these diet-related effects. Regardless, the concept of glycemic index continues to be explored even though it measures individual foods, not mixed meals within which the carbohydrate effect might vary. These concepts can be helpful for management of diabetes and hypoglycemia (Keim et al, 2014).

Nonetheless, consider the potential value of the glycemic index in the following situations. The glycemic index of a food may affect a person's blood glucose level, but that same food as part of a meal of several foods (a mix of high and low glycemic indexes) will have a different effect or glycemic load. If a person's dietary goal is to have an even blood glucose level, one could choose foods that provide an even response and, by consuming foods throughout the day, avoid a feasting or fasting experience. Certainly, this is what individuals with diabetes (abnormally high blood glucose levels) accomplish through counting carbohydrates and planning nourishment within intentional intervals. For those of us who are prone to hypoglycemia (abnormally low blood glucose level), consuming low glycemic index foods or meals with moderate glycemic loads may maintain adequate blood glucose levels. For the rest of us, having a stable level of blood glucose for energy from the foods we consume provides much-needed stamina. The bottom line to this issue for most of us is that we struggle enough with just preparing and finding time to eat adequate meals. Adding the layer of assessing glycemic index and glycemic loads to foods and meals may fine-tune maintaining stability of blood glucose levels—even within the stressors of our contemporary lifestyles (Box 4.2).

SIMPLE CARBOHYDRATES

Monosaccharides

Glucose, often called blood sugar, is the form of carbohydrate most easily used by the body. It is the simple carbohydrate that circulates in the blood and is the main source of energy for the central nervous system and brain. Glucose is rapidly absorbed into the bloodstream from the intestine, but it needs insulin to be taken into the cells, where energy is released.

Fructose is the sweetest of the sugars. Although fruits and honey contain a mixture of sugars, including sucrose, fructose provides the characteristic taste of fruits and honey. After absorption from the small intestine, fructose circulates in the bloodstream. When it passes through to the liver, liver cells rearrange fructose into glucose.

Galactose is rarely found in nature by itself but is part of the disaccharide lactose, the sugar found in milk. Absorbed like fructose, galactose is converted to glucose by the liver.

Disaccharides

Sucrose is formed from the pairing of units of glucose and fructose. We know it as table sugar. Sugarcane and sugar beets are two sources of sucrose, which is found naturally in fruits. Because it contains fructose, sucrose is quite sweet. Sucrose has a special place in our history of food consumption and is further explored in the following section.

Maltose is created when two units of glucose are linked. It is available when cereal grains are about to germinate, and the plant starch is broken down into maltose. The majority of

BOX 4.2 To Eat or Not to Eat?

"Carbs" are a part of everyday food talk, much as "fat" used to be. We thought that if only "fat" intake was lower we would be at healthy weights and free of heart disease and other chronic diseases. Not so. As a nation, we gained weight instead. Now, just replace "fat" with "carbs," and the myth continues.

Can Eating Fewer Carbs Lead to Weight Loss?

Yes, it can, but only if total caloric intake is lower. Weight will return, though, if calories and carbohydrate intake are again elevated. Reducing intake to very low levels, such as 20g a day, is not a long-term weight-loss approach. Our bodies function best when we consume some carbohydrates because daily, we must use about 100g of carbohydrates as glucose for brain function.

Isn't Eliminating Carbs Such as Doughnuts and Sweets a Healthy Approach to Weight Loss?

The answer depends on how carbs are decreased. Replacing carbohydrate calories with saturated fats found in animal proteins is not health promoting. But if nutrient-empty carbohydrate foods are replaced with low-carbohydrate salad greens and vegetables, health benefits may accrue. The key is portion size and calorie control. Moderate intake of all nutrient groups is best. Some of us may feel better with a higher carbohydrate intake, whereas others feel best with a greater proportion of protein (lean, of course) consumption.

What About Eating Lower Carb Products Such as Breads, Tortillas, and Pasta?

This issue, too, depends on how many calories of carbohydrates a person tends to consume and what kinds of carbohydrates. Whole-grain foods provide more health benefits than refined grain products. Lower carb products may be labeled as reduced in carbohydrate content because of the addition of dietary fiber to the ingredient formulation of the product. The label statement "reduced carbohydrate content" is based on "net carbs," which are not defined by the U.S. Food and Drug Administration. Manufacturers often present net carbs as equaling total carbohydrates minus dietary fiber and sugar alcohols (which do not quickly raise blood glucose levels). Consuming such products may increase fiber intake, but 100% whole-grain products are the best choice because they most likely contain dietary fiber and less processed ingredients.

For each of the nutrient categories studied in this book, a "ChooseMyPlate" section is included to emphasize the importance of portion sizes for the MyPlate food categories. For carbohydrates, the focus is on portions of grains.

maltose in human nutrition is created from the breakdown of starch in the small intestine. Maltose is of particular value in the production of beer and other malt beverages. When maltose ferments, alcohol is formed.

Lactose is composed of glucose and galactose. It is sometimes called milk sugar because it is the primary carbohydrate in milk.

Sugar: A Special Disaccharide

The term sugar is a word with many meanings. Sugar may refer to the simple carbohydrates (monosaccharides and disaccharides). Sucrose, the disaccharide naturally found in many fruits, is also called sugar. White table sugar refers to sucrose extracted from sugarcane and sugar beets. Sugar may also be an umbrella term used to cover numerous kcal-sweetening agents used in our food production system, although U.S. commercial law defines sugar as "sucrose." There is a distinction between how the term sugar is used on a label and how it is used by a biologist, chemist, or nutritionist. Often blood glucose levels are called blood sugar levels. It is important that we, as health professionals, be aware that our clinical use of the term may confuse clients. Concerns about sugar focus on the following three issues: sources in the food supply, consumption levels, and health effects.

Sources in the food supply. Sugar in our food supply may include the following nutritive sweeteners: refined white sugar, brown sugar, dextrose, crystalline fructose, high-fructose corn syrup (HFCS), glucose, corn sweeteners, lactose, concentrated fruit juice, honey, maple syrup, molasses, agave nectar, and reduced energy polyols or sugar alcohols (e.g., sorbitol, mannitol, xylitol) (Fitch & Keim, 2012) (Table 4.3). All forms of sugar are chemically similar; each provides kcal, and most do not contain any other nutrients. Blackstrap molasses does contain iron, but other more nutrient-dense sources of iron are easily available. Honey, which seems less processed than other sweeteners, provides only a trace of minerals and therefore is as nonnutritious as any other sweetener.

The U.S. Food and Drug Administration (FDA, 2017) categorizes some sweeteners as generally recognized as safe (GRAS) ingredients and others as food additives. For food additives, an acceptable daily intake (ADI) is determined as the amount that a person can safely consume daily over a lifetime without risk. Table 4.3 lists descriptions, regulatory status, and energy amounts provided by sweeteners.

Consumption levels. Our national intake of refined white sugar has declined, whereas consumption of HFCS has greatly increased since the 1970s. In the 1970s a process was perfected by which HFCS, very sweet-tasting syrup, could be made from corn syrup. HFCS is less expensive to produce than refined sugar and is sweeter. Used extensively in food manufacturing, it has replaced refined white sugar in many products, such as soft drinks.

Health effects. The health concerns regarding sugar consumption include nutrient displacement, dental caries, and the related issues of obesity and diabetes.

Does it matter to our bodies what the source of the sweet taste is? That depends. A major health concern is nutrient displacement. Displacement occurs when whole foods, which are minimally processed, are not eaten and are replaced by foods containing added sugars. If we eat candy, soda, and other sweet snack foods instead of a sandwich and juice for lunch, we lose a number of important nutrients (Fig. 4.4).

Foods and drinks with added sugars often contain empty kcal that provide few nutrients. Because all forms of sugar are chemically similar, the sucrose in fruits is actually the same as the sucrose in a cream-filled doughnut. The difference, however, is that naturally occurring vitamins, minerals, and fiber available in the fruit are not available in the doughnut. The doughnut's empty kcal can replace kcal from other foods that might contain a natural sweetener and also provide vitamins, minerals, protein, complex carbohydrates, and fiber. Consumption of excessively sugared food does not support wellness goals because it probably replaces other, more nutrient-dense foods.

Dental caries is related to eating concentrated sweets and sticky carbohydrates. Sugar supports the growth of bacteria,

TABLE 4.3 **Nutritive and Nonnutritive Sweeteners**

Sweetener	kcal/g	Regulatory Status	Other Names	Description
Sucrose	4	GRAS	Granulated: coarse, regular, fine; powdered; confectioners'; brown; turbinado, demerara; liquid: molasses	Sweetens; enhances flavor; tenderizes, allows browning, and enhances appearance in baking; adds characteristic flavor with unrefined sugar
Fructose	4	GRAS	High-fructose corn syrups: 42%, 55%, 90% fructose; crystalline fructose: 99% fructose	Sweetens; functions like sucrose in baking Some people experience a laxative response from a load of fructose ≥20 g May produce lower glycemic response than sucrose
Monosaccharide Polyols				
Sorbitol	2.6	GRAS (label must warn about a laxative effect)	Same as chemical name	50%–70% as sweet as sucrose Some people may experience a laxative effect from a load of sorbitol ≥50 g
Mannitol	1.6	Permitted for use on an interim basis (label must warn about a laxative effect)	Same as chemical name	50%–70% as sweet as sucrose May cause a laxative effect with a load of mannitol ≥20 g
Xylitol	2.4	GRAS	Same as chemical name	As sweet as sucrose
Erythritol	0.2	Independent GRAS determination	Same as chemical name	60%–80% as sweet as sucrose
Tagatose	1.5	Independent GRAS determination	Same as chemical name	75%–92% as sweet as sucrose
Nonnutritive				
Saccharin	0	Limited to <12 mg/fl oz in beverages, 20 mg/serving in individual packages, or 30 mg/serving in processed foods ADI: not determined	Sweet'N Low, Sugar Twin	300% sweeter than sucrose Noncariogenic and produces no glycemic response Synergizes the sweetening power of NSs and NNSs Sweetening power is not reduced with heating
Aspartame	4[a]	Approved as a general-purpose sweetener ADI: 50 mg/kg BW	NutraSweet, Equal	160%–220% sweeter than sucrose Noncariogenic and produces limited glycemic response New forms can increase its sweetening power in cooking and baking
Acesulfame K	0	Approved for use as a tabletop sweetener and as an additive in a variety of desserts, confections, and alcoholic beverages, except not in meat and poultry ADI: 15 mg/kg BW	Sunette[b]	200% sweeter than sucrose Noncariogenic and produces no glycemic response Sweetening power is not reduced with heating Can synergize the sweetening power of other NSs and NNSs
Sucralose	0	Approved for use as a tabletop sweetener and as an additive in a variety of desserts, confections, and nonalcoholic beverages	Splenda[c]	600% sweeter than sucrose Noncariogenic and produces no glycemic response Sweetening power is not reduced with heating
Stevia	0	GRAS Approved for use in a variety of food products ADI: 4 mg/kg BW	Truvia, Sun Crystals, Stevia in the Raw	250% sweeter than sucrose

[a]Provides limited energy to products because of its sweetening power.
[b]Hoechst Food Ingredients, Edison, NJ.
[c]McNeil Specialty Products Company, New Brunswick, NJ.
ADI, Acceptable daily intake; *BW*, body weight; *GRAS*, generally recognized as safe by the U.S. Food and Drug Administration; *NNS*, nonnutritive sweetener; *NS*, nutritive sweetener.
(Data from Fitch C, Keim KS: Academy of Nutrition and Dietetics: Position of the Academy of Nutrition and Dietetics: Use of nutritive and nonnutritive sweeteners, *Acad Nutr Diet* 112:739–758, 2012.)

which promotes the formation of plaque. Plaque leads to tooth decay. Ways to decrease the development of caries are to eat sweets at the end of meals—rather than between meals—and to monitor the quantity and frequency of sugar intake. Sticky, sugary foods are more cariogenic than sweet liquids. Optimal dental hygiene reduces plaque formation and promotes dental health.

A misconception is that obesity is caused by high sugar intake only. In fact, obesity may be caused by an excess intake of kcal from any of the energy nutrients, which is then stored as

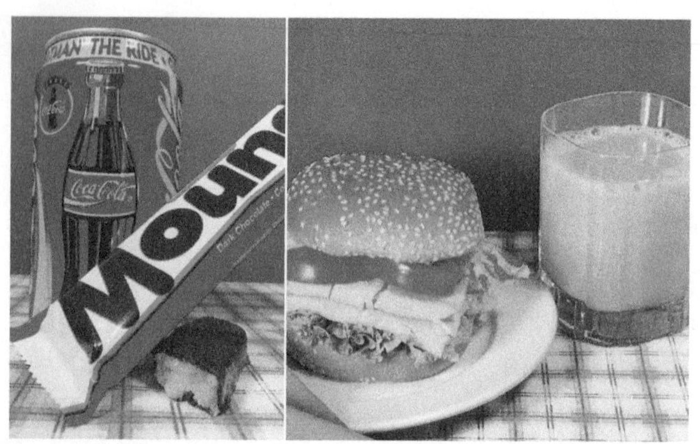

Fig. 4.4 Consuming products with added sugars *(left)* can displace more nutrient-dense foods *(right)*. (From Joanne Scott/Tracy McCalla.)

body fat. Many sugared foods are also high in fat. Because fat is the most energy-dense nutrient, fat intake may be more of a risk factor for obesity than sugar intake.

There is no confirmed relationship between the level of sugar intake and increased risk for the development of T2DM (NRC, 2006). Once the disorder is confirmed, people with diabetes are counseled to restrict their intake of concentrated sweets to assist the regulation of insulin needs. However, consumption of sweets does not cause the disorder. These issues become complicated because obesity is a risk factor for T2DM. Health concerns related to obesity and T2DM are explored in Chapters 9 and 15.

A myth that sugar consumption by children produces hyperactivity or attention-deficient/hyperactivity disorder (ADHD) continues to be perpetuated. Controlled research studies have consistently failed to support this assertion (Fitch & Keim, 2012). More than likely, excessively active behavior is related to the occasions at which sugared foods such as cake and candy are ingested. If children regularly consume excessive amounts of refined sugar, their overall dietary intake may be nutritionally deficient, possibly resulting in altered behaviors.

So how much sugar is acceptable? Moderate amounts may be all right when our diets are low in fat and high in fiber. The *Dietary Guidelines for Americans* suggests consuming sugars in moderation at less than 10% of caloric intake (see Chapter 2). Less added sugar intake ensures a dietary intake that is adequate in complex carbohydrates. The Nutrition Facts label now lists the number of added sugar grams that will provide additional information for consumers buying processed food products. By following recommendations to increase consumption of fruits and vegetables to at least five servings or 4½ cups a day and of grains to 6 ounces a day, we can reduce our intake of simple sugars.

Other Sweeteners

Other available sweeteners are sugar alcohols (polyols) and alternative sweeteners. **Sugar alcohols**, also called sugar replacers to avoid confusion with noncarbohydrate alcohol, are nutritive sweeteners because they provide 2 to 3 kcal/g but fewer than the 4 kcal/g of carbohydrates. They occur naturally in fruits and berries. Sorbitol, mannitol, and xylitol are the most commonly used sugar alcohols. **Alternative sweeteners** are nonnutritive substances produced to be sweet tasting; however, they provide no nutrients and few, if any, kcal. For food production purposes, sugar alcohols are synthesized rather than derived from natural sources (Fitch & Keim, 2012). Sucralose, aspartame, and saccharin are commonly used alternative sweeteners.

Products containing these sweeteners may be labeled as "sugar free," but this label does not mean "calorie free." Consumers still need to be aware of calories per serving as well as *trans* fat and saturated fat contents. Sometimes when "sugar" is removed, fats are added to improve the taste and texture of the product. This may be problematic for individuals with diabetes who monitor their carbohydrate and dietary fat intake.

Sugar alcohols have several advantages when used to replace sugar. They are less cariogenic than sucrose. In contrast to carbohydrate sugars, sugar alcohols do not encourage the growth of bacteria in the mouth that leads to tooth decay. In fact, xylitol may actually prevent cavity formation and may be protective when used in chewing gum. Although chemically related to carbohydrates, sugar alcohols are absorbed more slowly and incompletely than carbohydrates. The longer absorption time leads to a slower rise in blood glucose levels or reduced glycemic response. People with diabetes may be able to consume moderate amounts of these sweeteners and still control their blood glucose levels.

A disadvantage of sugar alcohols is that if large quantities are consumed, they may ferment in the intestinal tract because of their slower absorption rate. This fermentation may cause gas and diarrhea. The incomplete absorption results in a lower caloric value per gram, and thus less energy is available. Therefore, the sugar alcohols are called reduced-energy or low-energy sweeteners.

Alternative sweeteners, also called artificial sweeteners or nonnutritive sweeteners (NNSs), are manufactured to be used as sweetening agents in food products. Their function is to replace naturally sweet substances, such as sugar, honey, and other sucrose-containing substances. Alternative sweeteners most commonly used in the United States and approved by the FDA are aspartame, sucralose, acesulfame potassium (K), and saccharin. Often a combination of alternative sweeteners is used that results in an increased sweetness (Fitch & Keim, 2012).

Aspartame is formed by the bonding of the amino acids phenylalanine and aspartic acid. When consumed, aspartame is digested and absorbed as two separate amino acids. Although aspartame contains the same kcal as sucrose, much less aspartame is needed to get the same sweet taste because it is 160 to 220 times sweeter than sucrose. This provides so few kcal that aspartame can be considered a noncaloric sweetener. Approved in 1981 and used in a wide variety of products such as soft drinks, cereals, chewing gum, frozen snacks, and puddings, aspartame is consumed in more than 100 countries. In 1996 aspartame was approved as a general-purpose sweetener for all foods and beverages.

Several studies have shown aspartame to be safe, yet some individuals have reported side effects thought attributable to its consumption. These included allergic reactions such as rashes; edema of the lips, tongue, and throat; and respiratory difficulties. However, within controlled settings, these reactions were not replicated—meaning that aspartame consumption was not responsible for the allergic reactions (Fitch & Keim, 2012). The Internet has been used by some individuals to spread false information about aspartame, linking its consumption to disorders that range from multiple sclerosis to brain tumors to arthritis. Logically, one substance would not cause such an array of serious disorders. Investigation of the authors of the e-mails revealed sources that were not credible, and therefore the FDA maintains its approval of aspartame.

Individuals with the genetic disorder phenylketonuria (PKU) should not consume aspartame because their bodies cannot break down excess phenylalanine, resulting in a buildup that causes medical problems. All products containing aspartame have a warning label to alert individuals with PKU. This warning should apply to pregnant women as well. Because the fetus would be exposed to excess phenylalanine before the presence of PKU could be determined, the safest approach is to restrict consumption of aspartame during pregnancy.

The general adult population is advised to keep daily aspartame consumption (for a 132-pound person) at or less than 50 mg/kg body weight (the equivalent of 83 packets of Equal, an aspartame product) or 14 12-ounce cans of aspartame-sweetened soda (Fitch & Keim, 2012). Aspartame, when added to products, is often listed by its original brand names, NutraSweet and Equal.

Sucralose (trichlorogalactosucrose) was approved by the FDA in April 1998 for use in desserts, candies, and nonalcoholic beverages and as a tabletop sweetener. Made from chemically altered sucrose, sucralose provides no energy but is 600 times sweeter than sucrose. Because the body poorly absorbs it, sucralose passes through the digestive tract and is excreted in urine. An advantage of sucralose is that it can be used in baking and cooking. Sucralose is currently sold as Splenda.

Saccharin has had a stormy history since it was accidentally discovered more than 100 years ago. The storm began when some animal studies indicated an association between excessive saccharin consumption and the development of bladder cancer. In 1977 the FDA proposed a ban on saccharin. Many Americans were upset that the only available noncaloric sweetener was to be banned. The public outcry was so great that Congress, in an unusual move, created a moratorium to prevent the ban. In addition, Congress passed legislation requiring all products containing saccharin to clearly state a warning that the consumption of saccharin may be hazardous to health. This warning is no longer required.

The danger from saccharin is probably minimal. The risk of bladder cancer does not appear to apply to humans because no noticeable increase in the rate of bladder cancer has occurred. In addition, an association between cancers and saccharin is not supported by studies of individuals with diabetes, who tend to consume high amounts of saccharin. Consequently, the moratorium is no longer in effect because the FDA is not pursuing the ban on saccharin. Saccharin is now considered an interim food additive to be used in cosmetics, pharmaceuticals, and foods and beverages (Fitch & Keim, 2012). For food products, the amount of saccharin contained must be identified on the product label. Restrictions include that beverages may contain no more than 12 mg/ounce or less than 30 mg per food serving (FDA, 2017).

Compared with other alternative sweeteners, saccharin has a bitter aftertaste. To mask this flavor, it is often used in combination with other alternative sweeteners. Saccharin is still valuable because it is extremely sweet—300 times sweeter than sucrose. Trade names for saccharin include Sweet'N Low and Sugar Twin.

Acesulfame K received FDA approval in 1988. Synthetically produced, it tastes 200 times sweeter than sucrose, but it is not digestible by the human body and therefore provides no kcal. Acesulfame K is approved for use in a variety of products, from chewing gum to nondairy creamers, but so far, its use has been limited. One advantage of this product over aspartame is that it can be used for baking. Heat does not affect its sweetening ability, whereas heat destroys the sweet taste of aspartame. People who must severely limit potassium intake because of nutritional therapy for renal disorders should consult a registered dietitian/nutritionist (RDN) about acceptable levels of acesulfame K intake. The consumer brand name for acesulfame K is Sunette.

Another NNS is stevia, which is created from the leaves of a South American shrub. Stevia has been approved as a GRAS food additive by the FDA. Rebiana may be extracted from the stevia leaves and combined with other ingredients to create sweetening products such as Truvia, Sun Crystals, and Stevia in the Raw. Because stevia is used in very small quantities and has no caloric value (depending on other ingredients), individuals with diabetes may use it as another sweetener alternative.

Sweet Decisions

Should you consume foods with real sugar or artificial sugar? Which is the best? Which is the worst? There are no clear answers, but here is a way to decide. A concept used with food safety issues is a benefit-risk analysis. Does the benefit of consuming a substance outweigh the risk? This analysis can be applied to the decision whether to consume artificial sweeteners.

Benefits of consuming artificial sweeteners include experiencing a sweet taste with fewer kcal and a less cariogenic effect than sucrose. Many people believe these sweeteners are an important part of their weight-reduction effort. For most, though, the saved kcal are often replaced by consuming other kcal foods, thereby undermining their weight-loss efforts. Another concern is that recent studies suggest that because nonnutritive sweeteners mimic sweetness, physiologic responses may occur as if a caloric sweetener has been consumed. These responses may promote weight gain. Results have been mixed, so more research is needed. Nonetheless, with the significant consumption of artificially sweetened products, such as diet sodas, beverages, and foods, unforeseen health concerns may surface (Moriconi et al, 2020).

As noted, risks associated with the use of alternative sweeteners may involve safety concerns. This is a difficult issue to sort out. Because sucrose in the form of sugar cane juice and white table sugar have been used for thousands of years, we essentially have a large-scale study of its safety for humans. In contrast, alternative sweeteners have existed only for a century or less. Because alternative sweeteners are not naturally formed in plants or animals, their safety must be determined through research studies.

The research process is difficult. Rather than use humans as test subjects, researchers use animals. The test animals are given extremely large doses of the artificial sweeteners and are followed by researchers for several generations of their species. If the physiology of the animals is affected, particularly in regard to cancerous tumors, the substance may be regarded as too dangerous for consumption by humans. The difficulty is that the extremely large doses given to the animals do not replicate the amounts that would be typically consumed by humans. Concerns raised include whether the substance caused the tumor or whether the excessive quantity interfered with normal cell function. Also, how many animals need to be affected for a substance to be considered dangerous and in what animal generation of the experiment? Attention should also be paid to who funds such studies. If the company manufacturing the substance pays for the research, does that fact affect the interpretation of the results? These are difficult questions with which health scientists and FDA officials grapple.

This is an area, however, in which we can make a personal decision whether to consume products that contain alternative sweeteners. Based on our analysis of the benefits and risks, we can decide whether our wellness goals are better met by consuming a moderate amount of sucrose or a reasonable intake of alternative sweetened products.

COMPLEX CARBOHYDRATES: POLYSACCHARIDES

Polysaccharides are many units of monosaccharides held together by different kinds of chemical bonds. These types of bonds affect the ability of the body to digest polysaccharides and therefore account for the classification of polysaccharides as complex carbohydrates.

Starch

All starchy foods are plant foods. Starch is the storage form of plant carbohydrate. The strings of glucose that form starch are broken down by the digestive tract to provide glucose. Food sources of starch include grains, legumes, and some vegetables and fruits. Grains are the best source of starch. Grains provide more carbohydrates than any other food category. Grains are consumed in many forms and include wheat, oats, barley, rice, corn, and rye. The overall health value of processed grain products differs according to their sugar, fat, and fiber content (see the *Personal Perspectives* box "Eat Food, Not Too Much, Mostly Plants").

Breads, bagels, breakfast cereals, pasta, pancakes, grits, oatmeal, and other cooked cereals provide high-quality complex carbohydrates. These grain products may also contain fiber if made with whole grains. Depending on the spreads and toppings served, they may also be low in fat. Main dish items such as pizza, rice casseroles, and pasta mixtures create another category of complex carbohydrate food. Other foods such as crackers, cakes, pies, cookies, and pastries also provide carbohydrates but often contain considerable amounts of added sugar and fats; they should be eaten in moderation.

Legumes (beans and peas) are another significant source of complex carbohydrates. They are low in fat and are an excellent source of fiber, iron, and protein. Available dried, canned, or frozen, beans can be easily incorporated into commonly eaten foods.

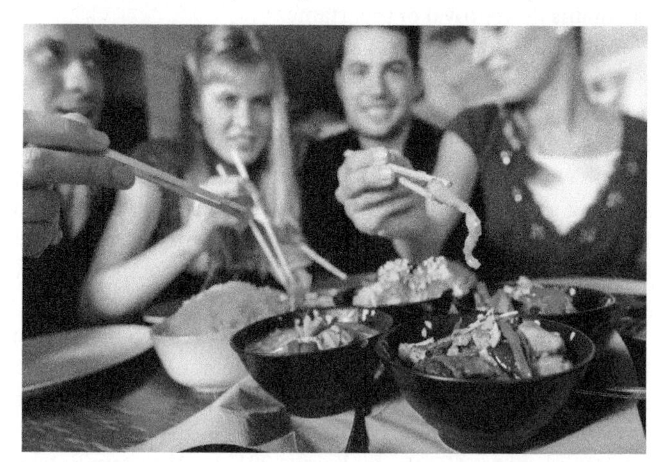

Thai (as above) and other ethnic cuisines can provide a source of complex carbohydrates and variety in the diet. (From www.thinkstockphotos.com)

Multicultural influences have expanded our exposure to inexpensive and versatile legumes. Mexican foods feature kidney beans as an ingredient of taco fillings and chili. Puerto Rican and Caribbean meals highlight rice and beans in savory sauces. Hearty Italian-style soups often depend on white and kidney beans combined with pasta. An African influence is reflected in dishes that combine black-eyed peas with meats or green vegetables. Hummus, a chickpea paste dip of Middle Eastern heritage, is often served with pita bread or vegetables.

Among vegetable sources of starch, potatoes lead the way. We consume potatoes in so many ways that we sometimes forget their humble "roots." As a root vegetable, the potato is a powerhouse of complex carbohydrates, fiber, vitamins, and even some protein. Unfortunately, some of the ways we prepare potatoes undo their positive health benefits. Most potatoes are processed into products loaded with fat and sodium. Nutritionally, potato chips have little in common with baked potatoes. The best health value is to eat potatoes in the least-processed form. Instead of French fries, choose a baked potato, or prepare mashed potatoes with skim milk and a small amount of margarine.

Other starchy root vegetables are parsnips, sweet potatoes, and yams. Sweet potatoes and yams provide the same nutrients as white potatoes plus significant amounts of beta carotene. Carrots and some varieties of squash, such as acorn and butternut, also provide starch and beta carotene. Beta carotene, a substance the body can convert into vitamin A, may have a protective effect against some forms of cancer.

Fiber

Fiber, like starch, consists of strings of simple sugars. Unlike starch, however, fiber cannot be broken down by human

PERSPECTIVES

"Eat Food, Not Too Much, Mostly Plants"

"Eat food. Not too much. Mostly plants" is the succinct nutrition/food consumption advice of author Michael Pollan for eating wisely. These seven words sum up his many years of extensive journalistic research about "What should I eat?" His results are presented in two of his best sellers: *The Omnivore's Dilemma* and *In Defense of Food: An Eater's Manifesto.* Mark Bittman, a journalist, a researcher, and a food lover, has also influenced attitudes about what to eat and how to prepare foods through his numerous best-selling cookbooks and writings. His latest books, *How to Cook Everything Vegetarian* and *The VB6 Cookbook: More Than 350 Recipes for Healthy Vegan Meals All Day and Delicious Flexitarian Dinners at Night,* provide "doable" strategies for consuming "more plants, fewer animals, and as little highly processed food as possible." Here are simple suggestions based on their writings that pertain to ecological, mindful, healthful, and satisfying consumption of carbohydrates and plants.

Eat Fewer Animal-Derived Foods; Eat More Plant Foods

Why

Production of animal-derived foods substantially affects the global environment, particularly climate change. For example, livestock production releases greenhouse gases into the atmosphere. The amount created accounts for 20% of all greenhouse gases produced. Animal-derived foods tend to be energy intensive. More energy is used to create these foods from animals than their actual food energy value. And finally, animal-derived foods tend to provide more saturated fats, dietary cholesterol, and energy than plant-based foods; these substances are potential risk factors for diet-related chronic disorders.

How

If less meat is eaten, more plant food easily takes its place. Smaller portion sizes are a good way to start. Rather than filling half the dinner plate with meat (beef, pork, chicken, fish, cheese, or eggs), restructure proportions to one-part meat (a quarter of the plate), two parts vegetables (half of the plate), and one-part grains (a quarter of the plate). Legumes (such as chickpeas, kidney beans, and black beans) can be used to replace some or all of the meat or added to the vegetables or grains.

Eat Real Food

Why

Real food is closest to the form found in nature. Foodstuffs may be cleaned of outer inedible parts, eaten raw or cooked, eaten alone or with other ingredients. But the plant or animal source is whole, not taken apart and put back together again with some parts containing nutrients removed (and not returned).

Avoid heavily processed foods. Why? The energy cost to create and package processed foods is substantial. Nutrients are lost during manufacturing. Often these nutrients are not returned to the product. Preservatives are added to maintain "freshness" so products can have a long shelf life, allowing processed foods to be shipped worldwide. The energy used for transportation adds to the actual cost of processed foods. Real food products, though, should not last forever!

How

We have lost the connection between the means of producing our food and our level of health. That a food product exists does not mean that it is worth consuming or is sufficiently valuable to expend our planet's limited energy and resources for its production.

We can take responsibility for our food intake. Michael Pollan, as described in *The Omnivore's Dilemma,* set out to procure all the ingredients for a meal, including participating in a hunt for a wild pig that he then helped eviscerate and cook as well as foraging for wild mushrooms in secretive forest areas in California. His intent was to realize the effect of his consumption on the earth in a very concrete manner.

Although we don't need to repeat his experience, we can take action by learning how to cook simple meals from scratch. We can return to our kitchens (and to simple cookbooks or Internet recipes) and begin planning and preparing real food. Bittman's advice is that with a little planning, we can alter our lifestyles to nourish our bodies while reducing our impact on the environment.

(Data from Bittman M: *Food matters: A guide to conscious eating,* New York, 2009, Simon & Schuster; Bittman M: *The VB6 cookbook: More than 350 recipes for healthy vegan meals all day and delicious flexitarian dinners at night,* New York, 2014, Clarkson Potter; Pollan M: *The omnivore's dilemma: A natural history of four meals,* New York, 2007, Penguin Group (USA) Inc.; and Pollan M: *In defense of food: An eater's manifesto,* New York, 2008, Penguin Group (USA) Inc.)

digestive enzymes. **Dietary fiber** consists of substances in plant foods, including carbohydrates and lignin, that for the most part cannot be digested by humans. We do not produce digestive juices strong enough to break down the bonds that hold the simple carbohydrates of most plant fibers, so fiber "passes through" our bodies without providing kcal or nutrients. Its texture provides bulk that thickens chyme and eases the work of the GI muscles that regulate movement of the food mass (Table 4.4).

Although human digestive juices cannot digest fiber, microflora that normally reside in the colon use fiber as a medium for microbial fermentation, resulting in the synthesis of vitamins and the formation of short-chain fatty acids (SCFAs). The bacteria that reside in the colon synthesize several vitamins, including vitamin K, biotin, B_{12}, folate, and thiamin. Only vitamin K and biotin can be absorbed in sufficient amounts from the colon to be significant; the other vitamins are absorbed from the small intestine so that the synthesized vitamins are not bioavailable. The SCFAs that are produced can be absorbed and used for energy by the mucosa of the colon, thereby maintaining the health of the colon epithelial cells (Sullivan et al, 2014). The effects of SCFAs also increase fecal matter bulk.

Dietary fiber actually refers to several kinds of carbohydrate substances from different plant sources; all serve similar functions in the human body. Dietary fibers are divided into two categories based on their solubility in fluids. **Soluble dietary fibers** dissolve in fluids, include pectin, mucilage, psyllium seed husk, guar gum, and other related gums. Soluble fiber thickens substances. **Insoluble dietary fibers** do not dissolve in fluids and therefore provide structure and protection for plants. Some insoluble dietary fibers are cellulose and hemicellulose. Lignin, considered a dietary fiber, is composed of chains of alcohol rather than carbohydrate.

Foods are sometimes classified according to the predominant type of fiber they contain. Oatmeal is a good source of soluble fiber because oat bran, part of the whole oatmeal grain, is particularly high in soluble fiber. But the whole grain

TABLE 4.4 Types, Composition, Sources, and Functions of Fibers

Type of Fiber	Major Chemical Component(s)	Sources	Major Function(s)
Less Soluble Fiber			
Cellulose	Glucose (β1–4 linkages)	Whole wheat, bran, vegetables	Increase water-holding capacity, thus increasing fecal volume and decreasing gut transit time
Hemicellulose	Xylose, mannose, galactose	Bran, whole grains	
Lignin	Phenols	Fruits and edible seeds, mature vegetables	Fermentation produces short-chain fatty acids associated with decreased risk of tumor formation
More Soluble Fibers			
Gums	Galactose and glucuronic acid	Oats, legumes, guar, barley	Cause gel formation, thus decrease gastric emptying, and slow digestion, gut transit time, and glucose absorption
Pectins	Polygalacturonic acid	Apples, strawberries, carrots, citrus	Also bind minerals, lipids, and bile acids, increasing excretion of each, thus decreasing serum cholesterol
Functional Fibers[a]			
Chitin	Glucopyranose	Supplement from crab or lobster shells	Reduces serum cholesterol
Fructans (including inulin)	Fructose polymers	Extracted from natural sources: chicory, onions, etc.	Prebiotics that stimulate growth of beneficial bacteria in gut; used as fat replacers
β-Glucans	Glucopyranose	Oat and barley bran	Reduces serum cholesterol
Algal polysaccharides (carrageenan)		Isolated from algae and seaweed	Gel forming—used as thickeners, stabilizers (can be toxic)
Polydextrose, polyols	Glucose and sorbitol, etc.	Synthesized	Used as bulking agents or sugar substitutes
Psyllium		Extracted from psyllium seeds	Has a high water-binding capacity (choking hazard)

[a]Isolated or extracted.
(Modified from Gallagher ML: The nutrients and their metabolism. In Mahan K, et al, eds: *Krause's food & the nutrition care process*, ed 13, St. Louis, 2012, Saunders.)

is a good source of insoluble fiber as well. Although Table 4.5 specifically lists foods containing soluble and insoluble dietary fiber, many fiber-rich foods contain some of each kind of fiber. For example, an apple is a source of the soluble dietary fiber pectin, which is part of the inside "stuff" of the apple. An apple also provides cellulose, an insoluble dietary fiber that forms the structure of the apple and gives it its characteristic shape (Fig. 4.5). Popcorn is another source of insoluble dietary fiber that has been with us for a long time (see the *Cultural Diversity and Nutrition* box The "Pop" Heard Through the Centuries).

TABLE 4.5 Dietary Fibers and Food Sources

Fibers	Food Sources
Insoluble	
Cellulose Hemicellulose Lignin	Whole grains, brown rice, buckwheat groats, whole-wheat flour, whole-wheat pasta, oatmeal, unrefined cereals, vegetables, wheat bran, seeds, popcorn, nuts, peanut butter, leafy green vegetables such as broccoli
Soluble	
Pectin Mucilage Guar and other gums	Kidney beans, split peas, lentils, chickpeas (garbanzo beans), navy beans, soybeans, apples, pears, bananas, grapes, citrus fruits (oranges and grapefruits), oat bran, oatmeal, barley, corn, carrots, white potatoes

Health Effects

All the health benefits of fiber improve the physical functioning of the human body. The benefits are not directly nutritional but instead allow the body to function at a more efficient level. Each of the following disorders listed may develop because of genetic predisposition, environmental factors, or lifestyle behaviors. However, the risk of developing these disorders seems to increase when consumption of dietary fiber is low. Because eating sufficient fiber appears to be a preventive factor, we consider the benefits of fiber for primary disease prevention. Primary prevention aims to avert the initial development of a disorder or health problem. The risk for the development of obesity, constipation, hemorrhoids, diverticular disease, and colon cancer may be decreased by regular consumption of sufficient amounts of fiber. Each of these topics is discussed in Part 4 of this book, Overview of Nutrition Therapy. A brief introduction to the relationship between fiber consumption and reduced risk of these disorders is given here.

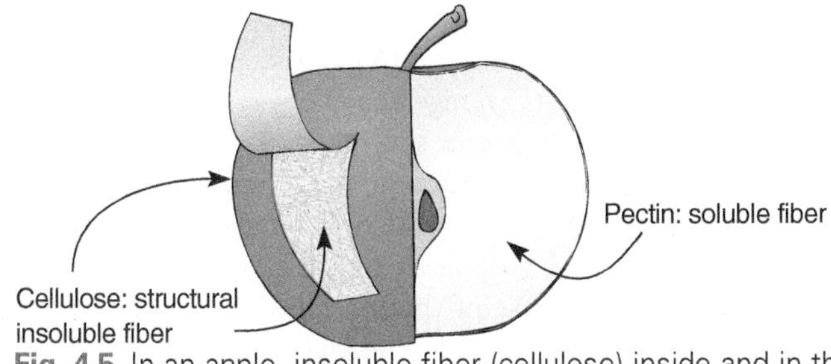

Fig. 4.5 In an apple, insoluble fiber (cellulose) inside and in the skin provides structure, and soluble fiber (pectin) inside adds substance.

CULTURAL DIVERSITY AND NUTRITION

The "Pop" Heard Through the Centuries

The next time you're at the movies digging into a giant tub of popcorn, be sure to appreciate one of the tastier contributions of Native Americans to our food supply: popping corn, first created over an open fire 5000 years ago. The delectable popcorn added variety to ways to prepare corn, a mainstay of the Native American diet. Gifts of popcorn necklaces and popcorn beer were made by the Indians of the Caribbean in the 1500s, and the Aztecs used popcorn in religious ceremonies. And what would Thanksgiving have been without some popped corn—compliments of the Wampanoag tribe?

Popcorn most likely originated in Mexico, but it was also grown in India, Sumatra, and China years before Columbus "discovered" America. Biblical stories of "corn" in Egypt were not entirely true. The term corn meant the most commonly used grain of a region. In Scotland and Ireland, corn referred to oats; in England, corn was wheat. In the Americas, the common grain was maize, and the two terms, corn and maize, became synonymous.

Today special varieties of corn have been developed for their "popping" characteristics. When a corn kernel is heated, water in it creates steam. This steam, unable to escape through the heavy skin of the kernel, causes an explosion that exposes the white starchy center. Fortunately, the skin remains attached to the starch, making popcorn an excellent source of dietary fiber.

Although all popcorn provides dietary fiber, some of the ways it is prepared negate this health benefit. Popcorn laden with butter and covered with salt is not a healthful snack, nor is a batch popped with the aid of oil, even if vegetable oil is used. Microwaveable packets of popcorn are equally deceiving because they contain oil and other additives. We also may easily be misled into eating more than we should because each bag contains four servings, which most of us devour singlehandedly.

Instead, return to the native style—fresh air-popped corn. Air-popping appliances and microwave containers eliminate the need for oil. Better toppings include sodium-reduced salt, garlic powder, and Cajun spices. While devouring your wholesome snack, remember to acknowledge the inventiveness of Native Americans.

(Data from Popcorn Institute: *Early popcorn history*, Chicago, 1996, Author; and National Agricultural Library, Special Collections: *Popcorn: Ingrained in America's agricultural history*, 2002 (updated October). Accessed 12 November, 2017, from specialcollections.nal.usda.gov/popcorn-exhibit.)

Obesity. Eating high-fiber foods seems to make weight control easier. The volume of such foods makes us feel fuller, so we consume less food. Often, high-fiber foods replace those that are higher in fat and kcal. Regularly eating foods high in fiber and low in fat may reduce or prevent obesity.

Constipation. Fiber, particularly insoluble fiber such as wheat bran and whole grains, prevents the dry, hard stools of constipation (see Chapter 13). A sufficient fiber intake plus adequate fluid intake ensures larger, softer stools that are easier to eliminate. Less straining during elimination also reduces the risk of hemorrhoids (enlarged veins in the anus) and diverticular disease.

Diverticular disease. Diverticular disease affects the large intestine. Pockets (diverticula) develop on the outside walls of the intestine. Low-fiber diets may create increased internal pressure from segmentation muscles attempting to move the food mass because the bulk of fiber is not available, which may then weaken intestinal muscles. Weakened muscles are more at risk for the formation of diverticula. If feces get caught in the pockets, bacteria may develop, multiply, and cause serious and painful inflammation (diverticulitis). Medical treatment and nutritional recommendations are necessary and are discussed in Chapter 13.

Cancer. Eating enough dietary fiber may also reduce the risk of colon cancer. Two potential risk factors for colon cancer related to fiber intake are a high dietary fat intake and exposure to carcinogenic substances in the GI tract (Keim et al, 2014). If we eat more fiber, we tend to eat less fat. High-fiber foods tend to replace foods that are high in fat. Because foods containing fiber are bulkier, they seem to fill the stomach quicker, providing satiety sooner and with fewer kcal than foods containing fat. Fiber-containing foods such as fruits and vegetables may contain other substances that may be protective for the colon.

Heart disease. Two heart disease risk factors are high blood cholesterol and increased lipid levels (see Chapter 17 for recommended levels). Increasing dietary fiber consumption can lower blood cholesterol and lipid levels in two ways: (1) High-fiber foods replace higher fat foods, particularly those containing dietary cholesterol and saturated fats; (2) soluble fiber such as pectin (citrus fruits and apples), guar gum (legumes), and oat gum (oat bran) binds lipids and cholesterol as they move through the intestinal tract and are then excreted with the fiber (Willis & Slavin, 2014).

Diabetes control. Dietary fiber intake may help people with diabetes to stabilize blood glucose levels. Diabetes mellitus affects the body's ability to regulate blood glucose levels. When fiber is consumed, particularly soluble fiber, glucose may be absorbed more slowly. The slower absorption rate of glucose may keep blood glucose within acceptable levels.

Potential Health Risks of Dietary Fiber

When the recommended increase of dietary fiber intake is fulfilled by fiber-containing foods, there tend to be few health risks. Problems may develop when fiber supplements or other forms of processed or purified fiber, such as oat or wheat bran, are consumed in large quantities. When used as a supplement, excessive quantities of purified fiber can overwhelm the GI tract and lead to blockages in the small intestine and colon (Willis & Slavin, 2014). This is a serious medical condition that fortunately is rare.

Bioavailability of minerals may be lowered by the presence of fiber-containing foods. Some fibers and substances in whole grains, such as phytates and oxalates, may bind minerals, making them unable to be absorbed. However, higher fiber dietary patterns tend also to be higher in mineral content; therefore, absorption of minerals remains adequate.

As fiber passes through the GI tract, it provides several health-promoting services that are still being analyzed. Some foods that contain fiber also contain an assortment of essential nutrients. That is why it is best to get fiber from real foods rather than from supplements.

Because some benefits do vary between soluble and insoluble fibers, should daily intakes of each kind of fiber be calculated? Not at all. Increase total dietary fiber to recommended levels slowly by gradually substituting whole-grain foods, fresh fruits, and vegetables for some lower fiber foods (see the *Teaching Tool* box What's Your Fiber Score Today?). This allows the body to adjust to the additional fiber, reducing the possible formation of intestinal gas.

TEACHING TOOL

What's Your Fiber Score Today?

Although the following foods are particularly good sources of dietary fiber, many other foods—all fruits and vegetables—contain smaller amounts that add up by the day's end. Does your typical intake meet the recommended levels of about 25 to 38 g per day?

Approximately 2g per Serving

Apricot	Grapefruit
Banana	Oatmeal
Blueberries	Peach
Broccoli	Pineapple
Cantaloupe	Rye crackers
Carrot	Whole-wheat bread
Cauliflower	Whole-wheat cereals

Approximately 3g per Serving

Apple with skin	Potato with skin
Corn	Raisins
Orange	Shredded wheat cereal
Pear	Strawberries
Peas	

Approximately 4g or More per Serving

Baked beans	Lentils
Bran cereals	Navy beans
Kidney beans	Whole-wheat spaghetti

(Data from U.S. Department of Agriculture, Agricultural Research Service: *USDA National Nutrient Database for Standard Reference* (Release 28, released September 2015, slightly revised May 2016). 2012, Nutrient Data Laboratory. Accessed 12 November, 2017, from https://ndb.nal.usda.gov/ndb/.)

FOOD SOURCES AND ISSUES

Although dietary fiber is not absorbed and does not serve a nutrient function in the body, the effects of fiber are important for optimum health. An adequate intake (AI) of dietary fiber is about 25 to 38 g per day, depending on age and gender (NRC, 2006). Most Americans consume much lower levels of fiber; adults often average less than 16 g of fiber per day, whereas children and young adults average 12 g (King et al, 2012).

This situation arises from several factors. First, many Americans do not consume enough fruits and vegetables on a daily basis. Somehow, high protein and fat dietary intakes have pushed fruits and vegetables out of our meal patterns. This is most likely because of the increased consumption of meals away from home tied with the fact that sugared beverages account for a significant percentage of daily caloric intake for many people.

Also, and possibly the most significant factor, is that many Americans regularly eat foods made with refined grains from which dietary fiber has been removed. Consumption of legumes and high-fiber cereal foods provides considerably more fiber. Fiber intake also differs by race and ethnicity (Fig. 4.6). Some of the difference is probably because of the fiber levels of traditional foods consumed. For example, Mexican American consumption of fiber is the highest, whereas Black Americans consumption of fiber is the lowest.

Unrefined Versus Refined Grains

Unrefined grains are prepared for consumption while they contain their original components. These grains are really seeds or kernels that include all the nutrients necessary to support plant growth and are segmented inside the kernel to be used when needed. **Whole-grain products** refer to food items made using all the edible portions of kernels.

In contrast, **refined grains** have been taken apart. Only portions of the edible kernel are included in refined grain products. Although both unrefined and refined grain products are good sources of complex carbohydrates, other nutritional qualities of the whole grain are lost when grains are refined. Grains most often refined are wheat, rice, oats, corn, and rye.

To better understand how the nutrients are lost, consider the wheat kernel shown in Fig. 4.7. The kernel consists of three nutrient-containing components. The outer layer, bran, is an excellent source of cellulose dietary fiber and contains magnesium, riboflavin, niacin, thiamin, vitamin B_6, and some protein.

The germ found in the base of the kernel contains a wealth of nutrients to support the sprouting of the plant. Some of these are thiamin, riboflavin, vitamin B_6, vitamin E, zinc, protein, and wheat oil (polyunsaturated vegetable oil). The endosperm, the largest component of the kernel, contains starch, the prime energy source for the sprouting plant. It also contains protein and riboflavin but much smaller amounts of niacin, thiamin, and B_6.

When flour is refined, the bran and germ are removed; the bran affects the physical lightness of the flour, and the oil in the germ may become rancid, reducing the shelf life of the flour. Only the starchy endosperm is used to mill refined flour. Because flour is the mainstay of grain products, the loss of nutrients for the population is significant. In the 1940s it was determined that deficiencies of thiamin, riboflavin, niacin, and iron occurred because of the refining process. To counteract

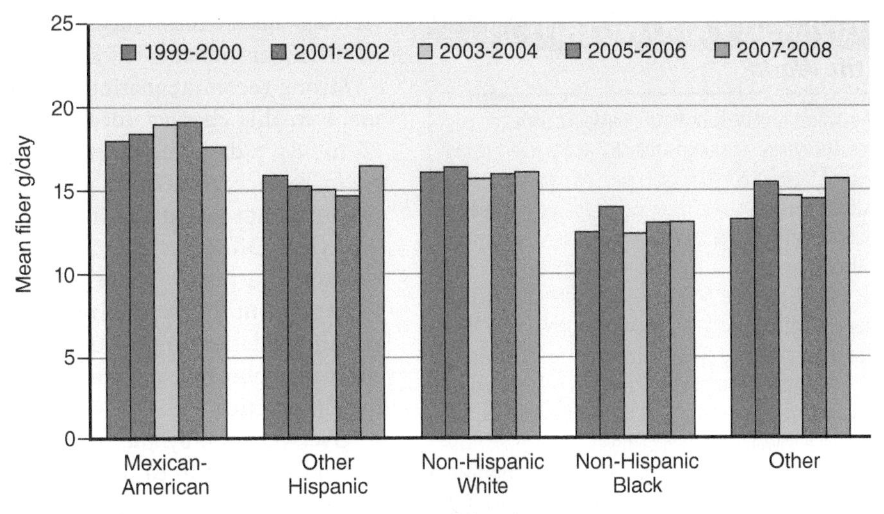

Fig. 4.6 Dietary fiber intake of Americans by race/ethnicity and year. *NHANES*, National Health and Nutrition Examination Survey. (From King DE, Mainous AG III, Lambourne CA: Trends in dietary fiber intake in the United States, 1999–2008, *J Acad Nutr Diet*, 112:642–648, 2012.)

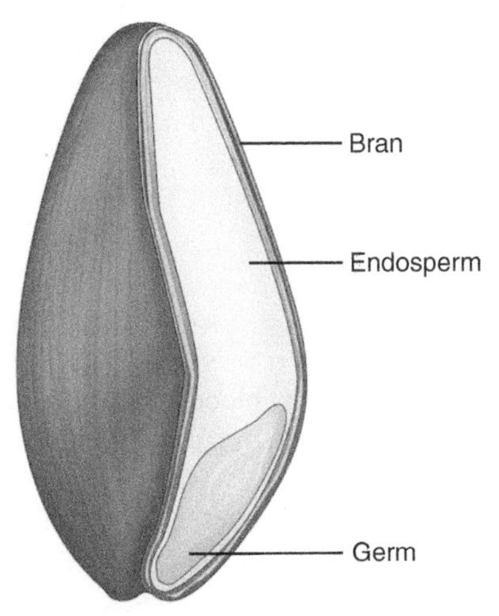

Fig. 4.7 Inside a wheat kernel.

this loss, those four nutrients were added back to flour. Now, flour with these specific nutrient additives is called enriched flour.

Enrichment is the replacement of nutrients to the level that was present before processing. Although the four lost nutrients are replaced in enriched flour, other vitamins, minerals, and fiber originally in whole wheat are not. Zinc, magnesium, vitamin E, and dietary fiber are not returned to the refined white flour. Consequently, any product made with enriched white flour is still nutritionally inferior to one made with whole-wheat flour (see the *Health Debate* box If Dietary Fiber Is So Important, Should Grain Products Be Allowed to Be Refined?).

HEALTH DEBATE

If Dietary Fiber Is So Important, Should Grain Products Be Allowed to Be Refined?

This chapter highlights the health benefits of eating the recommended levels of fiber. Also emphasized are nutrition losses that occur when fruits, vegetables, and grains are processed or refined. The process of refining can lead to the extensive loss of fiber and various nutrients. Although some nutrients are replaced, some, such as dietary fiber, are not.

If health benefits of dietary fiber and nutrients are so valuable, should there be government regulations to restrict or prohibit the removal of valuable nutrients and dietary fiber? Several of the diseases associated with low fiber intake are chronic. Treating these long-term diseases places a burden on the entire U.S. health care system.

Is it fair for all of us to bear the financial burden for those not consuming the most healthful form of foods available? Should there be a law against the processing of whole grains? Should white flour production be restricted? Or is the availability of white (or wheat) and whole-wheat products sufficient? Is it our "freedom of choice" to be able to select among different food products even though some are more beneficial to health than others?

What do you think?

The preference for refined complex carbohydrates may be changing. The health benefits of dietary fiber have been so newsworthy and the focus of such intensive advertising that consumer perception of fiber has evolved from a negative selling point to a positive one. Twenty years ago, if products claimed to be high in fiber or made from whole grains, sales would decline. Today, high-fiber food items are among the better sellers in categories such as cereals and breads (see the *Cultural Diversity and Nutrition* box Cereals Around the World).

CULTURAL DIVERSITY AND NUTRITION

Cereals Around the World

Hot cereals have been the mainstay of carbohydrate breakfast calories among cultures in colder climates. The adage "sticking to the ribs" foods refers to the warming and filling effects of freshly cooked cereals such as oatmeal, cream of wheat, and oat bran. Just as the Inuit have many words for snow to reflect its many variations in a climate often characterized by snow, Norway, another cold country, has many kinds of porridge or hot cereal. In Norway, porridges may include oats, wheat, barley, rye, and rice. Porridge is often eaten as a winter dinner and can be served cold as dessert pudding topped with fruit sauce. Porridge also has social significance. Extra-creamy porridge is served to women who just gave birth as a way to boost their nutrition. A lucky individual may refer to good luck as being "in the middle of a butter island," meaning the kind of melting butter found in a bowl of steaming porridge.

Consider your own cultural background. Is there a grain or carbohydrate food that has special significance to your family because of its ethnic or regional influence?

(Data from The Norwegian Table: *Some like it hot*, Norway, 2001.)

TOWARD A POSITIVE NUTRITION LIFESTYLE: TAILORING

Consider what a tailor does. A tailor takes a bolt of cloth and, by cutting, shaping, and sewing, fits a garment to a person's exact measurements. Tailoring as a behavior-change technique takes a health recommendation and, by "cutting," "shaping," and "sewing," fits the recommendation to the limitations or requirements of our individual lifestyles.

Strong recommendations to increase our fiber intake are made in this chapter. Ideally, fiber intake should be about 25 to 38 g a day. The most efficient means of intake would be to replace all refined grain products with whole-grain products. But is that possible if one considers contemporary lifestyles? Often, we are not able to control available food choices, and thus we have difficulty changing our behavior to implement this type of recommendation. By tailoring the recommendation or goal to our individual lifestyles, we can succeed. Following are some recommendations for "tailoring" in practice:

- Overwhelmed by the thought of eating only whole-grain foods? Decide to eat more whole-grain products for breakfast and dinner, which are eaten at home, where control is easier.
- No time to cook vegetables? Prepare or order salads and keep fresh fruits of any kind handy.
- Need to add fiber to your diet? When possible, choose fiber-rich foods for lunch. Be realistic, however, because foods available at the cafeteria or coffee shop are limited.
- Attending a family holiday dinner or special event or going on vacation? Enjoy what's served. Then resume a regular fiber-rich dietary pattern when back at work or school.

Although the goal is to increase fiber intake, the objective is to fit positive dietary choices and habits to the shapes of our nutrition lifestyles.

SUMMARY

- Carbohydrates are organic compounds composed of carbon, hydrogen, and oxygen in the form of simple carbohydrates.
  - There are three sizes of carbohydrates: monosaccharides (glucose, fructose, and galactose); disaccharides (sucrose, maltose, and lactose); and polysaccharides (starch, fiber, and glycogen).
  - Food carbohydrates are divided into two categories: simple carbohydrates (monosaccharides and disaccharides) and complex carbohydrates (polysaccharides, excluding glycogen).
  - Dietary recommendations for carbohydrates are as follows:
    - Dietary Reference Intake (DRI) for carbohydrates is 130 g/day for adults between 19 and 30 years of age.
    - Acceptable macronutrient distribution range (AMDR) is 45% to 65% of kcal intake per day as primarily complex carbohydrates.
    - *Dietary Guidelines* recommends emphasizing a plant-based diet including fruits, vegetables, cooked dried beans and peas, whole grains, and seeds.
- Carbohydrates are an abundant food source of energy and dietary fiber.
  - Energy circulates in the bloodstream as glucose.
  - Blood glucose levels are regulated and balanced through hormonal systems.
  - Hypoglycemia and diabetes mellitus may occur when these systems cannot regulate glucose within normal levels.
  - Dietary fiber does not provide energy; it is not digestible by humans.
  - Consuming adequate quantities of soluble and insoluble fiber has significant health benefits.
  - The DRI for dietary fiber is 25 to 38 g for adult women and men, respectively.
- Best carbohydrate food energy sources: grains, legumes, and starchy root vegetables.
- Best dietary fiber sources: fruits, vegetables, and whole-grain products.
- Nutrients are lost when unrefined (whole) grains are refined.
- *Dietary Guidelines* recommends increased consumption of complex carbohydrates:
  - MyPlate proposes 6 ounces of grains (with at least 3 ounces whole grains), 4½ cups of vegetables, and 2 cups of fruits.

THE NURSING APPROACH

Clinical Judgment and Next-Generation NCLEX® Examination-Style Questions

Case Study 1

Diverticulosis and Constipation

Mary, age 62, is in the nurse practitioner's (NP's) office for a routine annual physical examination. When collecting the health history, the NP finds that Mary often has had abdominal discomfort and constipation. Her medical history indicates a medical diagnosis of diverticulosis. The NP interviews Mary and performs an abdominal examination.

Assessment/Recognize Cues

Subjective (from Patient Statements)

- Small, hard, pebblelike stools, usually two times a day
- Uncomfortable straining with bowel movements
- Bloating and gas
- Drinks 4 to 6 glasses of water per day
- Prefers white bread and refined grains
- Eats few fruits and vegetables and peels those she does eat
- Does not exercise regularly

Objective (from Physical Examination)

- Abdomen distended, nontender
- Bowel sounds hypoactive

Diagnosis(Nursing)/Analyze Cues

1. Constipation related to low fiber and fluid intake, and lack of exercise as evidenced by hypoactive bowel sounds and patient statements about small, hard stools and uncomfortable straining with bowel movements
2. Chronic noncancer pain related to diverticulosis as evidence by patient's complaint of abdominal pain and uncomfortable straining

Planning/Prioritize Hypotheses

Patient Outcomes

Short term (at the end of this visit):

- Mary will identify foods high in fiber and develop plans to gradually include them in her diet.
- Mary will verbalize intention to drink at least 8 glasses of water and walk at least 15 minutes per day.

Long term (at the follow-up visit in 1 month):

- Mary will report she was able to follow her plan.
- Mary will report regular soft bowel movements with no discomfort or straining.

Nursing Interventions/Generate Solutions

1. Teach Mary about the causes of constipation and diverticulosis.
2. Teach Mary about lifestyle changes that will prevent constipation.

Implementation/Take Action

1. Explained causes of constipation and how constipation can lead to diverticulosis and diverticulitis.
   Common causes of constipation are insufficient fiber, fluids, and activity. Strained defecation increases intracolonic pressure and can weaken the muscles in the bowel, allowing outpouching of the intestinal wall (diverticulosis). If fecal matter gets caught in the diverticula, infection can result (diverticulitis). For diverticulosis, a high-fiber diet is prescribed. For diverticulitis, the patient may receive nothing by mouth temporarily or may consume only low-fiber foods and fluids to allow healing of the irritated bowel.
2. Encouraged Mary to add fiber gradually until she is eating at least six servings of whole-grain breads and cereals and five servings of fruits, vegetables, and legumes per day.
   Fiber adds bulk to stools and stimulates peristalsis. Increasing fiber intake too quickly can lead to bloating, gas, cramps, abdominal discomfort, and diarrhea. Generally, one high-fiber food can be added every 2 weeks, until the client is eating 25 to 38 g of fiber per day.
3. Provided written information on types and sources of fiber and explored food likes and preferences to determine high-fiber foods acceptable to Mary.
   Substituting high-fiber foods for low-fiber foods can prevent constipation, but the diet needs to be individualized. Examples of high-fiber foods are whole-wheat bread, bran cereal, kidney beans, prunes and other fruits with peelings, and broccoli.
4. Encouraged Mary to drink 8 to 12 glasses of fluid per day, especially water and fruit juices.
   Fluid softens stools and increases bulk, promoting peristalsis. As fiber is increased, fluids must be increased to prevent further constipation, intestinal blockage, and abdominal pain.
5. Encouraged Mary to exercise regularly—for example, start by walking for at least 15 minutes five times a week.
   Activity promotes peristalsis. It is recommended that adults get 2 hours 30 minutes of moderate-intensity aerobic activity every week and participate in muscle-strengthening activities 2 or more days per week.

Evaluation/Evaluate Outcomes

Short term (at the end of the visit):

Mary wrote down specific goals for lifestyle changes to correct constipation.

- Changes to make right away:
  - Substitute whole-wheat bread for white bread.
  - Eat three servings of fruits and vegetables per day.
  - Drink 8 glasses of water per day.
  - Walk for 15 minutes three times a week.
- Changes to make gradually, starting in 2 weeks:
  - Replace one low-fiber food with one new high-fiber food every 2 weeks.
  - Increase walking to 20 minutes five times a week.
- Changes not willing to make: drinking prune juice

Short-term outcomes achieved.

Mary set up an appointment for follow-up in 1 month.

Discussion Questions

At her follow-up appointment, Mary said her stools had been softer, better formed, and more comfortable to eliminate. She said she had eaten whole-wheat bread 3 days per week, had eaten three fruits per day, had drunk about five glasses of water per day, and had walked for 15 minutes twice a week. Last week she began eating raisin bran cereal 4 days per week.

1. How would you judge Mary's goal achievement (Evaluate Outcomes)—met, partially met, or not met at all? What was the basis for your answer?
2. If you were the nurse, what would you say to Mary about her report? What questions would you ask?

Continued

THE NURSING APPROACH—cont'd

Case Study 2

An emergency department (ED) nurse is assessing an elderly female client who has come to the ED with complaints of abdominal pain, severe constipation, and no bowel movement in 7 days. The client is alert and oriented and guarding her abdomen. Her bowel sounds are hypoactive. She lives with her daughter and family, eats three meals a day but admits to having low dietary fiber consumption. Her vital signs are temperature 98.8° F (37.1° C), pulse = 92 beats per minute, respiration = 24 breaths per minute, blood pressure = 132/78 mm Hg. Her pain level is 7/10 on a 10/10 scale.

Which of the following client assessment findings require **immediate follow-up** by the nurse?

Use an X to mark the client assessment findings that require immediate follow-up by the ED nurse. Select all that apply.

Assessment findings that require immediate follow-up

1. Alert and oriented
2. Abdominal pain is 7/10
3. Severe constipation with no bowel movement in 7 days
4. Pulse = 96 beats per minute
5. Respirations = 24 breaths per minute
6. Blood pressure = 132/78
7. Edematous abdomen
8. Hypoactive bowel sounds

APPLYING CONTENT KNOWLEDGE

You are at a restaurant having lunch with friends. After hearing you order a sandwich on whole-wheat bread, the friend comments, "Whole-wheat bread, white bread, what's the big deal? They're all complex carbohydrates." How would you respond?

WEBSITES OF INTEREST

American Public Health Association
www.apha.org
Promotes and protects the public's health to achieve a healthy global society.

Wheat Foods Council
www.wheatfoods.org
Provides nutrition and food preparation resources for incorporating more grains into the American diet.

USA Rice Federation
www.usarice.com
Offers information about rice production, preparation, research, and environmental issues.

REFERENCES

Dolan, J. P., & Adams-Smith, W. N. (1978). *Health and society: a documentary history of medicine*. New York: The Seabury Press.

Fitch, C., & Keim, K. S. (2012). Academy of nutrition and dietetics: position of the academy of nutrition and dietetics: use of nutritive and nonnutritive sweeteners. *Journal of the Academy of Nutrition and Dietetics, 112*, 739–758.

Gallagher, M. L. (2012). The nutrients and their metabolism. In K. Mahan (Ed.), *Krause's food & the nutrition care process* (13th ed.). St. Louis: Saunders/Elsevier.

Keim, N. L., et al. (2014). Carbohydrates. In A. C. Ross (Ed.), *Modern nutrition in health and disease* (11th ed.). Philadelphia: Wolters Kluver/Lippincott Williams & Wilkins.

King, D. E., et al. (2012). Trends in diet fiber intake in the United States, 1999-2008. *Journal of the Academy of Nutrition and Dietetics, 112*, 642–648.

Moriconi, E., et al. (2020). Neuroendocrine and metabolic effects of low-calorie and non-calorie sweeteners. *Frontiers in Endocrinology, 11*, 444.

National Research Council. (2006). *Dietary reference intakes: the essential guide to nutrient requirements*. Washington, DC: The National Academies Press.

Sullivan, S., et al. (2014). Nutritional physiology of the alimentary tract. In A. C. Ross (Ed.), *Modern nutrition in health and disease* (11th ed.). Philadelphia: Wolters Kluver/Lippincott Williams & Wilkins.

U.S. Department of Health Human Services (USDHHS), & U.S. Department of Agriculture (USDA), (December 2020). *2020–2025 Dietary Guidelines for Americans* (9th ed.). Home | Dietary Guidelines for Americans. Available at: https://www.dietaryguidelines.gov/sites/default/files/2020-12/Dietary_Guidelines_for_Americans_2020-2025.pdf. (Accessed 5 January 2021).

U.S. Food and Drug Administration (FDA). (2017). *Electronic code of federal regulations title 21*. Washington, DC: The Office of the Federal Register. From: <https://www.ecfr.govbin/searchECFR?ob=r&idno=&q1=GRAS&r=&SID=adc865fbc75522b06f14aba1ec8d98f2&mc=true>. (Accessed 11 November, 2017).

Willis, H. J., & Slavin, J. L. (2014). Dietary fiber. In A. C. Ross (Ed.), *Modern nutrition in health and disease* (11th ed.). Philadelphia: Wolters Kluver/Lippincott Williams & Wilkins.

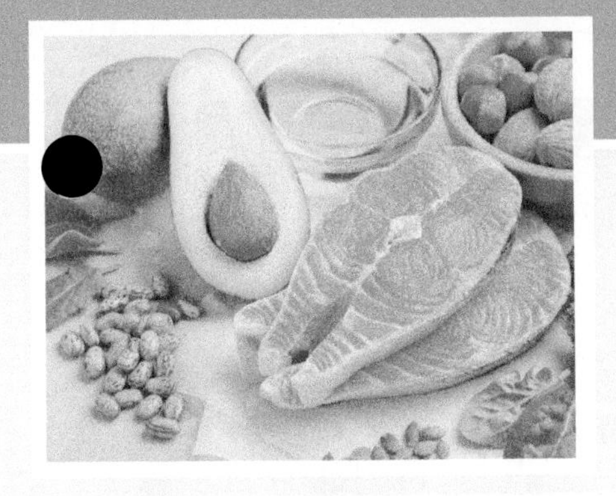

5

Fats

Fat is the densest form of stored energy in food and our bodies. This means that gram for gram, food fat—in the form of triglycerides—can produce more than twice the energy in kcal as that provided by carbohydrate or protein.

http://evolve.elsevier.com/GRODNER/FOUNDATIONS

LEARNING OBJECTIVES

- List the major functions of triglyceride in food and physiologically in the body.
- State the functions of phospholipids and cholesterol.
- Summarize the structures and sources of the three types of lipids.
- Discuss the function and sources of the linolenic and linoleic essential fatty acids.
- Explain the digestion, absorption, and transportation of lipids in the body.
- Identify the three different types of lipoproteins and their functions.
- Describe the potential health concerns and benefits related to dietary fat intake.

ROLE IN WELLNESS

It may be time for a truce about the consumption of dietary fat. Since the 1970s, consumption of fats gained a negative reputation as a possible source of diet-related disorders and a factor in the increasing waistlines of Americans. We are now recognizing that the types and amount of fats being consumed determine the impact on our bodies. Some dietary fats are essential, and others are not. Some actually confer additional health benefits, and a few, when eaten in large amounts, may increase the risk of certain diseases. This chapter explores these issues.

Fat is valuable and necessary to health. It is important to learn about fat in food, what the fat we eat does in our bodies, and how it can be both helpful and harmful to our health. Individual preference for fat is developed in either infancy or early childhood; innate preferences for sweet taste are observed at birth (Drewnowski, 2000). Thus, children learn to prefer tastes, flavors, and textures that are associated with foods that are rich in fat, sweet, or both. Aging may be associated with increasing acceptance of bitter tastes and consumption of more fruits, vegetables, and whole grains (Drewnowski, 2000). Nonetheless, reducing fat consumption takes time and effort, perhaps because of food selection habits, symbolic meaning associated with certain foods, and sensory values of fats in foods.

The six dimensions of health provide ways to think about the effects of changing dietary fat consumption. *Physical health* is maintained by consuming dietary fats that are necessary for essential fatty acids (EFAs), for energy, and for fat-soluble vitamins. Excessive intake of fats, though, may increase the risk of obesity and diet-related diseases. The *intellectual health* dimension encompasses the skills necessary to assess the type of dietary fat modification most appropriate for our patients' and our own health needs. How we emotionally approach nutritional lifestyle changes for our patients and ourselves affects success, which reflects the emotional health dimension. Can these emotions be expressed, or are changes simply disregarded because they make us feel uncomfortable? The social dimension is tested as change is initiated. Are relationships of family and friends based on sharing high-fat meals? Can you or your patients refuse to take part in social situations without jeopardizing relationships or making others feel defensive? Can you or your patients make food preparation suggestions to lower the fat content without seeming overly critical? Some religions maintain that taking care of one's body is necessary to achieve spiritual goals. Adopting a healthier fat intake supports these *spiritual health* dimension goals. The environmental health dimension may require seeking or making available foods that contain healthier fats. Some food stores and restaurants may better support one's dietary fat intake goals.

Fat actually refers to the chemical group called lipids. Lipids are divided into three classifications: fats (or triglycerides), and the fat-related substances phospholipids and sterols. Triglycerides, the largest class of lipids, may be in the form of fats (somewhat solid) or oils (liquids). Approximately 95% of the lipids in foods and in our bodies are in the triglyceride form of fat. Of the other two lipid classifications, lecithin is the best-known phospholipid, and cholesterol is the best-known sterol. All are organic—composed of carbon, hydrogen, and oxygen—and cannot dissolve in water.

FUNCTIONS

The functions of lipids may be divided into two categories: (1) specific characteristics of foods that arise from lipids and (2) maintenance of the physiologic health of our bodies.

Food Functions

Source of Energy

Fat is the densest form of stored energy in food and our bodies. This means that gram for gram, food fat—in the form of triglycerides—can produce more than twice the energy in kcal that carbohydrate or protein can. For example, a gram of nearly pure fat (9 kcal), such as butter, provides more than twice the kcal provided by a gram of nearly pure carbohydrate (4 kcal), such as sugar, or a gram of nearly pure protein (4 kcal), such as dried, lean fish.

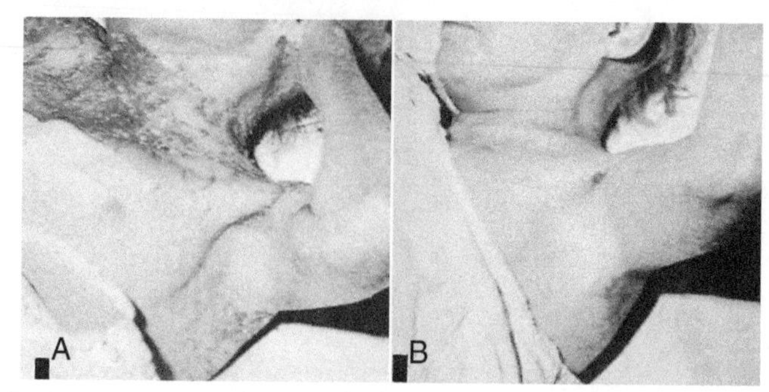

Fig. 5.1 Essential fatty acid deficiency. (A) Biochemical abnormalities and skin lesions have developed in a patient receiving fat-free parenteral nutrition. (B) Resolution in same patient after 2 weeks of treatment. (Courtesy Dr. M. C. Riella. From McLaren DS: *A colour atlas and text of diet-related disorders*, ed 2, London, 1992, Mosby.)

Palatability

Fat makes food smell and taste good. Deep-fat fried potatoes outrank all other vegetable choices among North Americans. Whether it's bread with butter (or margarine), salad with dressing, or desserts with cream, fat makes foods taste pleasant for many people. For patients who are anorexic because of illness, strategically adding small amounts of fats to meals may increase nutrient intake.

Satiety and Satiation

Fat helps prevent hunger between meals. Fat slows down digestion because of the hormones released in response to its presence in the gastrointestinal (GI) tract, causing us to feel full and satisfied; we call this feeling satiety. Satiation is another, different aspect of fat consumption that occurs during, not after, eating. In contrast to satiety, satiation tends to increase our desire to eat more fatty food, not less. The effect of fat on satiation is likely to be more important than its effect on satiety and may lead to overeating (Tso & Liu, 2004). A satiation that often occurs with the last slice of pizza provides a good example: You want it, you eat it, and half an hour later, you feel too full.

Food Processing

Certain qualities of lipids, besides their nutritional purposes, make them a valuable resource for the processing of foods. The use of processed hydrogenated fats helps keep the fat in food products from turning rancid. Lecithin, a phospholipid, has an extensive role as an emulsifier—a substance that works by being soluble in water and fat at the same time. These functions, which are described in more detail, also increase our overall intake of lipids by allowing their use in numerous processed foods.

Nutrient Source

Some fats contain or transport the fat-soluble nutrients of vitamins A, D, E, and K and the EFAs of linoleic and linolenic fatty acids.

These essential fatty acids (EFAs), components of fat triglycerides, are polyunsaturated fatty acids (PUFAs) that cannot be made in the body and must be consumed in the diet. EFAs are necessary materials for making compounds, such as prostaglandins, that regulate many body functions, including blood pressure, blood clotting through platelet aggregation, gastric acid secretions, and muscle secretions. The overall strength of cell membranes depends on EFAs.

Overt symptoms of EFA deficiency include skin lesions and scaliness (eczema) caused by increased permeability, which leads to membrane breakdown throughout the body (Fig. 5.1). Inflammation of epithelial tissue and increased susceptibility to infections throughout the body are also possible. Because the minimum amount of EFA required is contained in only about 2 teaspoons of polyunsaturated vegetable oil, deficiencies of EFAs were thought to be rare. However, deficiencies have been noted in (1) older patients with peripheral vascular disease (a potential complication of diabetes mellitus), (2) patients with fat malabsorption, such as cystic fibrosis, and (3) patients receiving treatment for protein malnutrition with low-fat, high-protein diets. Individuals recovering from serious accidents and burns are also at risk. It is possible that individuals who strive to achieve extremely low dietary fat intake for perceived health reasons or from disordered eating could experience EFA deficiencies.

Physiologic Functions

Stored Energy

Body fat cells contain nearly pure fat, also in the form of triglycerides. This means that a pound of FDA, the storage depot of body fat, could produce about 3500 kcal as energy. Because glucose stored in our bodies as glycogen is stored with water, carbohydrate is a bulkier form of stored energy than body fat. Adipose tissue provides important fuel during illness or times of food restriction and is a major energy source for muscle work.

Organ Protection

Stored fat safely cushions and protects body organs during bumpy activities, such as participating in impact aerobics and snowboarding.

Temperature Regulation

The fat layer just under our skin serves as insulation to regulate body temperature by minimizing the loss of heat.

Insulation

A substance composed largely of fatty tissue, called myelin, covers nerve cells. This covering provides electrical insulation that allows for transmission of nerve impulses.

Functions of Phospholipids and Sterols

So far, we have discussed the major roles of triglycerides. Phospholipids are also important because they form part of all cell membrane structure and serve as emulsifiers to keep fats dispersed in body fluids.

Lecithin is the main phospholipid. Lecithin is a constituent of lipoproteins—carriers or transporters of lipids—including fats and cholesterol in the body. This characteristic has earned lecithin a reputation for carrying fat and cholesterol away from plaque deposits in the arteries. Although lecithin does play a role in transporting fat and cholesterol, supplementary lecithin from sources outside the body does not help make the body's transportation system more efficient. Instead, dietary lecithin is simply digested and used by the body as any other lipid.

As a lipid group, sterols are critical components of complex regulatory compounds in our bodies and provide basic material to make bile, vitamin D, sex hormones, and cells in brain and nerve tissue. Cholesterol in particular is a vital part of all cell membranes and nerve tissues and serves as a building block for hormones. When exposed to ultraviolet light, a cholesterol substance in our skin can be converted to vitamin D by the kidneys and liver. The liver synthesizes cholesterol to make bile, the emulsifying substance necessary to absorb dietary lipids.

STRUCTURE AND SOURCES OF LIPIDS

Fats: Saturated and Unsaturated

Triglycerides are the largest class of lipids found in food and body fat. A **triglyceride** is a compound consisting of three fatty acids and one glycerol molecule (Fig. 5.2). The glycerol portion is derived from carbohydrate, but it is a small part compared with the fatty acids, which may be alike or different from each other. Fatty acids can be made of long or short chains of carbon atoms. Each carbon atom has four bonding sites or imaginary arms where it can attach to other atoms. To form a carbon chain, one site on each side of the carbon bonds to a neighboring carbon, as if one arm on each side were outstretched to form a chain. Because these atoms have four arms, the two extra arms each attach to a hydrogen atom, making the chain saturated with hydrogen.

If a hydrogen atom is removed from two neighboring carbons, freeing the extra arm on each, the carbons are bonded to each other at two sites. The two arms on the same side both clasp the two arms of the neighboring carbon, forming a double bond. We call this an unsaturated carbon chain because there is a possibility that hydrogen could come along and saturate the chain by breaking one set of clasped arms and attaching to them. In foods this is sometimes done artificially through the process of **hydrogenation**, which forces hydrogen atoms to break a double bond and attach to the carbons, creating a saturated fat (Fig. 5.3). Hydrogenation is discussed in the section on processed fats.

All natural fats are mixtures of different types of fatty acids. Plants contain mostly polyunsaturated fats, but most plant oils contain some saturated fatty acids (Fig. 5.4). Animal fats,

Three fatty acids join to glycerol in a condensation reaction to form a triglyceride.

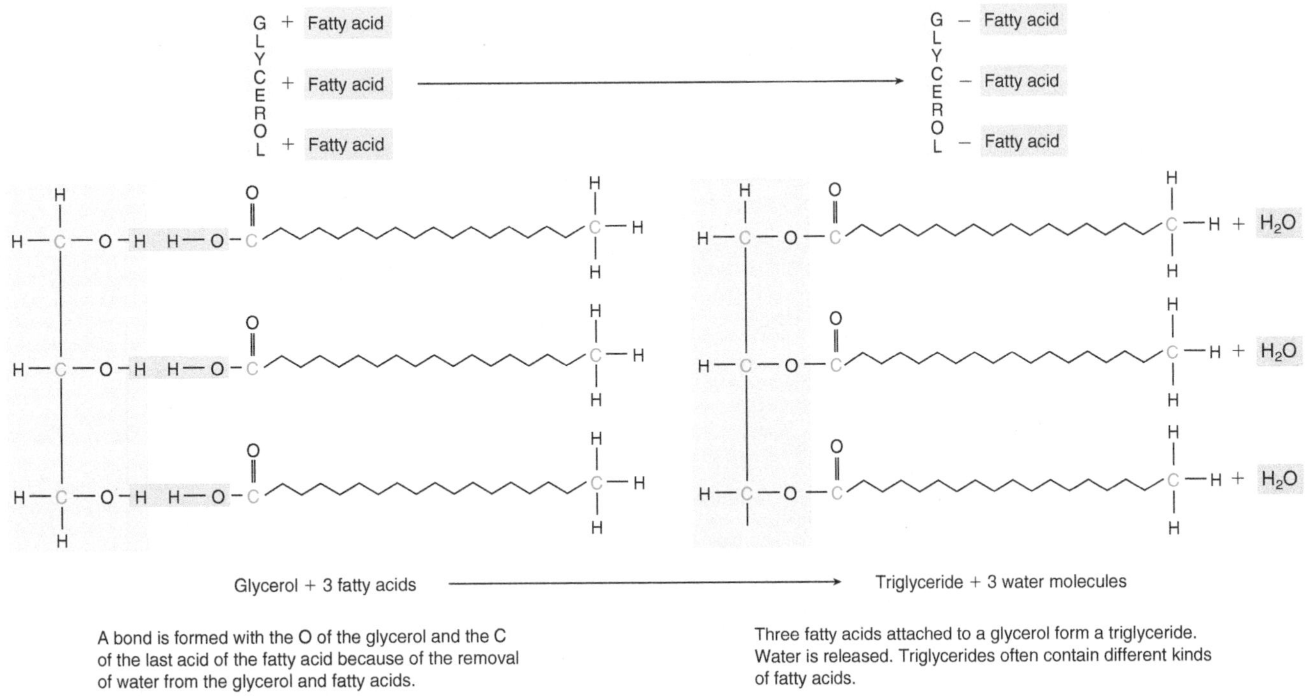

GLYCEROL + Fatty acid + Fatty acid + Fatty acid → GLYCEROL – Fatty acid – Fatty acid – Fatty acid

Glycerol + 3 fatty acids → Triglyceride + 3 water molecules

A bond is formed with the O of the glycerol and the C of the last acid of the fatty acid because of the removal of water from the glycerol and fatty acids.

Three fatty acids attached to a glycerol form a triglyceride. Water is released. Triglycerides often contain different kinds of fatty acids.

Fig. 5.2 Formation and structure of a triglyceride.

although high in saturated fats, contain amounts of polyunsaturated fats. The predominant type of fat in a food determines its category.

A saturated fatty acid has a single-bonded carbon chain that is fully saturated because hydrogen atoms are attached to all available bonding sites. Palmitic acid (16 carbon atoms) (Fig. 5.5A), a saturated fatty acid, is contained in meats, butterfat, shortening, and vegetable oils. Other saturated fatty acids are stearic acid (18 carbon atoms), myristic acid (14 carbon atoms), and lauric acid (12 carbon atoms). Additional food sources of saturated fatty acids are primarily animal, including beef, poultry, pork, lamb, luncheon meats, egg yolks, and dairy products (milk, butter, and cheeses); the only major plant sources are palm and coconut oils (often called tropical oils) and cocoa butter.

$$-\underset{\mathrm{H}}{\mathrm{C}}=\underset{\mathrm{H}}{\mathrm{C}}- + \mathrm{H_2} \rightarrow -\overset{\mathrm{H}}{\underset{\mathrm{H}}{\mathrm{C}}}-\overset{\mathrm{H}}{\underset{\mathrm{H}}{\mathrm{C}}}-$$

Fig. 5.3 Process of hydrogenation.

Each unsaturated fatty acid has one or more unsaturated double bond along the carbon chain. If a carbon chain has only one unsaturated double bond, it is a monounsaturated fatty acid (MUFA). Oleic acid (Fig. 5.5B) is the main MUFA in foods. Dietary sources include olive oil, peanuts (peanut butter and peanut oil), and canola oil.

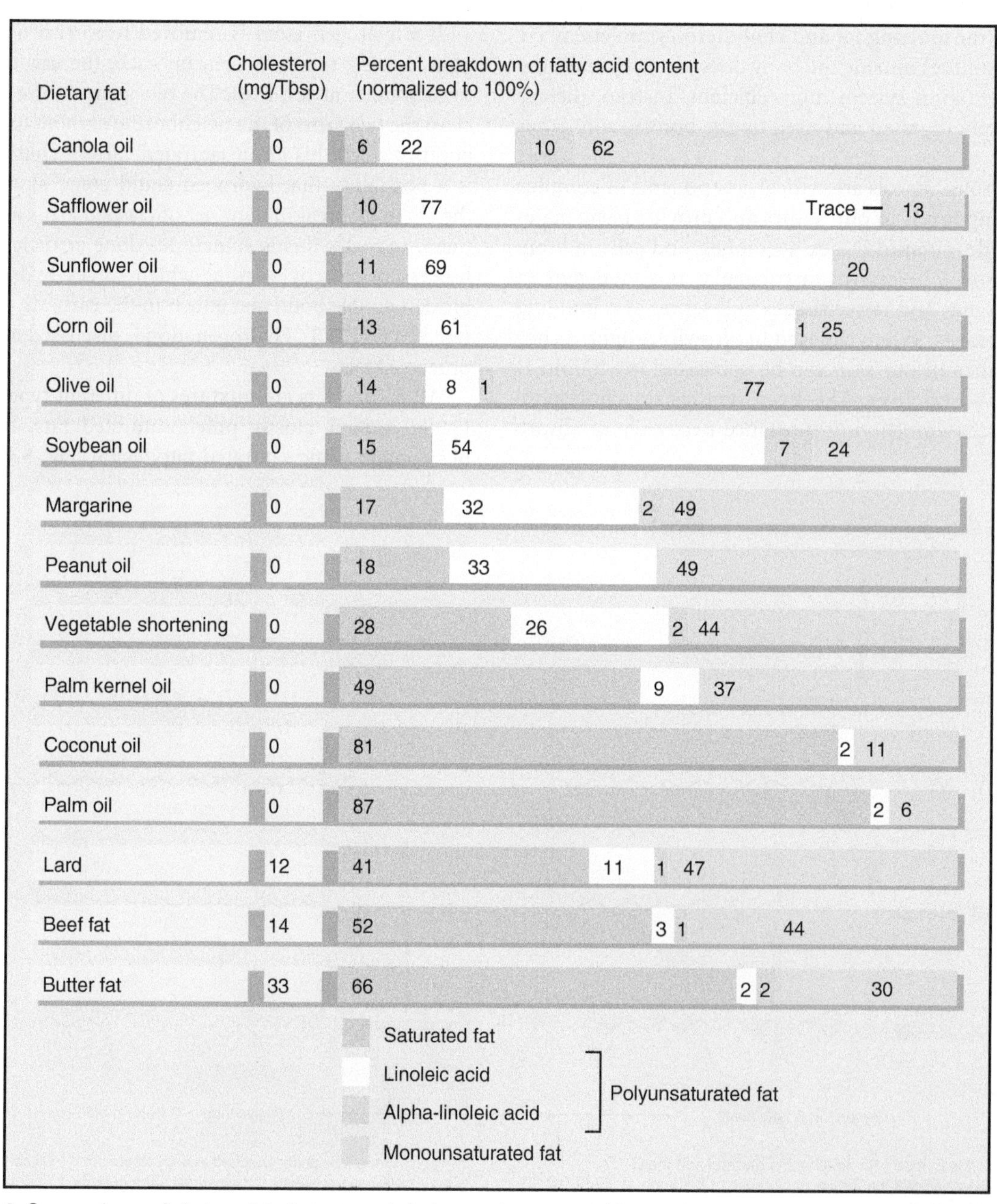

Fig. 5.4 Comparison of dietary fats in terms of cholesterol, saturated fat, and the most common unsaturated fats. *TBSP*, Tablespoon.

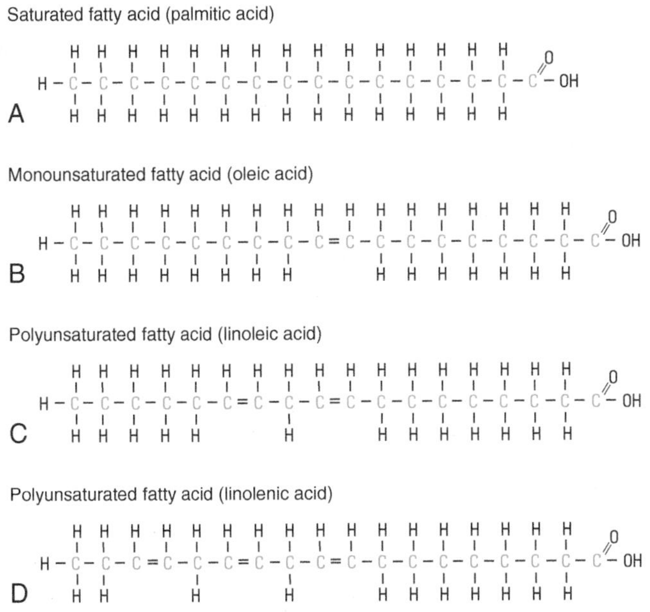

Saturated fatty acid (palmitic acid)

A

Monounsaturated fatty acid (oleic acid)

B

Polyunsaturated fatty acid (linoleic acid)

C

Polyunsaturated fatty acid (linolenic acid)

D

Fig. 5.5 Examples of fatty acids found in foods. Foods with these fatty acids include (A) animal-derived foods (beef, poultry, lamb, pork, eggs, dairy, tropical oils); (B) olive oil, peanuts (butter and oil), and canola oil; (C) vegetable oils (margarine and salad dressings), some animal fats, and prepared foods; and (D) fatter fish (bluefish, tuna, salmon, etc.), fish, and canola oil.

If a carbon chain has two or more unsaturated double bonds, it is a polyunsaturated fatty acid (PUFA). Food sources include vegetable oils (corn, safflower, wheat germ, canola, sesame, and sunflower), fish, and margarine.

PUFAs are categorized by the location of the unsaturation in the molecular structure of the fatty acid. Two categories of PUFAs, omega-6 and omega-3, contain two fatty acids (linoleic and linolenic) that our bodies cannot manufacture; these acids are EFAs and must be provided by dietary intake. The characteristic that distinguishes them from other PUFAs is the position of the final double bond in relation to the end of the carbon chain. The final double bond is at the sixth carbon from the omega end of the chain in linoleic acid (Fig. 5.5C), the main member of the omega-6 family. The first double bond is at the third carbon atom from the omega end in linolenic acid (Fig. 5.5D), the main member of the omega-3 family.

Americans consume an abundance of linoleic acid from consumption of large amounts of vegetable oils, such as margarine and salad dressing, and large amounts of prepared foods. Another source of linoleic acid may be animal foods; for example, although poultry fat is predominantly saturated, it also contains some PUFAs, including linoleic acid.

In contrast, American consumption of linolenic acid is not abundant at all. Linolenic acid is associated with fish consumption because that is how it was first recognized as important in health. A low incidence of heart disease among the native people of Greenland and Alaska, in spite of a very high-fat diet, was traced to the oils in deep-water fish, the staple in their diet (Harris, 1989). One of the main omega-3 fatty acids in fish is

TABLE 5.1 Food Sources of Omega-3 Fatty Acids

Fish sources	Salmon Mackerel Herring Tuna Rainbow trout Sardines
Plant sources	Canola oil Walnuts and walnut oil Soybean and soybean oil Flaxseed ground and oil Wheat germ and oat germ Green leafy vegetables

eicosapentaenoic acid (EPA), which is derived from linolenic acid. Fish are more efficient in this conversion of fatty acids than humans. Omega-3 fatty acids appear to lower the risk of heart disease by reducing the blood clotting process; clots can cause blockages in the arteries in the presence of plaques. Although consuming extra omega-3 fatty acids is likely to have little effect on blood cholesterol levels, it may reduce the risk of clots that may cause a myocardial infarction (heart attack) and appears to reduce risk of sudden death, such as from arrhythmias. According to prospective studies, reduced risk of cardiovascular disease (CVD) because of higher consumption of fish or omega-3 fatty acids appears applicable to men and women (Jones & Rideout, 2014). Chapter 17 further discusses the relationships between heart disease and fatty acids.

Certain fish provide more omega-3 fatty acids than others. Good sources are tuna, salmon, bluefish, halibut, sardines, and rainbow trout. Table 5.1 lists additional sources. Eating fish twice a week or using canola oil, another source of linolenic acid, should provide an adequate balance between sources of omega-6 and omega-3 fatty acids, although the best balance is still unknown.

Inuits consume 4 to 5 g of EPAs daily, about the amount in 1.5 to 3 pounds of certain deep-water fish (Harper & Jacobson, 2005). Because it is unlikely that most Americans will consume this quantity of fish, fish oil supplements of these fatty acids are manufactured. However, questions about proper dosages, safety, and side effects are still being researched. Large doses can decrease immunity. Therefore, supplements should be taken only when prescribed by a health care provider.

Phospholipids

Phospholipids are lipid compounds that form parts of cell walls and act as fat emulsifiers. Similar to triglycerides, phospholipids contain fatty acids, but they have only two fatty acids; the third spot contains a phosphate group. The body manufactures phospholipids, which are found in every cell; therefore, they are not essential nutrients. Lecithin, the main phospholipid, contains two fatty acids, with the third spot filled by a molecule of choline plus phosphorus (Fig. 5.6). In the body, lecithin's function as an emulsifier is to work by being soluble in water and fat at the same time.

Lecithin from soybeans is used in food processing to perform an emulsification role. Naturally found in egg yolks, lecithin is

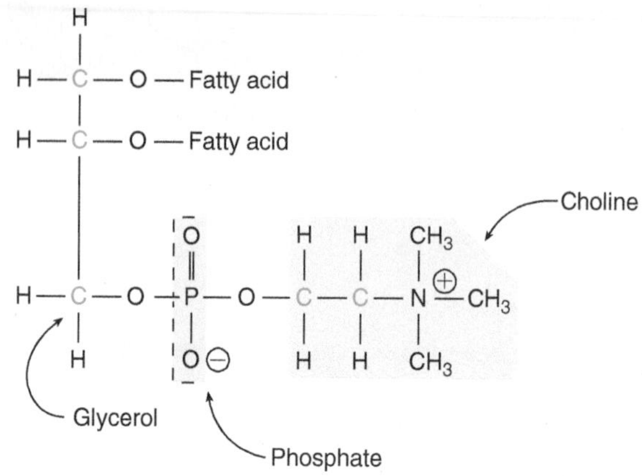

Fig. 5.6 A phospholipid: lecithin.

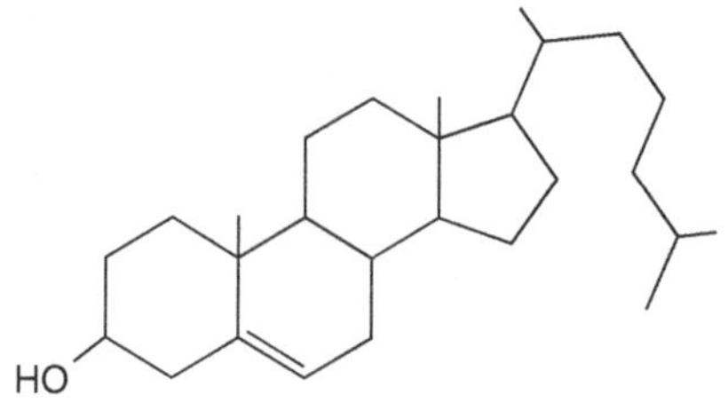

Fig. 5.7 A sterol: cholesterol. Foods containing cholesterol include animal-derived foods such as beef, pork, chicken, bacon, luncheon meats, eggs, fish, and dairy products.

the versatile ingredient in mayonnaise that prevents separation of vinegar and oil. Lecithin is also used in manufacturing chocolate to keep the cocoa butter and other ingredients combined and in cakes and other bakery products to maintain freshness.

Sterols

Sterols, a fatlike class of lipids, serve vital functions in the body. Sterol structures, including cholesterol, are carbon rings intermeshed with side chains of carbon, hydrogen, and oxygen, making them more complex than triglycerides (Fig. 5.7). Like phospholipids, sterols are synthesized by the body and are not essential nutrients. For example, if dietary cholesterol is not consumed, the liver will produce the amount required for body functions.

Generally, dietary cholesterol accounts for about 25% of the cholesterol in the body. The rest, which is made in the liver, seems to be produced in relation to how much is needed. The only food sources of cholesterol are animal and include beef, pork (bacon), chicken, luncheon meats, eggs, fish, and dairy products (milk, butter, and cheeses); plant foods do not contain cholesterol.

FATS AS A NUTRIENT IN THE BODY

Digestion

Mouth

The mouth's primary fat-digestive process is mechanical, as teeth masticate fatty foods. The glands of the tongue produce a fat-splitting enzyme (lingual lipase) released with saliva that begins digestion of long-chain fatty acids such as those found in milk.

Stomach

Mechanical digestion continues through the strong actions of peristalsis. Fat-splitting enzymes, such as gastric lipase, hydrolyze some fatty acids from triglycerides.

Small Intestine

Fats entering the duodenum initiate the release of cholecystokinin (CCK) hormone from the duodenum walls. CCK, as described in Chapter 3, then sparks the gallbladder to release bile into the small intestine. The bile emulsifies fats to facilitate digestion. Mechanical digestion through muscular action allows for increased exposure of the emulsified fat globules to pancreatic lipase. This enzyme is the primary digestive enzyme that breaks triglycerides into fatty acids, monoglycerides, and glycerol molecules. Note that fats may not be completely broken down. Some may also pass through without being digested or absorbed. Fig. 5.8 summarizes digestion of triglycerides.

Use of Medium-Chain Triglycerides

Triglycerides are composed of long chains of fatty acids. To aid fat digestion in those patients with malabsorption, synthetically manufactured medium-chain triglycerides (MCTs) may be incorporated into a patient's dietary intake. MCTs should not be used to completely replace dietary fats because they do not contain EFAs.

Absorption

Bile salts help fatty acids, monoglycerides, and cholesterol move from the lumen to the villi for absorption. Micelles, created by bile salts encircling lipids, aid diffusion through the membrane wall. Once through the membrane wall, fatty acids and glycerol combine back into triglycerides. These triglycerides are incorporated into chylomicrons, which are the first lipoproteins formed after absorption of lipids from food. They contain fats and cholesterol and are coated with protein. The protein coating allows them to travel through the lymph system to the blood circulatory system and then toward the hepatic portal system and the liver. Some glycerol and any short- and medium-chain fatty acids are absorbed directly into the blood capillaries leading to the portal vein and liver.

At the cell membranes, the triglycerides in the chylomicrons are broken down into fatty acids and glycerol, with assistance from an enzyme called lipoprotein lipase. Muscle cells, adipose cells, and other cells in the vicinity take up most of the fatty acids released by the breakdown of chylomicrons. Cells can either use the absorbed fatty acids immediately as fuel or reform them into triglycerides to be stored as reserve energy supplies.

Metabolism

Lipid metabolism consists of several processes. Catabolism (breakdown) of lipids for energy involves the hydrolysis of triglycerides into two-carbon units that become part of acetyl coenzyme A (acetyl CoA). Acetyl CoA is an important

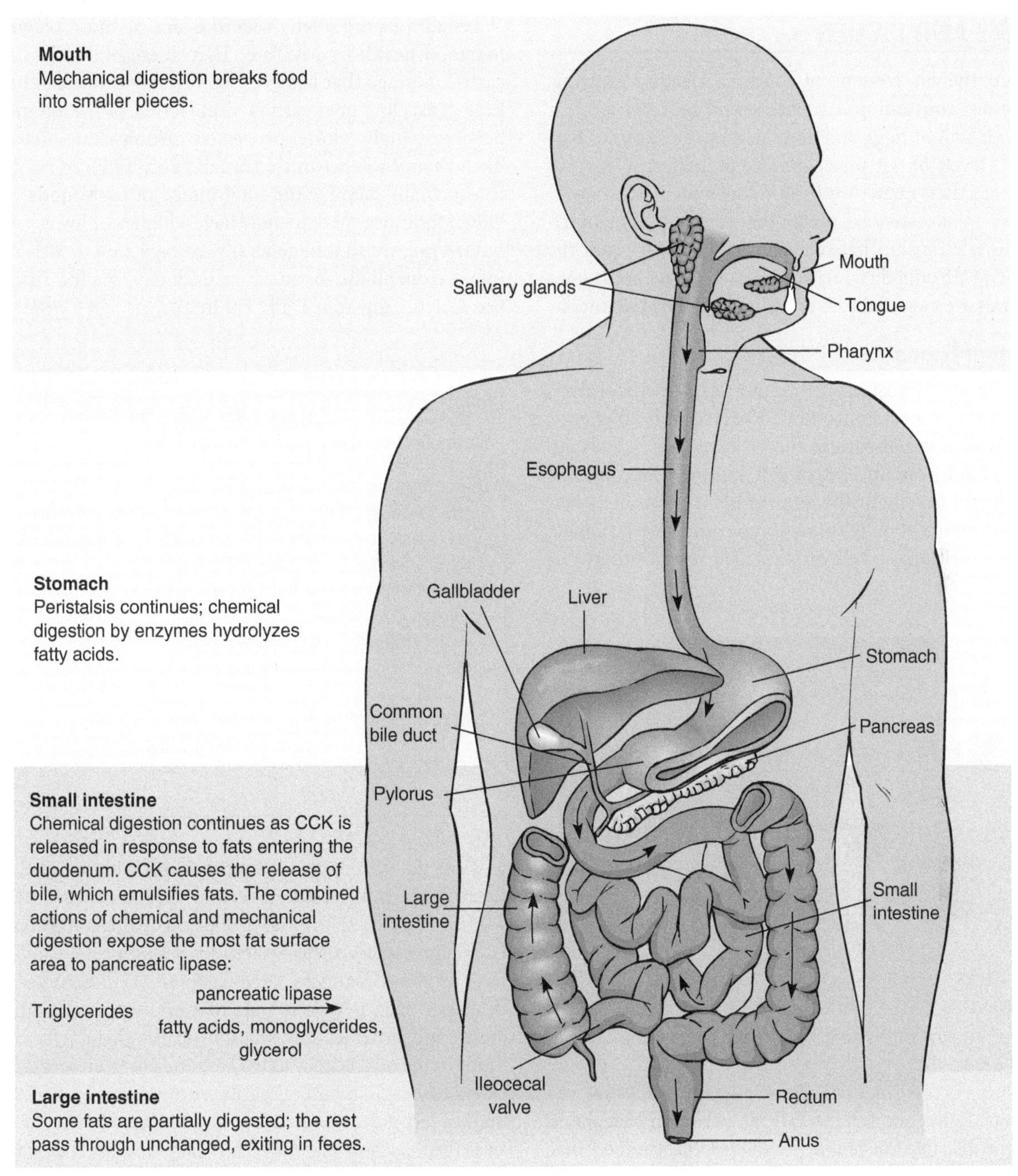

Mouth
Mechanical digestion breaks food into smaller pieces.
Stomach
Peristalsis continues; chemical digestion by enzymes hydrolyzes fatty acids.
Small intestine
Chemical digestion continues as CCK is released in response to fats entering the duodenum. CCK causes the release of bile, which emulsifies fats. The combined actions of chemical and mechanical digestion expose the most fat surface area to pancreatic lipase:
Triglycerides
pancreatic lipase
fatty acids, monoglycerides, glycerol
Large intestine
Some fats are partially digested; the rest pass through unchanged, exiting in feces.
Salivary glands
Mouth
Tongue
Pharynx
Esophagus
Gallbladder
Liver
Stomach
Common bile duct
Pancreas
Pylorus
Large intestine
Small intestine
Ileocecal valve
Rectum
Anus

Fig. 5.8 Summary of fat digestion and absorption. *CCK*, Cholecystokinin. (From Rolin Graphics.)

intermediate byproduct in metabolism formed from the breakdown of glucose, fatty acids, and certain amino acids. The acetyl CoA then enters the series of reactions called the TCA (tricarboxylic acid) cycle, eventually leading to the oxidation of the carbon and hydrogen atoms derived from fatty acids (or carbohydrates or amino acids) to carbon dioxide and water with the release of energy as adenosine triphosphate (ATP) (see Fig. 9.2). If fat catabolizes quickly because of a lack of carbohydrate (glucose) for energy, the liver cells form intermediate products from the partial oxidation of fatty acids called ketone bodies. These ketone bodies may excessively accumulate in the blood, causing a condition called **ketosis**.

Anabolism (synthesis) of lipids, or lipogenesis, results in the formation of triglycerides, phospholipids, cholesterol, and prostaglandins for use throughout the body. Triglycerides and phosphates form from fatty acids and glycerol or from excess glucose or amino acids. Extra carbon, hydrogen, and oxygen from any source can be converted to and stored as triglycerides in adipose tissues, so we can gain fat from foods other than fat.

Lipid metabolism is regulated mainly by insulin, growth hormone, and the adrenal cortex hormones; adrenocorticotropic hormone (ACTH), which stimulates secretion of more hormones; and glucocorticoids, which affect food metabolism.

FAT INTAKE AND ISSUES

Awareness of the fat content of foods is steadily growing. Whether we are consuming a sophisticated gourmet feast or chowing down on hot dogs and hamburgers at a summer barbecue, the fat levels of our meals may be of interest. Concerns about fat in our diets center on health issues such as excessive intake of energy, excessive fat intake that replaces other nutrients, and the relationship between dietary fat intake and the development of chronic diet-related diseases. Some lipids consumed in foods are essential to our bodies to achieve wellness.

Fat Content of Foods

High-fat foods are almost always high-calorie foods. This is because fats are the most concentrated source of food energy, supplying 9 kcal/g; carbohydrates and proteins supply 4 kcal/g. Because most foods contain a mixture of nutrients, we can identify the fat content of food by the number of fat grams in a serving or the percentage of daily value of recommended fat intake in a serving. Nutritional labels on packaged food contain this information.

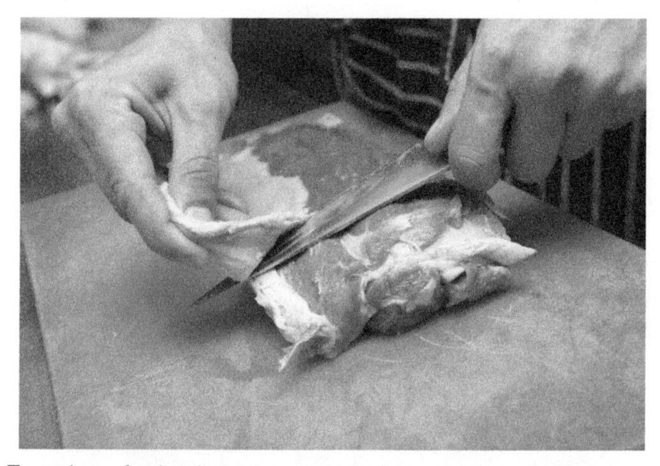

To reduce fat intake, trim meat before cooking. (From www.thinkstockphotos.com)

The Dietary Reference Intakes (DRIs), based on acceptable macronutrient distribution ranges (AMDRs), recommend that we eat 20% to 35% of our kcal intake from fats, with an increased consumption of n-3 PUFAs and a limit of 10% or less of kcal from saturated fats (Vannice & Rasmussen, 2014). According to the daily values, total fat intake for an average daily kcal intake of 2000 to 2500 kcal should range from about 40 to 97 g or less (≤400–875 kcal). Saturated fat should be 20 to 25 g or less (≤180–225 kcal).

Most Americans consume 35% to 40% of total energy intake as fat (Jones & Rideout, 2014), even though many believe they are avoiding or limiting high-fat foods. One reason may be that high-fat foods have both potent sensory qualities and high-energy density; overeating is then often more passive than active. Another reason is that people who eat a lot of high-fat foods are unsure whether their diets are high in fat because the rate of home cooking has fallen sharply; the cook no longer knows exactly what goes into each dish. Also, portion sizes at restaurants are often twice the size of those recommended for good health by MyPlate. Then there is the "less fat, more carbs" message that has been incorrectly translated into sweet, kcal-dense, low-fiber carbohydrate foods, so the low-fat diet has become a high-calorie, processed-carbohydrate diet. It is also likely that people are misled by labels on "reduced fat" foods and thus actually *increase* the total intake of such foods. The individual foods we eat daily may have a higher or lower fat content, but overall, we should generally average 25% to 30% of kcal fat intake from all the foods we eat each day (see the *Teaching Tool* box Calculating Your Daily Fat Intake).

TEACHING TOOL

Calculating Your Daily Fat Intake

Use the following steps to calculate your daily grams of fat:

1. Use the Recommended Energy Intake chart in Chapter 9 to determine your appropriate energy needs for the day. Multiply that number of kcal by 0.25 for 25% fat intake or by 0.30 for 30% fat intake.
2. Divide that number by 9, because each gram of fat has 9 kcal. For example, if you consume 1800 kcal a day and want to get 25% of those kcal from fat: $0.25 \times 1800 = 450$. Then divide 450 by 9 to get 50 g of fat. Energy needs for the day kcal × 0.30 = kcal fat intake/day. Kcal fat intake/day ÷ 9 kcal = g of fat/day.
3. Next, check food labels or use food composition tables (available at the Evolve website) for the grams of fat per food serving. Then compare the sum of the fat grams consumed with the recommended levels for your particular energy needs.

How do we measure the fat in foods without labels, such as fresh foods, home-cooked recipes, and restaurant items? One way is to classify foods into groups according to fat content. The Exchange List uses this system by listing protein foods on the basis of their "leanness" (see Chapter 2). In contrast, MyPlate devotes a section to oils (fats that are liquid at room temperature) and provides information on the dietary fat content of foods in the oil category as well as foods in fruit, meats, and bean categories that contain oils. Oils are not considered a food group but are recognized as needed for good health. MyPlate emphasizes the health-promoting oils from plants and fish, rather than the solid, more saturated fats from palm kernel oil and coconut oil and many animal foods and from hydrogenation of vegetable oils. As shown in Box 5.1, commonly consumed oils are canola, corn, olive, cottonseed, safflower, and soybean. Foods listed as good sources of oils are nuts, certain fish, avocado, and olives. Table 5.2 provides examples of fat in servings from different foods. Common solid fats include butter, lard (pork fat), shortening, beef fat (suet, tallow), stick margarine, and chicken fat.

Detecting Dietary Fat

Some fats are visible; others are invisible. Visible fat is fairly easy to find and control; just cut off the white fat on the outside of a steak and measure the butter or sour cream on the baked potato. Invisible fat is harder to measure. Fat in milk, cheese, and yogurt is nearly impossible to see, but many people learn to taste the difference between whole- and low-fat dairy products.

BOX 5.1 MyPlate: Oils

What Are "Oils"?

Oils are fats that are liquid at room temperature, like the vegetable oils used in cooking. Oils come from many different plants and from fish. Oils are not a food group, but they provide essential nutrients. Therefore, oils are included in the U.S. Department of Agriculture food patterns.

Some **commonly eaten oils** include canola, corn, cottonseed, olive, safflower, soybean, and sunflower oils. Some oils are used mainly as **flavorings**, such as walnut oil and sesame oil. A number of foods are naturally high in oils, like nuts, olives, some fish, and avocados.

Foods that are mainly oil include mayonnaise, certain salad dressings, and soft (tub or squeeze) margarine with no *trans* fats. Check the Nutrition Facts label to find margarines with 0 grams of *trans* fat. Amounts of *trans* fat are required to be listed on labels.

Most oils are high in monounsaturated or polyunsaturated fats, and low in saturated fats. Oils from plant sources (vegetable and nut oils) do not contain any cholesterol. In fact, no plant foods contain cholesterol. A few plant oils, however, including coconut oil, palm oil, and palm kernel oil, are high in saturated fats and for nutritional purposes should be considered to be solid fats.

Solid fats are fats that are solid at room temperature, like butter and shortening. Solid fats come from many animal foods and can be made from vegetable oils through a process called hydrogenation. Some common fats are butter, milk fat, beef fat (tallow, suet), chicken fat, pork fat (lard), stick margarine, shortening, and partially hydrogenated oil.

How Much Is My Allowance for Oils?

Some Americans consume enough oil in the foods they eat, such as the following:

- Nuts
- Fish
- Cooking oil
- Salad dressings

How Do I Count the Oils I Eat?

The following table gives a quick guide to the amount of oils in some common foods.

	Amount of Food	Amount of Oil Teaspoons/Gram	Calories from Oil Approximate Calories	Total Calories Approximate Calories
Oils				
Vegetable oils (such as canola, corn, cottonseed, olive, peanut, safflower, soybean, and sunflower)	1 tbsp	3 tsp/14 g	120	120
Foods Rich in Oils				
Margarine, soft (*trans* fat free)	1 tbsp	2½ tsp/11 g	100	100
Mayonnaise	1 tbsp	2½ tsp/11 g	100	100
Mayonnaise-type salad dressing	1 tbsp	1 tsp/5 g	45	55
Italian dressing	2 tbsp	2 tsp/8 g	75	85
Thousand Island dressing	2 tbsp	2½ tsp/11 g	100	120
Olives,[a] ripe, canned	4 large	½ tsp/2 g	15	20
Avocado[a]	½ med	3 tsp/15 g	130	160
Peanut butter[a]	2 tbsp	4 tsp/16 g	140	190
Peanuts, dry roasted[a]	1 oz	3 tsp/14 g	120	165
Mixed nuts, dry roasted[a]	1 oz	3 tsp/15 g	130	170
Cashews, dry roasted[a]	1 oz	3 tsp/13 g	115	165
Almonds, dry roasted[a]	1 oz	3 tsp/15 g	130	170
Hazelnuts[a]	1 oz	4 tsp/18 g	160	185
Sunflower seeds[a]	1 oz	3 tsp/14 g	120	165

[a]Avocados and olives are part of the Vegetable Group; nuts and seeds are part of the Protein Foods Group. These foods are also high in oils. Soft margarine, mayonnaise, and salad dressings are mainly oil and are not considered to be part of any food group.

(Modified from U.S. Department of Agriculture, Center for Nutrition Policy and Promotion: *Oils: What are "oils"?* Accessed 9 December, 2020, from www.choosemyplate.gov/eathealthy/oils.)

In addition, dairy foods are all labeled so fat content is known. Some foods give other clues that they contain fat. Press a napkin on a slice of pizza, a Danish pastry, or an egg roll. Look for oil around the edge of stir-fried Chinese food.

Be aware of general characteristics that signal the level of fat in foods. Some cooking methods, such as deep-frying, add fat. The way a prepared food is usually eaten may also increase fat intake, such as spreading butter or oil on bread rather than just dipping it in soup. Whether you are eating in or dining out, the amount of food regularly selected from high-fat animal sources such as meat and cheese compared with the amount of food consumed from low-fat grains, vegetables, and fruit affects total dietary fat consumption levels.

Government and consumer groups have encouraged restaurants and institutional food service operations to offer identifiable low-fat, low-calorie food choices. These choices allow patients to meet health promotion goals while maintaining social interactions. Encourage patients to identify healthy menu choices when eating away from home.

The cuisines of China and Italy are based on rice, pasta, and bread. When prepared with small amounts of fat and eaten with little fatty meat and plenty of vegetables, these cultural food

TABLE 5.2 Fat in Food Servings

Food	Serving Size	Fat Content
Butter/margarine	1 tbsp	11 g
Salad dressing	1 tbsp	7 g
Mayonnaise	1 tbsp	11 g
Cream cheese	1 tbsp	10 g
Carrots	½ cup	Trace
Broccoli	½ cup	Trace
Potato, baked	1	Trace
French fries	1 cup	8 g
Apple	1	Trace
Orange	1	Trace
Banana	1	Trace
Fruit juice	1 cup	Trace
Rice or pasta	½ cup	Trace
Bagel	1	Trace
Muffin	1 medium	6 g
Danish pastry	1 medium	13 g
Skim milk	1 cup	Trace
Low-fat milk	1 cup	5 g
Whole milk	1 cup	8 g
American cheese	2 oz	18 g
Cheddar cheese	1½ oz	14 g
Frozen yogurt	½ cup	2 g
Ice milk	⅓ cup	3 g
Ice cream	⅓ cup	7 g
Lean beef	3 oz	6 g
Poultry	3 oz	6 g
Fish	3 oz	6 g
Ground beef	3 oz	16 g
Bologna (2 slices)	1 oz	16 g
Egg	1	5 g
Nuts (⅓ cup)	1 oz	22 g

CULTURAL DIVERSITY AND NUTRITION

Choosing Lower Fat Ethnic Dishes

Perhaps you've grown up eating rice and beans, homemade gravy on lasagna, or Chinese takeout. Regardless of who prepares the food, Americans are consuming more international foods than ever before. We have a smorgasbord of ethnic food from which to choose. Chinese, Indian, Mexican, and Greek dishes have become commonplace.

We may assume, however, that because these foods are different and exotic, they are healthier for us. After all, aren't hamburgers and hot dogs—all-American favorites—the worst offenders for our health? However, although some ethnic dishes are lower in fat and higher in dietary fibers, others aren't much better than traditional American favorites.

The Chinese foods eaten in America would be considered far too rich (and high in fat) by the Chinese; they are reserved for banquets and even then, are eaten in moderation. To enhance the healthfulness of prepared Chinese foods, avoid fried dishes, especially egg rolls and deep-fried breaded meats or poultry. Top the rice with moderate portions of entrees of chicken or seafood mixed with vegetables.

Italian dishes of pasta and "gravy" (i.e., tomato sauce) are healthful but become problematic when teamed with sausage, meatballs, fried breaded meats, and layers of cheeses or when tomato sauce is replaced by a cream Alfredo sauce. Each adds substantial amounts of saturated fats. Be aware of portion sizes, and focus on large portions of pasta served with smaller servings of the high-fat foods.

Mexican and Latino foods are sometimes made with lard, a heavily saturated animal fat, and with fatty portions of pork. These negatives, however, are somewhat offset by the generous (and delicious) use of beans, rice, and soft tortillas made from corn or wheat. When possible, avoid or reduce the use of lard; vegetable oils are a good substitute. Generally, the less fat used, the healthier the entrée. For example, a taco made with a soft tortilla contains less fat than one made with a hard-fried tortilla. And be sure to pile on lots of lettuce, tomatoes, and salsa!

Application to nursing: Become familiar with the exotic tastes of international cuisines. By doing so, you'll be able to help patients understand the fat content of their ethnic favorites. Guide them to resources such as a dietitian to suggest strategies to prepare their meals with less dietary fat. Just remember that the palatability of fat is a worldwide phenomenon, so choose wisely.

patterns are excellent examples of healthful diets. Yet when Chinese and Italian foods are prepared to please the American palate, large amounts of fat are used in cooking the food, and portion sizes are larger than usual for specific ethnic tradition (see the *Cultural Diversity and Nutrition* box Choosing Lower Fat Ethnic Dishes).

Fast but High-Fat Foods

Contemporary lifestyles sometimes leave little room for meal planning and preparation. Often, we may find ourselves heading for the nearest fast-food restaurant or snack bar as we dash off to school or work. What impact do these meals have on our nutritional status? A positive trend among fast-food chains is the use of less saturated fat in fried potatoes and the addition of items such as salads and skim milk to the menu. On the negative side, between 40% and 50% of fast-food kcal comes from fat—far higher than the recommended 30%.

One may wonder why some foods that are fast to fix, such as apples, oranges, and bananas, are not considered fast foods, nor are they sold in fast-food restaurants. The answer probably has to do with the fact that fat lends a seductive flavor to fast-food favorites (see the *Teaching Tool* box But Fast Foods Are So Convenient!).

How can fat intake be lowered? First, start early to include children and the whole family in buying food, preparing it, and having low-fat foods on hand. Many people prefer fast food because they don't have fresh or partly prepared foods ready to cook. Teaching children cooking skills from simple recipes, from videos, and through friends establishes low-fat food preferences early. Individuals are more likely to adopt low-fat diets if eating partners or families do the same by modeling healthy eating patterns.

Second, most major secondary and tertiary health care settings have an active dietetic department, often geared to pediatrics and family practice. Programs offered may include healthy cooking classes for children and their parents or nutrition and wellness classes. Providing lists of such programs is a valuable resource for patients.

Third, never say never. It is okay to include some high-fat foods in food plans because they taste good. If a mixture of

> **TEACHING TOOL**
>
> ***But Fast Foods Are So Convenient!***
>
> Our advice to patients needs to be realistic, which means accepting the fact that most people occasionally eat at fast-food restaurants. Rather than attempting to dissuade them from going at all, we should give patients the following tools for helping to make lower-fat selections.
>
> Most menus now include healthier options. For restaurant chains, visit Internet sites to determine nutrition information and newer specialty items that are more nutrient dense and lower in overall calories and fat content.
>
> - Avoid breaded fried chicken and fish sandwiches. Chicken and fish, if grilled, can be lower in fat and cholesterol than beef, but a breaded and fried chicken or fish sandwich may provide more fat (and calories) than a hamburger.
> - Choose grilled chicken sandwiches and leave off the high-fat sauces.
> - Order a hamburger, plain, and add your own serving of ketchup or mustard.
> - If French fries are a necessity, order a small size. Today's small sizes were considered the large size in the past!
> - Realize that soda and sweetened iced tea contain empty calories. Therefore, the larger the container size, the more calories consumed. Better to enjoy the calories as filling food items than to guzzle sugary beverages.
> - Always order a side salad or add lettuce and tomatoes to sandwiches, when possible.
> - Salad bars can be deceiving. Salad greens are fine, but mayonnaise-based coleslaw and potato salad can pile on calories, especially when topped with creamy salad dressings. Selecting carrots, greens, other sliced vegetables, beans, and unprocessed fruits and consuming them with a small amount of dressing provide a filling side or main dish. Keep dressing use to a minimum by dipping a fork into dressing and then into the salad—same taste with less fat.

low-fat and high-fat foods is eaten, preferences for both are developed; this practice automatically controls overdoing the fatty foods. The *Teaching Tool* that discusses fast foods is packed with other strategies for fast-food, low-fat eating patterns.

Preserving Fats in Food

Processed Fats and Oils: Hydrogenated and Emulsified

A problem with unsaturated fats in foods is that oxygen attacks the unsaturated double bonds (oxidation), causing damage that makes them rancid; rancid fats have an odor and bad flavor and may cause illness. One way to reduce vulnerability to oxidation is to artificially saturate the fatty acids by adding hydrogen at the double bonds. This process of hydrogenation makes the fat solid and more stable, which provides cooking benefits. When vegetable oil, which is polyunsaturated, is completely hydrogenated, it becomes a white, waxy, or plastic-like substance called vegetable shortening. Because it is saturated with hydrogens, the body processes it as if it were a saturated fat.

The ingredient list on a product label can truthfully state that the product contains more unsaturated liquid oil, although it is mixed with the partially hydrogenated fat. Partially hydrogenated fats are used in a variety of food products.

Sometimes the solution to one problem causes another problem. Although it stabilizes fat, hydrogenation changes the structure of some of the fatty acids from cis fatty acids to *trans* fatty acids (Fig. 5.9). Most fatty acid double bonds in natural foods are in the *cis* form, but margarine and vegetable shortening may contain high concentrations of *trans* fatty acids (*trans* fats). *Trans* fatty acids have unusual double-bond structures caused by hydrogenated unsaturated oils. Most margarines are now processed to contain no *trans* fatty acids. Often manufacturers will note whether their margarine products are free of *trans* fatty acids. Controversy over the effect of *trans* fats in relation to cancer vulnerability and elevated blood cholesterol values has confused the public.

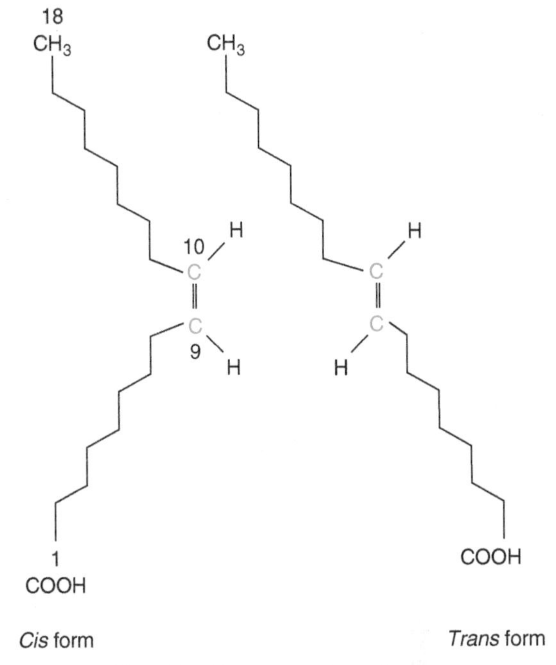

Fig. 5.9 *Cis* bond to *trans* bonds.

Many commercially produced foods, such as French fries, potato chips, and bakery products, are made from partially hydrogenated vegetable oils. Many margarines and other products are now offered as "*trans* free." On the other hand, of the average 35% of kcal consumed as fat by Americans, only about 2% to 7% of total kcal comes from *trans* fats (Jones & Rideout, 2014).

Nonetheless, *trans* fat consumption appears to increase risk for CVD. Risk is increased because the *trans* fat raises the blood cholesterol component (low-density lipoproteins [LDLs]) that delivers cholesterol throughout the body and, while doing so, may contribute to plaque formation in arteries. *Trans* fat also decreases the blood cholesterol component (high-density lipoproteins [HDLs]) that removes excess and used cholesterol from the body. Maintaining higher levels of this component decreases the risk of CVD. Considering these effects on blood cholesterol, total consumption of *trans* fatty acids formed from partially hydrogenated oils or naturally occurring in ruminant animal foods should be limited (Evidence Analysis Library, 2013).

Since January 2006, listing *trans* fatty acid content on nutrition labels has been mandatory. This requirement led manufacturers to reformulate products without *trans* fats. "Partially hydrogenated fat or oil" as an ingredient is another clue that *trans* fat is present in a product. When possible, *trans* fat should be replaced by a monounsaturated fat such as canola oil. Guidelines currently suggest as a priority to reduce overall food fat to 30% of total kcal; less fat means less *trans* fat as well. Depending on product formulation, this may mean eating less margarine, French fries, potato chips, cakes, and cookies, as well as less fried chicken, fried fish, fatty meat, and ice cream.

Ordinances banning the use of artificial *trans* fats in the preparation of foods for direct consumption by consumers in restaurants and other food outlets have been implemented in several cities in the United States. The U.S. Food and Drug Administration (FDA) has removed artificial *trans* fat from the generally recognized as safe (GRAS) list of ingredients because of its effect on blood cholesterol levels. The use of *trans* fat would be as a food additive requiring specific regulations to allow for its use. It is expected that artificial *trans* fat will be banned from use as an ingredient.

Antioxidants

Another way to preserve polyunsaturated fats without hydrogenation is through the use of antioxidant additives. These substances block oxidation, or the breakdown of double bonds by oxygen. Food manufacturers can use either natural or synthetic forms of antioxidants. Natural sources include vitamin E (tocopherol) and vitamin C (ascorbic acid). Their use not only helps preserve foods but also adds essential vitamins. Synthetic forms consist of the food additives butylated hydroxyanisole (BHA) and butylated hydroxytoluene (BHT). These forms are used in packaging as well to help prevent oxidation of the foods.

Food Cholesterol Versus Blood Cholesterol

Cholesterol is a waxy substance found in all tissues in humans and other animals; thus all foods from animal sources, such as meat, eggs, fish, poultry, and dairy products, contain cholesterol. The highest sources of cholesterol are egg yolks and organ meats (liver and kidney). No plant-derived food contains cholesterol, not even avocado or peanut butter, both of which are very high in fat. People often misunderstand this issue because they confuse food (dietary) cholesterol with blood cholesterol.

A high level of cholesterol in the blood is a risk factor for CVD. For an understanding of blood cholesterol levels, the role of lipoproteins—specialized transporting compounds—needs clarification. Lipoproteins are compounds that contain a mix of lipids—including triglycerides, fatty acids, phospholipids, cholesterol, and small amounts of other steroids and fat-soluble vitamins—that are covered with a protein outer layer (Fig. 5.10). The outer layer of protein allows the compound to move through a watery substance, such as blood. Lipoproteins transport fats in the circulatory system.

The amounts of fat and protein determine the density or weight of the lipoprotein. The more fat and lipid substances present, the lower the density of (or the lighter) the compound. Four forms of these compounds are most important for understanding the route of cholesterol in the body; they are chylomicrons, very low-density lipoproteins, LDLs, and HDLs.

Chylomicrons transport absorbed fats from the intestinal wall to the liver cells. Fats are then used for synthesis of lipoproteins.

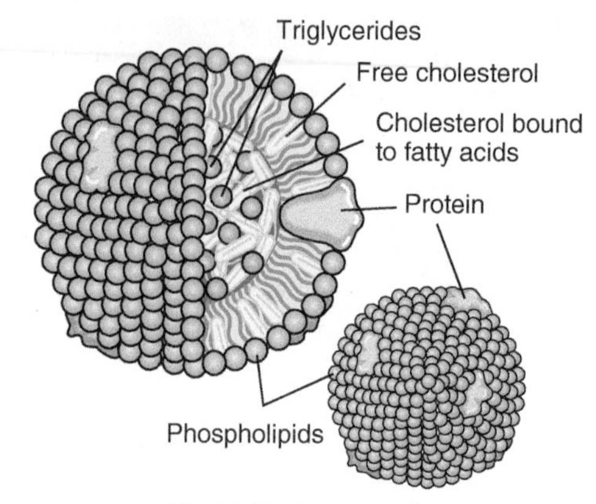

Fig. 5.10 Lipoprotein.

Very low-density lipoprotein (VLDL) leaves the liver cells full of fats and lipid components to transfer newly made (endogenous) triglycerides to the cells. LDL forms from VLDL because density is reduced as fats and lipids are released on their journey through the body. LDL carries cholesterol throughout the body to tissue cells for various functions.

In contrast to the delivery functions of the first three lipoproteins, HDL is formed within cells to remove cholesterol from the cell, bringing it to the liver for disposal.

A total blood cholesterol reading reflects the level of cholesterol contained in LDL and HDL. To get a clearer assessment of cholesterol activity in the body, the individual levels of LDL and HDL are valuable. The risk of CVD associated with blood cholesterol levels is presented in Table 17.1. LDL levels reflect the amount of cholesterol brought to cells that has the potential to be dropped off along the way to clog vessels and arteries, contributing to plaque formation. **Plaques** are deposits of fatty substances, including cholesterol, that attach to arterial walls. As this happens, HDLs remove cholesterol from the circulatory system. Removal of cholesterol is a positive action that reduces CVD risk.

Although past health guidelines generally recommended a dietary cholesterol intake of 300 mg or less per day, the *Dietary Guidelines, 2020–2025*, does not include a specific daily recommendation for dietary cholesterol. Dietary cholesterol does not significantly cause a rise of blood cholesterol levels. Table 5.3 lists the cholesterol content of selected foods. However, the major culprit that raises blood cholesterol is not dietary food cholesterol but too much food fat (dietary triglycerides), particularly saturated fats; food cholesterol alone makes a minor difference for most people. Too much food cholesterol becomes a problem when it is eaten in conjunction with very high-fat diets. Sometimes, this extra cholesterol in the blood may be dropped off, staying in the vessels and arteries. It may be a factor involved in the development of lesions that may block arteries, leading to CVD. This topic is discussed in detail in Chapter 17.

One reason for the confusion is the way food is cooked and eaten. Eggs, for example, are high in cholesterol and are often cooked and served with high-fat bacon or sausage. The combined meal of eggs and bacon then gets a bad reputation for raising blood cholesterol. The fact is that the large amount of fat

TABLE 5.3 Cholesterol Content of Selected Foods[a]

Food	Amount	Cholesterol (mg)
Milk, nonfat/skim	1 cup	4
Mayonnaise	1 tbsp	8
Cottage cheese, low-fat/2%	½ cup	10
Milk, low-fat/2%	1 cup	18
Cream cheese	1 oz	28
Hot dog[†]	1	29
Ice cream, 10% fat	½ cup	30
Cheddar cheese	1 oz	30
Butter	1 Tbsp	31
Milk, whole	1 cup	33
Clams, fish fillets, oysters	3 oz	50–60
Beef,[b] pork,[b] poultry	3 oz	70–85
Shrimp	3 oz	166
Egg yolk[b]	1	213
Beef liver	3 oz	410

[a]In ascending order.
[b]Leading contributors of cholesterol to U.S. diet.

in bacon and sausage is more likely to raise blood cholesterol than the food cholesterol in eggs. Shrimp are high in cholesterol but low in fat—that is, low in fat if the shrimp are steamed or broiled, not encased in a deep fat–fried coating. Of course, moderation is recommended for eating eggs and shrimp.

Another source of confusion is that cooking oils made from corn, safflower, and soybeans are often labeled as cholesterol free. Of course, they are cholesterol free; only foods from animals contain cholesterol. Yet vegetable oils are virtually 100% food fat, and large amounts of dietary fat can also raise blood cholesterol.

To be a savvy consumer (and teach your patients), read ingredient labels and be aware of some finer points of fat education:

- Hydrogenated vegetable oils—corn, soybean, and cottonseed—contain artificial *trans* fatty acids, and these cholesterol-forming saturated fats are often used to prepare potato and corn chips.
- Tropical oils of palm, palm kernel, and coconut are the only plant sources of naturally saturated fat. Found in many food products, they should be consumed only occasionally. (Popcorn popped in tropical oils came under fire; many movie theater chains now offer air-popped popcorn in addition to traditionally prepared popcorn.)
- Margarines are cholesterol free if made from vegetable oils but still contain the same number of calories as butter; both are about 100% lipid. Margarines, however, contain unsaturated fatty acids. Note that the level of hydrogenation used to form the margarine affects the amounts of *trans* and saturated fatty acids contained. Use label information to select the least saturated product.
- Advise patients to check the labels of foods they eat regularly; a cholesterol-free product might not be as healthy as it seems.

In addition to the amount of fat, another characteristic of food fat that causes it to affect blood cholesterol differently is whether the fat is saturated or unsaturated—that is, whether the fat contains mostly saturated or unsaturated fatty acids. Saturated fatty acids generally raise blood cholesterol by providing the liver with the best building blocks for making cholesterol.

A simple guideline followed by many people is that blood cholesterol is raised by eating solid saturated fats and lowered by eating unsaturated and monounsaturated liquid fats. However, this rule is oversimplified for two reasons. First, food fats are a mixture of the three types. Second, although saturated fatty acids as a group raise cholesterol, some individual ones do not. Therefore, although we classify food fats as cholesterol-raising (butter/saturated) and cholesterol-lowering (corn oil/PUFA and olive oil/monounsaturated), these guidelines are based on the proportion of specific fatty acids in each food and how much each fatty acid affects blood cholesterol. Total fat intake can also influence blood cholesterol levels regardless of the source. Table 5.2 and Fig. 5.5 clear up some confusion over the finer points of fat.

Synthetic Fats and Fat Replacers

Many people dream about eating brownies and ice cream that are magically stripped of fat but still richly satisfying in taste and texture. Although surveys show that sugar substitutes have not reduced the amount of sugar we consume, optimists hope fat substitutes will reduce fat in our diets. Scientists are working to develop reduced-fat or fat-free substances that replace fat yet retain the taste and mouth-feel of fat in foods.

Fat replacers, as they are called, are generally classified two ways: already existing in nature or synthesized in the laboratory. The naturally occurring ones do not change chemically and thus require less rigorous testing before the FDA allows them to be used in foods. Heating and then blending protein from milk or eggs in a process called microparticulation produces one type of fat replacer. Simplesse is an example. Food applications include ice cream, frozen yogurt, and salad dressings—but not baked or deep-fried foods.

Carrageenan, a carbohydrate extracted from seaweed, has been used for centuries to thicken foods. Added to lean ground beef, carrageenan yields moist, juicy cooked meat with the texture of higher fat beef. Similar gum like products from oats, corn, and potatoes are under development and would provide lower kcal fatlike properties in food.

Salatrim, which stands for short- and long-chain triglyceride molecules, is made in the laboratory and provides sensory qualities with reduced energy content (5 kcal/g vs. 9 kcal/g). Olestra is a fat replacer made in the laboratory that binds fatty acids to sugar in a nontraditional way so that enzymes in the digestive tract are not able to break away the fatty acids. Olestra resembles standard fats and oils in many ways, including the ability to withstand frying and baking at high temperatures. Several characteristics of olestra are attractive to manufacturers and consumers, including the sensory properties of taste and texture, the no-kcal value because of the body's inability to digest it, and the reduced absorption of fat and cholesterol from the intestine. Potato chips cooked in olestra have 75 kcal/oz—half that of regular chips. A disadvantage is that olestra passes through the gut swiftly, possibly causing abdominal cramping and loose stools and loss of fat-soluble nutrients such as vitamins and carotenoids.

As the story of fat replacers continues to unfold, we need to study their effect on people's food choices. Will we be misled into thinking that low- or no-fat foods automatically are low in kcal? Many fat-reduced foods have increased amounts of other ingredients, such as carbohydrates, and are not low-kcal items.

To what degree will products containing fat replacers stimulate mechanisms to compensate for reduction in fat? Some studies suggest that incorporating reduced-fat products into the diet results in total fat reduction. Yet diets reduced in fat may not result in a reduction of total kcal. Thus, fat-free foods help some people consume fewer kcal overall; other times people eat a fat-free food at one meal and then make up the kcal by eating more at the next. What about appetite guiding what we eat? If mouth-feel is maintained in reduced-fat foods, we may not distinguish between high- and reduced-fat foods. Then there is the "bargain" appeal. In studies in which people did not know which chips were regular and which were made with olestra, they ate similar amounts of each. When they did know, they ate significantly more olestra chips, thus mistakenly thinking they got two for the "fat price" of one.

Although fat replacers are widely available, the most prudent and health-promoting approach is for products to be reformulated or developed without the use of fat replacers so products contain lower fat ingredients without added sugars and still taste good. Consistently consuming a low-fat diet can lead to a decrease in the preference for fat. Is it possible that fat replacers could undermine this healthful change? Nutritionists and scientists undoubtedly will continue to seek answers to make our fat-free brownie and ice cream dreams come true—without side effects.

Energy Intake

Foods containing significant amounts of dietary fat will naturally provide more kcal than other lower-fat foods. Although high-fat treats are fine occasionally, indulging too often or not even realizing which foods are fat laden can result in consumption of too many kcal that may end up stored as body fat in adipose tissues.

Fat is even more efficient at being stored than carbohydrate and protein, which means that we may gain more body fat from eating fat kcal than eating the same number of carbohydrate kcal (see Fig. 9.2). The evidence for this effect comes from studying people who eat low-fat, high-calorie diets, as discussed earlier. A likely explanation is that the energy cost to convert dietary fat to body fat requires only 3% of the kcal consumed, whereas carbohydrate requires 23% of the energy consumed to be converted to body fat. Both storage and oxidation of fats differ from those of carbohydrates and protein.

Diets high in fat are not the primary cause for the high prevalence of excess body fat in our society. We have an "all-food-all-the-time" lifestyle coupled with an aversion to physical activity. Overeating and underactivity are likely reasons for the steady increase in overweight and obese Americans (see the *Personal Perspectives* box Hooked on Salt, Sugar, Fat). Another reason may be the ability to be aware of internal cues of hunger. Consider whether we mistake fatigue as a cue of hunger. Consumption of food becomes a way to relieve tiredness, which of course does not work. Still, for many individuals struggling with moderate or even excessive weight gain, awareness of their dietary fat intake sources can make a difference. If we gradually reduce fat intake—without increasing carbohydrate intake—energy intake decreases and weight maintenance becomes easier.

PERSONAL PERSPECTIVES

Hooked on Salt, Sugar, and Fat

As I spoke with scientists about the way fat behaves, I couldn't resist drawing an analogy to the realm of narcotics. If sugar is the methamphetamine of processed food ingredients, with its high-speed, blunt assault on our brains, then fat is the opiate, a smooth operator whose effects are less obvious but no less powerful.

Michael Moss, *Salt, sugar, fat: How the food giants hooked us* (New York, 2013, Random House, p 148)

Michael Moss, a Pulitzer Prize-winning author, conducted an extensive investigation of the marketing and research methods of giant food corporations. As a result of these methods, the American population, and increasingly the global population, has become "hooked" on industrially processed, ready-to-eat, prepared foods that are high in salt, sugar, and fat. The taste and the mouth feel of these three substances in unnaturally high quantities has become, for too many Americans, the standard for appealing food. Our health, and particularly that of our children, is suffering, as is our ability to appreciate the wholesome unadulterated food of our past.

Research has shown, through magnetic resonance imaging of the brain, that the same portion of the brain that experiences pleasure becomes excited when individuals consume sugar, fat, or a mixture of fat and sugar. For food manufacturers, adding more and more sugar (in all its various forms) and fat increases sales because we begin to crave such foods; hence the analogy of addiction to narcotics. Foods prepared without artificially high levels of salt, sugar, and fat begins to taste bland and unappealing. Such food products have lower sales and yield smaller profits. The goal of such corporations may be not to nourish our bodies but to expand their revenues.

Reduced Intake of Other Nutrients

Even if dietary fat consumption does not result in weight gain, foods high in fat tend not to contain much dietary fiber and may be low in other nutrients. Not consuming enough dietary fiber, as noted in Chapter 4 (and in Chapters 13 and 17), is a risk factor for several chronic conditions. The seductive nature of foods containing fats may lead us to crave these foods and neglect others (see the *Personal Perspectives* box Hooked on Salt, Sugar, and Fat). The best guarantee for achieving the goal of nutritional wellness is to consume a balanced intake of nutrients, based on recommended guidelines, through consumption of at least five to seven servings of naturally low-fat fruits and vegetables per day.

Dietary Fat Intake and Diet-Related Diseases

The presence in the American diet of too much fat is directly related to several chronic diseases, such as CVD and certain types of cancers. High-fat diets are indirectly related to type 2 diabetes mellitus and hypertension. Health guidelines to prevent and treat these diseases call for less dietary fat than the average American eats. The DRI daily recommendations are to eat a total fat intake of 30% or less of kcal, an intake of saturated fatty acid less than 10% of kcal, and less than 300 mg of cholesterol. The average intakes of Americans are actually above those levels. Considerations of how this intake affects the risk for these diet-related disorders are presented in Chapters 14, 15, 17, and 20.

TOWARD A POSITIVE NUTRITION LIFESTYLE: GRADUAL REDUCTION

It's the subject of TV situation comedies. One member of the family becomes a health food fanatic, serving blades of grass, sprouts, and weird mixtures of soybeans, nuts, and who knows what. And what is the immediate response of the sitcom family? Disgust and rebellion, of course.

As we make recommendations to our patients (and perhaps decide for ourselves and our families) to reduce or modify the type of fat consumed, we should consider that often the most effective way to achieve permanent change is through gradual reduction. That's the mistake made by the TV character: too many changes made too quickly. An action plan for gradual reduction of dietary fat intake could consist of the following steps:

1. For 1 week, record all food and beverages consumed.
2. On the basis of reading this chapter, assess which foods are likely to be high in fat.
3. Particularly note whether one high-fat food item, such as whole milk, is consumed often or whether a certain meal or snack regularly includes fatty foods. Perhaps scrambled eggs and bacon are eaten almost every morning for breakfast, and an afternoon coffee break always includes either a sweet Danish pastry or a huge, buttery muffin.
4. The next week, choose one item and either reduce its consumption or replace it with a lower fat substitute. Instead of whole milk, use 2% or 1% fat milk, or replace the coffee break treat with an English muffin with a bit of butter or margarine and jelly.
5. The following week, select another food item or meal and make a simple substitution. This process can continue with small changes—gradual reductions—resulting in major reductions in dietary fat intake.

SUMMARY

- Functions of lipids include specific characteristics of foods that arise from lipids and maintenance of the physiologic health of the body.
  - Triglycerides provide food functions of energy, palatability, satiety, food processing, and source of nutrients. Physiologic functions include form of stored energy; organ protection; temperature regulation; and insulation.
  - Phospholipids are a component of all cell membrane structures, emulsifiers of fluids within of the body, and part of the transport of lipids throughout the body.
  - Sterols are part of complex regulatory compounds within the body, a basic material to make bile, vitamin D, sex hormones, and cells in brain and nerve tissues. Cholesterol, a sterol, is a vital part of all cell membrane and nerve tissues and of building blocks for hormones.
- Lipids are organic, composed of carbon, hydrogen, and oxygen.
  - Triglycerides are composed of one glycerol molecule and three fatty acids.
  - Fatty acids may be saturated, monounsaturated, or polyunsaturated, depending on the number of double bonds.
  - Phospholipids are composed of one glycerol molecule with only two fatty acids; the third spot contains a phosphate group.
  - Sterol structures, including cholesterol, are carbon rings intermeshed with side chains of carbon, hydrogen, and oxygen.
- All three types of lipids can be manufactured by the body, except for linolenic and linoleic fatty acids (found in triglycerides), which therefore are essential nutrients.
- Digestion of lipids occurs mainly in the small intestine; absorption depends on the transportation of lipids through the lymph and blood circulatory systems.
  - Lipids travel through the body in lipoprotein packages containing triglycerides, protein, phospholipids, and cholesterol.
  - Lipoproteins differ according to the proportions or ratio of these ingredients. Very low-density lipoprotein (VLDL), low-density lipoprotein (LDL), and high-density lipoprotein (HDL) are found in the blood.
- Health concerns about dietary fat intake fall into several categories: appropriate energy intake, reduced intake of other nutrients because of excessive dietary fat consumption, and the relationship between dietary fat intake and diet-related disorders. Health benefits of monounsaturated and polyunsaturated fats may decrease risk of diet-related disorders.

THE NURSING APPROACH

Clinical Judgment and Next-Generation NCLEX® Examination-Style Questions

Case Study 1

High-Fat Diet and Heart Disease

John is a 35-year-old male who just had blood work done for his annual checkup. He lives a sedentary lifestyle and admits a majority of the meals he consumes are takeout or fast food. His father died from heart disease at the age of 55 years. He has two children and is concerned about his health and well-being. His doctor prescribed him a statin.

Subjective (From Patient Statements)/Recognize and Analyze Cues

- "I always feel tired."
- "My dad had high cholesterol and died young. I don't want my kids to grow up without a father."

Objective (From Physical Examination)/Recognize and Analyze Cues

- Height 5′9″, weight 200 pounds
- Blood pressure 130/90 mm Hg
- Total cholesterol 300 mg/dL, low-density lipoprotein (LDL) 220 mg/dL, high-density lipoprotein (HDL) 35 mg/dL, and triglycerides 200 mg/dL

Diagnosis/Prioritize Hypotheses

1. Hyperlipidemia and hypercholesterolemia related to unhealthy diet and familial history, as evidenced by total cholesterol of 300 mg/dL, LDL of 220 mg/dL, HDL of 35 mg/dL, and triglyceride level of 200 mg/dL
2. Potential for cardiovascular disease related to unhealthy diet, overweight, sedentary lifestyle, hyperlipidemia, and hypercholesterolemia as evidenced by blood pressure

Planning/Generate Solutions

Patient Outcomes

Short term (at the end of this visit):

- John will identify foods high in saturated fat and will state the relationship between saturated fat and blood cholesterol.
- He will commit to reading food labels and choose foods lower in fat.
- He will verbalize the importance of taking his medication as prescribed.

Long term (in 6 months):

- John will reduce his consumption of high-fat foods.
- He will lose 1 to 2 pounds per week until he is at his ideal body weight.
- Blood lipid values will be lowered.

Nursing Interventions/Generate Solutions

1. Teach him about general dietary and lifestyle changes to reduce his cholesterol.
2. Review medication information.

Implementation/Take Action

1. Taught John how to reduce total fat consumption and choose healthier fats.
   Saturated fats, which are primarily found in red meats and dairy products, increase LDL and total cholesterol. Trans fats, which are found in partially hydrogenated oils, increase LDL cholesterol while lowering HDL cholesterol. He should be encouraged to choose leaner cuts of meat, low-fat dairy, and monounsaturated fats, which are found in plant-based oils, avocados, peanut butter, and many nuts and seeds.
2. Recommended choosing grilled, broiled, or baked foods over fried foods when consuming takeout or fast food.
   John eats a majority of his meals away from home. By choosing options that are grilled, broiled, or baked, he can significantly reduce his intake of saturated fats, trans fats, and cholesterol. He should also be encouraged to avoid "super-sizing" his order to help cut down on fat.
3. Taught John how to read food labels.
   Learning and understanding how to read food labels can help John make healthier choices.
4. Provided medication teaching on statins.
   Statins lower cholesterol in the blood by blocking hydroxy-methylglutaryl-coenzyme A reductase (HMG-CoA reductase), which is responsible for making cholesterol. Too much cholesterol in the body contributes to the development of atherosclerosis (plaque buildup within arteries). Grapefruit interacts with some statins and should be avoided. Liver enzymes should be checked periodically. Common side effects include muscle cramping, diarrhea or constipation, stomach upset, and headache. The statin should be taken as prescribed by the provider.
5. Encouraged him to begin an exercise program, as approved by the doctor.
   Regular exercise can improve cholesterol by raising HDL cholesterol. It also helps with weight reduction.

Evaluation/Evaluate Outcomes

Short term (at the end of the visit):

- John identified foods high in saturated fat.
- He said he would try to be better about reading food labels and choosing healthier options when eating away from home.
- He agreed to take his statin every day as prescribed.

Long term (at the end of 6 months):

- John stated that he does not eat fried foods as much.
- He only lost 5 pounds.
- His blood lipid values were significantly reduced and almost within normal limits.
  Goals partially met.

Discussion Questions

1. Which foods contain saturated fats? Which animal products should be limited?
2. What are the Dietary Reference Intake daily recommendations for total fat and saturated fat intake?

Case Study 2

A 68-year-old female comes to the Medical Clinic with complaints of abdominal pain (7/10) and frequent waves of nausea. Today, her vital signs are temperature 98.8° F (37.1° C), apical pulse 104 beats per minute, respirations 22 breaths per minute, and blood pressure 152/94 mm Hg. Her weight is 162 pounds and she is 5 feet 3 inches tall. She has a history of high blood cholesterol and today her LDL level is 165. She is unsure what to order at the daily business lunches at work and has noticed that she has gained some weight lately. She wonders if this is caused by a lack of exercise or eating too much.

Highlight the assessment findings that require follow-up by the nurse.

A 68-year-old female comes to the medical clinic with complaints of abdominal pain (7/10) and frequent waves of nausea. Her vital signs are temperature = 98.8° F (37.1° C), apical pulse = 104 beats per minute, respiration = 24 breaths per minute, blood pressure = 152/94 mm Hg. Her weight is 162 pounds, and she is 5 feet 3 inches tall. She has a history of high blood cholesterol and today her LDL level is 165 mg/dl. She is unsure what to order at the daily business lunches at work and has noticed that she has gained some weight lately. She wonders if this is because of a lack of exercise or eating too much.

APPLYING CONTENT KNOWLEDGE

Disease prevention for chronic diet-related diseases depends on changes in lifestyle behaviors. Consider the lifestyle behaviors Henry Mason could adopt on the basis of his personal history. Henry Mason is a 20-year-old White man; his mother and father both have high cholesterol levels and family history of cardiovascular disease. Although John's cholesterol level is average for his age, what three disease prevention strategies could he pursue? Would these strategies be primary, secondary, or tertiary?

WEBSITES OF INTEREST

USDA Nutrient Database Laboratory (Food Composition Tables)
www.ars.usda.gov/Services/docs.htm?docid=8964
Creates and supports nutrient databases through the most advanced procedures to obtain, assess, collect, and distribute composition data on foods accessible in the United States.

Center for Science in the Public Interest (CSPI)
www.cspinet.org
Improving the American food supply through educative, legislative, regulatory, and judicial advocacy and by publication of the monthly *Nutrition Action Healthletter*.

Eating Well Online
www.eatingwell.com
Online version of the magazine *Eating Well: Where Good Taste Meets Good Health;* has information on nutrition, food, and low-fat cooking.

REFERENCES

Drewnowski. A. (2000). Sensory control of energy density at different life stages. *Proc Nutr Soc, 59*(2), 239–244.

Evidence Analysis Library 2013: What effect does consuming natural (ruminant) vs. synthetic (industrially hydrogenated) trans fatty acids have on LDL-, HDL- and non-HDL cholesterol?, Academy of Nutrition and Dietetics. From: <www.andeal.org/> (Accessed 24 November, 2017).

Harper, C. R., & Jacobson, T. A. (2005). Usefulness of omega-3 fatty acids and the prevention of coronary heart disease. *Am J Cardiol, 96*(11), 1521–1529.

Harris. W. S. (1989). Fish oils and plasma lipid and lipoprotein metabolism in humans: a critical review. *J Lipid Res, 30*, 785–807.

Jones, P. J. H., & Rideout, T. (2014). Lipids, sterols, and their metabolites. In A. C. Ross (Ed.), *Modern nutrition in health and disease* (11th ed.). Philadelphia: Lippincott Williams & Wilkins.

Tso, P., & Liu, M. (2004). Ingested fat and satiety. *Physiol Behav, 81*(2), 275–287.

Vannice, G., & Rasmussen, H. (2014). Position of the academy of nutrition and dietetics: dietary fatty acids for healthy adults. *J Acad Nutr Diet, 114*(1), 136–153.

6

Protein

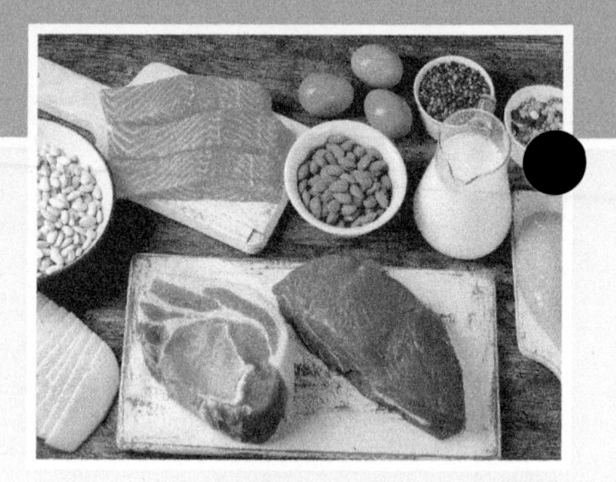

The proteins we consume in foods are not the same proteins used by our bodies. Actually, the only nutrient role protein in foods serves is to provide amino acids, the building blocks of all proteins.

http://evolve.elsevier.com/GRODNER/FOUNDATIONS

LEARNING OBJECTIVES

- Define the composition of protein.
- Describe how the composition of protein differs from that of carbohydrate and lipid.
- Define essential and nonessential amino acids.
- Distinguish between complete proteins and incomplete proteins.
- Discuss how protein is digested, is absorbed as amino acids, and becomes available to cells.
- List the functions of protein.

ROLE IN WELLNESS

In 1928 a political slogan promised "a chicken in every pot!" At that time, being able to afford animal protein on a daily basis was the mark of a high standard of living and an assurance of good health. Today the phrase might be "rice and beans for all of us!" We now know that there are many sources of protein available in our food supply. Some offer advantages over others by being lower in fat and higher in other nutrients such as complex carbohydrates and fiber.

Protein in food is our only source of amino acids, which are absolutely necessary to make the thousands of proteins that form every aspect of the human body. It is no wonder that protein, which is plentiful in our food supply, has gained the status of a super-nutrient for Americans. A common but inaccurate belief is that we expect that the more protein we eat, the stronger our immune system will be, the less we will weigh, and the more muscles we will develop.

Although proteins formed by our bodies do have a role in those functions, the amounts we consume are often greater than we need. Awareness of protein sources and portion sizes is important as we work toward achieving health promotion goals to decrease our risk of diet-related diseases (Box 6.1).

The six dimensions of health provide ways to think about the effects of protein consumption. Our overall physical health and well-being depend on our eating enough essential amino acids for body protein synthesis. The ability to comprehend and apply new approaches to protein consumption by adapting to different protein sources (e.g., legumes and grains) and reducing portion sizes depends on our intellectual health capacity to implement change. Protein is a super-status food for some Americans; favorite sources may provide emotional health security. Clients needing to make dietary changes, such as changing to lower fat sources of protein (e.g., cutting back on sausages), may need our advice on coping strategies. Because we and our clients follow different eating patterns, such as practicing vegetarianism or reducing consumption of animal protein, family and social dynamics may be affected when one member changes and thereby tests our level of social health. Religious and spiritual health beliefs lead individuals to nourish their bodies through a harmless philosophy that views humans as civilized enough to nourish their bodies without taking life. Environmental health concerns are being raised because of the ecologic impact of byproducts of production of animal sources, such as manure polluting farmlands.

STRUCTURE OF PROTEIN

Proteins are organic compounds formed by the linking of many smaller molecules of amino acids. Like glucose, **amino acids** are organic compounds made of carbon, hydrogen, and oxygen. However, amino acids also contain nitrogen, which clearly distinguishes protein from other nutrients.

There are 20 amino acids from which all the proteins that are required by plants and animals are made. The human body is able to manufacture some of the amino acids for its own protein-building function; however, 9 amino acids cannot be made by the cells of the body. Therefore, these **essential amino acids (EAAs)** must be eaten in food, digested, absorbed, and then

BOX 6.1 MyPlate: Protein Foods

What Foods Are in the Protein Foods Group?

All foods made from meat, poultry, seafood, beans and peas, eggs, processed soy products, nuts, and seeds are considered part of the Protein Foods Group. Beans and peas are also part of the Vegetable Group.

Select a variety of protein foods to improve nutrient intake and health benefits, including at least 8 ounces of cooked seafood per week. Young children need less, depending on their age and calorie needs. The advice to consume seafood does not apply to vegetarians. Vegetarian options in the Protein Foods Group include beans and peas, processed soy products, and nuts and seeds. Meat and poultry choices should be lean or low-fat.

How Much Food From the Protein Foods Group Is Needed Daily?

The amount of food from the Protein Foods Group you need to eat depends on age, sex, and level of physical activity. Most Americans eat enough food from this group but need to make leaner and more varied selections of these foods. Recommended daily amounts are shown in the following table.

DAILY RECOMMENDATION[a]		
Children	2–3 years old	2 ounce-equivalents
	4–8 years old	4 ounce-equivalents
Girls	9–13 years old	5 ounce-equivalents
	14–18 years old	5 ounce-equivalents
Boys	9–13 years old	5 ounce-equivalents
	14–18 years old	6½ ounce-equivalents
Women	19–30 years old	5½ ounce-equivalents
	31–50 years old	5 ounce-equivalents
	51+ years old	5 ounce-equivalents
Men	19–30 years old	6½ ounce-equivalents
	31–50 years old	6 ounce-equivalents
	51+ years old	5½ ounce-equivalents

[a]These amounts are appropriate for individuals who get less than 30 minutes per day of moderate physical activity, beyond normal daily activities. Those who are more physically active may be able to consume more while staying within calorie needs.

What Counts as an Ounce-Equivalent in the Protein Foods Group?

In general, 1 ounce of meat, poultry or fish, ¼ cup cooked beans, 1 egg, 1 tablespoon of peanut butter, or ½ ounce of nuts or seeds can be considered as 1 ounce-equivalent from the Protein Foods Group.

The following table lists specific amounts that count as 1 ounce-equivalent in the Protein Foods Group toward your daily recommended intake.

	Amount That Counts as 1 Ounce-Equivalent in the Protein Foods Group	Common Portions and Ounce-Equivalents
Meats	1 ounce cooked lean beef	1 small steak (eye of round, filet) = 3½ to 4 ounce-equivalents
	1 ounce cooked lean pork or ham	1 small lean hamburger = 2 to 3 ounce-equivalents
Poultry	1 ounce cooked chicken or turkey, without skin	1 small chicken breast half = 3 ounce-equivalents
	1 sandwich slice of turkey (4½ inches × 2½ inches × ⅛ inch)	½ Cornish game hen = 4 ounce-equivalents
Seafood	1 ounce cooked fish or shellfish	1 can of tuna, drained = 3 to 4 ounce-equivalents
		1 salmon steak = 4 to 6 ounce-equivalents
		1 small trout = 3 ounce-equivalents
Eggs	1 egg	3 egg whites = 2 ounce-equivalents
		3 egg yolks = 1 ounce-equivalent
Nuts and seeds	½ ounce of nuts (12 almonds, 24 pistachios, 7 walnut halves)	1 ounce of nuts or seeds = 2 ounce-equivalents
	½ ounce of seeds (pumpkin, sunflower, or squash seeds, hulled, roasted)	
	1 tablespoon of peanut butter or almond butter	
Beans and peas	¼ cup of cooked beans (such as black, kidney, pinto, or white beans)	
	¼ cup of cooked peas (such as chickpeas, cowpeas, lentils, or split peas)	1 cup split pea soup = 2 ounce-equivalents
	¼ cup of baked beans, refried beans	1 cup lentil soup = 2 ounce-equivalents
	¼ cup (about 2 ounces) of tofu	1 cup bean soup = 2 ounce-equivalents
	1 ounce of tempeh, cooked	1 soy or bean burger patty = 2 ounce-equivalents
	¼ cup roasted soybeans	
	1 falafel patty (2¼ inches, 4 oz)	
	2 tablespoons hummus	

(From U.S. Department of Agriculture, Center for Nutrition and Promotion: *What foods are in the Protein Foods Group?* 2017. Accessed 2 December, 2017, from https://www.choosemyplate.gov/protein-foods.)

BOX 6.2 Amino Acids

Essential Amino Acids	Nonessential Amino Acids
Histidine	Alanine
Isoleucine	Arginine
Leucine	Aspartic acid
Lysine	Cysteine
Methionine	Cystine
Phenylalanine	Glutamic acid
Threonine	Glutamine
Tryptophan	Glycine
Valine	Proline
	Serine
	Tyrosine

brought to cells by circulating blood. The remaining 11 are nonessential amino acids (NEAAs) (Box 6.2). The liver can create NEAAs as long as structural components, including nitrogen, from other amino acids are available.

Each cell constructs or synthesizes the proteins it needs. To build proteins, the cell must have access to all 20 amino acids. This available supply of amino acids is in the metabolic amino acid pool. The amino acid pool is a collection of amino acids that is constantly resupplied with EAAs (from dietary intake) and NEAAs (synthesized in the liver). The pool allows the cell to build proteins easily.

PROTEIN COMPOSITION

The functions of proteins are closely related to their structures. The complex composition of proteins is best understood through four structural levels: primary, secondary, tertiary, and quaternary (Fig. 6.1).

The primary structure of protein composition is determined by the number, assortment, and sequence of amino acids in polypeptide chains. Amino acids are linked together by peptide bonds to form a practically unlimited number of proteins. The peptide bond occurs at the point at which the carboxyl group of one amino acid is bound to the amino group of another amino acid (Fig. 6.2).

The 20 amino acids form chains that may contain any combination or assortment of amino acids, allowing for thousands of different proteins to be formed. Two proteins may contain the same assortment and number of amino acids yet still have different functions because of the sequencing or order of the amino acids.

The secondary structure level of proteins affects the shape of the chain of amino acids; they may be straight, folded, or coiled. The tertiary structure results when the polypeptide chain is so coiled that the loops of the coil touch, forming strong bonds within the chain itself. At the quaternary structural level, proteins contain more than one polypeptide chain.

A protein may not be able to perform its original function if its structure or shape changes. The shape may be changed by heat (cooking), ultraviolet light (exposure to sunlight), acids (vinegar), alcohol, or mechanical action. A protein has been denatured and physically changed when the shape of a protein is affected (e.g., a folded chain unfolding).

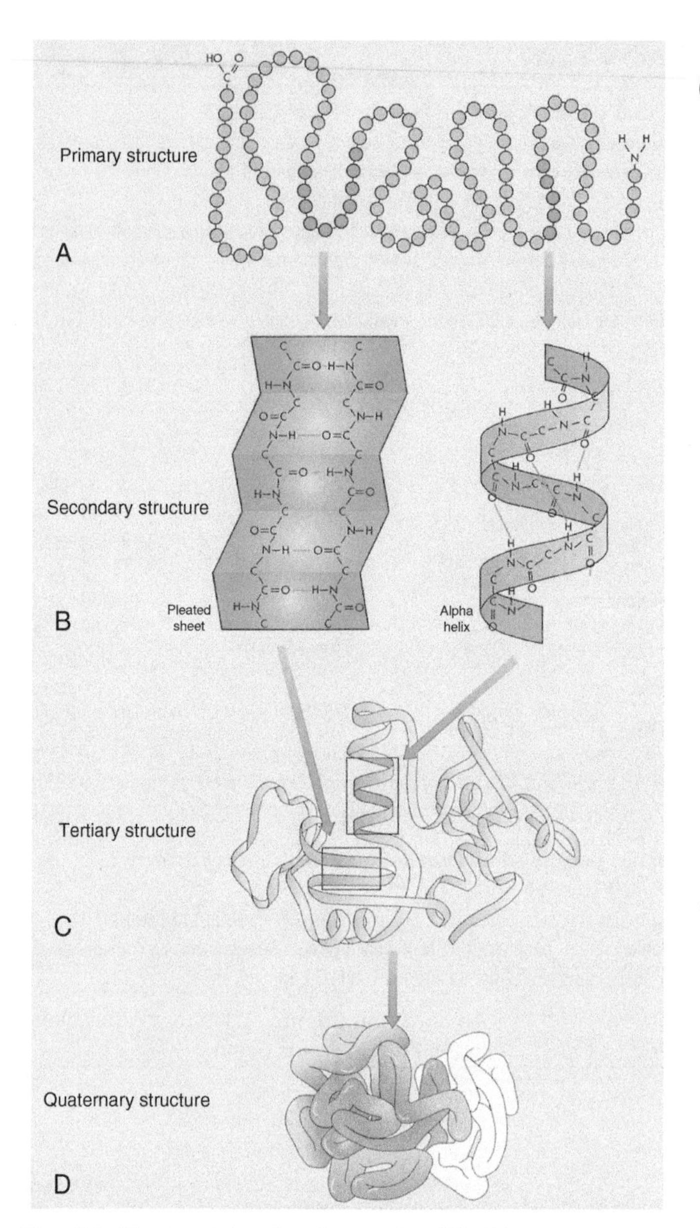

Fig. 6.1 Structural levels of protein. (A) Primary structure: determined by number, kind, and sequence of amino acids in the chain. (B) Secondary structure: hydrogen bonds stabilize folds of helical spirals. (C) Tertiary structure: globular shape maintained by strong intramolecular bonding and by stabilizing hydrogen bonds. (D) Quaternary structure: results from bonding between more than one polypeptide unit. (Courtesy Bill Ober. In Thibodeau GA, Patton KT: *Anatomy & physiology*, ed 4, St. Louis, 1999, Mosby.)

An example of denaturing a food protein is the change that occurs when the white of an uncooked egg (a clear liquid) is beaten. The clear liquid turns white, foamy, and stiff. Although the protein in the egg has been denatured, it is still a valuable source of amino acids. The amino acids are not affected; only the shape of the chain has been changed.

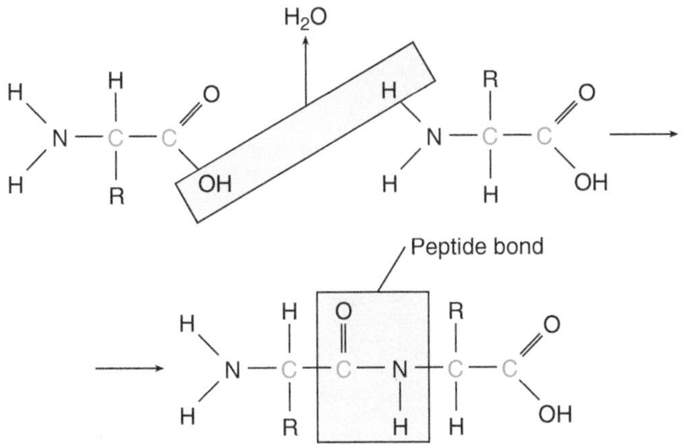

Fig. 6.2 Peptide bonds.

Inside the body, denaturing of proteins is controlled by mechanisms that keep the internal body environment from getting too basic or too acidic. Either extreme can lead to the denaturation of vital proteins within the body. Body temperature also affects the protein structure of the body. High fevers can become lethal when protein structures within the body become denatured. When body proteins are denatured, they cannot perform their original functions.

Although uncontrolled denaturation can be dangerous, it is helpful for digestion. Denaturing changes the three-dimensional structure of a protein, providing more surface area on which digestive juices act to release the amino acids of the food proteins.

PROTEIN AS A NUTRIENT IN THE BODY

The proteins we consume in foods are not the same proteins used by our bodies. Actually, the only nutrient role protein in foods serves is to provide amino acids, the building blocks of all proteins.

Digestion and Absorption

Because of the complex structure of proteins, a number of protein enzymes, or proteases, produced by the stomach and pancreas are required to hydrolyze proteins into smaller and smaller peptides until individual amino acids are ready for absorption (Fig. 6.3).

Mouth

Only mechanical digestion of protein occurs in the mouth. Mastication breaks protein-containing food into smaller pieces that mix with saliva passing through to the stomach.

Stomach

Pepsinogen, an inactive form of the gastric protease pepsin, is secreted by the stomach mucosa. Pepsin becomes activated when it mixes with hydrochloric acid, also produced by stomach secretions. Pepsin then begins the process of protein hydrolysis, breaking the bonds linking the amino acids of the protein peptide. The result is smaller polypeptides rather than single amino acids or dipeptides. The polypeptides pass through to the small intestine for further hydrolysis.

Rennin, an important gastric protease, is produced only during infancy. It functions with calcium to thicken or coagulate the milk protein casein; thickening slows the movement of milk nutrients from the stomach, allowing additional digestion time.

Small Intestine

In the small intestine, pancreatic and intestinal proteases continue the hydrolysis of polypeptides. As these smaller peptides touch the intestinal walls, peptidases are released that complete the hydrolysis of protein into absorbable units of individual amino acids and dipeptides.

The primary pancreatic enzyme is trypsin. It is first secreted as trypsinogen, an inactive form. The intestinal hormone enteropeptidase activates trypsinogen into trypsin, which continues the hydrolysis of polypeptides. Two other pancreatic enzymes assist in the hydrolysis process: chymotrypsin hydrolyzes polypeptides into dipeptides, and carboxypeptidase breaks polypeptides and dipeptides into amino acids. Two intestinal peptidases are aminopeptidase, which releases free amino acids from the amino ends of short-chain peptides, and dipeptidase, which completes the hydrolysis of proteins to amino acids.

Absorption of amino acids occurs through the intestinal walls by means of competitive active transport that requires vitamin B_6 (pyridoxine) as a carrier. Because amino acids are water soluble, they easily pass into the bloodstream.

Metabolism

To understand the importance of protein metabolism in the growth and maintenance of the body, consider that most protein functions are a result of protein anabolism (synthesis) in cells. Hormones have a major role in the regulation of protein metabolism. Anabolism is enhanced by the effect of growth hormone (from the pituitary gland) and the male hormone testosterone. Hormones affecting the catabolism (breakdown) of proteins are the glucocorticoids that are enhanced by adrenocorticotropic hormone (ACTH); these hormones are secreted from the adrenal cortex. This process releases proteins in the cells to break down to amino acids, and then the amino acids travel in the bloodstream, contributing to an available pool of amino acids (Fig. 6.4).

The liver cells begin the process of catabolism through deamination. Deamination results in the breaking off of an amino acid (NH_2) group from an amino acid molecule, resulting in one molecule each of ammonia (NH_3) and a keto acid. Liver cells convert most of the ammonia to urea, which is later excreted in urine. The keto acid may enter the tricarboxylic acid (TCA) cycle to be used for energy (see Fig. 9.2) or, through gluconeogenesis and lipogenesis, may be converted to glucose and fat (see Fig. 6.4).

Protein Excess

An excessive intake of protein results in increased deamination by the liver. The increased deamination may result in high

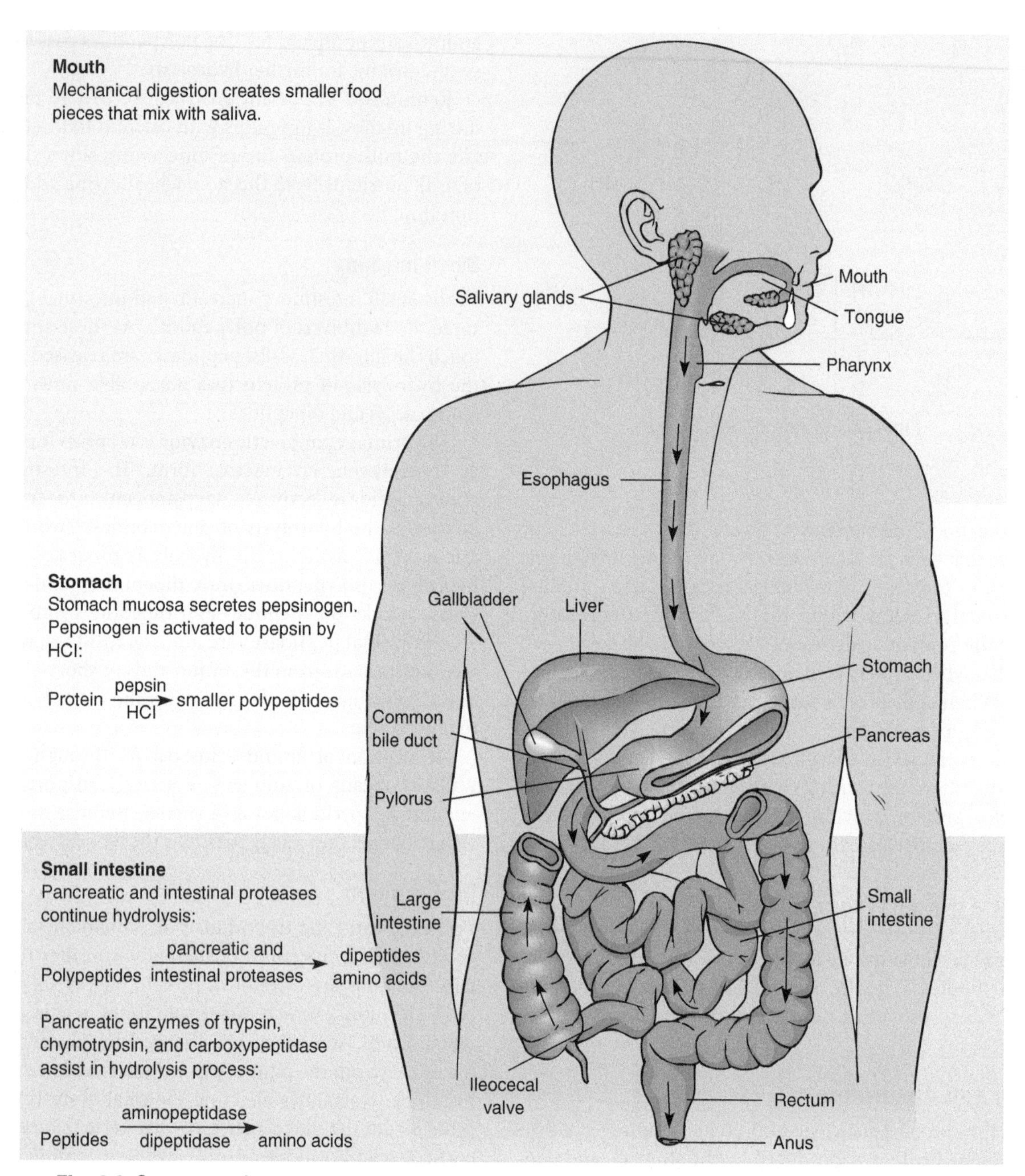
Mouth
Mechanical digestion creates smaller food pieces that mix with saliva.
Stomach
Stomach mucosa secretes pepsinogen. Pepsinogen is activated to pepsin by HCl:
Protein pepsin HCl smaller polypeptides
Small intestine
Pancreatic and intestinal proteases continue hydrolysis:
Polypeptides pancreatic and intestinal proteases dipeptides amino acids
Pancreatic enzymes of trypsin, chymotrypsin, and carboxypeptidase assist in hydrolysis process:
Peptides aminopeptidase dipeptidase amino acids
Salivary glands
Mouth
Tongue
Pharynx
Esophagus
Gallbladder
Liver
Stomach
Common bile duct
Pancreas
Pylorus
Large intestine
Small intestine
Ileocecal valve
Rectum
Anus

Fig. 6.3 Summary of protein digestion and absorption. *HCl,* Hydrochloric acid. (From Rolin Graphics.)

levels of keto acids, possibly putting the body into a state of ketosis. The increased urea is excreted by the kidneys. Because the liver and kidneys are involved with the deamination process, the increased stress on the organs could initiate an underlying disorder of these organs. There are no definitive benefits of excessive protein intake, so the general recommendation is to consume no more than twice the recommended dietary allowance (RDA) for protein.

In fact, the source of excess protein may be a health concern. Animal-derived protein sources such as meats may also be high in saturated fat and dietary cholesterol. Consuming excess amounts may increase the risk of cardiovascular disease (CVD) and some cancers. The relationship between protein intake and osteoporosis also has been considered. When protein intake is high, there is a slight increase of calcium excretion from the body, but calcium absorption is not affected. Studies have yielded mixed results about this effect on the risk of osteoporosis. Because osteoporosis is multifactorial, this specific relationship is difficult to determine. Recommendations to consume moderate amounts of protein and to meet the Dietary Reference Intake (DRI) levels for calcium are the best dietary approaches to decrease the risk of CVD and cancer. (See Chapter 8 for an in-depth discussion of osteoporosis.)

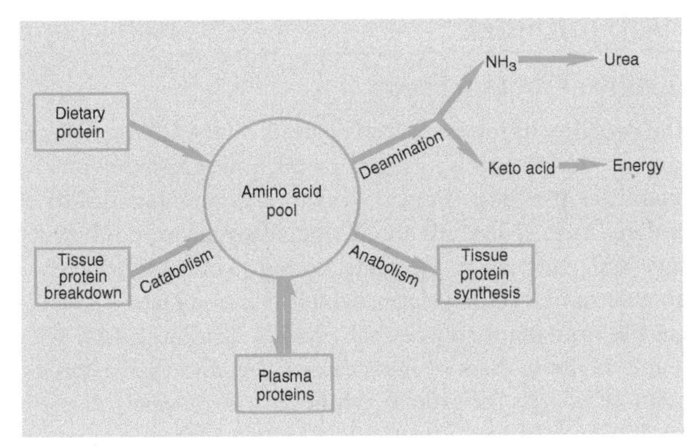

Fig. 6.4 The body's equilibrium depends on a balance between the rates of protein breakdown (catabolism) and protein synthesis (anabolism). (Modified from Williams SR: *Essentials of nutrition and diet therapy*, ed 7, St. Louis, 1999, Mosby.)

Nitrogen Balance

Nitrogen-balance studies are used to determine the protein requirements of the body throughout the life cycle and to assign value to the protein quality of foods to determine their biologic value. Because nitrogen (N) is a primary component of protein, the body's use of protein can be determined by nitrogen-balance studies that compare the amount of nitrogen entering the body in food protein with the nitrogen lost from the body in feces and urine.

Nitrogen lost or excreted from the body may be endogenous nitrogen (from catabolism of body protein), metabolic nitrogen (from intestinal cells), or exogenous nitrogen (from dietary proteins). Nitrogen in feces may be metabolic and exogenous (from cells and dietary proteins) and that in urine may be endogenous (catabolism of body protein) and exogenous (from dietary proteins).

An individual is in nitrogen equilibrium or zero nitrogen balance if the amount of nitrogen consumed in foods equals the amount excreted. This state occurs in normal, healthy adults when nitrogen in food protein entering (input) the body equals the nitrogen leaving the body (output). Because adults are no longer growing, the nitrogen that enters the body is not needed to build new tissue but is used simply to maintain the body.

Positive nitrogen balance occurs when more nitrogen is retained in the body than is excreted. The nitrogen is used to form new cells for growth or healing. This state occurs in growing children and in pregnant women who require additional nitrogen (and protein) for the growth of the fetus. Individuals recovering from illness or injury may be in positive nitrogen balance as the body heals. Negative nitrogen balance happens when more nitrogen is excreted from the body than is retained from dietary protein sources. It occurs when there is a breakdown of proteins within the body, such as in muscles and organs. Negative nitrogen balance may be caused by aging, physical illness, extreme stress, starvation, surgery, or eating disorders.

FUNCTIONS

Proteins created in our bodies perform numerous functions, including the following:

- Growth and maintenance
- Creation of communicators and catalysts
- Immune system response
- Fluid and electrolyte regulation
- Acid–base balance
- Transportation

Growth and Maintenance

Each body cell contains proteins. All growth depends on a sufficient supply of amino acids. The amino acids are needed to make the proteins required to support muscle, tissue, bone formation, and the cells themselves.

Maintaining our bodies also requires a constant supply of amino acids. There is a continual turnover of body cells, which are composed of protein. The cells break down and must immediately be replaced. Each replacement cell requires the formation of additional protein.

Also needed for growth and maintenance is the protein collagen, found throughout the body. Collagen forms connective tissues such as ligaments and tendons and acts as a glue to keep the walls of the arteries intact. In addition, collagen has a role in bone and tooth formation by forming the framework structure, which is then filled with minerals, such as calcium and phosphorus. Synthesis of scar tissue also depends on collagen. Wound healing depends on an adequate intake of protein. Other structures, such as hair, nails, and skin, are composed of similar protein substances.

Creation of Communicators and Catalysts

Many vital substances produced by our bodies are formed of protein. Some hormones are proteins. Hormones act as communicators to alert different parts of the body to changes or to regulate functions of organs. Insulin, a hormone that directs cells to take in glucose, is a protein. Enzymes are also proteins. Enzymes are catalysts that enable chemical reactions or biologic changes to occur within the body. Each enzyme has a specific target; consequently, numerous enzymes are continually formed.

Blood clotting depends on protein substances as well. Twelve blood clotting factors must be in place for blood to clot when injury has occurred; several of the factors, such as fibrinogen, are composed of protein.

Immune System Response

The defense system of our bodies depends on proteins produced in response to foreign viruses and bacteria that invade our bodies. The proteins, or antibodies, are specific to each intruder. If sufficient levels of amino acids are not available to form these antibodies, we may have difficulties maintaining our health. Our overall immunologic response—our resistance to disease—depends on proteins formed within our bodies.

Fluid and Electrolyte Regulation

Water is balanced among three compartments in the body: intravascular (within veins and arteries), intracellular (inside cells), and interstitial (between cells). Proteins and minerals attract water, creating osmotic pressure. As proteins circulate through our bodies, they maintain body fluid and electrolyte balance by keeping water appropriately divided among the three compartments.

Acid–Base Balance

Some reactions occurring within the body lead to the release of acidic substances; others cause basic matter to enter the fluids of the body. Blood proteins can buffer the effects of fluids to maintain a safe acidic level in body fluids. The ability of protein to regulate the balance between the acidic and base characteristics of fluids is called the buffering effect of protein. Because the chemical structure of amino acids combines an acid (the carboxyl group [COOH]) and base (amine), an amino acid can function as either an acid or a base, depending on the pH of its medium. This is why the buffering effect of blood proteins is possible. This function is crucial to protect all proteins in the body. If fluids become either too acidic or too basic, the shapes of proteins are altered or denatured. Denatured proteins are not able to perform their usual functions.

Many of the constituents of blood are protein based, and if protein functions are affected, the result can be lethal. Therefore, proteins maintain a delicate pH level to ensure the proper functioning of all body systems (Box 6.3).

Transportation

Throughout our bodies, proteins are able to transport nutrients and other vital substances. For individual cells, proteins act as pumps, assisting the movement of nutrients in and out of cells. Many nutrients, including lipids, minerals, vitamins, and electrolytes, are carried in the blood by proteins such as lipoproteins. This allows the nutrients to be available to all parts of the body. Hemoglobin, a special carrier composed of protein, transports oxygen in the blood. Oxygen is stored in our muscles in another protein carrier, myoglobin. These protein carriers, hemoglobin and myoglobin, are essential for a well-functioning body.

BOX 6.3 Genetic Disorders

Phenylketonuria (PKU) is a genetic disorder with a protein link. This disorder is characterized by the inability to use or break down excess phenylalanine, an essential amino acid. The excess phenylalanine circulating inside the body can cause various health problems. Infants with this disorder consume low-phenylalanine formulas, whereas children and adults with PKU follow a limited-protein diet to control the intake of phenylalanine.

Another genetic protein disorder is sickle cell disease, which affects the shape of red blood cells. Because of abnormalities of the hemoglobin molecule, the red blood cell is curved or sickle shaped rather than round. The sickle shape can cause these blood cells to clog small blood vessels. This clogging can be painful, may cause damage to internal organs such as the kidneys and heart, and may lead to frequent infections throughout the body. Early screening followed by long-term penicillin treatment can prevent secondary infections.

Having the sickle cell disease trait is not the same as having the disease itself. Both parents have to have the trait for a child to be at risk. Even then, there is only a 25% chance of development of the disorder. Sickle cell disease may occur in any ethnic group, but it is more common among people from Africa and Black Americans; some states screen all infants to determine susceptibility.

FOOD SOURCES

Quality of Protein Foods

The proteins in foods are categorized by the EAAs they contain. Complete protein contains all nine EAAs in sufficient quantities that best support growth and maintenance of our bodies. Animal-derived foods, including meat, poultry, fish, eggs, and most dairy products, contain complete protein. (A notable exception is gelatin, which is incomplete.) Soybeans are the only plant source that provide all nine EAAs. Foods that contribute the best balance of EAAs and the best assortment of NEAAs for protein synthesis and are easily digestible are high-quality protein foods. The two highest quality protein foods are eggs and human milk. The egg is of high quality because it contains all the necessary nutrients to support life. Human breast milk is the perfect food; its nutrient profile is ideal for human growth.

Incomplete protein lacks one or more of the nine EAAs. Incomplete proteins will not provide a sufficient supply of amino acids and will not support life (Box 6.4). Many plant foods contain considerable amounts of incomplete proteins. Some of the better sources are grains and legumes.

The EAAs that those incomplete proteins lack are called limiting amino acids. The limiting amino acid reduces the value of the protein contained in the food. Unless the limiting amino acid is consumed in other foods, the amino acid pools

BOX 6.4 Sources of Complete and Incomplete Proteins

Foods Containing Complete Proteins	Foods Containing Incomplete Proteins
Fish	Cereals:
Shellfish	Ready-to-eat
Chicken	Oatmeal
Turkey	Wheatena
Duck[a]	Grains:
Beef[a]	Wheat
Lamb[a]	Rice
Pork[a]	Corn
Eggs[a]	Oats/oatmeal
Soybeans (tofu)	Barley
Cheese:	Spaghetti/pasta
Hard cheeses:	Bagels
Cheddar	Bread
Muenster	Legumes:
Swiss	Black-eyed peas
Soft cheeses:	Lentils
Cottage cheese[b]	Beans
Ricotta[b]	Peanuts/peanut butter
Milk[b]	Chickpeas
Ice milk/reduced-fat ice cream	Split peas
Yogurt[b]	Broccoli
Frozen yogurt	Potatoes
	Green peas
	Leafy green vegetables

[a] Possible high-fat source of protein.

[b] Protein in skim, 2%, and whole milk products.

inside the cells would be missing some of the EAAs. Protein production within the cell would be affected, and fewer proteins could be formed. Consequently, limiting amino acids reduces the number of proteins our bodies can make. Generally, we consume a sufficient mix of complete and incomplete proteins; therefore, this is not a health problem. Only those who adopt a dietary pattern restricting certain types of protein foods are at risk for an imbalanced intake.

Complementary Proteins

If different kinds of plant foods are eaten throughout the day, the total protein intake will equal that of complete proteins found in animal-related products. The advantages to complementary proteins are that plant foods cost less and tend to contain less fat; consuming less dietary fat is a prevention strategy for several chronic diet-related diseases.

A balance of amino acids is required throughout the day for protein synthesis. A sufficient assortment of EAAs is provided without planning if both animal and plant protein foods are eaten. If animal foods are not eaten, more care is required to ensure that limiting amino acids are consumed. Combinations of plant foods that provide all the EAAs are grains (e.g., wheat or rice) with legumes (e.g., kidney beans or chickpeas) and grains or legumes with small amounts of animal protein from dairy, meat, poultry, or fish (Box 6.5).

Measures of Food Protein Quality

Many foods contain protein, but the value of specific foods as protein sources varies. Perhaps the protein contained is incomplete or is difficult to digest (bound tightly to fiber). If food proteins are not digested, the amino acids can't be absorbed to nourish our bodies.

Several methods are used to analyze the quality of proteins in food, including biologic value, amino acid score, and protein efficiency ratio. The **biologic value** measures how much nitrogen from a protein food is retained by the body after digestion, absorption, and excretion. This measurement of nitrogen balance reveals how available the protein of that food is to the human body. An egg has the highest reference protein score, 100; all of the egg protein can be used. It has become a standard against which all other food proteins are judged. Fish has a score of 75 to 90, and corn, which contains protein but also has lower amino acid ratios, has a score of 40 (Matthews, 2014).

The **amino acid score** is a simple measure of the amino acid composition of a food in comparison with a reference protein. The score is based on the limiting amino acid(s) of the food. Digestibility of the protein is not considered.

A third method for assessing protein quality is the **protein efficiency ratio (PER)**. With this method, rats are fed a set amount of protein, and then, on the basis of weight gain, the physiologic value of the food protein consumed is determined as follows (Matthews, 2014):

$$\text{PER} = \frac{\text{Weight gain}}{\text{Protein intake}}$$

BOX 6.5 Food Combinations That Provide Complete Proteins

Grains + Legumes = Complete Protein

- Peanut butter sandwich
- Tacos with refried beans
- Rice and beans
- Split pea soup with croutons
- Falafel (chickpea balls) on pita bread
- Lentil soup with rye bread
- Baked beans with bread

Grains or Legumes + Animal Protein (Small Amount) = Complete Protein

- Chili with beans and cornbread
- Ready-to-eat cereal with skim milk
- Cheese sandwich
- Pasta with cheese
- Rice pudding
- French toast
- Pancakes (made with milk and/or eggs)
- Tuna casserole

Protein Recommended Dietary Allowance

The RDA for protein provides for sufficient intake of the EAAs and enough total protein to provide the amino groups needed to build new NEAAs. Other factors that affect the RDA for protein are age, gender, physiologic state, and sources of protein.

Age affects protein requirements because when growth occurs, such as during childhood, a greater percentage of dietary intake of protein is needed than in adulthood. Growth results in additional muscle and tissues, all of which require the amino acids contained in dietary protein. Theoretically, older adults may require lower levels of protein because muscle mass is reduced as we age; protein use may also be affected by variables such as decreased physical activity, illness, and long-term use of medications. However, few studies exist to confirm a lower requirement, so the protein RDA for adults 50 years and older is the same as for younger adults (National Research Council [NRC], 2006). Gender differences also affect protein needs. Men tend to have more lean body mass or muscle than women. Lean body mass requires more protein for maintenance.

Certain physiologic states, such as pregnancy and lactation, require different amounts of nutrients. A pregnant woman should consume additional protein to meet the needs of the growing fetus as well as those of her own body. RDA recommendations for protein are 25 g protein/day higher for pregnant women (71 g). **Lactation**, the production of breast milk, also requires consumption of additional protein. Breast milk contains high-quality protein that is formed from amino acids provided by the woman. The protein RDA for lactation is the same as for pregnancy (71 g). Special circumstances—serious physical illness, wound healing, fevers (increased metabolic rate), and unusual stress—may also increase protein needs.

The type of food source also affects the amount of protein needed. In the United States, most of the protein eaten is complete protein from animal sources. These sources are considered when the RDA for protein is set. Other countries rely on more plant sources of incomplete proteins, so worldwide recommendations, such as those of the World Health Organization, differ from the U.S. guidelines.

The RDA for protein is 0.8 g/kg (or 2.2 pounds) (NRC, 2006). For an average adult man, the RDA is 56 to 63 g; for an average adult woman, the RDA is 46 to 50 g. Research suggests that recommended levels for athletes are 1.2 to 2.0 g protein/kg body weight, depending on whether a sport requires endurance or strength (Thomas, Erdman, & Burke, 2016). Because most Americans eat more protein than recommended, even athletes tend to easily meet protein recommendations. Determine your recommended protein intake using the formula in the *Teaching Tool* box Calculating Your Recommended Protein Intake.

TEACHING TOOL

Calculating Your Recommended Protein Intake

To determine your personal protein recommendation, compute the following:

1. Divide your body weight by 2.2 to determine your weight in kilograms (kg):

   Weight in lb ÷ 2.2 = Weight in kg

   Example:

   140 ÷ 2.2 = 63.63 kg
2. Multiply the kilogram weight by 0.8 g/kg to determine your protein recommended daily allowance (RDA) (i.e., weight in kg × 0.8 g/kg = g of protein/RDA).

   Example:

   63.5 kg × 0.8 g/kg = 50.9 g protein/RDA

The acceptable macronutrient distribution ranges (AMDRs) suggest that protein consumption accounts for between 10% and 35% of energy intake. Depending on the percentage of protein energy consumed, consumption of energy from carbohydrates and lipids should be adjusted accordingly.

Vegetarianism

Vegetarianism, particularly veganism, has recently gained more acceptance as awareness grows of the values resulting from plant-based food plans. Advantages include health benefits such as reduced risk of diet-related disorders, protection of environmental resources, and recognition of the ethical treatment of animals, including avoiding the use of hormones and antibiotics to enhance animal food production. Instead of animal protein sources, vegetarian dietary categories focus on plant proteins to provide EAAs (Table 6.1). The vegan dietary pattern consists of only plant foods, including grains, legumes, fruits, vegetables, seeds, and nuts; no animal-derived products are eaten. The lacto-vegetarian dietary pattern is a food plan composed of only plant foods plus dairy products. It contains all the vegan foods plus dairy products such as milk, cheese, yogurt, and butter. The ovo-lacto-vegetarian dietary pattern or food plan consist of plant foods plus dairy products and eggs. It incorporates eggs into the lacto-vegetarian assortment of foods.

The Benefits of Vegetarianism

Vegetarian dietary patterns may be followed to achieve health, spiritual, economic, and environmental benefits. When well planned, vegetarian dietary patterns result in health benefits that are similar to those of a low-fat, high-fiber diet and consist of reduced risks for obesity, CVD, T2D mellitus, hypertension, gastrointestinal disorders, and certain cancers such as lung and colorectal cancers (Melinda, Craig, & Levin, 2016).

Because animal foods are our primary source of saturated fat and our only source of cholesterol, plant-based vegetarian dietary patterns tend to be lower in total fat and cholesterol. This reduced intake, combined with the high fiber content of plant foods, often results in lower blood cholesterol levels. Other nutrients that are usually higher in vegan diets are magnesium, folic acid, vitamins C and E, iron, and phytochemicals (Melinda et al., 2016). In addition, the body weights of individuals following vegetarian dietary patterns are generally lower. This effect also reduces the risk for development of hypertension and diabetes.

The spiritual rationale for some individuals who are vegetarians is based on the belief in nonharming. Several religions, including Hinduism and Seventh Day Adventists, see the consumption of animal flesh as being unhealthy or polluting to the body. Other vegetarians do not follow a formal religion but believe strongly in the protection of animal rights and are opposed to the slaughter of animals for human consumption. Information about the treatment of animals before and during the slaughtering process is now more available to the public because of increased exposure through Internet videos and websites.

The economic approach addresses the belief that animal-related products cost more than plant protein foods, not only financially but in terms of costs to our natural environment as well. Livestock and other domesticated animals are inefficient producers of protein. Although protein foods from cattle and chicken are of high quality, many pounds of grains are used by

TABLE 6.1 Vegetarian Categories

Vegan	Includes all plant foods (grains, legumes, fruits, vegetables, seeds, and nuts)	Excludes all animal-derived foods
Lacto-vegetarian	Includes all plant foods plus dairy products (milk, cheese, yogurt, and butter)	Excludes animal meat (meat, fowl, and fish) and eggs
Ovo-lacto-vegetarian	Includes all plant foods, dairy products, and eggs	Excludes animal meat
Pescatarian	Includes all plant foods, dairy products, eggs, and fish	Excludes meat and fowl
Flexitarian	Includes all plant foods, dairy, and eggs, with occasional consumption of meat, fowl, or fish	No exclusions but minimal consumption of animal meat

these animals to produce 1 pound of edible food. Some people maintain that eating from lower on the food chain—that is, eating more plant foods—involves less waste and has limited environmental impact on our natural resources and climate change.

The Drawbacks of Vegetarianism

The vegetarian dietary pattern has several drawbacks. Most may affect vegans. The vegan dietary pattern can provide all the essential nutrients except vitamins D and B_{12}, calcium, and omega-3 fatty acids. These will need to be consumed through carefully selected fortified foods or consumption of supplements as needed.

Most dietary vitamin D is consumed through milk fortified with the vitamin. Because vegans do not consume any dairy products, this source of vitamin D is unavailable. Vitamin D is also available through synthesis during exposure of the skin to direct sunlight; however, many individuals (even those consuming a traditional animal-derived intake) have inadequate levels of vitamin D and should rely on vitamin D–fortified foods or supplements. Factors such as regional limitation to sun exposure, darker skin pigmentation, elderly age, cultural clothing customs that conceal the body, and regular use of sunscreen increase the risk of vitamin D deficiency for child and adult vegans.

Reliable sources of vitamin B_{12} are all animal related. Excluding animal-derived foods, including milk, means that sources of B_{12} are simply not available. Even ovo-lacto-vegetarians may have low levels of vitamin B_{12}. Symptoms of vitamin B_{12} deficiency take years to appear and may cause permanent damage to the central nervous system. Individuals who restrict their intake of or exclude animal foods should take B_{12} supplements or consume foods fortified with vitamin B_{12} such as fortified soy milk to ensure adequate intake.

Other nutrients that could be deficient in vegans are iron and zinc, minerals usually consumed in meat, fish, and poultry. Calcium levels may also be low if dairy products are excluded; few plants are good sources of calcium. These nutrients are available in a well-planned vegan diet of whole foods. Nonetheless, care must be taken to consume sufficient amounts of calcium during pregnancy and growth periods; supplements will be necessary. If the vegan dietary pattern is poorly implemented and depends on refined and processed foods, nutrients may be lacking.

Ensuring that a vegetarian dietary pattern is healthful necessitates learning about protein complementing and new ways of preparing meatless dishes. Simply replacing meat with a lot of cheese won't have any health benefits. In fact, the fat content of a cheese dish is probably higher than that of a lean meat dish. The most helpful approach is to read vegetarian cookbooks that not only provide recipes but also include vegetarian nutrition information. MyPlate includes support for vegetarian dietary patterns. The food group recommendations for age, sex, and activity levels provide adequate energy and nutrient intake for vegetarianism if a variety of nutrient-dense foods are chosen. Guidance is available at the MyPlate website (www.choosemyplate.gov).

Contemporary Vegetarianism

Other terms have evolved to describe semivegetarian dietary patterns. The most inclusive term is the flexitarian approach. Flexitarians primarily consume vegetarian foods, with occasional meat, chicken, or fish consumption. This pattern enables an individual to decrease meat consumption without totally eliminating it. Another approach is pescatarian, which adds fish to vegetarian selections. These concepts do not reflect the original ideals of vegetarianism. Instead, they represent new, contemporary dietary patterns evolving in response to current health issues. These health issues center on the risk for development of one or more of the chronic diet-related diseases: CVD, cancer, T2D mellitus, and hypertension. Risk is reduced as dietary fat intake is lowered. A major source of fat in our diets is our consumption of animal protein foods. Reducing levels of this category of dietary fat lowers risk for chronic diet-related diseases. Doing so allows one to achieve the health promotion goals of *Healthy People 2020*.

DIETARY PATTERNS OF PROTEIN

So, what should we eat for protein? No longer do we need to be confined to a meat and potatoes mentality when it comes to protein. The healthiest approach is to eat mixed sources of protein—animal and plant sources. (See the *Cultural Diversity and Nutrition* box Rituals for Animal-Derived Protein for a discussion of the religious aspects of protein consumption.) The mix provides an excellent assortment of EAAs, plus sufficient building block materials for constructing NEAAs. Eating fewer animal protein foods reduces dietary fat intake, and eating more plant protein foods increases dietary fiber.

Restructuring the Dinner Plate

If you were asked to plan a balanced meal, what would the plate look like? Perhaps it would have animal protein (meat, fish, or poultry), vegetables (broccoli, potato, and a salad), and a grain (bread). But how much room on the plate would each portion take?

Before learning about MyPlate, a person's plate would most likely look like that in Fig. 6.5. Notice how meat is the centerpiece and takes up the most space on the plate. Such a large portion of chicken, however, is not necessary. A 6-ounce serving of chicken provides about 53 g of protein. Add to that amount the protein in the bread (3 g), potato (4 g), broccoli (2 g), salad (1 g), and skim milk (8 g), and the total protein intake from one meal alone is 71 g. Because we eat protein throughout the day, no one meal needs to provide all our protein. Instead, the balance of the meal needs to be restructured. Because each component of the meal contains protein, whether from animal or plant sources, portion sizes can shift and still provide plenty of protein. An adequate serving of meat is about the size of a deck of cards or the size of an adult's palm. Notice in Fig. 6.6 how the chicken, now reduced to 3 ounces, is no longer the focus of the plate. All items occupy more equal spaces on the plate. The protein total is still high at 48 g.

Spreading protein intake throughout the food groups allows the objectives of MyPlate to be met. The first plate (see Fig. 6.5) provides the following:

- 1 oz (whole) grains
- 3 cups vegetables
- 0 cups fruit
- 1 cup milk (low-fat or fat-free)
- 6 oz meat and beans
- The second plate (see Fig. 6.6) provides the following:
- 2 oz (whole) grains
- 4 cups vegetables
- ½ cup fruit
- 1 cup milk (low-fat or fat-free)
- 3 oz meat and beans

CULTURAL DIVERSITY AND NUTRITION

Rituals for Animal-Derived Protein

Most religions identify foods with specific holidays and rules regarding consumption. Two predominantly Western religions, Judaism and Islam, have rules regarding the daily preparation and consumption of foods; most of these directions focus on consumption of animal-derived protein foods.

Kashrut: Jewish Dietary Laws

The rules of *kashrut* were presented in the Torah, or bible of the Jewish people. *Kosher* means "fit" and is the concept referring to the Jewish dietary laws. Although most of the rules can be explained on the basis of physical health benefits, the foundation and observance of the restrictions are driven by spiritual health rather than physical. By observing the kosher dietary laws, one is respecting God, oneself, and other Jews. There are about eight laws regarding consumption of animal-derived protein. They are briefly described as follows:

1. Only certain animals may be eaten. Only mammals with cloven hooves that chew the cud may be eaten and their milk consumed; this allows cattle, deer, goats, and sheep to be consumed but not pigs. Birds must also meet specific criteria; acceptable birds (and their eggs) include chickens, ducks, geese, and turkey. In addition, fish must have fins and scales to be consumed; therefore, all shellfish, eel, and catfish are not permitted. Acceptable foods are viewed as coming from "clean" animals, and unacceptable foods are viewed as "unclean."
2. Animals must be slaughtered in a specific manner that is quick and painless and that causes most blood to drain from the carcass.
3. Slaughtered animals must be free of any bruises or diseases to be consumed.
4. Only certain parts of permitted animals may be consumed. Animal blood from any animal and layers of solid fat may not be consumed.
5. Meat must be prepared for consumption in specific procedures. Blood must be completely drained, and cuts of meat must avoid certain nerves and animal parts. Specially trained "kosher" butchers prepare animals foods according to *kashrut*.
6. Meat and dairy are not consumed together. Consequently, separate cooking utensils, plates, and eating utensils are maintained for meat consumption and dairy consumption. Some foods are considered neither meat nor dairy and may be eaten with either category. These foods are called *pareve*.
7. Products from unclean animals may not be consumed. The exception is honey. Although bees may not be consumed, honey is acceptable.
8. Foods are examined for insects and worms that may not be consumed but may be on vegetables, fruits, and grains.

To ensure that these rules are followed, product preparation is supervised by rabbis (spiritual teachers), after which point the product may then display special logos to that effect. Most often it is a "K" that appears on product packaging.

Halal: Islamic Dietary Laws

The Islamic rules of *halal* or permitted foods, presented in the Koran (the bible of Islam), regard food consumption as an aspect of worship. Consequently, eating is viewed as a way to keep one's body healthy. Food should not be consumed excessively and is to be shared with others. All food is permitted unless specifically prohibited. Specific rules concerning foods that may not be consumed include the following:

- Swine (pigs) and birds of prey may not be consumed.
- Animals that are not slaughtered according to specific Muslim procedures may not be consumed. These rules are similar to those of Jewish laws regarding the exact means of slaughter and blood drainage.
- Alcoholic beverages and drugs that affect consciousness, unless required for medicinal purposes, may not be consumed. Coffee and tea, because they contain the stimulant caffeine, are discouraged.

Application to Nursing

In nursing practice, it is valuable to be knowledgeable and thereby respectful of the possible dietary restrictions of clients. Assistance can then be given as to the best dietary pattern to ensure wholesome nutrient intakes and the alternative medications or treatment available. For example, because observant Jews and Muslims do not consume pigs or products derived from pigs, the source of insulin (usually from pigs) may be problematic for Jewish or Muslim patients with diabetes.

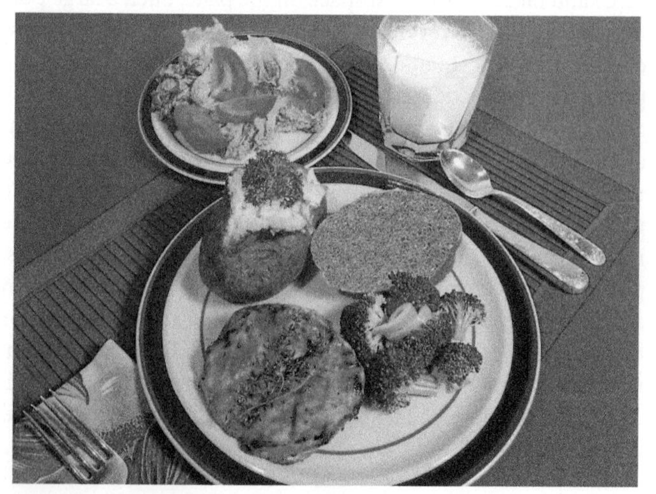

Fig. 6.5 A balanced meal. (From Joanne Scott/Tracy McCalla.)

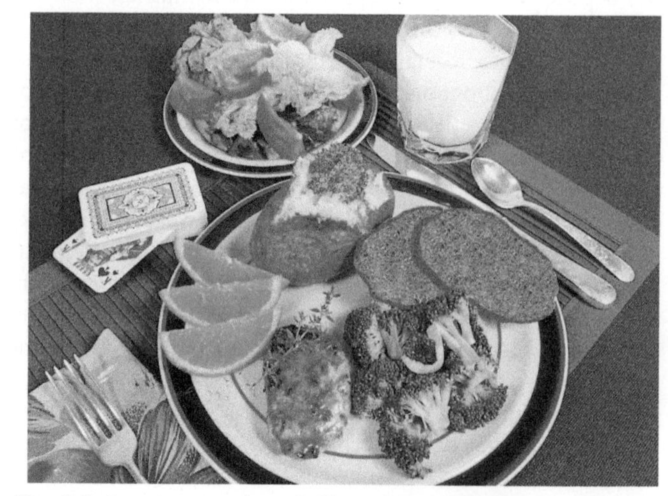

Fig. 6.6 A restructured meal. (From Joanne Scott/Tracy McCalla.)

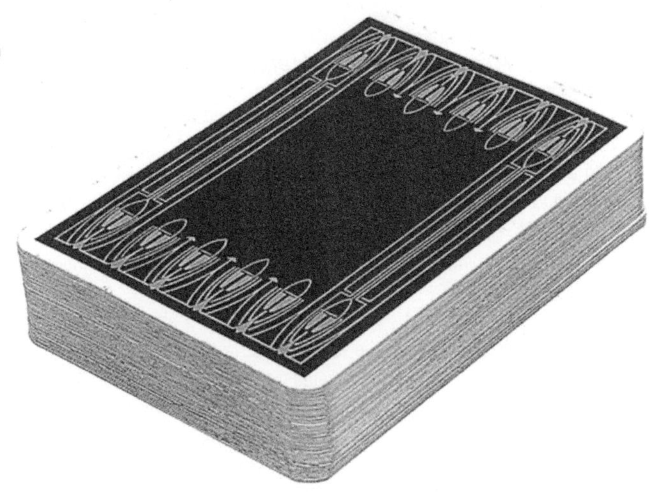

Fig. 6.7 A deck of cards is a simple visual tool to judge the size of a protein food.

The new plate provides more complex carbohydrates from grains, fruits, and vegetables, while still providing sufficient amounts of protein.

Use the concept of the deck of cards and the restructured meal to visually display appropriate animal-protein portion sizes for clients (Fig. 6.7).

PROTEIN AND MALNUTRITION

Malnutrition, the imbalance of nutrient intake, encompasses conditions that range from overconsumption of nutrients to extreme underconsumption. This discussion concerns the conditions related to underconsumption of nutrients, particularly protein. Underconsumption can result in nutrient deficiencies that range from marginal to severe starvation. Marginal deficiencies occur when lower than recommended levels of nutrients are regularly consumed. Although obvious signs of specific nutrient deficiencies may not be visible, the level of wellness and the ability to function at an optimum level are compromised. As the other nutrient categories of vitamins and minerals are studied in Chapters 7 and 8, specific symptoms of deficiencies will be explored.

Starvation has become a catch-all term. Although we may say "I'm starving" when we've missed a meal, our starvation in no way compares with that experienced by those who truly do not have access to sufficient quantities of high-quality food. The technical term for starvation is protein energy malnutrition (PEM). PEM is an umbrella term for malnutrition caused by the lack of protein, of energy, or both.

In young children, PEM can cause permanent disabilities because most brain growth occurs during the early years of life. Extreme PEM results in the conditions marasmus and kwashiorkor (Fig. 6.8). These disorders can be fatal because of decreased resistance to infections; the body, lacking protein, is unable to create sufficient quantities of antibodies to support the immune system. A brief discussion of marasmus and kwashiorkor follows.

Marasmus is malnutrition caused by a lack of sufficient energy (kcal) intake. An individual with marasmus is extremely thin; skin seems to hang off the skeletal bones. Fat stores that normally fill out the skin have been used for energy to maintain minimum body functioning. Muscle mass is also reduced, having also been used for energy, and nutrients are not available to rebuild it. If the condition continues, damage may occur to major organs, such as the heart, lungs, and kidneys. Children experiencing marasmus will not grow. If the condition occurs between 6 and 18 months of age, the time during which the most brain development occurs, permanent brain damage may result.

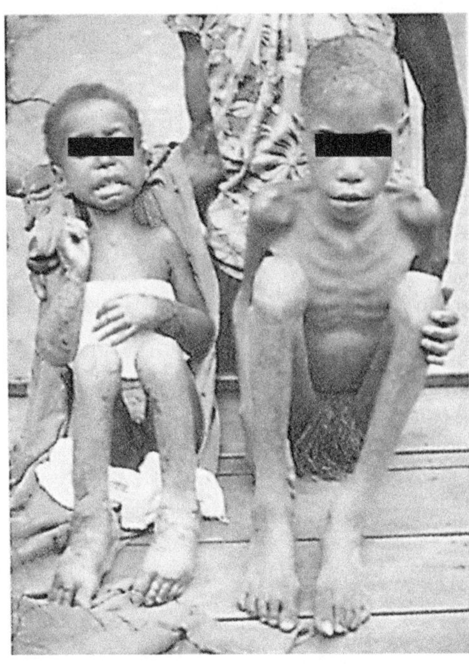

Fig. 6.8 Children suffering from kwashiorkor *(left)* and marasmus *(right)* as a result of inadequate energy intake. (Courtesy Professor R. Hendricksen. In McLaren DS: *A colour atlas and text of diet-related disorders*, ed 2, London, 1992, Mosby Europe Limited.)

In contrast to marasmus, the symptoms of kwashiorkor give the appearance of more than sufficient fat stores in the stomach and face. Kwashiorkor is defined as malnutrition caused by protein deficiency even though adequate energy is consumed. The swollen belly and full cheeks of kwashiorkor are caused by edema (water retention). Edema occurs because protein levels in the body are so low that protein is not available to maintain adequate water balance in the cells, and fluid accumulates unevenly. When adequate nutrition is provided, the fluid is no longer retained. Instead of a full belly and round cheeks, the loss of fat stores becomes apparent, and the skin hangs loosely, similar to marasmus. Without sufficient protein, lipids produced by the liver are unable to leave and thus accumulate there. The liver becomes fatty and unable to function well. An individual with kwashiorkor is apathetic and experiences muscle weakness and poor growth.

Although the extremes of PEM are rare in the United States, health care professionals may encounter patients experiencing nutritional risk from hunger related to lack of access to sufficient quantities of food or malnutrition caused by physiologic stress from injury or illness. Clinical issues related to patient care are discussed in Chapter 11.

Malnutrition Factors

Malnutrition is often caused by several factors that affect food availability. Although poverty tends to be a dominant influence, other forces also affect the development of malnutrition. These include biologic, social, economic, and environmental factors (Box 6.6).

BOX 6.6 Malnutrition Factors

Biologic Factors
- Maternal malnutrition before or during pregnancy and/or lactation
- Infections that may affect nutrient absorption
- Chronic diarrhea as both a cause and an effect of malnutrition
- Toxins such as aflatoxin
- Lack of food, particularly protein

Social Factors
- Ignorance of nutrient needs of children, resulting in inappropriate weaning foods
- Child abuse and neglect
- Eating disorders, particularly anorexia nervosa
- Drug abuse affecting the ability to care for oneself appropriately
- Social isolation of older adults, leading to an inability to purchase and prepare adequate quantities of food
- Alcoholism (kcal from alcohol replace consumption of nutrient-dense foods)
- Wars/civil strife disrupting normal social and food production systems

Economic Factors
- Poverty and socioeconomic status
- Unemployment
- Little education
- Political strife affecting distribution of wealth and land ownership
- Environmental factors
- Polluted water, which reduces food production and directly affects the health of populations
- Famine caused by droughts or crop failures
- Improper farming techniques

Biologic factors affect the ability of the body to use nutrients. Economic effects encompass the ability to purchase food and also consider the structure of a country's economy and access to employment. Environmental factors directly affect the availability of food as related to crop production and food safety. Lack of education, social isolation, and the rippling effects of underemployment seem to be malnutrition factors throughout the world, regardless of the overall wealth of nations. Health and economic support systems provided throughout the life cycle may prevent the development of factors affecting food availability.

Groups at Risk in North America

Most people in North America are well nourished, although growing numbers of homeless individuals living in shelters or other temporary sites are at risk for varying levels of malnutrition. Without access to cooking facilities or the funds to purchase adequate quantities of foods, these individuals are at nutritional risk. In response to this crisis, food pantries and soup kitchens have been established by nonprofit and charitable groups to distribute food and meals (see the *Social Issues* box Hunger All Around: How to Help). Also at risk are the working poor, whose incomes barely cover the basic expenses of housing, utilities, and health care, leaving little for food purchases. Programs providing support services to these populations also can arrange nutrition education on making healthier choices when buying and preparing economical meals. Societal and personal changes may interrupt family ties, causing the loss of recipes and opportunities to share skills of preparation of low-cost, nutritious meals.

SOCIAL ISSUES

Hunger All Around: How to Help

"Finish all that food on your plate. Children around the world are starving." Parents often said this to their children at the dinner table, causing countless numbers of children to try to figure out how finishing their own vegetables would help feed the children in a faraway land. Of course, parents wanted their children not to waste food and to appreciate their good fortune. However, many children probably believed that by finishing their food they were somehow helping those hungry children.

Because of today's technology, we can have no illusions about the plight of others. We get complete, immediate reports of devastation caused by global pandemics (COVID-19), natural climate-related disasters (Australian megafires of 2019–2020), famines (either climate or war-related) and ongoing wars. Reports of hunger among the homeless, older adults, unemployed individuals and even among income earning individuals and families are televised. All of these factors combined may push 265 million people toward severe food insecurity. To respond to these contemporary global events, individuals, communities, and societal groups need to delineate beliefs and goals to create a more aware, sustainable, and resilient social order (Perroni, 2020). If only finishing the food on our plates would help.

Key findings noted in *Not enough to Eat: COVID-19 Deepens America's Hunger Crisis*, a report commissioned by the Food Research & Action Center (FRAC) reveal that:
- More than 1 in 5 Black and Latinx adults with children did not have enough food to eat; this is double reports of white and Asian households during July 2020.
- Families experiencing limited food supplies range from the poorest families to 1 in 4 of those having usual incomes above $50,000 a year.
- Widespread unemployment and/or reduced income because of decreased working hours resulted in limited funds to afford sufficient food supplies.
- 16% of those with a high school diploma or less didn't have enough to eat, compared with only 3% of those with a college degree.

Although these crises are escalating serious food insecurities around the world, they may lead to a humanitarian drive to work together to develop sustainable solutions to these overwhelming situations. (Perroni, 2020)

So, what can we do? Here are some ideas:

As Individuals
- Be well informed. Learn about hunger in your neighborhood. All communities have people who are in need.
- Volunteer to help in a local soup kitchen.
- Create a food drive at holidays; donate foods to a food bank.
- Let local politicians know of your concerns; give a voice to the voiceless. Send an e-mail to local and state officials.

Campus Organizations (Political, Social, and Religious)
- Include a service component in the group's mission.
- Create a food pantry to provide needed food for your campus community. College students experience hunger as well, with limited funds and high expenses.
- Support World Food Day, which is sponsored by the United Nations and other organizations.
- Ask representatives from local antihunger agencies to speak to campus groups.
- Incorporate volunteer time as part of an initiation process or as a commitment of all members of sororities, fraternities, and social clubs.

(Data modified from Food First, Institute for Food and Development Policy: *Hunger at home: The growing epidemic*, Oakland, CA, 2006, Author; Perroni E: *Times of Crisis Demand Counterstories for Change: Food First*, 30 May, 2020. Accessed 14 December, 2020, from: https://foodfirst.org/times-of-crisis-demand-counterstories-for-change/; Schanzenbach DW: *Not Enough to Eat: COVID-19 Deepens America's Hunger Crisis*, Washington, DC, December 2020, Food Research & Action Center. Accessed 14 December, 2020, from: https://frac.org/news/frac-covid-report.)

Older adults also are at risk. Although their nutritional concerns are covered in depth in Chapter 10, consider that the physical and financial limitations of older adults may reduce their ability to purchase and prepare wholesome meals. When these issues are compounded by social isolation, the situation of older adults becomes serious.

Chronic Hunger

Although famines and wars affect the nutritional status of people throughout the world, the population of North America has not experienced these extremes of deprivation. Instead, chronic hunger, defined as a continual experience of undernutrition (not enough food to eat), has become the norm for a subset of our population. This subset is growing as the economies of North America tighten, causing government food and welfare programs to be unable to provide an appropriate safety net to prevent and alleviate chronic hunger. Instead, more individuals and families are faced with a consistent lack of opportunities to improve their standard of living and, most important, their health.

TOWARD A POSITIVE NUTRITION LIFESTYLE: CHAINING

Chaining refers to the linking of two behaviors. If two actions consistently occur together, they often become linked or tied to each other. They become one behavior and a habit. Many of us already practice chaining; unfortunately, the results often have a negative impact on our dietary intake patterns. Frequently eating potato chips while studying can link these two actions—eating chips and studying. The chain requires that whenever studying takes place, chips need to be eaten. Chaining, however, can also be used to improve nutritional status.

Consider the following chains:

- When you eat a sandwich, eat some fruit too. Instead of linking chips and a sandwich (or hoagie, grinder, or sub), this practice links a sandwich to some fruit.
- Have a glass of skim milk with the midday meal regularly to increase calcium intake. Skim milk becomes chained to lunch.
- At home, weigh portions of meat, fish, and poultry. Compare the size of an appropriate portion to the size of a deck of cards. Are they similar? Weigh portions regularly, and consciously compare sizes. Animal protein portion sizes will be linked to the deck of cards, and portion control can be achieved without weighing.

These are just a few chains related to protein consumption. Chaining can be applied to other nutrition and wellness situations of our clients as well.

PERSONAL PERSPECTIVE

More Than Just School Breakfast and Lunch

More than 22 million children participate in the National School Lunch Program and the National School Breakfast Program, receiving free or reduced-price meals. For a number of those children, these meals may be their only food for the day.

But What Happens After School?

When school is over for the day, there is a federal child nutrition program that provides afterschool meals programs that serve wholesome meals and snacks to children in need in a safe, supervised location. Organizations like No Kid Hungry strive to let children, families, and educators take advantage of this program. Over a million children receive afterschool suppers on an average day. The meals may be served at school districts or sponsored by approved government agencies, and private nonprofit organizations located at schools, recreation centers, YMCAs, Boys & Girls Clubs, and other sites where afterschool programs are offered to children.

What About Over the Weekend?

Several organizations, such as Feeding America, have developed BackPack programs that provide nourishing and simple-to-prepare food for children to eat during the weekend. Children are given backpacks filled with foods; the backpacks are an inconspicuous way for the food to be sent home. The Feeding America BackPack Program has, over the past 15 years, distributed food through more than 160 local food banks to over 450,000 children.

During the COVID-19 pandemic when schools were closed and/or learning was hybrid or remote, meals were distributed from school sites, providing nourishment throughout the week, with many programs providing meals for all family members.

- To check out the advocacy efforts of No Kid Hungry organization: www.nokidhungry.org.
- To find a local Feeding America Food Bank that runs a BackPack Program: Food Bank Locator www.feedingamerica.org/find-your-local-foodbank/.
- To locate meals for kids when school is out, use FIND MEALS 4 KIDS Interactive: www.fns.usda.gov/meals4kids

(Data from Feeding America from www.feedingamerica.org/our-work/hunger-relief-programs/backpack-program/. Accessed 15 January, 2021; Food Research & Action Center (FRAC): Facts, The Afterschool Meal Program, February 2019. Accessed 15 January, 2021; No Kid Hungry from https://www.nokidhungry.org/who-we-are/hunger-facts. Accessed 15 January 2021.)

SUMMARY

- Proteins consist of chains of organic compounds composed of carbon, hydrogen, oxygen, and nitrogen called amino acids.
- All proteins are made from 20 amino acids.
- Nonessential amino acids (NEAAs) can be created by the liver.
- Essential amino acids (EAAs) must be consumed in food.
- All amino acids are available to cells through the amino acid pool to allow proteins to be synthesized.
- Complete proteins contain all nine EAAs, whereas incomplete proteins lack one or more EAAs.
- During digestion, food protein is broken down to amino acids. Once absorbed, the amino acids circulate in the blood to build new proteins.
- The new proteins perform numerous functions, including growth and maintenance, creation of essential substances, immune system response, fluid regulation, acid–base balance, and transportation of nutrients and other substances in the body.
- Chronic hunger and malnutrition, such as **protein energy malnutrition** (marasmus and kwashiorkor), continue to be of global concern.

THE NURSING APPROACH

Clinical Judgment and Next-Generation NCLEX® Examination-Style Questions

Case Study 1

Protein (Wound Healing)

Roy, a 69-year-old homeless male, came to a neighborhood mobile van health clinic with a leg ulcer. Roy said the ulcer had been there for several months, and it had gradually gotten bigger. He said he ate what he could find on the street and sometimes went to the city food center for a hot meal. The nurse cleaned Roy's leg ulcer, and the physician ordered laboratory tests.

Assessment/Recognize Cues

Subjective (from patient statements):

- Minimal intake of meat, eggs, or other protein foods
- Fatigue and weakness
- Objective (from physical examination):
- Height 6′2″, weight 140 pounds
- Muscle atrophy in extremities bilaterally
- Decreased muscle strength
- Poor skin turgor
- Hair is dull and thin
- Slight ankle edema bilaterally
- Left lower leg ulcer irregular in shape, 2cm deep, 4cm in diameter, rolled edges, reddened base, with moderate amount of foul drainage
- Serum albumin 2.7 g/dL (norm 3.4–4.8 g/dL)

Diagnoses (Nursing)/Analyze Cues

1. Weight loss related to lack of food availability, as evidenced by minimal intake of protein foods, 74% ideal body weight (IBW), albumin 2.7 g/dL, delayed healing of lower left leg ulcer
2. Pressure ulcer related to inadequate nutrition, as evidence by left lower leg ulcer, present for several months and increasing in size
3. Potential for infection related to impaired skin integrity

Planning/Prioritize Hypotheses

Patient Outcomes

Short term (at the end of this visit):

- Roy will identify foods high in protein, appropriate portion sizes (such as a deck of cards), and state the importance of protein in healing wounds.
- Roy will verbalize intention to eat high-protein foods at least once each day.
- Roy will demonstrate how to clean and dress his wound.
- He will agree to come to clinic for follow-up twice a week.

Long term (after 2 months):

- Roy will report he ate several appropriate portions of high-protein foods each day.
- Roy's ulcer will heal within 2 months.
- He will gain 4 pounds in 2 months.

Nursing Interventions/Generate Solutions

1. Teach Roy about the importance of protein in wound healing.
2. Discuss resources for obtaining high-protein food.
3. Provide wound care as ordered by the physician.

Implementation/Take Action

1. Discussed with Roy the role of protein in wound healing.
   Protein is needed for tissue repair and resistance to infection. Sufficient kcal are needed to spare use of proteins for energy.
2. Discussed dietary sources of protein.
   Soy and foods from animals contain complete proteins. Plant foods must be combined to provide complete proteins.
3. Supplied Roy with cans of high-protein and vitamin supplements at each clinic visit.
   Adequate protein, calories, water, and vitamins are needed for tissue repair. Vitamins A and C and zinc are particularly helpful in wound healing. Vitamin C is needed for collagen formation. Vitamin A is an antioxidant and an important helper in wound healing. Zinc increases tensile strength of the healing wound.
4. Taught Roy how to clean wound with soap and water, apply an antibiotic ointment to wound base, cover the wound with gauze, and wrap it with a reusable wrap bandage. Instructed him to change the dressing daily or whenever drainage is visible.
   Keeping the wound clean, applying antibiotic ointment, and maintaining the dressing help to prevent infection. The gauze helps absorb the drainage, and the wrap bandage can be washed and reused because the client has limited funds.
5. Encouraged Roy to move into a homeless shelter affiliated with the clinic until the leg ulcer heals.
   A shelter can provide cleanliness, rest, and nutritious food, an environment conducive to healing.
6. Encouraged Roy to eat at least one meal per day in the shelter.
   Nutritious food can help an individual heal wounds and regain weight.

Continued

THE NURSING APPROACH—cont'd

Evaluation/Evaluate Outcomes

Short term (at the end of the first visit):

- Roy identified several foods high in protein and thanked the nurse for the supplements to help his ulcer heal.
- He said he would try to eat at least one meal per day at the shelter.
- Roy said he would return to the clinic twice a week for follow-up.
- Short-term goal met.

Long term (in 1 month):

- Roy said he had eaten at least one meal each day at the shelter on most of the days and was thinking about moving to the shelter.
- His leg ulcer measured 2 cm in diameter and 1 cm deep.
- He had gained 2 pounds.
- Long-term goal partially met.

Discussion Questions

1. What resources are available in your community to help the homeless and hungry?
2. If Roy has little money for food, what should he buy? Consider nutrient density, food needed, and cost.

Case Study 2

At a medical clinic, a nurse is caring for a female client who says she is a committed vegetarian. The nurse is aware of what potential nutrition concerns of a vegetarian dietary pattern?

Highlight the correct potential nutrition concerns of a vegetarian dietary pattern. Select all that may apply.

1. Vitamin D deficiency
2. Large amounts of zinc
3. Replaces meat with a lot of cheese
4. Focuses on increased amount of vitamin B_{12}
5. Lacks intake of milk and fortified milk replacements.
6. Contains high levels of calcium
7. Limits exposure to the sun
8. Lacks omega-3 fatty acids

APPLYING CONTENT KNOWLEDGE

Karen and her husband, Roger, want to reduce their intake of fat and increase their fiber intake. Both grew up in families that prided themselves as being the "meat and potatoes" type. Suggest three strategies they could adopt to restructure their dinner plates to add plant-based meals and/or alternative sources of protein to meet MyPlate goals.

WEBSITES OF INTEREST

Nutrition.gov
www.nutrition.gov
Functions as an entry for consumers to trustworthy food and nutrition information from all federal websites and agencies.

Physicians Committee for Responsible Medicine
www.pcrm.org
A nonprofit research and advocacy organization endorsing plant-based dietary patterns, preventive medicine and alternatives to animal research while encouraging "higher standards of ethics and effectiveness in research."

National Academy of Medicine
nam.edu/
Offers impartial and respected recommendations based on evidence from studies conducted for the government and independent organizations regarding health decisions affecting the nation. Functions as an independent, nonprofit organization.

REFERENCES

Melinda, V., Craig, W., & Levin, S. (2016). Position of the academy of nutrition and dietetics: vegetarian diets. *Journal of the Academy of Nutrition and Dietetics, 116*, 1970–1980.

Matthews. D. E. (2014). Proteins and amino acids. In C. A. Ross (Ed.), *Modern nutrition in health and disease* (11th ed.). Philadelphia: Lippincott Williams & Wilkins.

National Research Council. (2006). *Dietary reference intakes: the essential guide to nutrient requirements*. Washington, DC: The National Academies Press.

Thomas, D. R., Erdman, K. A., & Burke, L. M. (2016). Position of the academy of nutrition and dietetics, dietitians of canada, and the american college of sports medicine: nutrition and athletic performance: vegetarian diets. *Journal of the American Dietetic Association, 116*, 501–528.

7

Vitamins

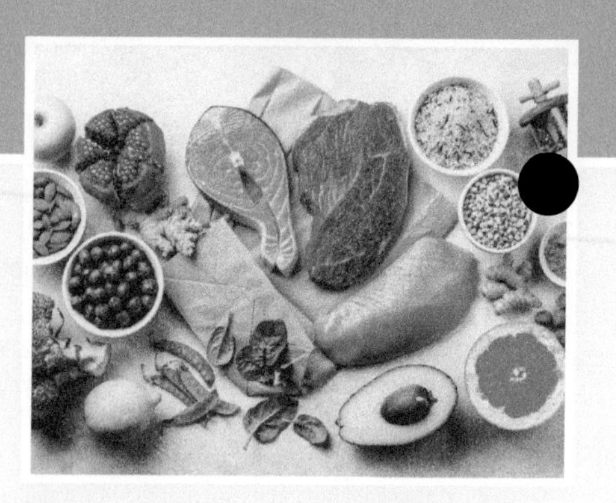

Knowledge of the existence of vitamins is recent; the discovery of vitamins slowly evolved, beginning in the early part of the twentieth century.

http://evolve.elsevier.com/GRODNER/FOUNDATIONS

LEARNING OBJECTIVES

- Define vitamins.
- Describe the differences between water-soluble and fat-soluble vitamins.
- List the water-soluble vitamins and their functions.
- List the fat-soluble vitamins and their functions.
- Discuss how water-soluble and fat-soluble vitamins are absorbed.
- Explain the level of risk from consuming an excess of water-soluble vitamins and fat-soluble vitamins from foods and from supplements.

ROLE IN WELLNESS

Vitamins seem to have a magical aura. Take enough and you will have more energy and be healthier, smarter, and even better looking. If only it were that easy. Although vitamins are essential for life, they are only one of many factors required for wellness.

Knowledge of the existence of vitamins is recent; the discovery of vitamins slowly evolved, beginning in the early part of the twentieth century. The focus of research was to discover the amounts of vitamins needed to prevent deficiency symptoms and diseases that undermine the health and well-being of populations throughout the world.

The scientific view of vitamins, however, is in flux. Additional effects of vitamin use are surfacing as more is learned about the functions of vitamins as antioxidants and hormone-like substances. Some vitamins and related substances such as carotenoids may reduce the risk for development of certain chronic diseases. New information points to relationships between consuming foods high in vitamins and a lower incidence of certain diseases.

The Dietary Reference Intake (DRI) considers the concern of providing nutrient requirements necessary to prevent deficiencies and toxicity from overdoses and accounting for the value of nutrient intake as a means of reducing disease risk (National Research Council [NRC], 2006). Recommendations within the DRI documents include the use of fortified foods or supplements for particular nutrients, such as folic acid for women of childbearing age, to ensure proper neural tube formation of the fetus during pregnancy.

Vitamins are organic molecules required in very small amounts for cellular metabolism. Each vitamin performs a specific metabolic function. Vitamins, except for vitamin D, are not synthesized by our bodies and thus are essential nutrients that must be provided through dietary intake (see the *Personal Perspectives* box A Candy Bar or an Apple: Healthy Corner Store Initiative). Vitamin D is the only vitamin created by the human body.

Vitamins are vital to life and therefore to the physical, intellectual, emotional, social, spiritual, and environmental dimensions of health. Vitamins are essential nutrients without which the body cannot continue functioning within the physical dimension. Dietary recommendations to eat at least five fruits and vegetables per day throughout the life span are made to reduce the risk of diet-related diseases in the future. Intellectual health skills are used to envision future benefits that accrue from food choices today. Deficiencies of several B vitamins can produce irritability, confusion, and paranoia, thereby affecting the emotional health dimension. Older adults may be at risk for deficiencies because of their inability to get to the store to buy fruits and vegetables; the physical health of older adults may depend on their social health in relation to neighbors who may provide assistance with shopping needs. Sometimes following religious teachings may jeopardize health, as noted by the development of rickets, the vitamin D deficiency disorder, among some Black children of families following the dietary and dress customs of the Islamic faith. Spiritual health is interdependent with the other dimensions of health. Because the best sources of vitamins are a variety of foods, the environmental health

PERSONAL PERSPECTIVES

A Candy Bar or an Apple: Healthy Corner Store Initiative

The student runs out the door at the end of the school day and goes straight to the nearest corner store to buy snacks. Will they choose a candy bar or an apple? Wait, there are no fresh apples in the corner store. Candy bar it is!

An innovative program approaches this situation from several determinants of food choice. Instead of just teaching children about why they should choose apples, this program aims to make that apple easily available in their built environment. As part of the Childhood Obesity Declines Project in Philadelphia, the Food Trust developed and continues to implement the Healthy Corner Store Initiative, grant-funded by the Robert Wood Johnson Foundation (RWJF). The purpose of the program is to improve healthy food choices in convenience stores (often on street corners of large cities) by modifying the built environment (the convenience stores) to better meet health goals.

The stores are selected by their location near schools in low-income neighborhoods. Store owners are provided business training and technical assistance as to how to modify their inventories to include healthy food items, while still making a profit. This training includes procuring such products, marketing (support for installing small shelving and refrigeration), displaying (signage in several languages), and pricing the healthy food merchandise. Participating owners agree to offer a larger healthy food selection, including fruits, vegetables, low-fat dairy, lean proteins, and whole-grain products. Incentives for participation are provided for the store owners as well as for their customers. More than 600 corner stores within the Philadelphia area are participating.

The stores have become not only a means to provide healthy foods for the children, but also hosts for adult in-store nutrition education lessons and even health screenings. Thus the "corner stores" validate the goals of the nutrition and health curriculum offered in schools by providing environments to support those goals.

Today, when the student runs out the door at the end of the school day and goes straight to the nearest corner store to buy snacks, will they choose an apple, a banana, or a snack pack of carrots and hummus?

(Data from ICF Macro: *Signs of progress in childhood obesity declines: Site summary report*, Philadelphia, 2015, Robert Wood Johnson Foundation. Updated June 2016. Accessed 17 December, 2020, from http://www.nccor.org/downloads/CODP_Site%20Summary%20Report_Philadelphia_public_clean1.pdf; The Food Trust: *Philadelphia's Healthy Corner Stores Initiative*. Philadelphia, 2012, Author. Accessed 17 December, 2020, from hcsi-y2report-final.original.pdf (thefoodtrust.org).)

dimension includes having adequate access to grocery stores and the financial means to purchase wholesome foods.

As vitamins are discussed, note that some are referred to by specific names or by letters and numbers. Each vitamin has a history that affects how we refer to it today. In 1929 Henrik Dam in Copenhagen, Denmark, discovered vitamin K. It was the only substance capable of halting a hemorrhagic disease in which blood does not coagulate. Dam named the vitamin *K* for the Danish word koagulation.

In another case, several B vitamins were isolated into the same test tube labeled *B*, and we therefore have vitamins numbered B_1, B_2, and B_3. In the 1970s the science community decreed that all vitamins should be called by their formal biochemical titles. The public and many health professionals still refer to the simpler letter and number names for vitamins. Both the formal and informal names are used in this chapter.

This chapter lists vitamin DRIs. Because *DRI* is an umbrella term that includes recommended dietary allowance (RDA), adequate intake (AI), and tolerable upper intake level (UL), applicable standards will be identified. Because RDAs and AIs differ with age, gender, and physiologic need, only those for men and women aged 19 to 30 years are included for each vitamin, unless special circumstances surrounding the need for a vitamin warrant discussion. The DRI tables can be accessed from www.nal.usda.gov/fnic/dietary-reference-intakes.

A primary deficiency of a vitamin occurs when the vitamin is not consumed in sufficient amounts to meet physiologic needs. A secondary deficiency develops when absorption is impaired or excess excretion occurs, limiting bioavailability. Most deficiencies are detected through clinical and biochemical assessment; specific diagnostic and laboratory procedures are beyond the scope of this text, and their descriptions are available elsewhere (Pagana et al., 2016).

Although vitamin deficiencies are no longer common among Americans, subgroups are at risk. Because of their greater needs, pregnant women are often at risk for marginal deficiencies of essential vitamins. Older adults may also be at risk because of decreased absorptive ability and limited economic and physical resources affecting food availability. Poverty has an overwhelming negative effect on the nutritional status of children and adults. Chronic alcohol and drug abuse not only alters psychologic and mental capacities, but also limits the body's ability to absorb and use essential vitamins.

Health professionals can also consider other special circumstances that may initiate vitamin deficiencies. Individuals dealing with long-term chronic disorders that affect the total body response, such as acquired immunodeficiency syndrome (AIDS) and liver and kidney disorders, have special vitamin concerns because the metabolic processes of the body may be compromised by these disorders and by the medications prescribed. Deficiencies have been documented that were possibly caused by the effects of cancer treatment, use of multiple alternative therapies, and lifestyle behaviors. These deficiencies were at first misdiagnosed because vitamin deficiencies were no longer thought to occur (Fain et al., 1998; Gessner et al., 1997; Wood et al., 1998).

Toxicities of vitamins rarely occur naturally from food consumption. Instead, inappropriate use of supplements may be toxic to our bodies. Vitamins have been studied for their physiologic effect or because of the basic need for health maintenance (Box 7.1). The recommended levels reflect this knowledge. Use of vitamin supplements at megadose levels is equivalent to a pharmacologic effect, with potential druglike physical responses. Some vitamins have ULs; for others, a megadose (i.e., 10 times the RDA for a specific nutrient) of a vitamin is considered the highest amount of the nutrient that will not cause adverse health effects. Because most vitamins have not been studied to determine function and safety at these megadose levels, their extensive use without guidance can be problematic.

BOX 7.1 Considering Vitamins and Minerals Through Function

Vitamins and minerals are discussed as two separate nutrient categories in Chapters 7 and 8. Although each is discussed individually, they are not grouped on the basis of their functions in the body. Following are the vitamins and minerals required for the specific body functions blood health, bone health, energy metabolism, and fluid and electrolyte balance. Additional functions of individual vitamins and minerals may be found in Tables 7.3, 7.6, 8.3, and 8.4.

Blood Health

Blood is *the* body fluid, supplying tissues with oxygen, nutrients, and energy through circulation within the cardiovascular system. It is composed of water, red and white blood cells, oxygen, nutrients, and other formed substances. Always moving, blood gathers and distributes nutrients and oxygen to all cells and disposes of waste products. Deficiency of any of these nutrients will affect overall blood health. Only the blood-related functions of the vitamins and minerals are listed.

Vitamin*	Function
Cobalamin (B_{12})	Transport/storage of folate needed for heme and cell formation and other functions
Folate (folic acid, folacin, pteroylglutamic acid [PGA])	Coenzyme metabolism (synthesis of amino acid, heme, deoxyribonucleic acid [DNA], ribonucleic acid [RNA]) and other functions
Pyridoxine (B_6)	Hemoglobin synthesis and other functions
Vitamin K Active form: menaquinones	Cofactor in synthesis of blood-clotting factors; protein formation

Mineral†	Function
Iron	Distributes oxygen in hemoglobin and myoglobin
Zinc	Cofactor for more than 200 enzymes, including enzymes to make heme in hemoglobin, genetic material, and proteins
Copper	Helps with iron use

Bone Health

As living tissue, bone requires nutrients to maintain cellular structure. Blood circulates through bone capillaries, delivering nutrients while removing waste materials no longer needed by cells. Hormones regulate the use of minerals either for storage and structural purposes in bone or for controlling body processes. Specific vitamins and minerals are indispensable for these functions to occur.

Vitamin*	Function
Vitamin D Precursor: 7-dehydrocholesterol Active form: cholecalciferol	Bone mineralization
Vitamin K Active form: menaquinones	Protein formation for bone mineralization; cofactor for blood clotting factors
Vitamin A Precursors: carotenoids Preformed vitamin: retinoids	Bone growth; maintains epithelial cells; regulation of gene expression

Mineral†	Function
Calcium	Bone and tooth formation
Phosphorus	Bone and tooth formation (component of hydroxyapatite)
Magnesium	Bone structure
Fluoride	Bone and tooth formation; increases stability of bone

Energy Metabolism

To metabolize carbohydrates, lipids, and protein for energy and other needs, the body depends on many nutrients to support the process, create new cells, and implement various related functions.

Vitamin(s)*	Function
Thiamin (B_1)	Coenzyme energy metabolism; muscle nerve action
Riboflavin (B_2)	Coenzyme energy metabolism
Niacin (B_3) (nicotinic acid and niacinamide) Precursor: tryptophan	Cofactor to enzymes involved in energy metabolism; glycolysis and tricarboxylic acid (TCA) cycle synthesis
Pyridoxine (B_6)	Forms coenzyme pyridoxal phosphate (PLP) for energy metabolism
Folate (folic acid, folacin, pteroylglutamic acid [PGA])	Coenzyme metabolism (synthesis of amino acid, heme, deoxyribonucleic acid [DNA], ribonucleic acid [RNA])
Cobalamin (B_{12})	Metabolism of fatty acids/amino acids
Pantothenic acid	Part of coenzyme A
Biotin	Metabolism of carbohydrate, fat, and protein

Mineral(s)†	Function
Iodine	Thyroxine synthesis (thyroid hormone) regulates growth and development; basal metabolic rate (BMR) regulation
Chromium	Carbohydrate metabolism, part of glucose tolerance factor
Phosphorus	Energy metabolism (enzymes)
Sulfur	Component of protein structures
Iron	Distributes oxygen in hemoglobin and myoglobin
Zinc	Carbohydrate metabolism (insulin function); cofactor to more than 200 enzymes

Fluid and Electrolyte Balance

Life systems depend on fluid and electrolyte balance within the body. Electrolytes consist of mineral salts that maintain cellular fluid balance. The acid–base balance of body fluids is buffered by other minerals.

Mineral†	Function
Sodium	Major extracellular electrolyte for fluid regulation; body fluid levels; acid-base balance; nerve impulse and contraction; blood pressure/volume
Potassium	With sodium and chloride, major intracellular electrolyte for fluid regulation; muscle function
Chloride	Acid–base balance
Phosphorus	Acid–base balance

*See text for additional information on vitamins.
†See Chapter 8 for additional information on minerals.

VITAMIN CATEGORIES

Vitamins are divided into two categories on the basis of their solubility in solutions. Water-soluble vitamins dissolve or disperse in water; they are the B complex vitamins (thiamin, riboflavin, niacin, pyridoxine, folate, vitamin B12, biotin, and pantothenic acid), choline, and vitamin C. Fat-soluble vitamins dissolve in fatty tissues or substances; they are vitamins A, D, E, and K.

Solubility characteristics affect how vitamins are absorbed and transported in the body. Water-soluble vitamins are easily absorbed in the small intestine and then pass into the bloodstream for circulation throughout the body. Fat-soluble vitamins follow the more complicated route of other fat-containing substances; bile is required for their absorption from the small intestine. Fat malabsorption problems may also lead to potential deficiencies of fat-soluble vitamins.

The water solubility of the B vitamins and vitamin C allows for minimal storage of any excess vitamin consumed; tissues may be saturated with these vitamins, but they usually are not stored. Deficiencies can develop quickly—within weeks—so we need to consume these vitamins on a daily basis. Excesses are generally not toxic and are simply excreted in urine. However, damage may result if vitamin levels are high over the long term because of supplementation.

If we consume more than the daily requirement of a fat-soluble vitamin, our bodies store the excess rather than excrete it (Box 7.2). The DRIs for fat-soluble vitamins consider this storage capacity. Although storage is expected in organs such as the liver and spleen, other fatty tissues in the body can also retain excessive amounts of fat-soluble vitamins. Overloading the storage capabilities can be toxic and produce illness; toxicity comes rarely from excessive dietary intake but rather from improper use of vitamin supplements.

FOOD SOURCES

Vitamins are in almost all foods, yet no one food group is a good source of all vitamins. Fresh fruits and vegetables are particularly rich sources. Others are legumes, whole grains, and animal foods—meat, fish, poultry, eggs, and dairy products. Even the almost pure fats of vegetable oils and butter provide vitamins E and A, respectively. Although this does not mean we should consume these products for their vitamin content, it does mean we have a wide range of foods from which to choose for our vitamin nutrition.

It is always best to consume vitamins from food sources. Although synthetic forms of vitamins will perform vitamin functions, there may be other factors in foods that provide benefits. For instance, broccoli and other cruciferous vegetables contain a wide variety of chemicals, including sulforaphane, which is a phytochemical (Box 7.3). Phytochemicals are nonnutritive substances in plant-based foods that appear to have disease-fighting properties. Sulforaphane appears to block the growth of tumors in animals. Broccoli, along with onions and grapes, also contains flavonoids, which seems to reduce the risk of cardiovascular disease (CVD) and cancer, while having an antiinflammatory effect (Rodriguez-Casado, 2016).

WATER-SOLUBLE VITAMINS

Thiamin (B_1)

For centuries a mysterious disease afflicted people of all ages and status throughout Asia. The disease so wasted muscles that Thai sufferers who tried to stand would cry out, "*Beri, beri*," meaning "I can't! I can't!" This phrase became the name of a serious disease, beriberi, caused by thiamin deficiency. In the 1890s it was discovered that beriberi resulted from consumption of hulled (white) rice and that eating unhulled (brown) rice prevented or cured it. Later, researchers found that the thiamin in the hulls of whole grains prevents or cures beriberi.

Function

The main function of thiamin is to serve as a coenzyme, a substance that activates an enzyme, in energy metabolism; it also has a role in nerve functioning related to muscle actions.

Recommended Intake and Sources

The RDA for thiamin is 1.2 mg for men and 1.1 mg for women. The amount of thiamin required increases as the metabolic rate rises. Those engaged in rigorous physical activity burn more energy, so they require more thiamin.

Lean pork, whole or enriched grains and flours, legumes, seeds, and nuts are good sources of thiamin. Because it is a water-soluble vitamin, some thiamin can be lost in food processing or when foods are cooked at home. Thiamin may be leached into cooking fluid or destroyed by heat. Generally, however, most of us consume sufficient amounts of thiamin.

Deficiency

Thiamin deficiency alters the nervous, muscular, gastrointestinal (GI), and cardiovascular systems. In beriberi a severe chronic deficiency results, characterized by ataxia (muscle weakness and loss of coordination), pain, anorexia, mental disorientation, and tachycardia (rapid beating of the heart). Wet beriberi manifests as edema, affecting cardiac function by weakening the heart muscle and vascular system. Dry beriberi affects the nervous system, producing paralysis and extreme muscle wasting. Marginal deficiencies may occur, producing psychological disturbances, recurrent headaches, extreme tiredness, and irritability (Bemeur & Butterworth, 2014).

Beriberi still occurs in areas of the world, such as Asia, where the staple food is highly polished rice, which is low in thiamin. The practice of repeatedly washing the milled rice results in further loss of thiamin. Very high intakes of raw fish can also produce beriberi. Raw fish naturally contains an enzyme, thiaminase, that destroys thiamin. The presence of this enzyme does not affect those of us who occasionally enjoy sushi or sashimi, Japanese specialties of raw fish.

In the United States, enrichment of refined flour has virtually eliminated thiamin deficiency. However, thiamin deficiency may develop in people who are chronic alcohol users because of decreased food intake and reduced intestinal absorption coupled with an additional need for thiamin by the liver to detoxify alcohol (see the *Cultural Diversity and Nutrition* box Cuban Crisis).

BOX 7.2 MyPlate: Fruits

The health benefits of eating fruits overlap with those of eating vegetables. Both the fruit and vegetable categories of MyPlate provide rich sources of vitamins and are valuable components of an overall healthy diet, providing nutrients essential for the health and maintenance of our bodies (see also Box 8.5). Health benefits of eating fruits and vegetables as part of an overall healthy diet include reduced risk for stroke, coronary artery disease, and T2D mellitus; protection against some cancers (mouth, stomach, colorectal); and, as an excellent source of fiber, possible decreased risk of several chronic diet-related disorders. The recommendation is to eat at least 2 cups of fruits every day.

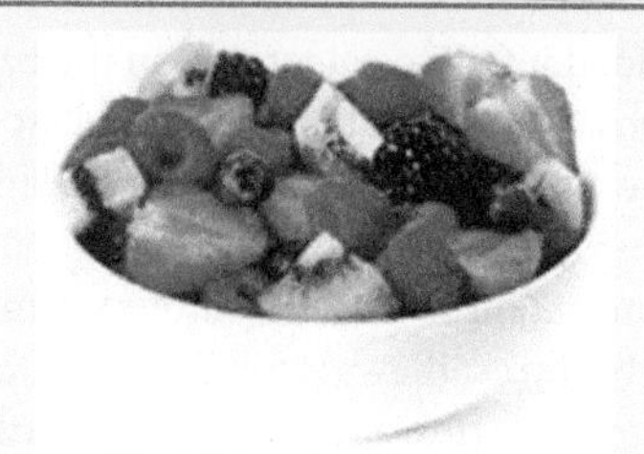

What Counts as a Cup of Fruit?

In general, 1 cup of fruit or 100% fruit juice, or ½ cup of dried fruit can be considered 1 cup from the fruit group. The specific amounts listed in the following table count as 1 cup of fruit (in some cases equivalents for ½ cup are also shown) toward your daily recommended intake.

Fruit	Amount That Counts as 1 Cup of Fruit	Amount That Counts as ½ Cup of Fruit
Apple	3¼ large (3¼-inch diameter)	½ cup sliced or chopped, raw or cooked
	1 small (2½-inch diameter)	
	1 cup sliced or chopped, raw or cooked	
Applesauce	1 cup	1 snack container (4 oz)
Banana	1 cup sliced	1 small (less than 6 inches long)
	1 large (8–9 inches long)	
Cantaloupe	1 cup diced or melon balls	1 medium wedge (⅛ of a medium melon)
Grapes	1 cup whole or cut-up grapes	
	32 seedless grapes	16 seedless grapes
Grapefruit	1 medium (4-inch diameter)	½ medium (4-inch diameter)
	1 cup sections	
Mixed fruit (fruit cocktail)	1 cup diced or sliced, raw or canned, drained	1 snack container (4 oz), drained = ⅜ cup
Orange	1 large (3¹⁄₁₆-inch diameter)	1 small (2⅜-inch diameter)
	1 cup sections	
Orange, mandarin	1 cup canned, drained	
Peach	1 large (2¾-inch diameter)	1 small (2-inch diameter)
	1 cup sliced or diced; raw, cooked, or canned; drained	1 snack container (4 oz), drained = ⅜ cup
	2 halves canned	
Pear	1 medium (2½ per lb)	
	1 cup sliced or diced; raw, cooked, or canned; drained	1 snack container (4 oz), drained = ⅜ cup
Pineapple	1 cup chunks; sliced or crushed; raw, cooked, or canned; drained 1 cup sliced, raw or cooked	1 snack container (4 oz), drained = ⅜ cup
Plum	3 medium or 2 large	1 large
Strawberries	Approximately 8 large	
	1 cup whole, halved, or sliced; fresh or frozen	½ cup whole, halved, or sliced
Watermelon	1 small wedge (1 inch thick)	6 melon balls
	1 cup diced or balls	
Dried fruit (raisins, prunes, apricots, etc.)	½ cup dried fruit is equivalent to 1 cup fruit (½ cup raisins, ½ cup prunes, ½ cup dried apricots)	¼ cup dried fruit is equivalent to ½ cup fruit (1 small box raisins [1½ oz])
100% fruit juice (orange, apple, grape, grapefruit, etc.)	1 cup	½ cup

Modified from U.S. Department of Agriculture, Center for Nutrition and Promotion: *ChooseMyPlate.gov: What counts as a cup of fruit?* Accessed 19 December, 2020, from www.choosemyplate.gov/eathealthy/fruits.

A severe deficiency of thiamin may cause a cerebral form of beriberi called Wernicke-Korsakoff syndrome. It is the most common disorder of the central nervous system, being the neuropsychiatric effect of chronic excessive alcohol intake on nutritional status. Individuals with severe GI disease, those with human immunodeficiency virus (HIV), and those receiving improper parenteral glucose solutions are also at risk for this syndrome (Bemeur & Butterworth, 2014). The effects of this thiamin deficiency syndrome may cause the loss of memory, extreme mental confusion, and ataxia exhibited by people with chronic excessive alcohol ingestion. Clinically, care must be taken when a malnourished person is given parenteral fluids containing dextrose. Parenteral fluids should contain a mix of B vitamins, otherwise the marginal thiamin levels of nutritionally

BOX 7.3 Phytochemicals and Functional Foods: The Value of Food

Nutrition tends to focus on the nutrients found in foods that are required for the health and well-being of the human body. Other food components exist that may have other health benefits but do not qualify as a nutrient.

Phytochemicals are nonnutritive substances in plant-based foods that appear to have disease-fighting properties. The health-promoting value of these substances is best obtained by eating a diverse assortment of vegetables, fruits, legumes, grains, and seeds. Green tea, soy, and licorice also contain phytochemicals with healthful qualities. *Functional foods* provide physiologic health benefits beyond the nutrients they contain. This includes whole foods as well as foods fortified, enriched, or enhanced to provide additional nutritional and health benefits.

Phytochemicals and functional foods are of great interest because they may assist in preventing or treating chronic diseases such as diabetes, coronary artery disease, cancer, and hypertension. Even osteoporosis, arthritis, and neural tube defects may be reduced by adequate consumption of these substances. Onions and garlic not only taste good but also contain allylic sulfides—phytochemicals—that improve immune function, enhance excretion of cancer-inducing substances, decrease blood cholesterol levels, and reduce spread of tumor cells—quite a long list of benefits for foods that taste so good. Tomatoes provide lycopene, which appears to have the ability to limit the spread of cancer cells. Consequently, consumption of cooked tomatoes has been related to a decreased risk of certain cancers. Soy contains isoflavones, which also decrease blood cholesterol levels and flavonoids that may reduce menopausal symptoms.

A number of products already use soy-derived ingredients, and others are in development. Consumers can gain health benefits while consuming familiar foods that have added soy ingredients. The availability of other functional food products continues to expand. Factors influencing this expansion consist of increasing health care costs, aging population, changing food regulations; increasing sense of self-efficacy and health care autonomy; and enhancing personal health among the general population.

Perhaps a significant means of disease prevention has always been available to us: consumption of adequate amounts of whole foods such as fruits and vegetables, along with less processed grains and legumes, possibly topped off with a few cups of green tea.

Data from Crowe KM, Francis C: Academy of Nutrition and Dietetics: Position of the Academy of Nutrition and Dietetics: Functional foods, *Acad Nutr Diet* 113:1096–1103, 2013; Rodriguez-Casado A: The potential of fruits and vegetables phytochemicals: Notable examples, *Crit Rev Food Sci Nutr* 56(7):1097–1107, 2016.

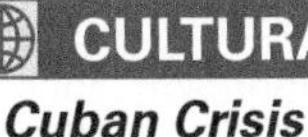

CULTURAL DIVERSITY AND NUTRITION

Cuban Crisis

In the spring of 1993, a harsh economy and natural disasters played havoc with Cuba's food supply. The breakup of the Soviet Union dissipated a valuable trade network for Cuba. This event, combined with the devastating effects of a tropical storm, severely limited the variety of foods available. The consequence? A disease resulting in vision loss and a numbness caused by nerve damage spread primarily among men. The *New York Times* headlines were startling: "26,000 Cubans Partly Blinded."

There is speculation that the epidemic was caused by nutritional deficiencies of thiamin and/or folate. These deficits were exacerbated by consumption of home-brewed rum. Thiamin was required to detoxify the alcohol from the rum consumption, further decreasing the thiamin available for body functions. Folate levels declined as supplies of folate-containing foods diminished. Increased reliance on naturally available foods, such as cassava root, and the popularity of cigarettes among 95% of Cuban men further affected folate availability. Both cassava root and cigarettes are high in cyanide, the processing of which uses up folate stores in the body. The epidemic was eventually brought under control when the Cuban government distributed vitamin supplements to provide the missing nutrients.

A follow-up epidemiologic study revealed that the Cuban male population is still at risk for vitamin B deficiencies, suggesting the need to continue recommendation of preventive vitamin supplementation and increased consumption of fruits and vegetables containing an assortment of B vitamins.

Application to Nursing

Unusual circumstances may precipitate unexpected conditions. We often expect disorders to be the result of new variations of bacteria or viruses, but sometimes simple deficiencies may be the cause. Note that this chapter also discusses instances of unexpectedly occurring rickets (vitamin D deficiency disorder) and pellagra (niacin deficiency disorder). All factors affecting health should be considered in the determination of the true cause of symptoms.

(Data from Altman LK: 26,000 Cubans partly blinded; cause is unclear, *New York Times*, 21 May, 1993, A7; Arnaud J, et al: Vitamin B intake and status in healthy Havanan men, 2 years after the Cuban neuropathy epidemic, *Br J Nutr* 85(6):741–748, 2001; Community Nutrition Institute: Epidemic, *Nutrition Week Newspaper* 22:8 (June 11), 1993.)

depleted individuals, combined with a sudden increase of glucose to the brain, can initiate Wernicke-Korsakoff syndrome, regardless of the level of alcohol intake.

Others at risk for thiamin deficiency include patients who are undergoing dialysis because of renal disease, who are receiving parenteral nutrition, who are HIV positive or have AIDS, or who have persistent vomiting (hyperemesis gravidarum), anorexia nervosa, gastrectomy, or genetic disorders that affect thiamin use (Bemeur & Butterworth, 2014). As the number of gastric bypass procedures increases, instances of peripheral neuropathy from thiamin deficiency may increase as well.

Toxicity

Excess thiamin is excreted in urine. Although thiamin is nontoxic, there is no rationale for supplementation in healthy people. In acute care settings, supplemental thiamin and other B vitamins may be recommended for individuals with chronic excessive alcohol consumption. In general, the best advice is to take a daily multivitamin containing B vitamins.

Riboflavin (B_2)

Have you ever wondered why milk is sold in opaque cardboard or nontransparent plastic containers? These containers protect riboflavin from exposure to light. Riboflavin is sensitive to ultraviolet rays in sunlight and artificial light; much of the riboflavin is destroyed if milk, an excellent source of riboflavin, is sold in clear glass or clear plastic receptacles. Why risk loss of a valuable vitamin?

Function

Like that of thiamin, the main function of riboflavin is as a coenzyme in the release of energy from nutrients in every cell of the body.

Recommended Intake and Sources

The RDA for riboflavin is 1.3 mg for men and 1.1 mg for women. The body's need is related to total kcal intake, energy needs, body size, metabolic rate, and growth rate. Conditions requiring increased protein also require increased riboflavin, such as during wound healing and the growth periods of childhood, pregnancy, and lactation.

Riboflavin is found in both plant and animal foods. In the United States, however, milk is a major source, with small amounts coming from other foods such as enriched grain. Good plant sources are broccoli, asparagus, dark leafy greens, whole grains, and enriched breads and cereals. Rich sources of animal origin include dairy products, meats, fish, poultry, and eggs.

As mentioned, riboflavin is sensitive to light and irradiation. It also can be lost in cooking water but is heat stable.

Deficiency

Ariboflavinosis is the name for a group of symptoms associated with riboflavin deficiency. The lips become swollen, and cracks develop in the corners of the mouth (cheilosis). The tongue becomes inflamed, swollen, and purplish red (glossitis), a common symptom of deficiency of riboflavin and other B vitamins. Seborrheic dermatitis, a skin condition characterized by greasy scales, may occur in the regions of the ears, nose, and mouth. Riboflavin deficiency may also affect the availability and use of pyridoxine and niacin.

Nutritional deficiencies tend to be multiple rather than single, and it is difficult to separate symptoms. If an individual is deficient in a nutrient such as riboflavin, more than likely a deficiency of other nutrients is also present. For example, esophageal cancer is associated with deficiencies of riboflavin and zinc, particularly in Africa, Iran, and China. In the United States, riboflavin deficiency may be related to congenital heart disease, chronic excessive alcohol ingestion, and some cancers (Said & Ross, 2014) as well as to anorexia nervosa and lactose intolerance—all of which are associated with potential multiple nutritional deficiencies.

Toxicity

Toxicity to riboflavin has not been reported. Absorption of riboflavin tends to be limited under normal circumstances; excessive absorption is extremely unlikely (Said & Ross, 2014).

Niacin (B_3)

Niacin occurs naturally in two forms: nicotinic acid and niacinamide. It is hard to imagine, but before niacin was identified, people who were actually suffering from niacin deficiency were so psychologically disoriented that they were sent to mental institutions for treatment. Niacin deficiency can bring on a psychosis that dissipates once sufficient quantities are consumed.

Function

Niacin is involved as a coenzyme for many enzymes, especially those involved in energy metabolism; it is critical for glycolysis and the tricarboxylic acid (TCA) cycle.

Recommended Intake and Sources

Niacin is available in foods as the active vitamin or as its precursor, the amino acid tryptophan. That is, tryptophan can be converted to niacin, and some niacin can be provided this way. Diets adequate in protein tend to be adequate in niacin.

Niacin requirements are measured in niacin equivalents (NEs), reflecting the body's ability to convert tryptophan to niacin. To form 1 mg of niacin, 60 mg of tryptophan is needed, both of which equal 1 mg NE. The RDA recommends that men and women consume 16 mg NE and 14 mg NE per day, respectively. The DRI for niacin includes a UL of 35 mg NE per day because of the adverse reactions experienced when excess amounts are taken in supplement form (see later section titled "Toxicity").

Protein-containing foods are good sources of both niacin and tryptophan. Meats, poultry, fish, legumes, enriched cereals, milk, and even coffee and tea are sources of niacin.

Deficiency

Pellagra, the niacin deficiency disorder, is characterized by the three Ds, as follows (Kirkland, 2014):

- Dermatitis: A symmetric scaly rash occurs only on skin exposed to the sun (Fig. 7.1).
- Dementia: As the central nervous system becomes affected in severe deficiencies, confusion, anxiety, insomnia, and paranoia develop.
- Diarrhea: Damage to the GI tract affects digestion, absorption, and excretion of food, leading to glossitis, vomiting, and diarrhea.

In the early 1900s, pellagra was common in the southern United States among the poor, who subsisted on corn-based diets. The niacin in corn is in a bound form unavailable for absorption, and many people subsisting on low incomes had such a limited intake of protein food that neither tryptophan nor preformed niacin was available. In addition, consumption of white flour increased deficiencies of niacin. The incidence of pellagra decreased dramatically when refined wheat flour (white flour) was required to be enriched with niacin. Niacin is naturally found in whole wheat flour but is lost when processed into refined white flour.

In the United States, health professionals need to be vigilant to recognize the symptoms of vitamin deficiencies among patients undergoing specialized treatments or experiencing disorders that may negatively affect their nutritional status. For example, pellagra may develop among people with chronic excessive alcohol ingestion, particularly if combined with homelessness and failure to eat regularly (not using shelter-based meal programs) (Terada et al., 2015). Several cases have been reported in which dermatitis was not recognized as a symptom of pellagra. In one situation the simultaneous use of several alternative remedies initiated pellagra, although the individual consumed sufficient dietary niacin (Wood et al., 1998). Pellagra may even occur secondary to anorexia nervosa (Prousky, 2003). In contrast, in Africa and Asia, pellagra still occurs among the general population.

Toxicity

The UL for niacin is 35 mg NE per day. When preformed niacin and nicotinic acid (but not niacinamide) are consumed in levels greater than the UL, the vascular system is affected, producing a

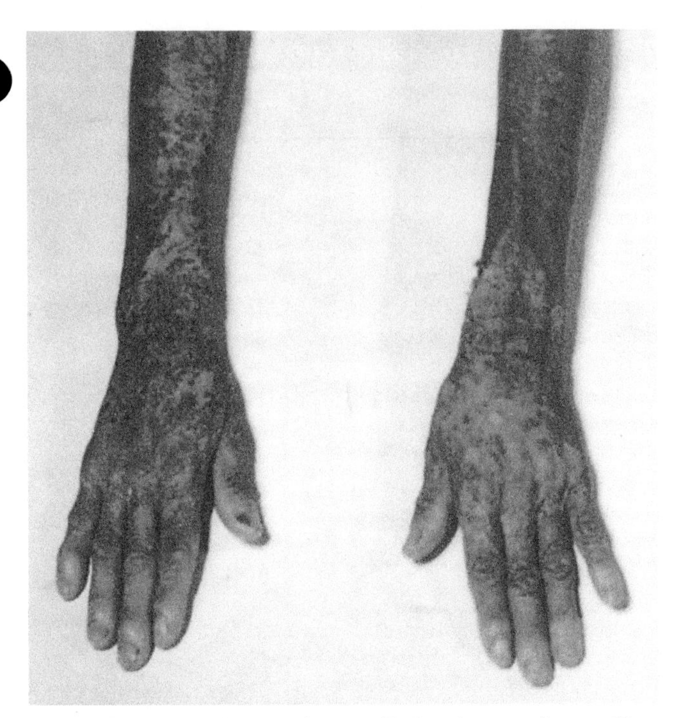

Fig. 7.1 Dermatitis in a patient suffering from pellagra. (From McLaren DS: A colour atlas and text of diet-related disorders, ed 2, London, 1992, Mosby.)

flushing effect throughout the body. Niacin has been used therapeutically because megadoses may lower total cholesterol and low-density lipoprotein (LDL) cholesterol and increase high-density lipoprotein (HDL) cholesterol (Kirkland, 2014). These therapeutic doses, however, must be medically administered to guard against liver damage and related gout and arthritic reactions.

The assumption that increasing HDL is beneficial for cardiovascular risk reduction is being reconsidered. Several large studies have found that therapeutic niacin treatment does not decrease the risk of cardiovascular events and may cause harm (Mani & Rohatgi, 2015). Further studies are expected to be implemented.

Pyridoxine (B_6)

Vitamin B_6 and pyridoxine are generic terms representing a group of related chemicals. The three main members are pyridoxine, pyridoxal, and pyridoxamine. All three forms can be converted to the coenzyme pyridoxal phosphate (PLP) for use in the body.

Function

The major function of vitamin B_6, in the form of PLP, is to act as a coenzyme in the metabolism of amino acids and proteins. These reactions are involved in the formation of neurotransmitters and are essential for proper functioning of the nervous system. PLP is essential for hemoglobin synthesis. It is required for the conversion of tryptophan to niacin. It also serves as a coenzyme for fatty acid and carbohydrate metabolism.

Recommended Intake and Sources

The RDA for vitamin B_6 is 1.3 mg for men and women. These amounts are based on protein intake. Vitamin B_6 is found in a wide variety of foods. Particularly good sources are whole grains and cereals, legumes, and chicken, fish, pork, and eggs.

Deficiency

A deficiency of vitamin B_6 rarely occurs alone; it normally accompanies low intakes of other B vitamins. Symptoms include dermatitis, altered nerve function, weakness, poor growth, convulsions, and microcytic anemia (small red blood cells deficient in hemoglobin).

Of the numerous drugs affecting the bioavailability and metabolism of vitamin B_6, oral contraceptive agents (OCAs) may be among the most widely used. Prolonged use of drugs such as isoniazid (for tuberculosis), penicillamine (for lead poisoning, cystinuria, Wilson's disease, sclerosis, and rheumatoid arthritis), cycloserine (for tuberculosis), and hydralazine (for hypertension) may require vitamin B_6 supplements to reduce neurologic side effects and prevent deficiency during treatment (DaSilva et al., 2014).

Toxicity

Vitamin B_6 has sometimes been prescribed to relieve the symptoms associated with premenstrual syndrome (PMS); however, there are no adequate data to support this treatment. Although doses of 10 mg, an amount often prescribed, are most likely not harmful (even considering the RDA, 1.3 mg), long-term supplementation in megadose gram quantities has been reported to cause ataxia and sensory neuropathy. The UL of B_6 is 100 mg/day.

Folate

Folate, like other B vitamins, actually consists of several similar compounds. One of these compounds was originally extracted from spinach and was given the name folic acid, from the Latin word folium, meaning "leaf." Folic acid was discovered in 1945 during the search for the nutritional factor responsible for control of pernicious anemia. We now know that vitamin B_{12}, rather than folate, is the nutrient that cures pernicious anemia. Folate and its related compounds, however, play a role in other essential biologic processes. The terms folate, folic acid, folacin, and pteroylglutamic acid (PGA) are often used interchangeably. Folate is the form of this vitamin found naturally in foods. Folic acid is a synthetic form used in vitamin supplements and for food fortification. Folic acid is actually more available for absorption by the body.

Function

Folate acts as a coenzyme in reactions involving the transfer of one-carbon units during metabolism. As such, it is required for the synthesis of amino acids, which are the building blocks of protein, and for the synthesis of deoxyribonucleic acid (DNA) and ribonucleic acid (RNA). Blood health also depends on folate to form the heme portion of hemoglobin. For the active form of folate to be maintained for use in the body, vitamin B_{12} must be available.

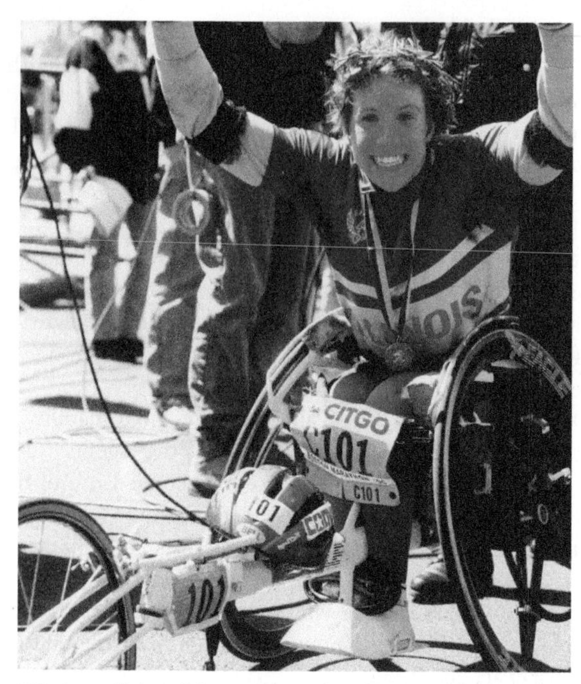

Fig. 7.2 Jean Driscoll is an Olympian, Paralympian, author, and advocate for persons with disabilities around the world who happened to be born with spina bifida. (More information about Jean Driscoll can be found on her website, https://usopm.org/jean-driscoll/.) (Copyright 1995 Paralyzed Veterans of America, Sports 'N Spokes.)

TABLE 7.1 Food Sources of Folate

Food	Serving Size	Amount (µg)	% Daily Value[a]
Chicken liver	3.5 oz	770	193
Breakfast cereals	½ to ½ cups	100–400	25–100
Braised beef liver	3.5 oz	217	54
Lentils, cooked	½ cup	180	45
Chickpeas	½ cup	141	35
Asparagus	½ cup	132	33
Spinach, cooked	½ cup	131	33
Black beans	½ cup	128	32
Burrito with beans	2	118	30
Kidney beans	½ cup	115	29
Baked beans with pork	1 cup	92	23
Lima beans	½ cup	78	20
Tomato juice	1 cup	48	12
Brussels sprouts	½ cup	47	12
Orange	1 medium	47	12
Broccoli, cooked	½ cup	39	10
Fast-food French fries	Large order	38	10
Wheat germ	2 tbsp	38	10
Fortified white bread	1 slice	38	10

[a]Based on daily value for folate of 400 µg.
(Data from US Department of Agriculture, Agricultural Research Service. 2016. *Nutrient Data Laboratory*. USDA National Nutrient Database for Standard Reference, Release 28 (Slightly revised). Version Current: May 2016. Accessed 18 December, 2020, from www.ars.usda.gov/nea/bhnrc/mafcl.)

Folate has a role in the proper formation of fetal neural tubes. Neural tube birth defects affect brain and spinal cord development, resulting in the disorders spina bifida and anencephaly. **Spina bifida** is a congenital neural tube defect caused by the incomplete closure of the fetus's spine during early pregnancy. It may involve incomplete development of the brain, spinal cord, and their protective coverings, resulting in a range of disabilities, including paralysis and incontinence (Fig. 7.2). In cases of **anencephaly**, a congenital defect in which the brain does not develop, death may occur shortly after birth. Although these disorders result from a combination of genetics and environment, adequate folate levels during the first month after conception appear to greatly reduce their incidence. Unfortunately, women of childbearing age are sometimes marginally deficient in folate. They may not know they are pregnant during the first few crucial weeks, when the neural tube of the fetus forms.

Recommended Intake and Sources

The RDA reflects that some folate is stored in the liver, but generally, daily supplies are needed. The RDA is 400 µg for men and women. Physiologic state greatly affects folate need. During pregnancy, a woman's blood supply increases. This increase of blood and the growth of other tissues necessitate a greater need for folate. Consequently, the RDA jumps to 600 µg during pregnancy. During lactation, nutrient needs are elevated because of the nutrient content of the human milk being produced. Therefore, the RDA for folate is 500 µg for lactation needs.

It is recommended that women of childbearing age increase their folate intake to include 400 µg of synthetic folic acid to reduce the risks of birth defects, including spina bifida. The increased levels could be provided by natural sources, fortified foods, or supplements (Table 7.1). To ensure adequate access to folic acid, the U.S. Food and Drug Administration (FDA) mandates that cereal-grain products be fortified with 140 µg folic acid per 100 g of enriched flour and uncooked cereal grains. This means that manufacturers of enriched breads, flours, cornmeal, rice, pastas, and other grain products are required to add folate to their products (Stover, 2014). Fortified product labels may include the claim that adequate intake of folic acid may reduce the risk of neural tube defects.

Although this folic acid fortification assists in meeting the recommended levels for women of childbearing age, health care professionals must be prepared to individualize nutrition guidance to ensure daily optimal consumption of folate and folic acid. Clients and patients need to understand that simply consuming fortified cereals and grains does not necessarily provide sufficient amounts of folate. Dietitians should be consulted to ensure the appropriateness of dietary recommendations.

Concern has been expressed regarding the risks and benefits of this fortification to other age groups. In particular, the effects on older adults may be an issue because an excess of folate can mask a B_{12} deficiency, for which older adults are at risk. Requiring vitamin supplements that contain folic acid to also contain vitamin B_{12} can reduce this risk. This decreases the risk that the larger folate intakes would overshadow possible deficiencies of B_{12}. Overall, the benefits appear to outweigh the risk.

Folate is widely available in foods, particularly in leafy green vegetables, legumes, ready-to-eat cereals, and some fruits and juices. Folate is affected by heat, oxidation, and ultraviolet light; processing and cooking of fresh foods reduce the amount of folate available. Folate is found in many foods that contain ascorbic acid (vitamin C), such as oranges and orange juice. Ascorbic acid protects folate from oxidation. Diets deficient in folate often are deficient in vitamin C, and vice versa.

Deficiency

Cells whose normal activities require rapid cell growth and division are particularly sensitive to folate deficiency. Examples include red blood cells and the cells that line the GI tract. Folate deficiency results in megaloblastic anemia. This is a form of anemia characterized by large red blood cells that cannot carry oxygen properly. Other deficiency symptoms are glossitis, diarrhea, irritability, absentmindedness, depression, and anxiety (Stover, 2014).

Deficiency may result from any condition that requires cell division to speed up, including infection, cancer, burns, blood loss, GI damage, growth, and pregnancy. Currently, about one third of pregnant women worldwide are affected by folate deficiency. Other groups at risk include people with limits on intake and variety of food, including older adults with low incomes and people with chronic excessive alcohol ingestion. Alcoholic cirrhosis often results in both liver damage (which interferes with storage and metabolism of folate) and excessive losses of the vitamin in feces and urine (Stover, 2014).

Numerous medications may affect folate absorption or may be antagonistic to folate. These drugs include anticonvulsants, oral contraceptives, aspirin, cancer chemotherapy agents, sulfasalazine, nonsteroidal antiinflammatory drugs, and antacids. Long-term use of any medication may affect the body's use of nutrients; folate is one that is particularly vulnerable.

Before folic acid supplementation is administered, the absence of vitamin B_{12} deficiency must be established. Therapy with folic acid in the presence of vitamin B_{12} deficiency will favorably improve blood profiles, decreasing megaloblastic anemia, while damage to the central nervous system from lack of B_{12} continues.

Toxicity

Excess folate or folic acid intake is not recommended or warranted. Consuming amounts beyond the UL of 1000 μg folic acid (for men and women) has not been studied. Such high levels may mask the presence of pernicious anemia, discussed later in the next section.

Cobalamin (B_{12})

Cobalamin and vitamin B_{12} are used as generic terms to refer to a group of cobalt-containing compounds. The common pharmaceutical name, used widely in supplements, is cyanocobalamin.

Function

Two cobalamins function as vitamin B_{12} coenzymes in humans. Vitamin B_{12} plays a role in folate metabolism by modifying folate coenzymes to active forms to support metabolic functions, including the synthesis of DNA and RNA. The metabolism of fatty acids and amino acids also requires vitamin B_{12}. In addition, this vitamin develops and maintains the myelin sheaths that surround and protect nerve fibers.

Recommended Intake and Sources

Absorption of vitamin B_{12} relies on an intrinsic factor. The intrinsic factor is produced by stomach mucosa. Both vitamin B_{12} and the intrinsic factor must be present for absorption. Recommended vitamin B_{12} levels take into account that some of the vitamin is stored in the liver. The RDA for young adults is 2.4 μg. Foods of animal origin are the only reliable sources of vitamin B_{12}; meat, fish, poultry, eggs, and dairy products are all good sources. For example, one glass of skim milk provides 0.93 μg of vitamin B_{12}. The vitamin has been reported to be found in legumes (nodules on roots) because of bacteria formation in soil, but they are not a reliable source. Vegans must increase their intake with vitamin B_{12} supplements or use fortified products.

Deficiency

Deficiencies of B_{12} are usually secondary. Pernicious anemia (from lack of intrinsic factor for vitamin B_{12} absorption) or megaloblastic anemia (from related folate dysfunction) occurs. Additional neurologic effects develop because of damage to the spinal cord as the breakdown of myelin sheath synthesis affects brain, optic, and peripheral nerves (Carmel, 2014).

Older adults are more at risk for deficiency because of a naturally occurring reduction in production of the intrinsic factor by the stomach mucosa. Most older adults, however, maintain vitamin B_{12} levels within normal range. For those who do become deficient, injections to bypass intestinal absorption are warranted. Particularly noted in this population are neuropsychiatric symptoms, including delusions and hallucinations, which may occur in the absence of anemia. These symptoms can be misdiagnosed as senility or other illnesses. To alleviate this risk, the recommendations include that adults older than 50 years consume foods fortified with vitamin B_{12} or take a B_{12} supplement to ensure adequacy of the RDA for B_{12}. Vitamin B_{12} is more absorbable in this form because it is already separated from food.

As discussed, folate levels may disguise a vitamin B_{12} deficiency. Hematologic damage is masked by folate, but neurologic damage continues.

Toxicity

Toxicity of vitamin B_{12} has not been noted, but there are no benefits to large doses unless deficiency exists.

Biotin

Humans need biotin, a member of the B vitamin complex, in tiny amounts.

Function

Biotin assists in the transfer of carbon dioxide from one compound to another, playing an important role in carbohydrate, fat, and protein metabolism.

Recommended Intake and Sources

Biotin is synthesized in the lower GI tract by bacterial microorganisms. However, the amount produced, and its bioavailability are unknown. Although biotin is produced in the body, it is still an essential nutrient. (The human body does not produce biotin, but bacteria hosted in the gut do.) It must also be consumed in foods.

The AI for biotin is 30 μg per day. Biotin is widespread in foods. The richest sources are liver, kidney, peanut butter, egg yolks, and yeast.

Deficiency

Deficiency of biotin is unknown among people eating a typical North American diet. When it is experimentally produced, symptoms include a scaly red rash, hair loss, loss of appetite, depression, and glossitis (Mock, 2014).

Biotin deficiency has been produced by consumption of large amounts of avidin, a protein in raw egg whites that binds biotin. A person would need to consume many raw egg whites for this to occur; salmonella poisoning would probably strike first. Avidin is denatured by heat, so cooked egg whites pose no problem to biotin status.

Antibiotics are known to reduce the number of biotin-producing bacteria. In addition, clients receiving long-term intravenous feeding are at risk for biotin deficiency; therefore, their feeding mixtures should contain biotin.

Toxicity

There is no known toxicity for biotin. Nonetheless, dietary supplementation of biotin adversely alters certain laboratory test results (Box 7.4).

BOX 7.4 U.S. Food and Drug Administration Alert: Biotin Supplements May Interfere With Laboratory Results

The U.S. Food and Drug Administration (FDA) issued a safety communication in November 2017 concerning individuals who consume high levels of supplemental biotin. Biotin in blood and other samples can have significant adverse effects on laboratory test results, particularly on thyroid function tests. The results may be falsely positive or negative or possibly misleadingly high or low. An increased number of adverse results have been reported, including one death, as a result of biotin supplementation interaction with the testing process. Biotin and certain medications can interact, whereas other medications, such as anticonvulsants, can negatively impact biotin levels in the body. Health care providers should be consulted when medications are taken regularly.

Biotin dietary supplements are marketed for skin, nail, and hair enhancement. Some of these products may be up to 650 times the AI for biotin (30 μg per day). Because biotin is widespread in foods, there is no health reason to supplement beyond the levels found either in foods or in most vitamin and mineral supplements (containing 100% or less of the Dietary Reference Intakes). High levels may be recommended by physicians for specific conditions such as multiple sclerosis but should be monitored for potential effects on laboratory testing.

Application to Nursing

Patients and health care providers may not be cognizant of the effects of biotin on laboratory testing or not aware that patients are taking supplements of biotin and in what quantities. The FDA is monitoring the adverse effects of biotin supplements and will provide the public with updates as needed. In the meantime, health care providers can question patients as to any supplements (and quantities) being taken, even for nontherapeutic purposes such as hair and nail improvement. It is possible that excessive intake of other nutrients may also affect other laboratory testing or therapeutic treatment.

Adverse events or side effects can be reported to FDA's MedWatch Safety and Adverse Event Reporting Program online (https://www.accessdata.fda.gov/scripts/medwatch/index.cfm).

Data from: Office of Dietary Supplements (ODS), NIH: Biotin Fact Sheet for Health Professionals, Washington, DC, Updated June 3, 2020, Author. Accessed 19 December, 2020, from ods.od.nih.gov/factsheets/Biotin-HealthProfessional/.

Pantothenic Acid

Pantothenic acid gets its name from its presence in all living things (from the Greek *pantothen*, meaning "from all sides").

Function

The principal active form of pantothenic acid functions as part of coenzyme A (CoA); therefore, it is required for the metabolism of carbohydrates, fats, and protein.

Recommended Intake and Sources

The AI for pantothenic acid is 5 mg/day. Pantothenic acid is widespread in foods and easily consumed in whole grain cereals, legumes, meat, fish, and poultry.

Deficiency

Deficiencies in pantothenic acid do not naturally occur in humans.

Toxicity

Doses of up to 10 g daily have been administered with no ill effects. Researchers have reported that daily doses of 10 to 20 g may produce diarrhea or water retention.

Choline

Function

Choline is needed for the synthesis of acetylcholine, a neurotransmitter, and lecithin, the phospholipid.

Recommended Intake and Sources

The body can actually make choline from the amino acid methionine, but this process does not produce enough choline to meet the needs of the body. Consequently, food sources are still required. This requirement qualifies choline as an essential nutrient. The AI is 550 mg/day for men and 425 mg/day for women, with a UL of 3500 mg/day for adults.

Food sources include many commonly consumed foods with rich sources, such as milk, eggs, and peanuts.

Deficiency

Deficiency of choline is rare.

Toxicity

Symptoms of choline toxicity include sweating, fishy body odor, vomiting, liver damage, reduced growth, and low blood pressure (hypotension).

Vitamin C

Vitamin C is almost a household word. It is hard to believe that it was isolated as a nutrient only around 1930. The discovery of vitamin C is associated with the search for the cause of scurvy, a potentially fatal disease that weakens the body's connective tissues and causes inflammation of them. As early as the eighteenth century, it was known that eating certain foods, particularly citrus fruits, could control scurvy, but the actual substance responsible for "gluing" the cells together was not determined until Albert Szent-Gyorgyi and Glen King isolated it in 1928 and 1930, respectively (Levine & Padayatty, 2014). One of the two active forms of vitamin C is ascorbic acid (ascorbic meaning "without scurvy").

Function

Vitamin C functions as an antioxidant and as a coenzyme. It can perform different functions in various situations. Collagen formation for bone matrix, teeth, cartilage, and connective tissue depends on ascorbic acid. Vitamin C provides the cement that holds structures together. Wound healing, which necessitates the formation of new tissue, also requires vitamin C.

As an antioxidant, vitamin C protects folate, vitamin E, and polyunsaturated substances from destruction by oxygen as they move throughout the body. An antioxidant is a compound that guards others from damaging oxidation by being oxidized itself. Vitamins C and E also work together as antioxidants to destroy substances released as cells age, are oxidized, or become damaged. Their work may prevent damage by free radicals to vascular walls, thereby limiting the development of atherosclerotic plaques.

Among its other functions, vitamin C enhances the absorption of nonheme iron, which is found in plant foods. Thyroid and adrenal hormone synthesis requires vitamin C. Several conversion processes depend on vitamin C; these include tryptophan to serotonin, cholesterol to bile, and folate to its active form.

Vitamin C may have a role in reducing the risk of cancer development. Epidemiologic studies have uncovered an association between levels of dietary intake of vitamin C and incidence of cancer in the stomach, esophagus, and colon. Because these studies are of dietary intakes of populations, it is not yet known whether the effects are caused by vitamin C or by other, as yet unidentified, components of foods containing vitamin C.

It is a common myth that vitamin C can prevent the common cold. Unfortunately, the bulk of evidence does not support the theory that vitamin C reduces the incidence of the common cold. Taking supplemental vitamin C for a limited time, however, can decrease the duration and reduce the severity of the symptoms. The UL, though, should always be observed.

Recommended Intake and Sources

The RDA for vitamin C has varied from 45 mg to 60 mg for adults. Currently, the RDA is 90 mg for men and 75 mg for women. Recommendations vary worldwide; the minimum daily requirement to prevent symptoms of scurvy is 10 mg. However, the amount recommended daily to provide enough circulating vitamin C for tissue saturation for good health is open to interpretation.

As more is learned about vitamin C functions, recommendations customized to specific diseases and lifestyle behaviors will be determined. For example, cigarette smokers have lower circulating levels of vitamin C than nonsmokers, regardless of their dietary intake of vitamin C. The metabolic use of vitamin C by smokers is twice that of nonsmokers. Recognition of this deficit has led to the advice that smokers increase their vitamin C intake from the 90-mg RDA to 125 mg daily.

Fruits and vegetables provide 95% of the vitamin C we consume. Many foods are excellent sources; some of them are citrus fruits, red and green peppers, strawberries, tomatoes, potatoes, broccoli, and other green leafy vegetables. Serving sizes to meet the RDA are listed in Table 7.2.

Some foods and drinks are fortified with vitamin C. Ready-to-eat cereals have added vitamin C (about 25% of the daily values) and other vitamins not naturally found in grains. Additional vitamin C, often 100% of the daily values, is added to the small amounts naturally found in apple and grape juice.

Vitamin C is destroyed by air, light, and heat. Fruit juices should be stored in an airtight container that holds only the amount that can be consumed in a short time. The vitamin C contents of cooked foods can be maximized by cooking in the minimal amount of water or, even better, by microwaving (see the *Teaching Tool* box Vegetable Victories).

Deficiency

Although vitamin C deficiency is rare in developed countries in the West, it may still occur among chronic alcohol and drug users, smokers, and those whose dietary intakes are poor. Older

TABLE 7.2 Recommended Dietary Allowance Serving Sizes of Vitamin C[a]

Food	Serving Size	Vitamin C (mg)
Orange juice	¾ cup	93
Orange	1 medium	80
Kiwifruit	1 medium	75
Cantaloupe	1¼ cups	68
Peppers, green or red	¾ cup	64
Strawberries	1 cup	64
Broccoli	¾ cup	58
Brussels sprouts	¾ cup	48
Grapefruit	½ fruit	47

[a]Recommended Dietary Allowance=75–90 mg.

(Data from US Department of Agriculture, Agricultural Research Service. 2016. *Nutrient Data Laboratory.* USDA National Nutrient Database for Standard Reference, Release 28 (Slightly revised). Version Current: May 2016. Accessed 18 December, 2020, from www.ars.usda.gov/nea/bhnrc/mafcl.)

TEACHING TOOL

Vegetable Victories

Every health recommendation proposes that we (and our clients) significantly increase our intake of vegetables. But how? This *Teaching Tool* provides several resources to be shared with clients, by providing information about websites to locate local farmers' markets, community-supported agriculture (CSA), teaching handouts about buying and preparing vegetables, and more.

Local Harvest; www.localharvest.org: Website that provides information about locations of local farmers' markets and CSAs (a group of individuals or families joining together to purchase shares of the harvest of a nearby farmer); offers additional strategies for preparing produce for immediate consumption or for storing through the winter.

ChooseMyPlate; www.choosemyplate.gov/myplatekitchen/resources: Access to recipe resource, food safety strategies, and seasonal produce guide, including the U.S. Department of Agriculture National Farmers Market Directory.

Have a Plant: Produce for Better Health Foundation; fruitsandveggies.org: A health initiative to increase Americans' consumption of fruits and vegetables; includes tools for buying fruits and vegetables, recipes, and expert advice.

adults may have marginal intake because of difficulty in obtaining and preparing fresh foods. These at-risk groups may experience other vitamin and mineral deficiencies as well.

Scurvy represents the extreme result of vitamin C deficiency. The symptoms are tied to the functions of vitamin C in the body. When the glue-like substance collagen is not replaced, tissues throughout the body degenerate. Gingivitis causes gums to bleed and teeth to come loose. Joints and limbs ache from muscle degeneration and lack of new connective tissue formation. Bruising and hemorrhages occur as the vascular system weakens, and plaques form as a result of the vascular damage. Death ultimately occurs as functioning of all body systems disintegrates.

Marginal deficiency may manifest as gingivitis, with soreness and ulcerations of the mouth, poor wound healing, inadequate tooth and bone growth or maintenance, and increased risk of infection as the integrity of tissues throughout the body becomes compromised.

Toxicity

Toxicity from foods high in vitamin C does not occur even if we consume cups of fresh strawberries washed down with a quart of orange juice. Long-term supplement intakes of megadoses from 1 to 15 g may result in cramps, diarrhea, nausea, kidney stone formation, and gout. The effects of anticlotting medication may also be affected (NRC, 2006).

Taking supplements of vitamin C seems benign, but the body adapts to protect itself from harm. If continually inundated with excessive vitamin C, the body develops a mechanism that destroys much of the extra vitamin C circulating within it. A rebound effect may occur if, after taking megadoses for several months or more, an individual abruptly stops supplementation and consumes a quantity closer to the RDA. The protective mechanism of the body is still in gear and continues to destroy vitamin C. An individual may experience symptoms of scurvy even though consuming the RDA. A newborn exposed to vitamin C megadoses in utero may experience this rebound effect. Although the rebound effect may not occur in every case, withdrawal from vitamin C megadoses should be gradual, over a period of 2 to 4 weeks. Consequently, there is a UL of 2000 mg for adults and 400 to 1800 mg for children and adolescents.

Table 7.3 provides a quick reference to water-soluble vitamins.

FAT-SOLUBLE VITAMINS

Vitamin A

Each year approximately 250,000 children enter a world of permanent darkness. The cause? Vitamin A deficiency. Extreme vitamin A deficiency is so damaging to corneas that blindness occurs. Although this could be prevented with just a few cents' worth of vitamin A per year, there is little money for preventive health measures in areas of the world where food is scarce.

Function

Vitamin A is a group of compounds that function to maintain skin and mucous membranes throughout the body. Specific activities depending on vitamin A are vision, bone growth, functioning of the immune system, and normal reproduction. Our eyes depend on visual purple, technically called rhodopsin, to be able to adjust to light variations. Rhodopsin is formed from retinal, a vitamin A substance, and opsin, a protein. Without enough vitamin A, rhodopsin cannot be formed, and the retina cannot easily respond to light changes. As a result, night blindness develops. Bone growth involves a process of remodeling that reshapes and enlarges the skeleton. Reshaping requires vitamin A to undo existing bone. Vitamin A also maintains the integrity of epithelial tissues throughout the body, providing protection against infections and ensuring optimum function. Hormone-like effects of vitamin A appear to be tied to cell synthesis for reproductive purposes.

Recommended Intake and Sources

Vitamin A is measured as retinol activity equivalents (RAE). The RDA, based on providing optimum storage of vitamin A in the liver, is 900 μg RAE for men and 700 μg RAE for women. RAE incorporates both the preformed, active forms of vitamin A, called retinoids (found in animal foods), and the precursor forms of vitamin A, called carotenoids (found in plant foods). The carotenoid beta carotene is the primary source of vitamin A from plant foods.

Because vitamin A (a fat-soluble vitamin) is stored in the body, daily doses are not necessary, but they are desirable. Deficiency of other nutrients affects the absorption and use of vitamin A (Ross, 2014). Nutrients are interdependent, and imbalances of specific nutrients affect the functioning of others.

Natural preformed vitamin A is found only in the fat of animal-related foods; these include whole milk, butter, liver, egg yolks, and fatty fish. Carotenoids are found in deep green, yellow, and orange fruits and vegetables. The best sources are broccoli, cantaloupe, sweet potatoes, carrots, tomatoes, and spinach

TABLE 7.3 Water-Soluble Vitamins

Vitamin	Function	Clinical Issues (Deficiency/Toxicity)	Recommended Daily Intakes	Food Sources
Thiamin (B_1)	Coenzyme energy metabolism; muscle nerve action	Deficiency: beriberi (ataxia, disorientation, tachycardia); wet beriberi (edema); dry beriberi (nervous system); Wernicke-Korsakoff syndrome Marginal deficiency: headaches, tiredness	Men: 1.2 mg Women: 1.1 mg	Lean pork, whole or enriched grains and flours, legumes, seeds, and nuts
Riboflavin (B_2)	Coenzyme energy metabolism	Deficiency: ariboflavinosis with cheilosis, glossitis, seborrheic dermatitis	Men: 1.3 mg Women: 1.1 mg	Milk/dairy products; meat, fish, poultry, and eggs; dark leafy greens (broccoli); whole and enriched breads and cereals
Niacin (B_3) (nicotinic acid and niacinamide) Precursor: tryptophan	Cofactor to enzymes involved in energy metabolism; glycolysis and TCA cycle	Deficiency: pellagra Toxicity: vasodilation, liver damage, gout, and arthritic reactions	Men: 16 mg NE Women: 14 mg NE UL: 35 mg NE	Meats, poultry, and fish; legumes; whole and enriched cereals; milk
Pyridoxine (B_6)	Forms coenzyme pyridoxal phosphate (PLP) for energy metabolism; CNS; hemoglobin synthesis	Deficiency: dermatitis, altered nerve function, weakness, anemia; OCAs decrease B_6 levels Toxicity: ataxia, sensory neuropathy	Men: 1.3 mg Women: 1.3 mg UL: 100 mg	Whole grains/cereals legumes, poultry, fish, pork, eggs
Folate (folic acid, folacin, PGA)	Coenzyme metabolism (synthesis of amino acid, heme, DNA, RNA); fetal neural tube formation	Deficiency: megaloblastic anemia; many drugs affect folate use Toxicity: megadoses may mask pernicious anemia	Men: 400 µg Women: 400 µg Pregnancy: 600 µg Lactation: 500 µg UL: 1000 µg	Widely available leafy green vegetables, legumes, ascorbic acid-containing foods
Cobalamin (B_{12})	Transport/storage of folate; metabolism of fatty acids/amino acids	Deficiency: pernicious anemia, CNS damage	Adults: 2.4 µg	Animal sources
Biotin	Metabolism of carbohydrate, fat, and protein	Deficiency: produced by avidin and long-term antibiotics	Adults: 30 µg AI	Liver, kidney, peanut butter, egg yolks, intestinal synthesis
Pantothenic acid	Part of coenzyme A	Deficiency: not possible	Adults: 5 mg AI	Widespread in foods
Choline	Synthesis of acetylcholine and lecithin	Deficiency: rare Toxicity: body odor, liver damage, hypotension	Men: 550 mg Women: 425 mg UL: 3500 mg	Widespread—milk, eggs, peanuts
Vitamin C	Antioxidant, coenzyme, collagen formation, wound healing, iron absorption, hormone synthesis	Deficiency: scurvy Toxicity: cramps, nausea, kidney stone formation, gout (1–15 g), rebound scurvy	Men: 90 mg Women: 75 mg UL: 2000	Fruits/vegetables (citrus fruits, tomatoes, peppers, strawberries, broccoli)

AI, adequate intake; *CNS*, central nervous system; *DNA*, deoxyribonucleic acid; *NE*, niacin equivalent; *OCAs*, oral contraceptive agents; *PGA*, pteroylglutamic acid; *RNA*, ribonucleic acid; *TCA*, tricarboxylic acid; *UL*, tolerable upper intake level.

(Table 7.4). High consumption of carotenoids, particularly beta carotene, has been associated with decreased risk of certain cancers and other chronic diseases. This may be attributed to their action as antioxidants. Table 7.5 lists other nutrients that also function as antioxidants.

When fats are removed from animal-related foods, preformed vitamin A is also lost. To maintain traditional sources of the vitamin, low-fat, skim, and nonfat milks are fortified with vitamin A. Other fortified products include margarine (which often replaces butter, a natural source of vitamin A) and ready-to-eat cereal, a staple food product commonly fortified with many nutrients.

Deficiency

Vitamin A deficiency is either primary, caused by lack of dietary intake, or secondary, the result of chronic fat malabsorption. As liver storage becomes depleted, symptoms develop. The effects are closely tied to vitamin A functions. Ocularly, **xerophthalmia** incorporates a range of problems, from **night blindness** (the inability of the eyes to readjust from bright to dim light) progressing to a hard, dry cornea (keratinization) or **keratomalacia**, resulting in complete blindness. The degeneration of the epithelial tissues protecting the eye itself leads to the effects of xerophthalmia. Compromised epithelial tissues also result in the development of hard white lumps of keratin on hair follicles

TABLE 7.4 Vitamin A/Beta Carotene Sources[a]

Food	Serving Size	Carotene (RAE)
Liver (beef)	3½ oz	10,000
Sweet potato	1 whole, baked	2488
Carrots	1 whole, raw	2025
	½ cup, cooked	1915
Spinach	½ cup, cooked	737
Butternut squash	½ cup, cooked	714
Cantaloupe	1 cup	516
Red pepper	1 whole	422
Apricots	3 medium	277

(Data from US Department of Agriculture, Agricultural Research Service. 2016. *Nutrient Data Laboratory*. USDA National Nutrient Database for Standard Reference, Release 28 (Slightly revised). Version Current: May 2016. Accessed 18 December, 2020, from www.ars.usda.gov/nea/bhnrc/mafcl.)
RAE, Retinol activity equivalent.
[a]Recommended dietary allowance=900 RAE for men; 700 RAE for women.

(hyperkeratosis), respiratory infections, diarrhea, and other GI disturbances. Overall, the immune system is endangered; for deficient children especially, a minor illness or a bout of measles may be deadly. Growth is inhibited because of lack of vitamin A-dependent proteins for bone growth.

In North America, individuals experiencing chronic fat malabsorption are at risk for vitamin A deficiency and deficiencies of other fat-soluble vitamins. These nutrients are incorporated into their overall nutrition plans. Although marginal vitamin A deficiency is possible, overt deficiencies are rare.

Deficiency is a health threat in parts of the world where food availability is limited. To counteract this threat in areas where rice is a staple food, Golden Rice has been genetically transformed to accumulate increased amounts of provitamin A (Gayen et al., 2016). Public health efforts are being made to distribute Golden Rice to farmers and to further increase the nutrient value of the grain (Dubock, 2014).

Toxicity

Hypervitaminosis A occurs only from preformed vitamin A from either a short- or long-term intake of supplements. Most food sources of preformed A do not contain high enough levels to ever result in toxicity. The only exception noted is polar bear liver and the livers of other large animals. Explorers who feasted on polar bear liver experienced hypervitaminosis A; in fact, the way we learned about the toxic effects of vitamin A was through their misfortune. Apparently, the livers of hibernating animals store an extraordinary quantity of vitamin A to provide sufficient amounts for a long winter without nourishment. When humans consume the preformed vitamin A of these livers, the quantity is toxic.

Toxicity does not occur from the carotenoid precursor in foods. If carotenoids are consumed in excess, either from foods or supplements, the skin takes on an orange hue, which dissipates when carotenoid consumption is reduced.

Immediate symptoms of vitamin A toxicity include blistered skin, weakness, anorexia, vomiting, headache, joint pain, irritability, and enlargement of the spleen and liver; long-term effects include bone abnormalities and liver damage (Ross, 2014).

Vitamin A supplements taken internally will not cure or improve acne and are toxic in excess. Even prescription medications can be problematic. The acne medications sotretinoin (Accutane) and isotretinoin (oral forms) are nonnutritive sources of vitamin A that cause birth defects when used by pregnant women. Women who take either of these drugs should be advised to use a highly reliable method of birth control.

TABLE 7.5 Antioxidants

Antioxidant	Antioxidant Functions	Major Food Sources	Adult RDA	Daily Recommended Supplementation
Beta carotene (provitamin A, vitamin A)	May decrease risk of some cancers and CVD	Sweet potatoes, winter squash, carrots, red bell peppers, dark green vegetables, apricots, mangos, cantaloupe	No RDA (1 sweet potato = 15 mg, 1 carrot = 10 mg)	6–15 mg; nontoxic; higher doses may give skin a harmless orange cast (not recommended for smokers)
Vitamin C	May decrease risk of certain cancers and CVD	Kiwi, citrus fruits, berries, cantaloupe, honeydew, bell peppers, tomatoes, cabbage family vegetables	75–90 mg (1 kiwi=150 mg, 1 cup broccoli=115 mg, 1 orange=70 mg)	250–500 mg, more may cause diarrhea (UL 2000 mg)
Vitamin E	May decrease risk of cancer; may also prevent or delay cataracts	Vegetable oil, nuts, seeds, margarine, wheat germ, olives, leafy greens, avocado, asparagus	15 mg α-TE (1 tbsp oil = 9 mg, 1 tbsp margarine or 1 oz nuts = 2 mg)	300–600 mg (200–400 international units) daily[a] for all adults; higher doses may cause headaches and diarrhea (UL 1000 mg)
Selenium	Prevents cell and lipid membrane damage	Meat, fish, eggs, whole grains	55 μg	Same as RDA; not more than 200 μg; higher levels very toxic, causing severe liver damage, vomiting, diarrhea, metallic aftertaste (UL 400 μg)

α-TE, Alpha-tocopherol; *CVD*, cardiovascular disease; *RDA*, recommended dietary allowance; *UL*, tolerable upper intake level.
aContraindicated for those who have hypertension or who take warfarin (Coumadin) and other drugs to inhibit blood clots.

Vitamin D

With sufficient exposure to ultraviolet light or sunshine, the body can manufacture its own supply of vitamin D. The exposure of skin to ultraviolet light begins the conversion process of the vitamin D precursor 7-dehydrocholesterol (found in our skin) to cholecalciferol, the active form of vitamin D. Because the body can produce vitamin D, it is technically a hormone. However, when vitamin D is supplied by the diet, it is technically a vitamin. Regardless of how it is classified, vitamin D is a substance necessary for a variety of the body's regulating processes as well as normal development of bones and teeth.

Function

Intestinal absorption of calcium and phosphorus depends on the action of vitamin D. This vitamin also affects bone mineralization and mineral homeostasis by helping to regulate blood calcium levels.

Vitamin D also has potential effects on growth and regulation, cardiovascular function, and immunologic performance.

Recommended Intake and Sources

The RDA for vitamin D is 15 μg (600 international units [IU]). For newborns through 1 year, an AI of 10 μg (400 IU) is recommended. The RDA for people aged 70 years and older jumps to 20 μg (800 IU). This level reflects the lesser efficiency of older adults to synthesize vitamin D from sun exposure. If these amounts are not consumed from foods or obtained from sunlight, supplement use may be appropriate. The UL for vitamin D is 100 μg (4000 IU). The effects of intakes higher than the UL are discussed in the section on toxicity.

The current recommendations for optimal vitamin D intakes are based on preventing bone disease and providing sufficient biologically active vitamin D for the other potential effects.

Vitamin D is available through body synthesis or from dietary sources. Cholecalciferol, the active form of vitamin D, can be synthesized. Ultraviolet irradiation from sunlight affects the vitamin D precursor 7-dehydrocholesterol in our skin, and this cholesterol derivative is transformed by the liver and kidneys into its hormonal form, calcitriol. The amount of vitamin D produced depends on length of exposure to ultraviolet irradiation, atmospheric conditions, and skin pigmentation. Geographic regions and seasons that are particularly cloudy and rainy diminish the quantity of vitamin D synthesized. Darker skin pigmentation also reduces the effect of radiation on the skin, as do sunscreen and concealing clothing. Aging may lessen the amount of vitamin D formed from sunlight exposure.

The few sources of natural preformed vitamin D are the fat of the animal-related foods butter, egg yolks, fatty fish, and liver. Milk, although containing fat, is not a good source; it is, however, a good vehicle for vitamin D fortification because it contains calcium and phosphorus, which need vitamin D for absorption. Because vegans consume no animal foods, they may require supplements or regular sunlight exposure to ensure formation of cholecalciferol. Appropriate guidance should be sought from a primary health care provider or dietitian.

Deficiency

A deficiency of vitamin D can lead to the disorder rickets (Fig. 7.3) and osteomalacia; the extent of vitamin D deficiency among children and adults in the United States may be more widespread than previously suspected (Jones, 2014). Because of insufficient mineralization of bone and tooth matrix, rickets in children leads to malformed skeletons, characterized by bowed legs unable to bear body weight, oddly angled rib bones and chests, and abnormal tooth formation. In adults, osteomalacia, or "bad bones," is characterized by soft demineralized bones that are at risk for fractures. It may be caused by vitamin D or calcium deficiency.

It has been thought that rickets occurs rarely among well-nourished populations. However, reports now reveal that the risk of rickets has increased among breastfed dark-skinned infants and toddlers of African and Asian descent, especially in northern areas such as Canada and Alaska. The increased risk for these children is caused by several factors, including darker pigmentation, use of heavier clothing by children that limits exposure of the skin to vitamin D synthesis, and limited consumption of dietary sources of fortified vitamin D dairy products by children or by women who are breastfeeding infants (Jones, 2014). Consequently, Canadian and U.S. pediatric medical associations recommend vitamin D supplementation of 10 μg (400 IU) per day. Use of rice milk or soy milk, neither of which may be fortified

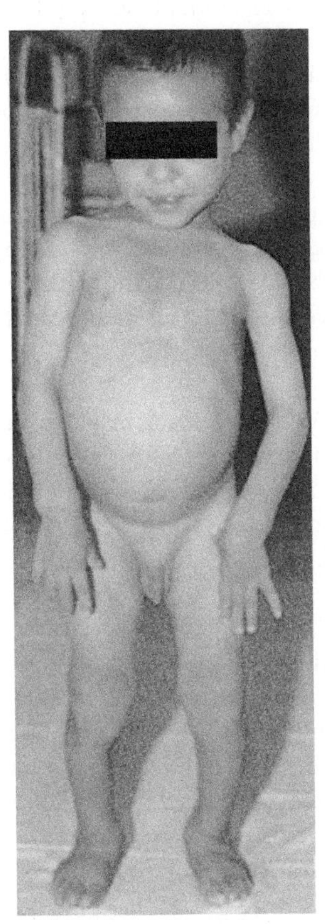

Fig. 7.3 Rickets. This child has characteristic bowed legs. (From McLaren DS: *A colour atlas and text of diet-related disorders*, ed 2, London, 1992, Mosby.)

with vitamin D and other nutrients found in human breast milk from well-nourished mothers and in infant formulas, may lead to severe nutrient deficiencies such as rickets. Children are also at risk for rickets as a result of chronic lipid malabsorption or continuous anticonvulsive therapy (Hollick, 2006).

Among older adults who may have a diminished ability to produce vitamin D, osteomalacia may develop when marginal intakes of vitamin D or calcium exist for a number of years. Calcium absorption may also be affected by the aging process and may contribute to osteomalacia risk. Older women are more at risk than older men because of the effects of repeated pregnancies and lactation on bone density. Symptoms of osteomalacia include weakness, rheumatic-like pain, and an awkward gait. Because bones are weakened, fractures of the spine, hips, and limbs may occur.

Another disorder of the skeleton is osteoporosis. Osteoporosis is a condition in which bone density is reduced and the remaining bone is brittle and breaks easily. Because vitamin D is crucial for absorption of calcium and the mineralization of bone, chronic vitamin D deficiency may be one of the risk factors for this disorder. Osteoporosis is discussed in detail in Chapter 8.

Vitamin D deficiency is associated with increased risk of CVD, rheumatoid arthritis, cancers, T1D mellitus, and multiple sclerosis.

Outright deficiency of vitamin D is thought to be rare in the United States because milk and related food products are fortified. But the amounts recommended for dietary consumption assume that greater amounts are produced by our bodies. Deficiency, however, is a concern when a lack of exposure to sunlight occurs as a result of (1) environmental limitations, (2) cultural clothing customs that conceal the body, or (3) the inability of older adults or people with disabilities to get outdoors or to the store, resulting in malnourishment. These conditions may require vigilance in the consumption of fortified dietary sources, or supplements may be appropriate. When dietary intake and blood levels of vitamin D are assessed, many more Americans are found to have marginal vitamin D status.

Toxicity

High intakes of vitamin D can result in hypercalcemia (high calcium level in blood) and hypercalciuria (high calcium level in urine), which affect kidneys and may cause cardiovascular damage. Toxicity symptoms occur when dietary intake of vitamin D is just above the UL of 100 μg, or 4000 IU.

Vitamin E

During the 1970s, vitamin E supplements were a popular aphrodisiac. Male virility, in particular, was thought to be enhanced by taking extra vitamin E. There was only one problem. Vitamin E increased the libido of male rats but not that of humans. Research conducted on rats about the effects of vitamin E noted that the rats were able to reproduce better with additional intake of vitamin E. Although research conducted on rats is often applicable to humans, in this instance the results could not be generalized to humans. However, vitamin E is an essential nutrient that performs vital functions; we are still learning about its role in relation to disease prevention.

Function

Vitamin E acts as an antioxidant, protecting polyunsaturated fatty acids and vitamin A in cell membranes from oxidative damage by being oxidized itself. This function is particularly important in protecting the integrity of lung and red blood cell membranes, which are exposed to large amounts of oxygen. Other antioxidative functions of vitamin E are performed as part of a system in conjunction with selenium and ascorbic acid (vitamin C).

Recommended Intake and Sources

Plants contain a family of compounds called tocopherols. Vitamin E requirement is met by a particular tocopherol, alpha-tocopherol, which is the most widely occurring form and the most active. The RDA for vitamin E is 15 mg for men and women (the older measurement, IU, may still be in use on dietary supplements: one IU equals 0.67 mg alpha-tocopherol). A positive relationship exists between dietary intake of polyunsaturated fats and vitamin E requirements. As our dietary intake of polyunsaturated fats increases, we need more vitamin E to protect the integrity of these fats from oxidation.

The best sources of vitamin E are vegetable oils (e.g., corn, soy, safflower, canola, and cottonseed) and margarine. Whole grains, seeds, nuts, wheat germ, and green leafy vegetables also provide adequate amounts of vitamin E. Processing of these foods may decrease the final vitamin E content.

Deficiency

A primary deficiency of vitamin E is rare. Secondary deficiencies occur in premature infants and in other people who are unable to absorb fat normally. Some chronic fat absorption disorders in which deficiencies may occur are cystic fibrosis, biliary atresia (blocked bile duct), other disorders of the hepatobiliary system, and liver transport problems. Symptoms of vitamin E deficiency are neurologic disorders resulting from cell damage and anemia caused by hemolysis of red blood cells (hemolytic anemia) (Traber, 2014).

Toxicity

There is no evidence of toxicity associated with excessive intake of vitamin E. Intakes of about 70 to 530 mg (100–800 IU) per day appear to be tolerated, but the value of such doses has not been determined. Megadoses of vitamin E can exacerbate the anticoagulant effect of drugs taken to reduce blood clotting; vitamin E supplementation is not recommended in people who are undergoing anticoagulant therapy, have a coagulation disorder, or have a vitamin K deficiency. A UL of 1000 mg alpha-tocopherol has been set.

Vitamin K

As previously mentioned, vitamin K was discovered by a Danish scientist and was called koagulationsvitamin for its blood clotting properties. Later research revealed that vitamin K is several related compounds with similar functions in the body.

Function

Vitamin K's main function is as a cofactor in the synthesis of blood clotting factors, including prothrombin. Protein formation in bone, kidney, and plasma also depends on the actions of vitamin K.

Recommended Intake and Sources

The AI for vitamin K is 120 µg per day for men and 90 µg for women. This amount provides for sufficient storage of vitamin K in the liver. Vitamin K actually consists of compounds in different forms in plant and animal tissues. All are converted by the liver to the biologically active form of menaquinone called vitamin K.

Vitamin K is available through dietary sources and can be synthesized by microflora in the jejunum and ileum of the digestive tract. From plants, vitamin K is consumed as phylloquinone; bacterial synthesis produces vitamin K homologues as forms of menaquinones. As noted, phylloquinone and vitamin K homologues are converted to the active form of menaquinone (vitamin K) by the liver.

Vitamin K is still an essential nutrient, although bacteria residing in the intestinal tract can synthesize it. The key distinction is that bacteria hosted by the human body produce the vitamin. Additionally, not enough vitamin K is produced by the microflora to ensure adequate levels for total blood clotting needs; dietary intake is still required (Suttie, 2014).

Primary food sources for vitamin K are dark green leafy vegetables. Lesser amounts are found in dairy products, cereals, meats, and fruits.

Deficiency

Deficiency of vitamin K inhibits blood coagulation. Deficiencies may be observed in clinical settings related to malabsorption disorders or medication interactions. Long-term intensive antibiotic therapy destroys the intestinal microflora that produce vitamin K. As with the other fat-soluble vitamins, any barrier to absorption affects the quantity of fat-soluble vitamin absorbed.

Premature infants and newborns are unable to immediately produce vitamin K; their guts are too sterile, free of the microflora necessary to produce vitamin K. Hospitals in the United States routinely give newborns an intramuscular dose of vitamin K to prevent hemorrhagic disease. Infants born in nonhospital settings (such as at home) may not receive the recommended dose of vitamin K. Intracranial bleeding and other symptoms consistent with abuse may actually be caused by vitamin K deficiency (Brousseau et al., 2005).

Because vitamin K also has a role in bone metabolism, research is investigating whether vitamin K has a function in the treatment of osteoporosis. Although insufficient data exist to support vitamin K as a formal treatment component for osteoporosis (Suttie, 2014), they do highlight the need to regularly consume at least the AI.

Toxicity

Consumption of foods containing vitamin K produces no problems of toxicity. Certain medications may be affected by vitamin K. The effectiveness of anticoagulant medications such as warfarin (Coumadin) and other blood-thinning drugs can be reduced by high intakes of vitamin K from either foods or supplements. Clients should be advised to moderate their consumption of foods containing vitamin K.

Vitamin K supplements should be used only if advised by a registered dietitian/nutritionist or primary health care provider. Because vitamin K has a role in blood clotting, excess amounts may decrease clotting time, thereby increasing the risk for stroke.

Table 7.6 provides a summary of fat-soluble vitamins.

CONSIDERING VITAMIN SUPPLEMENTATION

Why do vitamins capture our attention? We generally do not suffer from vitamin deficiencies, and any problems of vitamin toxicity tend to be self-imposed. Considered through a wellness perspective, vitamin consumption is just one of many factors for achieving optimum health. Yet sales of dietary supplements continue to significantly increase. More than half the adult American population uses these products (Marra & Bailey, 2018).

Perhaps vitamins are an easier target on which to focus when one is emphasizing good health. If a person is concerned about vitamin intake, they can always take a vitamin pill. That is a lot easier than the dietary and behavior modifications required to meet other health factors, such as decreasing fat intake or increasing physical activities. There are, however, circumstances that may warrant supplementation.

Rethinking Vitamin Supplementation

Recommendations for vitamin supplementation intend to improve the nutritional status of at-risk groups of the population. These have included adolescent girls, pregnant and lactating women, individuals with limited economic resources, older persons, alcohol-dependent individuals, and possibly those following vegetarian or vegan food patterns. Additionally, individuals with increased nutrient needs as a result of medication interaction with nutrients or chronic health conditions may require vitamin supplementation. Another subgroup at risk are people experiencing food insecurity, whose intake may have nutrient gaps. Folate, vitamins A and C, and the minerals iron, calcium, and zinc tend to be consumed in inadequate amounts by these at-risk groups.

The purpose of recommendations for these groups is to address basic deficiency issues. If adequate levels are not consumed as a result of social, cultural, or economic reasons, then it is the role of health professionals to provide guidance as to how to achieve these levels.

Recommendations are beginning to move beyond the level of nutrient adequacy to issues of health promotion and prevention of disease. For example, folate requirements are vitally important for the development of a healthy fetus. Should the whole population receive folic acid through fortification when only potentially pregnant women have the additional requirement?

The DRI addresses the issue of availability of vitamin B_{12} and older adults. It recommends that adults older than 50 years use a vitamin B_{12} supplement or foods fortified with the vitamin to ensure adequate bioavailability to prevent potential deficiencies. But what foods should be fortified that older adults are sure to eat? The DRI has also recommended that the level of vitamin D be increased above the levels usually consumed, suggesting the

TABLE 7.6 Fat-Soluble Vitamins

Vitamin	Function	Clinical Issues Deficiency/ Toxicity	Requirements	Food Sources
Vitamin A Precursors: carotenoids Preformed vitamin: retinoids	Maintains epithelial tissues (skin and mucous membranes); rhodopsin formation for vision; bone growth; reproduction	Deficiency: xerophthalmia; night blindness; keratomalacia; degeneration of epithelial tissue; inhibited growth (respiratory and gastrointestinal disturbances) Toxicity: hypervitaminosis A (from supplements) with blistered skin, weakness, anorexia, vomiting, enlarged spleen and liver	Men: 900 μg RAE Women: 700 μg RAE UL: 3000 μg RAE	Deep green, yellow, and orange fruits and vegetables; animal fat sources: whole milk, fortified skim, and low-fat milk; butter; liver; egg yolks; fatty fish
Vitamin D Precursor: 7-dehydrocholesterol Active form: cholecalciferol	Calcium and phosphorus absorption; bone mineralization	Deficiency: bone malformation, rickets (children), osteomalacia (adults) Toxicity: hypercalcemia, hypercalciuria	Adults: 5 μg AI (<51 years 10 μg) (<70 years 15 μg) UL: 50 μg	Animal (fat) sources: butter, egg yolks, fatty fish, liver, fortified milk; body synthesis
Vitamin E α-Tocopherol	Antioxidant for polyunsaturated fatty acid and vitamin A; antioxidant with selenium and ascorbic acid	Deficiency: primary deficiency rare; secondary deficiency (caused by fat absorption) neurologic disorders Toxicity: none, but supplements contraindicated with anticoagulation drugs	Adults: 15 mg α-TE UL: 1000 mg α-TE	Vegetable oil, whole grains, seeds, nuts, green leafy vegetables
Vitamin K Active form: menaquinones	Cofactor in synthesis of blood clotting factors; protein formation	Deficiency: blood coagulation inhibited; hemorrhagic disease (infants) Toxicity: therapeutic vitamin K (menadione form) reactions in neonates, causing hemolytic anemia and hyperbilirubinemia	Men: 120 μg AI Women: 90 μg AI	Green leafy vegetables, intestinal synthesis

α-TE, Alpha-tocopherol equivalent; *AI*, adequate intake; *RAE*, retinol activity equivalent; *UL*, tolerable upper intake level.

use of vitamin D supplements. This recommendation marks a significant change in philosophy because supplements of vitamin D had been discouraged because of toxicity issues. Other important questions for health professionals to consider are how will older adults know of these vitamin B_{12} and vitamin D recommendations, and how should the recommendations be implemented?

Nutrition education regarding the use of functional (fortified) foods and appropriate use of supplements is one means of teaching a target population about nutrient needs. When such education is implemented on a broad scale to the public at large, other segments of the population learn of the nutrient value. For example, women should be taught the value of folic acid during pregnancy, but men can also be aware of this value so that they can support the implementation of the folic acid goal by the women in their lives. In addition, younger women can become aware of the special nutrient needs of the pregnancy years before they enter them, so that the importance of nutrition during pregnancy is not something new or an afterthought when they are older.

Functional foods may increase the amount of a nutrient in the food supply. Through careful selection of the foods to which specific nutrients are added, increased consumption of the nutrient can be achieved with little effort by the target group. This is a public health approach that affects the community at large. Folic acid fortification provides a safety net for women of childbearing age but only if they consume foods containing the additional folic acid. Supplements may still be warranted.

A third approach to nutrient supplements is an individualized one. Individuals take the supplements on their own. Ideally a qualified health professional such as a registered dietitian/nutritionist, licensed nutritionist, or primary health care provider guides the individual as to the need and quantity of the nutrient supplements to be regularly taken. This approach requires the individual to take the responsibility for continued consumption of the supplement, if appropriate.

The optimal strategy is the use of all three approaches to achieve nutrient adequacy that takes into account the special needs of subgroups.

Role of the Health Practitioner

Recommendations for the use of nutrient supplements should be determined by dietetic professionals such as registered dietitians or by informed primary health care providers. Their counseling evaluates the client's current nutrient intake and assesses their dietary supplementation practices and possible interactions with prescribed medical treatments and medications. Foremost in importance is that dietary adequacy should first be met by eating a diverse selection of whole foods while following the basic dietary guidelines of MyPlate with awareness of portion (moderation) sizes.

The role of other health professionals, such as nurses, is to guide the client to the appropriate nutritional counseling to determine the client's actual nutrient status. After counseling has been completed, nurses can support the recommendations of the dietitian through teaching strategies such as how to incorporate more fruits and vegetables into the diet and how to reinforce the understanding of potential drug-nutrient interactions.

TOWARD A POSITIVE NUTRITION LIFESTYLE: SOCIAL SUPPORT

Social support extends throughout the life span; it goes beyond having friends and family with whom to socialize. For families with young children, social support may be cooperative meals when illness strikes (e.g., during a flu epidemic) and cooking time becomes compromised. The term cooperative may mean cooking double portions to feed a friend's family during bouts of the croup or childhood ear infections. The kindness would then be reciprocated in the future. Both families gain nutritious meals at times when merely thinking about cooking seems overwhelming.

Support for older adults, as mentioned earlier in this chapter, may mean assistance with food shopping or food delivery. Neighbors or relatives may provide this social support. In some communities, local Red Cross chapters and other charitable organizations have developed car or bus services specifically to provide transportation for older residents. This measure enables individuals to safely shop in food stores and have the convenience of being driven to their homes and helped with carrying groceries into their kitchens. Health care professionals working with older clients should be aware of these services or perhaps help community organizations initiate similar programs.

SUMMARY

- Vitamins are divided into water soluble and fat soluble.
  - Solubility of vitamins affects the processes of their absorption, transportation, and storage in our bodies.
- Water-soluble vitamins are vitamin C, choline, and the B complex vitamins (thiamin, riboflavin, niacin, folate, pyridoxine [B_6], vitamin B_{12}, pantothenic acid, and biotin).
  - B vitamins function as coenzymes.
  - Choline is part of a neurotransmitter and lecithin.
  - Vitamin C serves as an antioxidant in addition to its coenzyme ability.
- Water-soluble vitamins are easily absorbed into blood circulation.
  - Excesses are excreted; toxicity is less likely; however, it may occur with pyridoxine and vitamin C.
- Fat-soluble vitamins are vitamins A, D, E, and K.
  - These serve structural and regulatory functions.
- Fat-soluble vitamins are absorbed the same as lipids; bile is required, and the nutrients enter the lymphatic system.
  - These are retained in fatty substances of the body; toxicity from supplemental fat-soluble vitamin intakes is possible.

NURSING APPROACH

Clinical Judgment and Next-Generation NCLEX® Examination-Style Questions

Case Study 1

Vitamins and Chronic Alcohol Use

Brad, aged 24, works in a manufacturing plant. His supervisor has been concerned about his frequent absences from work, declining productivity, and noticeable weight loss. When Brad came to work today, he looked unkempt and thin. With alcohol on his breath, he was slurring his words and having difficulty with balance. His coworker reported that Brad had a longtime drinking problem. His supervisor, worried about safety, took Brad to the occupational nurse on site.

Assessment/Recognize Cues

Subjective (From Patient Statements)

- "Maybe I drank a little too much last night, but I am not an alcoholic."
- "I can't remember how long I have worked here. Am I in trouble because I was late today? Where am I anyway?"
- Complained of headache
- Says he has lost weight, is not interested in eating because food doesn't taste good and his mouth is sore

Objective (From Physical Examination)

- Height 5′10″, weight 135 lbs
- Blood pressure 110 mm Hg systolic/70 mm Hg diastolic, temperature 98° F, pulse 92 beats per minute, respirations 21 breaths per minute
- Ataxia (muscle weakness and loss of coordination)
- Alcohol on breath, speech slurred
- Stomatitis (inflamed mouth and gingiva)
- Pale conjunctiva

Diagnoses (Nursing)/Analyze Cues

1. Weight loss related to probable chronic alcohol use and inadequate food intake as evidenced by alcohol on breath, reported weight loss, 81% ideal body weight (IBW), ataxia, stomatitis, and pale conjunctiva
2. Decreased functional ability related to chronic alcohol use as evidenced by being late for work, ataxia, and slurred speech

Planning/Prioritize Hypotheses

Patient Outcomes

Short term (at the end of this visit):

- Brad will eat at least two meals per day and take a multiple vitamin with minerals each day.
- He will identify foods he can eat without irritation to his mouth.

Long term (at follow-up visit in 1 month):

- Brad will report that he took a multiple vitamin with minerals every day, and he will participate in a more thorough nutrition assessment.
- He will weigh at least 2 more pounds.
- He will have no alcohol on his breath, stable balance, less inflammation in his mouth, and pink conjunctiva.

Nursing Interventions/Generate Solutions

1. Encourage Brad to decrease or avoid alcohol intake.
2. Encourage him to increase food intake and take a multiple vitamin with minerals every day.

Continued

THE NURSING APPROACH—cont'd

Implementation/Take Action

1. Sent a blood sample to the laboratory for complete blood cell count (which includes hemoglobin and hematocrit), ferritin, and a comprehensive metabolic panel (which includes albumin and electrolytes).
   Pale conjunctiva could indicate anemia. Weight loss and muscle weakness could be a result of inadequate food intake and toxicity from alcohol. Electrolyte abnormalities are common because of fluid balance issues and nutritional deficiencies.
2. Recommended that Brad stop drinking alcohol and start taking a multiple vitamin with minerals every day.
   Alcohol inhibits the absorption of thiamin while increasing the need for it. Insufficient thiamin can lead to decreased mental alertness, short-term memory loss, and ataxia (muscle weakness and loss of coordination). Lack of riboflavin can cause stomatitis. Lack of vitamin B6, folate, and iron can cause anemia. Vitamin supplements ensure adequate intake of vitamins when diets are not consistently well balanced.
3. Encouraged him to eat small, frequent meals high in protein, vitamins, and calories.
   Small, frequent meals are more easily absorbed than large meals and are easier to tolerate when a person has anorexia. Protein, vitamins, and sufficient calories are needed for healing and weight gain.
4. Gave him a list of nonirritating dietary sources of protein and vitamins (especially B vitamins).
   Milk products are high in protein. Cold, smooth foods are soothing to a sore mouth: puddings, eggnog, milkshakes, ice cream, yogurt, cottage cheese, instant breakfast drinks, and supplements like Ensure. Soy milk could be substituted if Brad has lactose intolerance. Other foods that would help provide vitamins include bland fruits without the peels; soft-cooked vegetables; refined enriched breads, cereals, and pasta; and tender pork, tuna, and chicken.
5. Set up an appointment for a follow-up visit in 1 month.
   Follow-up is needed to evaluate health status and changes made.
6. Provided Brad with a list of alcohol abuse programs and treatment centers. Encouraged him to see a counselor to help him reduce his alcohol intake.
   An alcohol rehabilitation program is likely indicated.

Evaluation/Evaluate Outcomes

Short term (at the end of the visit):

- Brad said he could take a vitamin each day and eat ice cream more often. He couldn't remember any other dietary recommendations but did take the list of foods.
- He declined to see a counselor about his alcohol intake but said he would come back in a month to see the nurse again.

Short-term goals partially met. Brad did not return for a follow-up visit in the nurse's office.

Discussion Questions

1. What additional information would the nurse need to obtain to confirm or rule out her nursing diagnoses?
2. How does alcoholism contribute to malnutrition? What food could provide the vitamins that Brad may be lacking?

Case Study 2

The nutritionist is lecturing to a group of nursing students about water-soluble vitamins.

What are the characteristics of water-soluble vitamins?

Put an X next to all that apply.

Characteristics	Place X if applies
1. Serves structural and regulatory functions	
2. Include vitamins A, D, E, and K	
3. Absorbed in the small intestine and then pass into the bloodstream for circulation	
4. Absorbed the same as lipids	
5. Are vitamin C and the B complex vitamins	
6. Excesses are excreted in urine	
7. The main function of thiamin (B_1) is to serve as a coenzyme,	
8. Deficiencies take months to develop	

APPLYING CONTENT KNOWLEDGE

Mark, age 3 years, is having his yearly health examination. His mom, rather proudly, tells you that Mark eats one apple and carrot sticks every day. She says that means he gets all the vitamins he needs. How do you respond?

WEBSITES OF INTEREST

MedlinePlus

www.nlm.nih.gov/medlineplus/

Provides reliable data about diseases, conditions, and wellness including nutrition. Created by the National Institutes of Health as a service of the U.S. National Library of Medicine.

U.S. Food and Drug Administration Center for Food Safety and Applied Nutrition

www.fda.gov/aboutfda/centersoffices/officeoffoods/cfsan/

Supplies FDA policies, rules, and *FDA Talk Papers* pertaining to supplements and health claims on foods.

WebMD

www.webmd.com

Offers strategies for managing health by providing accurate health and medical reference information, including online community interaction.

REFERENCES

Bemeur, C., & Butterworth, R. F. (2014). Thiamin. In A. C. Ross (Ed.), *Modern nutrition in health and disease* (11th ed.). Philadelphia: Lippincott Williams & Wilkins.

Brousseau. T. J., et al. (2005). Vitamin K deficiency mimicking child abuse. *The Journal of Emergency Medicine, 29*(3), 283–288.

Carmel. R. (2014). Cobalamin (vitamin B_{12}). In A. C. Ross (Ed.), *Modern nutrition in health and disease* (11th ed.). Philadelphia: Lippincott Williams & Wilkins.

DaSilva. V. R., et al. (2014). Vitamin B_6. In A. C. Ross (Ed.), *Modern nutrition in health and disease* (11th ed.). Philadelphia: Lippincott Williams & Wilkins.

Dubock. A. (2014). The politics of Golden Rice. *GM Crops Food, 5*(3), 210–222.

Fain. O., et al. (1998). Scurvy in patients with cancer. *British Medical Journal, 316*, 1661–1662.

Gayen. D., et al. (2016). Metabolic regulation of carotenoid-enriched Golden Rice line. *Front Plant Sci, 7*, 1622.

Gessner. B. D., et al. (1997). Nutritional rickets among breast-fed black and Alaska Native children. *Alaska Med, 39*(3), 72–74.

Hollick. M. F. (2006). Resurrection of vitamin D deficiency and rickets. *Journal of Clinical Investigation, 116*(8), 2062–2072.

Jones. G. (2014). Vitamin D. In A. C. Ross (Ed.), *Modern nutrition in health and disease* (11th ed.). Philadelphia: Lippincott Williams & Wilkins.

Kirkland. J. B. (2014). Niacin. In A. C. Ross (Ed.), *Modern nutrition in health and disease* (11th ed.). Philadelphia: Lippincott Williams & Wilkins.

Levine, M., & Padayatty, S. J. (2014). Vitamin C. In A. C. Ross (Ed.), *Modern nutrition in health and disease* (11th ed.). Philadelphia: Lippincott Williams & Wilkins.

Mani, P., & Rohatgi, A. (2015). Niacin therapy, HDL cholesterol, and cardiovascular disease: is the HDL hypothesis defunct? *Current Atherosclerosis Reports*, *17*(8), 43.

Marra, M. V., & Bailey, R. L. (2018). Academy of nutrition and dietetics: position of the academy of nutrition and dietetics: micronutrient supplementation. *The Journal of the Academy of Nutrition and Dietetics*, *18*(11), 2162.

Mock. D. M. (2014). Biotin. In A. C. Ross (Ed.), *Modern nutrition in health and disease* (11th ed.). Philadelphia: Lippincott Williams & Wilkins.

National Research Council (NRC). (2006). *Dietary reference intakes: The essential guide to nutrient requirements*. Washington, DC: The National Academies Press.

Pagana. K. D., et al. (2016). *Mosby's diagnostic and laboratory test reference* (13th ed.). St. Louis: Mosby.

Prousky. J. E. (2003). Pellagra may be a rare secondary complication of anorexia nervosa: a systematic review of the literature. *Alternative Medicine Review*, *8*(2), 180–185.

Rodriguez-Casado. A. (2016). The health potential of fruits and vegetables phytochemicals: notable examples. *Critical Reviews in Food Science and Nutrition*, *56*(7), 1097–1107.

Ross. A. C. (2014). Vitamin A. In A. C. Ross (Ed.), *Modern nutrition in health and disease* (11th ed.). Philadelphia: Lippincott Williams & Wilkins.

Said, H. M., & Ross, A. C. (2014). Riboflavin. In A. C. Ross (Ed.), *Modern nutrition in health and disease* (11th ed.). Philadelphia: Lippincott Williams & Wilkins.

Stover. P. J. (2014). Folic acid. In A. C. Ross (Ed.), *Modern nutrition in health and disease* (11th ed.). Philadelphia: Lippincott Williams & Wilkins.

Suttie. J. W. (2014). Vitamin K. In A. C. Ross (Ed.), *Modern nutrition in health and disease* (11th ed.). Philadelphia: Lippincott Williams & Wilkins.

Terada. N., et al. (2015). Wernicke encephalopathy and pellagra in an alcoholic and malnourished patient. *BMJ Case Rep, 2015* bcr2015209412.

Traber. M. G. (2014). Vitamin E. In A. C. Ross (Ed.), *Modern nutrition in health and disease* (11th ed.). Philadelphia: Lippincott Williams & Wilkins.

Wood. B., et al. (1998). Pellagra in a woman using alternative remedies. *Australasian Journal of Dermatology*, *39*(1), 42–44.

8

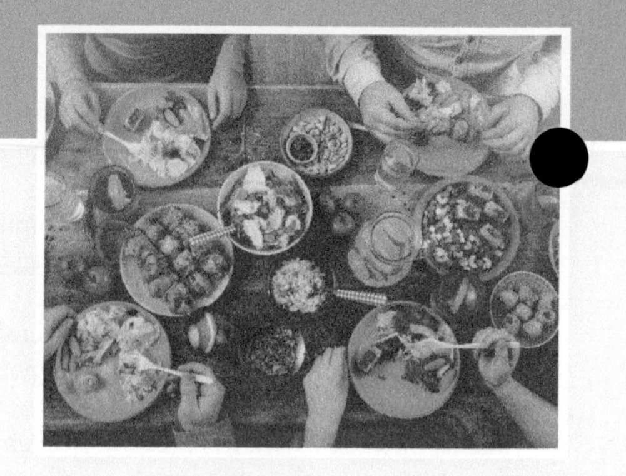

Water and Minerals

An ever-circulating ocean of fluid bathes all the cells in our bodies; this fluid allows for chemical reactions, transmission of nerve impulses, and transportation of nutrients and waste products throughout the body.

http://evolve.elsevier.com/GRODNER/FOUNDATIONS

LEARNING OBJECTIVES

- List the functions of water.
- Describe dietary sources of water.
- Explain the diverse roles of minerals.
- List and define major and trace minerals.
- Discuss plant and animal food sources of minerals.
- Explain the different levels of bioavailability of the food sources of minerals.

ROLE IN WELLNESS

An ever-circulating ocean of fluid bathes all the cells in our bodies; this fluid allows for chemical reactions, transmission of nerve impulses, and transportation of nutrients and waste products throughout the body. The fluid is not simply water, although water is its primary constituent. Some fluid in the body is used to form blood, lymph, and structure for cells. Minerals circulating in our body fluids create the setting for biochemical reactions to occur.

Water and minerals affect every system of our bodies, as well as our six dimensions of health. The physical health dimension depends on adequate levels of these nutrients. The intellectual health dimension is compromised when iron levels are low; iron deficiency affects cognitive abilities and thus diminishes the ability to learn. Emotional health may rely on our being sufficiently hydrated with fluids; cases of fluid volume deficit or dehydration have been mistaken for senility when the thirst acuity of older adults diminishes. The social health dimension may be affected if older adults become debilitated by bone fractures or osteoporosis caused by chronic calcium deficiencies; social mobility may be limited as their physical movement is inhibited. Vegans who consume no animal-derived foods because of spiritual health beliefs need carefully designed eating plans that provide adequate levels of zinc, iron, and calcium to avoid deficiencies. The environmental health dimension affects access to safe and plentiful sources of water, a nutrient essential to health.

Although water and minerals are primary components of body fluids, they perform other functions as well. This chapter explores water and minerals in the context of their nutritional requirements and physiologic roles in achieving nutritional wellness.

WATER

We can live several weeks without food but can survive only a few days without water or fluids. Although our bodies use stored nutrients to fuel energy needs, a minimum intake of water is required for cell function and as a solution through which waste products of the body are excreted in urine.

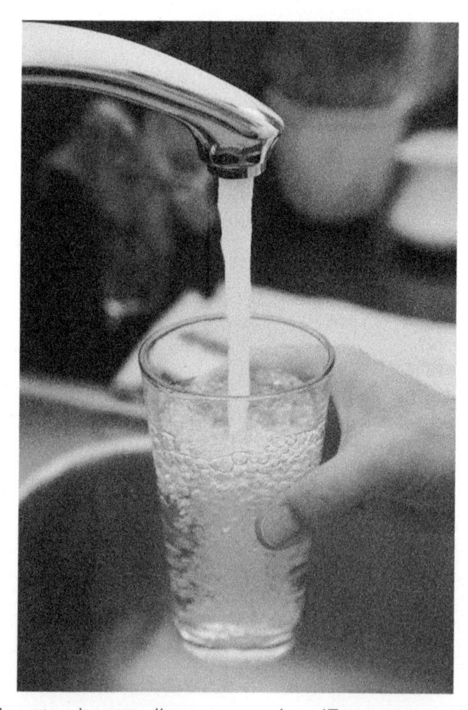

We need water in our diets every day. (From www.thinkstockphotos.com)

Food Sources

If we drank only water and no other liquids, we could meet our body's need for fluid. Most of us, however, consume fluids in addition to water throughout the day. Some fluids also contain other nutrients. Consider the wealth of nutrients found in milk (skim or whole), fruit juices, and soups. Some fruits and vegetables contain as much as 85% to 95% water. Watermelon, grapes, oranges, lettuce, tomatoes, and zucchini have high water content. Most foods contain water, but some are better sources of fluids than others. Generally, we depend on beverages as our main source of fluids.

The adequate intake (AI) recommendations for water are about 13 cups a day for men and 9 cups a day for women. This amount is in addition to fluids from foods consumed throughout the day, such as fruits and vegetables (National Research Council [NRC], 2006). Although the minimum amount needed by healthy adults may be about 4 cups, higher amounts are optimum, considering an individual's physiologic status and energy output.

Our primary source of water should be the liquids we drink (Table 8.1). Notice that coffee, tea, alcohol, and soft drinks are not listed as primary sources. Although they do contain water, coffee, tea, and alcohol act as diuretics, which cause an increase in water loss via the kidneys as urine. Soft drinks add fluid to the body, but they contain solutes (sugar, salt, various chemicals) that must be diluted as they enter the bloodstream. Drinking a soda increases the concentration of these solutes in the blood. The body responds by pulling fluid from the cells into the bloodstream to dilute the sugar and salt. The body loses the increased fluid in the bloodstream when it is excreted as urine. In addition, the body responds to the increased solutes and decreased fluid content by once again triggering the thirst mechanism.

Bottled water has become a mainstay in U.S. beverage selections and an economic force. Sales of bottled water have reached to more than $12.8 billion (Statista, 2017). Products range from imported sparkling mineral waters to spring waters to waters treated from nearby reservoirs. Although the price range is equally broad, the common denominator is that Americans enjoy the convenience of water as a beverage when available in portable containers and single portions.

TABLE 8.1 Foods as Sources of Water (by Percentage)

Food	Percentage Water
Dairy Products	
Milk	88–91
Cheddar cheese	37
Cottage cheese	79
Ice cream, ice milk	61–66
Fruits	
Apples	84
Grapefruit (whole or juice)	90
Grapes	81
Melons	90
Oranges (whole or juice)	88
Vegetables	
Asparagus	91
Carrots	88
Cucumber	96
Lettuce	96
Potato	75
Spinach	90
Sweet potato	73
Tomatoes	94
Miscellaneous	
Beans (cooked)	60–70
Bread	30–40
Fruit punch	88
Gelatin	84
Meats	50–60
Oatmeal (cooked)	85
Poultry	65
Soups	85–98

(Data from US Department of Agriculture, Agricultural Research Service. 2016. *Nutrient Data Laboratory*. USDA National Nutrient Database for Standard Reference, Release 28 (Slightly revised). Version Current: May 2016. Accessed 24 December, 2020 from www.ars.usda.gov/nea/bhnrc/mafcl.)

Water Quality

The minerals found naturally in water vary. **Hard water** refers to water that contains high amounts of minerals such as calcium and magnesium. Drinking this water can provide a significant amount of these nutrients. Non–nutrition-related problems from hard water can develop; mineral deposits may damage appliances and other machinery that interacts with water, and soap suds are reduced. To diminish these problems, a filtration process can be installed to soften water by replacing some minerals with sodium chloride (salt). **Soft water** containing sodium, however, can be a problem for sodium-sensitive individuals, such as those at risk for hypertension. To prevent health problems, water softeners may be used on only the hot tap in kitchens, leaving the cold tap unsoftened for consumption.

Another aspect of water quality is contamination. For example, many older buildings have pipes with lead solder joints that can release lead into the water that sits in or runs through them. If the level of lead in water is more than 15 parts per billion (ppb), pregnant women, infants, and children are advised to drink bottled water because even low levels of lead can seriously impair normal development. The local health department can recommend a competent laboratory that tests household water quality.

To reduce the chance that lead will leak into drinking and cooking water, do the following:

- Run the water for 2 minutes after it has been standing in the pipes.
- Use only cold water for drinking, cooking, and preparing baby formula (cold water absorbs less lead than hot).

Water treatment processes can remedy some contamination concerns. Others, such as industrial pollution, can be difficult to identify. Complications of bacterial contamination or inadvertent exposure of water to carcinogenic industrial substances can lead to health problems that range from simple gastroenteritis to cancer. Municipal and regional water processing plants take great care to ensure the safest water supply possible. Some water sources (private wells, surface water, springs, and cisterns), however, may exceed the maximum contaminant levels set by the Environmental Protection Agency (EPA).

The most severe water-related threats, such as cholera and typhoid, are no longer public health hazards in North America. Other potential industrial and environmental pollutants, however, can enter our water supply and endanger our health. Small suppliers may not have the financial means to improve technologic surveillance.

Poorer countries throughout the world continue to struggle with unsafe water supplies. Without the financial and technologic knowledge and resources, many people become ill by consuming bacteria-contaminated water. An increased incidence of stomach cancer is associated with exposure to *Helicobacter pylori*, which is sometimes found in contaminated waters. But even in the United States, incidences of contamination of municipal water supplies occurs, as happened in Flint, Michigan in 2014, and more recently in Newark, New Jersey (see the *Personal Perspectives* box Do Not Take Water for Granted).

Water as a Nutrient in the Body

Structure

The structure of water—two hydrogen atoms bonded to one oxygen atom—allows it to provide a base for biochemical reactions in the body and to easily move through the various compartments of cells and body systems. As the basis of body fluids, water can host other substances of different electrical charges and characteristics. **Intracellular fluids** (within the cell) are composed of water plus concentrations of potassium and phosphates. **Interstitial fluids** (between the cells) contain concentrations of sodium and chloride. **Extracellular fluids** consist of interstitial fluid and encompass all fluids outside cells, including plasma and the watery components of body organs and substances (Box 8.1).

Digestion and Absorption

Because water is inorganic, it is not digested. It passes quickly to the small intestine. Once there, most water is absorbed; the

PERSONAL PERSPECTIVES

Do not Take Water for Granted

When you are thirsty, what do you drink? If water, are you concerned about the safety of the tap water at home or at work? Or do you choose bottled water? Why? Are you well hydrated? Or underhydrated? Most likely, you may not have thought about these concerns, but not everyone feels that their water supply is safe, nor do they consider their hydration levels.

The United Nations (UN) considers access to clean drinking water a human right (UN, 2010). We tend to take this for granted, but recently, the towns of Flint, Michigan and Newark, New Jersey learned otherwise.

After the General Motors factory closed in Flint, the town fell into financial difficulties, and eventually the municipality of Flint came under the financial control of the state of Michigan. Under state control, attempts were made to limit spending as much as possible to meet new budget guidelines. Officials decided that one way to achieve significant savings was to transfer the source of municipal water from Lake Huron, also used by the much larger city of Detroit, to the Flint River. With appropriate treatment, Lake Huron provides a safe water supply; the Flint River, in contrast, was and is contaminated by industrial waste requiring extensive treatment to provide nontoxic water. Before the lack of proper treatment protocol was discovered, residents noticed that their tap water was turning brown and had an off taste and unusual odor. Flint's children began showing unusual symptoms. Ultimately the cause was found to be corrosive industrial chemicals in the tap water, which was not only toxic to humans but was corroding the aging lead pipes connecting the water supply to the homes of Flint. Lead was released into homes' water supply. The adults and children of Flint were experiencing lead poisoning, symptoms of which can be lifelong.

After almost 3 years of controversy and legal wrangling, the water of Flint finally had lower levels of lead, but the confidence of residents in their local government and state services was diminished, and they and their children may experience continuing effects of lead poisoning. The concerns are still ongoing as the lead pipe replacements to individual homes are still being completed.

Unfortunately, a similar situation is happening in Newark, the largest city in New Jersey, where about 50% of the population is Black, 30% Latino, and more than 25% live in poverty (Nathanson, 2020). In 2015, high lead levels in the water supply were reported. By 2016, the levels were so high that Newark Public schools closed access to drinking water in 30 schools. Further investigations of water quality throughout Newark revealed issues about the integrity of lead-lined water pipes to homes and other structures. These pipes depend on added chemical compounds to prevent lead from leaching into the water. In Newark, two factors resulted in lead contaminated water. First, Newark's ongoing financial challenges hindered the rehabilitation of the aging water distribution infrastructure. The second factor was that the city did not remedy a defective chemical compound that keeps lead from contaminating the water being distributed to homes and other community buildings such as schools. Although residents had been told for months by government officials that the problem was being remedied, the water was not safe for consumption. No level of lead in water is safe.

Instead, large portions of the city, predominantly Black American and low-income neighborhoods, are still receiving contaminated water into their homes. In an attempt to temporarily provide safer water for consumption, the city provided free faucet water filters, but the filters were not removing lead sufficiently. Consequently, Newark citizens are still receiving cases of bottled water for drinking and food preparation. The struggle to educate the community and to rectify the situation to provide safe water to all citizens is still on-going.

What would you do if concerned about the water quality of your tap water? Whom would you contact? What water would you drink? How would you prepare food? Wash the dishes? Shower? It all becomes personal when it is happening to you.

(Data from Corasaniti N et al: Lead Crisis in Newark Grows, as Bottle water distribution is bungled, *The New York Times*, 14 August, 2019. Accessed 24 December, 2020, from: Lead Crisis in Newark Grows, as Bottled Water Distribution Is Bungled - The New York Times (nytimes.com); Nathanson R: Newark's lead crisis isn't over: "People are still drinking water that they shouldn't, *The Intercept*, 15 March, 2020. Accessed 26 December, 2020, from: https://theintercept.com/2020/03/15/newark-new-jersey-lead-water-crisis/; U.N. General Assembly resolution 64/292. *The human right to water and sanitation*. 28 July, 2010.)

BOX 8.1 Body Fluid Compartments

Intracellular Fluid (65% of Body Water)	Extracellular Fluid (35% of Body Water)
Enzymes	Antibodies
Hemoglobin	Bicarbonate ions
Magnesium	Blood proteins
Minerals	Carbohydrates
Phosphorus	Chloride
Potassium	Glucose
Proteins	Minerals
	Proteins
	Lipids
	Lipoproteins
	Sodium

BOX 8.2 Functions of Water

Provides shape and rigidity to cells
Helps regulate body temperature
Acts as a lubricant
Cushions body tissues
Transports nutrients and waste products
Acts as a solvent
Provides a source of trace minerals
Participates in chemical reactions

rest is regulated by the colon and is either absorbed or excreted with feces.

Metabolism

Although not metabolized or broken down by gastrointestinal (GI) tract processes, water is an integral component of metabolic processes. In some reactions, the water of metabolism is water released as a byproduct of oxidative reactions; in others, water may be a part of the process to release energy from adenosine triphosphate (ATP), which is discussed in greater detail in Chapter 9. The released water may be excreted as waste or used elsewhere in the body. Glycogen in muscle and the liver contains water in the structure of glycogen molecules. When glycogen is used for energy, the water becomes available for body functions.

Functions

Water performs a variety of vital functions in the body (Box 8.2). It is an important structural component of the body, giving shape and rigidity to cells. It assists in regulating body temperature. Water conducts heat, absorbing and distributing it throughout the body, keeping body temperature stable from day to day. Water also helps cool the body by evaporating invisibly from the lungs and the surface of the skin, carrying off excess heat. This type of water loss is called **insensible perspiration**.

Water acts as a lubricant in the form of joint fluid and mucous secretions. It forms a shock-absorbing fluid cushion for body tissues such as the amniotic sac, spinal cord, and eyes.

Water is a major component of blood, lymph, saliva, and urine. As such, it delivers nutrients and removes waste products. Acting as a **solvent**, it enables minerals, vitamins, glucose, and other small molecules to be moved throughout the body.

Water may also supply trace minerals such as fluoride, zinc, and copper. Sometimes it is a source of too many minerals, including potentially toxic metals, such as lead, cadmium, and incidental substances from pesticides and industrial waste products.

In addition to serving as a medium for biochemical reactions, water also participates as a reactant. A **reactant** is a substance that enters into and is altered during a chemical reaction. For example, large molecules such as polysaccharides, fats, and protein are split into smaller molecules; water participates in and is changed by the process.

Ultimately, no growth or cell renewal occurs without water; it is part of every cell and is necessary as a medium for reactions and transporter of supplies.

Regulation of Fluid and Water in the Body

Our bodies have delicate but efficient mechanisms for maintaining appropriate fluid levels. The intake of fluids is balanced with the output through urine, sweat, feces, and insensible perspiration (Fig. 8.1). Regulation of fluid in the body is of physiologic importance because water makes up 50% to 60% of the weight of an average adult; the percentage is even higher for an infant; whose body weight is 75% to 80% water (Fig. 8.2). Fortunately, all we need to do is take in enough fluids, and our bodies' natural systems take care of the rest.

Homeostasis (physiologic equilibrium) is maintained by electrolytes that include minerals and blood proteins. Two of

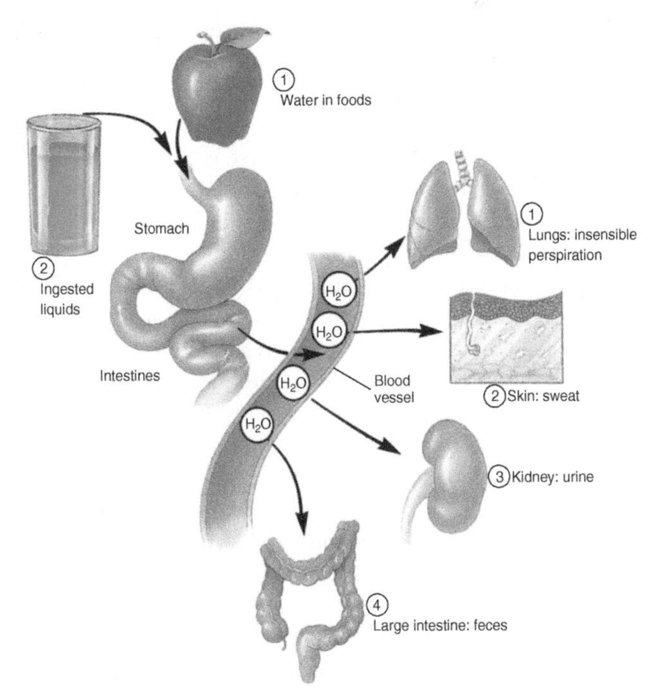

Fig. 8.1 Intake of fluids is balanced with output. (Courtesy Joan Beck. Modified from Thibodeau GA, Patton KT: *The human body in health and disease*, ed 2, St. Louis, 1997, Mosby.)

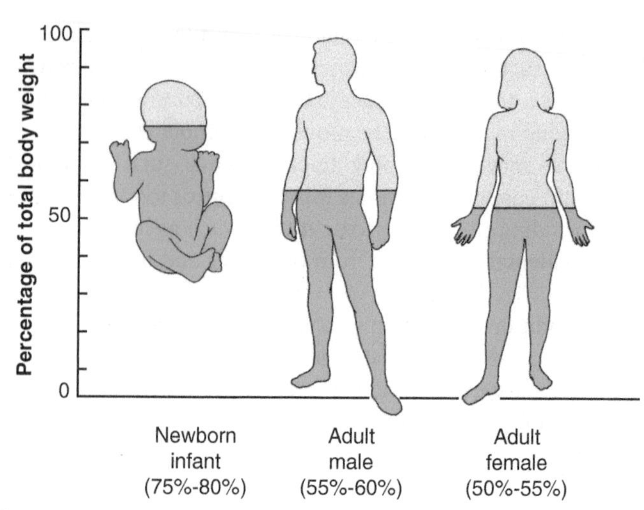

Fig. 8.2 Percentage of body weight represented by water in infants compared with that in adults. (From Rolin Graphics. In Thibodeau GA, Patton KT: *Structure and function of the body*, ed 10, St. Louis, 1997, Mosby.)

the most important minerals are sodium and potassium. The extracellular distribution of fluid depends on sodium, and potassium influences intracellular water. Water moves within and between the cells in interstitial fluids in response to the levels of these minerals. An imbalance is corrected by mechanisms that cause thirst and regulate the ability of the kidneys to release or retain fluids.

Thirst, a dryness in the mouth, stimulates the desire to drink liquids. We often ignore our thirst until mealtimes. The thirst mechanism is controlled by the hypothalamus and involves several steps. The sodium and solute levels in blood rise as the water level in the body gets low. This causes water to be drawn from the salivary glands to provide more fluid for the blood. The mouth then feels dry because less saliva, which keeps the mouth moist, is produced. This sensation, thirst, stimulates the drinking process. If the thirst mechanism is faulty, as it may be during illness, physical exertion, or aging, hormonal mechanisms also help conserve water by reducing urine output.

The mechanisms of the kidneys regulate the amounts of water excreted. Obligatory water excretion of at least 500 mL (1 pint) must be performed daily, regardless of the amount ingested, to clear the body of waste products. The mechanism relies on the combined actions of the brain, kidneys, pituitary gland, and adrenal gland. When fluid in the body becomes low, the hypothalamus stimulates the pituitary gland to release antidiuretic hormone (ADH). ADH is secreted in response to high sodium levels in the body or too-low blood pressure or blood volume. The target organ of the hormone is the kidney. The kidneys then conserve water by decreasing excretion of water, and the retained fluid is recycled for use throughout the body.

When the sodium concentration in the kidneys gets high (too much fluid excreted), another process kicks in to counteract the lowered blood volume and pressure. The kidneys release renin, an enzyme that activates the blood protein angiotensin. Angiotensin raises blood pressure by narrowing blood vessels; it is a vasoconstrictor. Angiotensin also prompts the adrenal gland to release the hormone aldosterone. The target organ of aldosterone is the kidney. The effect is to decrease excretion of sodium, causing the kidneys to respond by retaining fluid in the body.

Fluid and Electrolytes

Dissolved in body fluids are minerals and other organic molecules required for the regulation of both intracellular and extracellular fluid distribution. Fluids follow salt concentrations; this means that cells can control fluid balance by directing the movement of mineral salts.

Electrolytes are minerals that carry electrical charges or ions (particles) when dissolved in water. These minerals separate into positively charged ions (cations) or negatively charged ions (anions). The primary extracellular electrolytes in body fluids are sodium (Na^+/cation) and chloride (Cl^-/anion), and the primary intracellular electrolyte is potassium (K^+/cation). To maintain fluid balance, cells control the movement of electrolytes. Water will follow sodium concentration. Moving electrolytes in and out of the cell membrane requires transport proteins. The sodium/potassium pump is a transport protein that works to exchange sodium from within the cells for potassium. Other ions are also exchanged.

In addition to water regulation, the kidneys also regulate electrolyte levels. If body levels of sodium are low, aldosterone directs the kidneys to reabsorb or retain more sodium. This in turn results in excretion of potassium so the balance of electrolytes is maintained.

Imbalances

What happens when our regulatory mechanisms are unable to maintain the balance? Abnormal shifts in fluid balance may cause a deficit or excess in fluid volume.

Fluid volume deficit. In fluid volume deficit (FVD), a person experiences vascular, cellular, or intracellular dehydration. FVD can occur from diarrhea, vomiting, or high fever—symptoms often experienced with stomach and intestinal viral infections and influenza. Other causes of excessive fluid loss are sweating, diuretics, and polyuria (excessive urination). Whenever we lose fluid and have difficulty taking in additional fluids, we are at risk for FVD.

Determining whether symptoms are caused by dehydration or illness can be difficult. Characteristics of FVD include infrequent urination, decreased skin elasticity, dry mucous membranes, dry mouth, unusual drowsiness, lightheadedness or disorientation, extreme thirst, nausea, slow or rapid breathing, and sudden weight loss. The person with FVD is less able to maintain blood pressure immediately after rising from a sitting or lying position (called orthostatic hypotension). A primary health care provider should be consulted for any illness that lasts more than a few days and causes loss of body fluids. In moderate or severe FVD, intravenous (IV) therapy is indicated to replace fluids.

FVD can also happen when we are not ill. Strenuous physical activity, either athletic or work related, that causes excessive sweating can lead to FVD. Hot, dry weather also can overwork the body's cooling mechanisms. Drinking fluids throughout the day despite a low level of thirst sensation can alleviate these risks.

Older adults and infants are the groups most at risk for FVD. Older adults have decreased fluid reserves and diminished thirst mechanism acuity. FVD symptoms may be misdiagnosed as senility. Reminding older clients to drink even when they are not thirsty is appropriate to ensure adequate intake of fluids. In infants, water makes up a larger percentage of body weight than in adults, and a greater percentage is extracellular fluid; dehydration from fluid loss can occur rapidly. In addition to other signs of FVD, an infant may have a depressed fontanelle (soft spot) in the skull.

Fluid volume excess. Fluid volume excess is a condition in which a person experiences increased fluid retention and edema. It is associated with a compromised regulatory mechanism, excess fluid intake, or excess sodium intake.

Edema is excess accumulation of fluid in interstitial spaces caused by seepage from the circulatory system, which results in the retention of about 10% more water than normal. Some of us may notice that when we eat meals that are particularly high in sodium, we feel bloated, and our weight may even rise a few pounds the next day. This weight gain is not true weight gain but simply water retention that occurs in response to the excess intake of sodium. Within a few days, weight and water levels in the body return to their usual levels.

Edema can be a symptom of a health risk in certain situations. Sodium-sensitive individuals not only retain fluid when consuming high levels of sodium but also experience an increase in blood pressure, leading to hypertension. Reducing excess water retention through a reduction in sodium consumption is a first step in treating this type of hypertension. A more serious form of edema occurs in victims of kwashiorkor when the protein levels in the body are so low that cellular fluid levels are imbalanced. Inappropriate levels of interstitial fluid accumulate in the stomach, face, and extremities.

Water intoxication refers to the consumption of large volumes of water within a short time, which results in a dilution of electrolytes in body fluids. It causes muscle cramps, decreased blood pressure, and weakness. Water intoxication is also possible if there is extensive loss of electrolytes because of dehydration, and rehydration is accomplished using only water, without the addition of replacement electrolytes. This condition is relatively rare but tends to occur when athletes continually hydrate without equivalent loss of fluid while participating in slower paced events such as runs lasting longer than 4 hours or extended triathlons, or they rehydrate after a strenuous event with excessive amounts of water. Nonetheless, fluid volume deficit, dehydration, is much more common and more dangerous for athletes.

Minerals

Minerals serve a variety of functions in our bodies (Box 8.3). Structurally, minerals provide rigidity and strength to the teeth and skeleton; the skeletal mineral components also serve as a storage depot for other needs of the body. Minerals, allowing for proper muscle contraction and release, influence nerve and muscle functions. Other functions of minerals are acting as cofactors for enzymes and maintaining proper acid-base balance in body fluids. Minerals are also required for blood clotting and for tissue repair and growth.

Mineral Categories

On the basis of the amount of each mineral in the composition of our bodies, the 16 essential minerals are divided into two categories: major and trace minerals. To maintain body levels of major minerals, the minerals must be consumed daily from dietary sources in amounts of 100 mg or higher. In contrast, trace minerals are required daily in amounts of 20 mg or less (Box 8.4). Although the required amounts differ greatly between the major and trace minerals, each is absolutely necessary for good health.

BOX 8.3 Considering Vitamins and Minerals Through Function

Vitamins and minerals are discussed as two separate nutrient categories in Chapter 7 and this chapter. Although each essential vitamin and mineral is discussed individually, they are not grouped together on the basis of their functions for the body. The information here provides vitamins and minerals required for the specific body functions blood health, bone health, energy metabolism, and fluid and electrolyte balance. Additional functions of individual vitamins and minerals may be found in Tables 7.3, 7.6, 8.3, and 8.4.

Blood Health

Blood is the body fluid supplying tissues with oxygen, nutrients, and energy through circulation within the cardiovascular system. It is composed of water, red and white blood cells, oxygen, nutrients, and other formed substances. Always moving, blood gathers and distributes nutrients and oxygen to all cells and disposes of waste products. Deficiency of any of these nutrients will affect overall blood health. Only the blood-related functions of the vitamins and minerals are listed.

Vitamin[a]	Function	Mineral [b]	Function
Cobalamin (B_{12})	Transport/storage of folate needed for heme and cell formation and other functions	Iron	Distributes oxygen in hemoglobin and myoglobin
Folate (folic acid, folacin, PGA)	Coenzyme metabolism (synthesis of amino acid, heme, DNA, RNA) and other functions	Zinc	Cofactor for more than 200 enzymes, including enzymes to make heme in hemoglobin, genetic material, and proteins
Pyridoxine (B_6)	Hemoglobin synthesis and other functions	Copper	Helps with iron use
Vitamin K Active form: menaquinones	Cofactor in synthesis of blood clotting factors; protein formation		

Continued

BOX 8.3 Considering Vitamins and Minerals Through Function—cont'd

Bone Health

As living tissue, bone requires nutrients to maintain cellular structure. Blood circulates through bone capillaries, delivering nutrients while removing waste materials no longer needed by cells. Hormones regulate the use of minerals, either for storage and structural purposes in bone or for controlling body processes. Specific vitamins and minerals are indispensable for these functions to occur.

Vitamin[a]	Function	Mineral[b]	Function
Vitamin D Precursor: 7-dehydrocholesterol Active form: cholecalciferol	Bone mineralization	Calcium	Bone and tooth formation
Vitamin K Active form: menaquinones	Protein formation for bone mineralization; cofactor for blood clotting factors	Phosphorus	Bone and tooth formation (component of hydroxyapatite)
Vitamin A Precursors: carotenoids Preformed vitamin: retinoids	Bone growth; maintains epithelial cells; regulation of gene expression	Magnesium Fluoride	Bone structure Bone and tooth formation; increases stability of bone

Energy Metabolism

To metabolize carbohydrates, lipids, and protein for energy and other needs, the body depends on many nutrients to support the process, create new cells, and implement various related functions.

Vitamin(s)[a]	Function	Mineral[b]	Function
Thiamin (B_1)	Coenzyme energy metabolism; muscle nerve action	Iodine	Thyroxine synthesis (thyroid hormone) regulates growth and development; basal metabolic rate regulation
Riboflavin (B_2)	Coenzyme energy metabolism	Chromium	Carbohydrate metabolism, part of glucose tolerance factor
Niacin (B_3) (nicotinic acid and niacinamide) Precursor: tryptophan	Cofactor to enzymes involved in energy metabolism; glycolysis and tricarboxylic acid (TCA) cycle synthesis	Phosphorus Sulfur Iron	Energy metabolism (enzymes) Component of protein structures Distributes oxygen in hemoglobin and myoglobin
Pyridoxine (B_6)	Forms coenzyme pyridoxal phosphate (PLP) for energy metabolism		
Folate (folic acid, folacin, PGA)	Coenzyme metabolism (synthesis of amino acid, heme, DNA, RNA)		
Cobalamin (B_{12})	Metabolism of fatty acids/amino acids	Zinc	Carbohydrate metabolism (insulin function); cofactor to more than 200 enzymes
Pantothenic acid	Part of coenzyme A		
Biotin	Metabolism of carbohydrate, fat, and protein		

Fluid and Electrolyte Balance

Life systems depend on fluid and electrolyte balance within the body. Electrolytes consist of mineral salts that maintain cellular fluid balance. The acid–base balance of body fluids is buffered by other minerals.

Mineral[b]	Function
Sodium	Major extracellular electrolyte for fluid regulation; body fluid levels; acid–base balance; nerve impulse and contraction; blood pressure/volume
Potassium	With sodium and chloride, major intracellular electrolyte for fluid regulation; muscle function
Chloride	Acid–base balance
Phosphorus	Acid–base balance

DNA, Deoxyribonucleic acid; *PGA*, pteroylmonoglutamic acid; *RNA*, ribonucleic acid.
[a]See Chapter 7 for additional information on vitamins.
[b]See text for additional information on water and minerals.

The Dietary Reference Intakes (DRIs) listed in this chapter for minerals are those for young adults ages 19 to 30 years (NRC, 2006). Levels for other groups are noted when special mention is needed. Keep in mind that because nutrition is a relatively young science, new functions of minerals as nutrients in the human body are still being discovered. The DRI tables can be accessed at https://ods.od.nih.gov/HealthInformation/Dietary_Reference_Intakes.aspx.

Food Sources

The prime sources of minerals are both plant and animal foods. Valuable sources of plant foods include most fruits, vegetables, legumes, and whole grains. Animal sources consist of beef, chicken, eggs, fish, and milk products. The discussions of individual minerals highlight the best food choices (Box 8.5).

In contrast to vitamins, minerals are stable when foods containing them are cooked. As inorganic substances, they are

BOX 8.4 Essential Minerals in the Human Body

Major	Trace
Calcium	Chromium
Chloride	Copper
Magnesium	Fluoride
Phosphorus	Iodine
Potassium	Iron
Sodium	Manganese
Sulfur	Molybdenum
	Selenium
	Zinc

indestructible. Minerals may leach into cooking fluids but can still be absorbed if the fluid is consumed.

Although plants may contain an abundance of various minerals, some minerals in plants are not easily available to the human body. Bioavailability refers to the level of absorption of a consumed nutrient and is of nutritional concern. Binders such as phytic and oxalic acids may bind some minerals to the plant fiber structures. Binders are substances in plant foods that combine with minerals to form indigestible compounds, making them unavailable for our use. The amount of plant minerals available for absorption may depend on minerals in soils in which the plants are grown.

BOX 8.5 MyPlate: Vegetables

As noted in Chapter 7, the health benefits of eating vegetables overlap with those of eating fruits. Both fruit and vegetable MyPlate categories provide rich sources of minerals and are valuable components of an overall healthy diet, providing nutrients essential for the health and maintenance of our bodies (also see Box 7.2). The health benefits of eating vegetables and fruits as part of an overall healthy diet include reduced risk for stroke, cardiovascular disease, and T2D mellitus; protection against some cancers (mouth, stomach, colorectal); and, because they are excellent sources of fiber, possible decrease in risk of several chronic diet-related disorders. The recommendation is to eat at least 2½ cups of vegetables every day.

What Counts as a Cup of Vegetables?

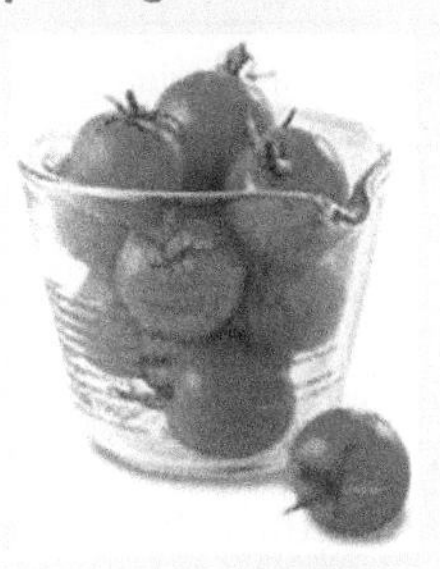

In general, 1 cup of raw or cooked vegetables or vegetable juice or 2 cups of raw leafy greens can be considered 1 cup from the vegetable group. the following lists specific amounts that count as 1 cup of vegetables (in some cases equivalents for ½ cup are also shown) toward your recommended intake.

		Amount That Counts as 1 Cup of Vegetables	Amount That Counts as ½ Cup of Vegetables
Dark green vegetables	Broccoli	1 cup, chopped or florets 3 spears 5 inches long raw or cooked	
	Greens (collards, mustard greens, turnip greens, kale)	1 cup, cooked	
	Spinach	1 cup, cooked 2 cups, raw	1 cup, raw
	Raw leafy greens: spinach, romaine, watercress, dark green leafy lettuce, endive, escarole	2 cups, raw	1 cup, raw
Red and orange vegetables	Carrots	1 cup, strips, sliced, or chopped, raw or cooked 2 medium 1 cup baby carrots (about 12)	1 medium carrot About 6 baby carrots
	Pumpkin	1 cup, mashed, cooked	
	Red peppers	1 cup, chopped, raw, or cooked 1 large pepper (3 inches diameter, 3¾ inches long)	1 small pepper
	Tomatoes	1 large raw whole (3 inches) 1 cup, chopped or sliced, raw, canned, or cooked	1 small raw whole (2¼ inches diameter) 1 medium canned
	Tomato juice	1 cup	½ cup
	Sweet potato	1 large baked (2¼ inches or more diameter) 1 cup, sliced or mashed, cooked	
	Winter squash (acorn, butternut, Hubbard)	1 cup, cubed, cooked	½ acorn squash, baked = ¾ cup
Beans and peas	Dry beans and peas (such as black, garbanzo, kidney, pinto, or soy beans, or black-eyed peas or split peas)	1 cup, whole or mashed, cooked	
Starchy vegetables	Corn, yellow or white	1 cup 1 large ear (8–9 inches long)	1 small ear (about 6 inches long)
	Green peas	1 cup	
	White potatoes	1 cup, diced, mashed 1 medium boiled or baked potato (2½–3 inches diameter)	

Continued

BOX 8.5 MyPlate: Vegetables—cont'd

		Amount That Counts as 1 Cup of Vegetables	Amount That Counts as ½ Cup of Vegetables
Other vegetables	Bean sprouts	1 cup, cooked	
	Cabbage, green	1 cup, chopped or shredded raw or cooked	
	Cauliflower	1 cup, pieces or florets raw or cooked	
	Celery	1 cup, diced or sliced, raw or cooked 2 large stalks (11–12 inches long)	1 large stalk (11–12 inches long)
	Cucumbers	1 cup, raw, sliced or chopped	
	Green or wax beans	1 cup, cooked	
	Green peppers	1 cup, chopped, raw or cooked 1 large pepper (3 inches diameter, 3¾ inches long)	1 small pepper
	Lettuce, iceberg or head	2 cups, raw, shredded or chopped	1 cup, raw, shredded or chopped
	Mushrooms	1 cup, raw or cooked	
	Onions	1 cup, chopped, raw or cooked	
	Summer squash or zucchini	1 cup, cooked, sliced or diced	

(Modified from U.S. Department of Agriculture, Center for Nutrition and Promotion: *ChooseMyPlate.gov: What counts as a cup of vegetables?* Accessed 24 December, 2020, from www.choosemyplate.gov/vegetables.)

Minerals from animal foods do not have the same bioavailability issues. In fact, minerals from animal foods can be absorbed more easily than those from plants. However, fat content may be an issue for some animal foods. Lower-fat sources of dairy and meat products are usually available and provide the same levels of minerals at a higher nutrient density. Liver is often cited as a good source of minerals such as iron and zinc. But liver is also high in cholesterol and saturated fats and may contain toxins to which the animal may have been exposed. These factors, combined with liver's somewhat unusual taste, often leave the impression that good nutrient intake depends on eating healthy food that tastes bad. Other sources of each nutrient may be more appealing and equally as nutritious.

Food processing may reduce the amount of minerals available for absorption. Processing oranges into orange juice does not affect potassium levels naturally contained in oranges. However, processing whole-wheat flour into white flour does cause significant loss of minerals because the whole grain is not used. Iron is the only mineral returned to white flour through enrichment; zinc, selenium, copper, and other minerals are permanently lost.

Because we have difficulty obtaining high enough levels of some minerals naturally, fortification of manufactured foods has become commonplace. It is through fortification that food processing can serve the nutrient needs of consumers while still addressing the issues of convenience and taste appeal. Salt fortified with iodine is available; dry cereals have added minerals such as iron and an assortment of vitamins and other minerals.

Minerals as Nutrients in the Body

Structure

Minerals are inorganic substances. As elements, they are found in the rocks of the earth. Their tendency to gain or lose electrons makes them electrically charged. Thus, they have special affinities for water, which itself carries positive and negative charges. As we consume plant and animal foods containing minerals, we can incorporate them into our body structures (bones), organs, and fluids.

Digestion and Absorption

During the process of digestion, minerals (as inorganic substances) are separated from the foodstuffs in which they entered our bodies. Digestion does change the valence states of some minerals, thereby changing their ability to be absorbed. However, their structure is not changed, so they can be absorbed.

As noted, bioavailability affects the level of minerals we actually absorb. Generally, consuming a variety of whole foods ensures an adequate intake of minerals. Mineral deficiencies for which Americans tend to be at risk are those of iron, calcium, and zinc. Concerns and strategies for consuming appropriate amounts of these nutrients are discussed later in this chapter.

Metabolism

Because minerals are inorganic and do not provide energy, they are not metabolized by the human body. Instead, some minerals assist as cofactors of metabolic processes.

MAJOR MINERALS

Calcium

Function

Calcium is the most abundant mineral in the body. Almost all the calcium in the body, about 99%, is found in our bones, serving structural and storage functions. The other 1% of body calcium is released into body fluids when blood passes through bones; this constant interaction of blood with bone allows calcium to be distributed throughout the body. Other functions that depend on calcium include (1) the central nervous system, particularly nerve impulses; (2) muscle contraction and relaxation, when needed; (3) formation of blood clots; and (4) blood pressure regulation. Continuing research supports that increased levels of calcium (and vitamin D) intakes may be protective for colorectal cancer (Meng, et al., 2019).

Regulation

Our dietary intake of calcium influences the deposition of calcium in our bones. Blood calcium levels, however, do not depend on a daily dietary calcium intake. Instead, the skeletal supply of calcium provides the source of calcium to be distributed throughout the body through the circulatory system. If calcium blood levels get too low, three actions can occur to reestablish calcium homeostasis: bones release calcium, intestines absorb more calcium, and kidneys retain more calcium.

Hormones that regulate the level of calcium in body fluids control the release of calcium from bones. Hormones affecting blood levels include parathormone (parathyroid hormone), calcitriol (active vitamin D hormone), and calcitonin. Parathormone is secreted by the parathyroid gland in response to low blood calcium levels. It raises blood calcium levels by stimulating all three ways of providing calcium to body fluids. Vitamin D has a hormone-like effect as calcitriol and increases blood calcium levels by acting on all three systems. The third hormone involved, calcitonin, is released by the special C cells of the thyroid gland. Calcitonin reacts in response to high blood levels of calcium by lowering both calcium and phosphate in the blood.

Reactions of very low or extremely high blood levels can occur if regulatory mechanisms are hindered by a lack of vitamin D or hormone malfunction. If calcium blood levels get too high, calcium rigor (with symptoms of hardness or stiffness of muscles) may occur. Conversely, if levels are too low, a person may experience calcium tetany, with spasms caused by muscle and nerve excitability.

Recommended Intake and Sources

Calcium recommended dietary allowance (RDA) for men and women ranges from 1300 mg/day (ages 9 through 18 years) to 1000 mg (ages 19 through 50 years). Levels increase to 1200 mg for men and women older than 50 years. The RDA during pregnancy and lactation is 1000 mg.

Concerns have been raised regarding the calcium intake of those most at risk for deficiency: youths aged 11 through 24 years and pregnant and lactating women. During adolescence, pregnancy, and lactation, calcium needs are still high, although actual consumption of calcium may decrease. For many Americans, meeting these recommendations means increasing the number of servings of calcium-rich foods to at least three or more a day (Box 8.6). Other issues surrounding calcium intake and children are discussed in Chapter 10.

BOX 8.6 MyPlate: Dairy

MyPlate focuses on the dairy group of foods as a source of the minerals calcium and potassium and vitamin D and protein. These nutrients can also be obtained from non–dairy-derived foods, but milk products are rich sources and are a traditional part of the dietary intake of most Americans.

The health benefits of consuming foods in the dairy group include assisting the building and maintaining of bone mass during the life span, particularly during childhood and adolescence; possible reduced risk of osteoporosis; and overall higher quality of nutritional intake. The recommendation is to consume 3 cups or servings daily of milk or dairy products. If milk products are not consumed because of lactose intolerance, lactose-reduced products, calcium-fortified foods, and other naturally good sources of calcium can be chosen instead. Nondairy products made from almond, soy, coconut, and rice should always be checked for added nutrients to equal or exceed the nutrient values of dairy products. Nutrients of concern include calcium, vitamin D and vitamin A.

What Counts as a Cup of Dairy?

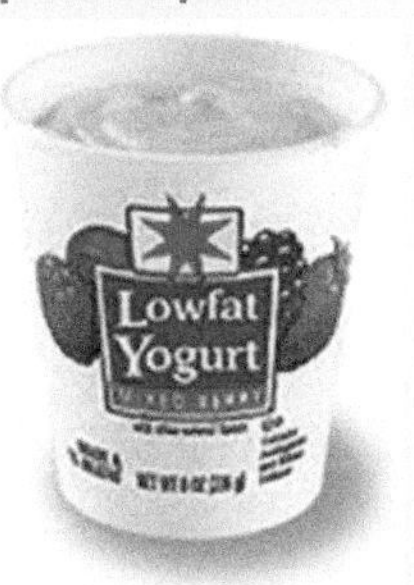

In general, 1 cup of milk, yogurt, or soy milk (soy beverage), 1½ ounces of natural cheese, or 2 ounces of processed cheese can be considered as 1 cup from the dairy group. The following table lists specific amounts that count as 1 cup in the dairy group toward your daily recommended intake.

	Amount That Counts as 1 Cup in the Dairy Group	Common Portions and Cup Equivalents
Milk (choose fat-free or low-fat milk)	1 cup milk	
	1 half-pint container milk	
	½ cup evaporated milk	
Yogurt (choose fat-free or low-fat yogurt)	1 regular container (8 fluid ounces)	1 small container (6 ounces) = ¾ cup
	1 cup yogurt	1 snack size container (4 ounces) = ½ cup
Cheese (choose reduced-fat or low-fat cheeses)	1½ ounces hard cheese (Cheddar, mozzarella, Swiss, Parmesan)	1 slice of hard cheese is equivalent to ½ cup milk
	⅓ cup shredded cheese	
	2 ounces processed cheese (American)	1 slice of processed cheese is equivalent to ⅓ cup milk
	½ cup ricotta cheese	
	2 cups cottage cheese	½ cup cottage cheese is equivalent to ¼ cup milk
Milk-based desserts (choose fat-free or low-fat types)	1 cup pudding made with milk	
	1 cup frozen yogurt	
	1½ cups ice cream	1 scoop ice cream is equivalent to ⅓ cup milk
Soy milk (soy beverage)	1 cup calcium-fortified soy milk	
	1 half-pint container calcium-fortified soy milk	

(Modified from U.S. Department of Agriculture, Center for Nutrition and Promotion: *ChooseMyPlate.gov: What counts as a cup in the dairy group?* Accessed 24 December, 2020, from www.choosemyplate.gov/dairy.)

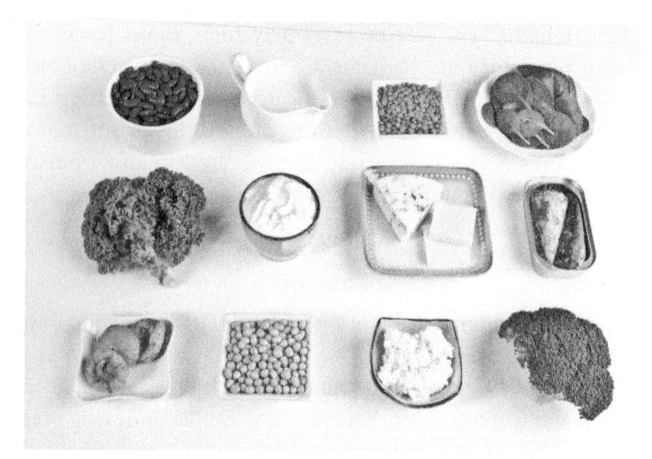

Fig. 8.3 Calcium can be consumed in many different foods, including beans, milk (animal-derived or fortified), yogurt, cheese, canned sardines and salmon, broccoli, kale, and other leafy greens. (From www.thinkstockphotos.com)

BOX 8.7 Suggestions for Boosting Calcium Intake

Dairy

Melted cheese added to broccoli
Calcium-fortified milk and cottage cheese
Powdered milk added to baking mixes, soups, puddings, gravies, hamburgers, and meatloaves
Eating cheese wedges with sliced apples and pears
Smoothies (fruit drinks made with milk, yogurt, and fruits)
Soups made with low-fat or skim milk

Nondairy

Bean burritos
Bean soups (split pea or lentil soup)
Breads fortified with calcium
Chicken cacciatore (chicken with bones cooked in tomato sauce; acid of tomatoes pulls calcium from bones)
Juices fortified with calcium
Soy milk and soy products fortified with calcium
Tofu (made with calcium carbonate), fresh or in frozen meals and desserts

Primary sources of calcium are dairy products, mainly milk (whole, low-fat, and skim) and milk-based products such as ice cream, ice milk, yogurt, frozen yogurt, cheeses, and puddings (Fig. 8.3). Although butter, cream cheese, and cottage cheese are dairy products, they are not good sources of calcium; butter and cream cheese are predominantly fat, and cottage cheese loses calcium through processing. Nondairy sources include green leafy vegetables (broccoli, kale, and mustard greens), small fish with bones (sardines and salmon canned with processed edible bones), legumes, and tofu processed with calcium. In addition, a variety of calcium-fortified foods are available, ranging from fortified orange juice to bread products. Box 8.7 lists foods that boost calcium intake, and the *Teaching Tool* box Visualizing the Calcium Values of Foods provides calcium education strategies for working with clients who have low literacy skills.

Some leafy green vegetables—in particular, spinach, collards, Swiss chard, and escarole—contain oxalic acid, a binder that reduces the calcium absorbed. Plant foods containing oxalic acid cannot be considered a trustworthy source of calcium but are good sources of other nutrients. Tea contains oxalic acid as well as tannins (also found in coffee), both of which may affect the absorption of calcium in foods consumed with tea. With the increased consumption of iced tea beverages, this effect should be considered, particularly for female adolescents and young adults.

TEACHING TOOL

Visualizing the Calcium Values of Foods

Food charts that show the calcium values of different foods may be helpful to most people, but they may be meaningless to clients who cannot read English or have minimal literacy skills. Consider this innovative teaching strategy for visualizing the calcium content of commonly consumed foods (e.g., skim milk, yogurt, hard cheese), as follows:

1. Select four calcium-rich foods (e.g., broccoli, pinto beans) and four low-calcium foods (e.g., cottage cheese).
2. Fill plastic resealable bags with small marshmallows to represent the calcium content of each of the selected foods. Each marshmallow can represent 10 mg of calcium. In addition, fill a large plastic resealable bag with 100 marshmallows (1000 mg or 100% Daily Value) as a reference.
3. Match the bag of "calcium" with the appropriate food model (or picture). Have the participants do the matching.
4. Distribute a pictorial representation of this activity with additional foods along with their bags of "calcium."

(Courtesy Gayle Coleman, M.S., R.D., when employed at State University Extension, East Lansing, Michigan.)

Many adults are lactose intolerant. Lactose intolerance occurs when the body does not produce enough lactase, an enzyme necessary for the digestion of lactose, the carbohydrate found in milk. (Lactose intolerance is detailed in Chapter 4.) People experiencing lactose intolerance need to regularly incorporate sources of calcium other than dairy products into their dietary patterns. For some people, calcium supplements may be indicated; a registered dietitian nutritionist or qualified nutritionist may be consulted.

Some calcium supplements are poorly absorbed because they don't dissolve in the stomach. If a calcium tablet does not readily dissolve when stirred into cider vinegar, it probably will not dissolve in the body.

Absorption Factors

Our bodies absorb calcium on the basis of physiologic need. During childhood growth phases, we may absorb up to 75% of calcium consumed, compared with absorption rates of 30% to 60% once we complete our primary growth years. Similarly, during pregnancy and lactation, percentages of absorption are higher as dictated by physiologic need (Weaver & Heaney, 2014). In addition to physiologic need, other factors also seem to enhance the levels of calcium absorbed, including the following (Box 8.8):

- Lactose: Found naturally in milk (an excellent source of calcium), lactose appears to increase calcium absorption.
- Sufficient vitamin D: Vitamin D is involved in the synthesis of a protein that allows calcium to pass through the intestinal wall into the bloodstream.

BOX 8.8 Factors Favoring and Hindering Calcium Absorption

Factors Favoring Calcium Absorption
Acidity of digestive mass
Body's need for higher amounts (as in pregnancy)
Lactose
Sufficient vitamin D

Factors Hindering Calcium Absorption
Aging
Binders such as phytic acid and oxalic acid
Dietary fat
Dietary fiber
Drug use
Excessive phosphorus intake
Laxative use
Sedentary lifestyle

- Acidity of digestive mass: Calcium is more soluble in acidic substances, so it is better absorbed when ingested as part of a meal. Generally, enough hydrochloric acid passes from the stomach to the intestine for calcium absorption. As we age, the amount of hydrochloric acid in digestive juices may decrease, causing less calcium to be absorbed.
- Binders: Naturally occurring substances in plant foods may bind with calcium in plant foods; two common calcium binders are phytic and oxalic acids (also called phytates and oxalates, respectively). Human digestive processes may be unable to separate calcium from the binder; both are then excreted, reducing the calcium available for absorption.
- Dietary fat: Dietary fat can form insoluble soaps with calcium; the insoluble soaps are harder to digest, making calcium less accessible for absorption. Moderate and low dietary fat intakes discourage the formation of this insoluble mass.
- High-fiber intake and laxatives: Excessive fiber consumption or laxative abuse results in foodstuff moving through the GI tract too quickly for minerals, particularly calcium, to be absorbed.
- Excessively high intakes of phosphorus or magnesium: Excessively high intakes of these minerals disturb the balance of calcium in the body. Calcium is best absorbed when moderate or recommended levels of phosphorus and magnesium are ingested in proportion to calcium intake.
- Sedentary lifestyle: Being a couch potato has its consequences. A physically inactive lifestyle leads to less bone density. In contrast, weight-bearing exercise that pulls the muscle against the bone enhances calcium deposits in the bone matrix. This action occurs during running, brisk walking, biking, and strength training.
- Drugs: Some medications, including anticonvulsants, tetracycline, cortisone, thyroxine, and aluminum-containing antacids, are associated with reduced calcium absorption.

Deficiency

Deficiency of calcium primarily affects bone health. During the growing years, inadequate intake of calcium reduces the density of bone mass and, if severe, can stunt growth. For adults, long-term calcium deficiency may be one of the risk factors for osteoporosis, a multifactorial systemic skeletal disorder. This condition takes many years to develop, and overt symptoms appear late in life. Osteoporosis is a condition in which bone density is reduced and the remaining bone is brittle and breaks easily.

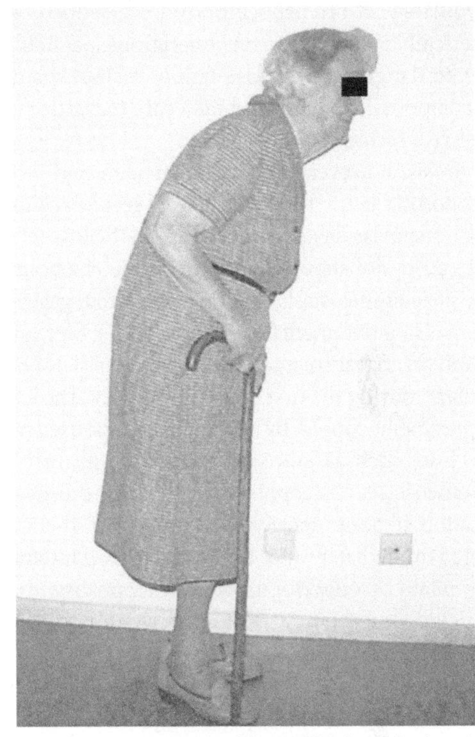

Typical posture in osteoporosis. (From Shipley M: *A colour atlas of rheumatology*, ed 3, London, 1993, Mosby-Year Book Europe Limited. By permission of Mosby International Ltd.)

One of the most recognizable characteristics of osteoporosis is the dowager's hump; as vertebrae in the spine collapse from weakness, the spine is no longer able to support the weight of the head. The back bows and the head angles down. Most significantly, the internal organs affected by the curvature are unable to function efficiently, and other health difficulties develop.

In contrast to osteomalacia, osteoporosis is multifactorial, and all the factors are tied to bone mineral density. These factors include genetics, diet, and lifestyle determinants. Bone density builds through early adulthood. Peak bone density is reached by about age 20 years, although some additional bone mineralization continues into the 30 s. The more density built early in life, the less potential risk encountered. Factors that affect bone density but cannot be modified include genetic determinants of race and gender and family history, as follows:

- Race: Osteoporosis is more common in White and Asian women than among African and Black American women. The reason is racial differences in the skeletal density, possibly caused by hormonal differences.
- Gender: Men have greater bone density than women and enter the later years, when bone demineralization begins, with a larger storage of calcium. The fact that men have more

lean body mass or muscularity may cause more calcium to be deposited and retained in comparison with women. Women lose greater amounts of bone calcium during the first few years after menopause. The drop in estrogen levels appears to initiate the calcium loss. To slow the loss, medications including hormone (estrogen) replacement therapy (each with potential risks) may be prescribed for postmenopausal women, depending on individual risk factors.

- Family history: A predisposition to lower bone density may be genetically passed between generations, particularly from mother to daughter. If a close family member is diagnosed with osteoporosis, one should take care to reduce the effects of other risk factors.

Osteoporosis, however, does occur in men and women. For men, osteoporosis tends to be a result of secondary causes that affect peak bone mass development or speed the loss of bone density. These causes are steroid therapy, chronic alcoholism, hypogonadism, skeletal metastasis, multiple myeloma, gastric surgery, and anticonvulsant treatment (Bethel et al, 2017). Men and women who undergo organ transplantation are more at risk for osteoporosis, particularly during the first year after surgery. The loss of bone density is probably caused by the medications used to prevent organ rejection, such as glucocorticoids, that disturb bone and mineral homeostasis. Osteoporosis prevention can begin before transplantation if bone density is marginal, or therapy can be implemented immediately after transplantation (Fratianni, 2016).

Factors related to development of osteoporosis that can be adjusted include nutrition, particularly calcium intake, and lifestyle determinants, as follows:

- Nutrition/calcium intake: Dietary calcium intake is of concern throughout the life span. In particular, the growth years (when calcium is deposited in the bone matrix) and the postmenopausal years of bone mineralization loss are periods when calcium intake appears crucial. Although the RDA for calcium provides sufficient amounts, many individuals consume less than these levels. Female adolescents often consume levels of kcal and nutrients well below the RDA while attempting to control body weight. These eating patterns often continue through adulthood. This long-term marginal deficiency of calcium may set the stage for future bone disorders. The issue is even more complicated for older adults. When they consume calcium-containing foods, they may absorb less calcium because of decreased gastric acidity and lower levels of available vitamin D.
- Alcohol: Long-term excessive intake of alcohol appears to reduce bone density. Alcohol may directly depress bone formation or may take the place of more nutritious foods, producing marginal deficiencies.
- Smoking: Cigarette smoking has been associated with a higher risk of osteoporosis. Smokers tend to be of lower weight (less bone density) than nonsmokers, and women who smoke appear to lose more bone mineralization after menopause than those who don't.
- Caffeine: Caffeine consumption has been tied to urinary excretion of calcium. Reasonable use of caffeinated beverages, however, may be acceptable. More than likely, the relationship of caffeine to lower levels of body calcium concerns replacement by caffeinated beverages of those containing calcium, such as skim milk and other calcium-fortified beverages. Although caffeinated coffee consumption may affect bone density of postmenopausal women, adequate calcium intake can overcome these effects (Tucker et al., 2014).
- Sedentary lifestyle: A physically active lifestyle not only enhances calcium absorption, but also helps maintain bone matrix mineralization. However, excessive exercise that results in extremely low body fat levels for women may be detrimental to bone density. If amenorrhea (abnormal cessation of menses) occurs because of excessive exercise, the resulting premature drop in estrogen may limit or decrease bone mineralization during the prime growth periods. Similarly, girls and women experiencing anorexia nervosa lose significant bone density within a year of onset and have a greater risk of hip fracture later in life. Boys and men with anorexia nervosa are at similar risk for osteoporosis and its complications (Coughlin et al., 2014).

Although the risk factors for osteoporosis may seem overwhelming, several can be reduced by following basic recommendations for achieving wellness. Consuming the serving amounts recommended by MyPlate and engaging in regular physical exercise can minimize most of the risk. The *Teaching Tool* box Calcium: By Any Means Possible provides tips on educating clients on appropriate calcium intake.

Low levels of calcium intake are also associated with an increased risk of colon cancer and hypertension.

Toxicity

Calcium toxicity from consuming foods that contain calcium is not a concern. Problems may occur when supplements of calcium and other nutrients are used instead of foods. Oversupplementation may cause constipation, urinary stone formation affecting kidney function, and reduction in absorption of iron, zinc, and other minerals (Weaver & Heaney, 2014). The general guideline for calcium supplements is that levels should not exceed the DRI for calcium. In addition, a tolerable upper intake level (UL) of 2500 mg has been established.

Phosphorus

Function

Most of the phosphorus in the body (85%) is in our bones and teeth as a component of hydroxyapatite, a natural mineral structure. The other 15% of body phosphorus has functions (1) in energy transfer; (2) as part of the genetic material of deoxyribonucleic acid (DNA) and ribonucleic acid (RNA); (3) as a buffer in the form of phosphoric acid, which balances body acid–base levels; and (4) as a component of phospholipids used for transportation and structural functions.

Recommended Intake and Sources

The RDA for phosphorus is 700 mg/day for men and women aged 19 years and older. Phosphorus is widely available in foods. Particularly good sources are protein-rich foods such as dairy foods, eggs, meat, fish, poultry, and cereal grains. Because of the processing of convenience foods and soft drinks, both are also sources of phosphorus.

TEACHING TOOL

Calcium: By Any Means Possible

The RDA for calcium ranges from 1000 to 1300 mg/day, depending on a person's age. The best sources are calcium-rich foods. But what if a client is lactose intolerant or just doesn't like many calcium-containing foods?

Because the potential ramifications of chronic calcium deficiency are serious—fractures and other complications of osteoporosis—calcium supplementation may be appropriate. Following are some suggestions and cautions for client education:

- Calcium supplementation may increase the dietary intake of calcium, but it does not alleviate other risk factors associated with osteoporosis. Other nutrients and lifestyle behaviors also affect the level of risk. Popping a calcium pill does not mean a person is osteoporosis free.
- Many people have problems with compliance; the regularity of calcium intake, not an occasional dose, builds dense bones. It is better to rely on food sources.
- The source of calcium affects the amount of actual calcium available. Tablets composed of calcium carbonate contain more elemental calcium (often 500–600 mg) than those made of calcium citrate or lactate (usually 200 mg per tablet), and it takes fewer pills to achieve the Recommended Dietary Allowance. Calcium citrate, however, is more easily absorbed by the digestive tract, even if more pills are needed.
- Be aware that calcium is always combined with another substance to form the tablet. A tablet may contain 1200 mg of calcium carbonate but only 500 mg of elemental calcium. The supplements to avoid are those made from dolomite, bone meal, and oyster shell; they may be contaminated with lead and other toxic metals.
- Although the tablets are supplementing dietary intake, it's best to take them with meals. The acid of the digestive process also helps in the breakdown and absorption of the calcium tablet(s) and tying the supplement to meals works as a reminder system. This also helps spread supplementation throughout the day. One large dose will not be absorbed as well as two or three smaller doses.
- Calcium supplements often contain added vitamin D. Vitamin D recommendation doubles after age 50 years and triples after age 70 years, so the added vitamin D may be age appropriate. If other sources provide sufficient amounts of vitamin D, such as multivitamin/mineral supplements or foods or cereals fortified with 100% of the daily value for vitamin D, then the added D is not necessary.
- Before starting a supplement, keep track of sources and amounts of dietary calcium for several days. Intake may be adequate. If not, first contemplate ways to increase intake with foods, and then consider supplementation.

Deficiency

Deficiency of phosphorus is unknown. It is part of the genetic material of every cell of the body.

Toxicity

Excessive amounts of phosphorus, usually possible only from phosphorus supplements, cause calcium excretion from the body. Very high phosphorus intakes could affect the calcium/phosphorus ratio, possibly reducing the amount of calcium absorbed. This is a problem only if calcium intake is inadequate. Because phosphorus-containing soft drinks and convenience foods have replaced milk beverages and less-processed foods for many American teens and adult women, this may be a dietary concern. A UL of 4000 mg has been determined for phosphorus.

Magnesium

Function

As with calcium and phosphorus, most of the magnesium in the body is found in our bones, providing structural and storage functions. Magnesium assists hundreds of enzymes throughout the body. It also regulates nerve and muscle function, including the actions of the heart, and has a role in the blood clotting process and in the immune system.

Recommended Intake and Sources

The RDAs for magnesium are 400 mg/day for men (420 mg for men aged ≥31 years) and 310 mg/day for women (320 mg for women aged ≥31 years). Many commonly eaten foods contain magnesium. Particularly good sources are most unprocessed foods, including whole grains, legumes, broccoli, leafy green vegetables, and other vegetables. Hard water can be a significant source of magnesium.

Deficiency

Magnesium deficiency tends to be related to secondary causes rather than because of a primary lack of magnesium consumption. These secondary causes include excessive vomiting and diarrhea caused by pathologic conditions. A GI tract disorder may affect magnesium absorption, or kidney disease may inhibit retention of the mineral. Malnutrition and alcoholism may also have a negative impact on magnesium levels in the body. Similarly, drug interference or artificial feeding solutions deficient in magnesium may influence total body levels of magnesium. Whenever body fluids are lost, so is magnesium. Individuals on long-term regimens of diuretic agents are also at risk for deficiency.

In addition, if magnesium intake levels are borderline and intake of calcium is high, such as from calcium supplements, magnesium absorption may be limited.

Symptoms of magnesium deficiency include twitching of muscles, muscle weakness, and convulsions. In children, magnesium deficiency also may be associated with growth failure.

Toxicity

Toxic effects of magnesium are rare but serious and are attributed to nondietary sources, such as supplements and mineral salts. A UL of 350 mg pertains to nonfood sources. Self-supplementation with calcium tablets containing magnesium while also taking magnesium supplements adds up to an excess that is not seriously toxic but is excessive enough to cause long-term diarrhea and deficient fluid volume (dehydration). This situation is an example of why all medications and dietary supplements should be reported to health care providers before invasive or costly procedures are conducted to determine the cause of symptoms. Simply stopping the magnesium supplementation will most likely restore proper function of the large intestine.

Sulfur

Function

Sulfur is a component of protein structures. It is present in every cell of the body and is part of several amino acids, thiamine, and biotin. Sulfur is also involved in maintaining the acid–base balance of the body.

Recommended Intake and Sources

No DRI has been established for sulfur. Diets adequate in protein provide sufficient amounts of sulfur. Sulfur is found in all protein-containing foods.

Deficiency

Deficiencies of sulfur do not occur; sulfur is so basic to the structure of the human cell that deficiencies cannot develop.

Toxicity

Toxicity of sulfur is not a health issue.

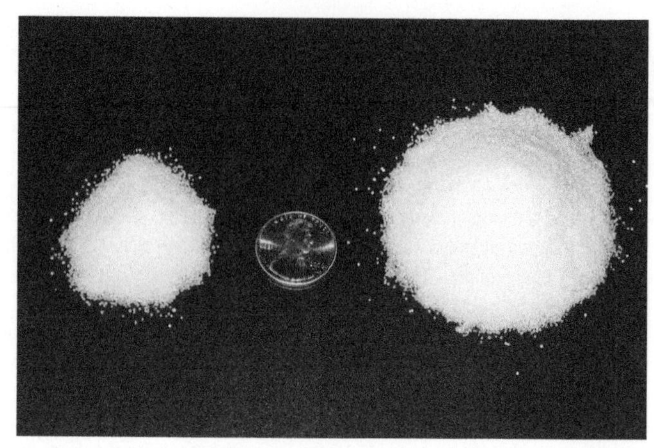

Fig. 8.4 Daily salt intakes: Adequate Intake of sodium (1500 mg) equals ¾ tsp salt *(left)*; excessive consumption of processed and fast-food products may result in an intake of sodium that equals 3 tsp salt (6000 mg) *(right)*. The Tolerable Upper Intake Level for sodium (2300 mg) equals about 1 tsp, whereas the average American intake (3300 mg) equals 1½ tsp salt.

Electrolytes: Sodium, Potassium, and Chloride

Electrolytes are minerals circulating in blood and other body fluids that carry an electrical charge. Maintaining a balance of these minerals is important because of their effect on body processes, such as the amount of water in the body, blood pH, and muscle action. Electrolytes travel in blood as acids, bases, and salts and include sodium, calcium, potassium, chlorine, magnesium, and bicarbonate. Laboratory studies of blood serum determine electrolyte values.

Sodium, potassium, and chloride are major electrolytes of the body. As electrolytes, these minerals serve specific functions. The acid-base balance of body fluids depends on regulated distribution of these minerals, proteins, and other electrolytes. Electrolytes also have a role in the normal functioning of nerves and muscles. In addition, each mineral serves other specific functions in the body.

Sodium

Function

Sodium performs a variety of important functions in the body. Blood pressure and volume are maintained by the characteristics of sodium as the major cation in extracellular fluid. Transmission of nerve impulses relies on body sodium levels. As the major extracellular electrolyte, sodium has a role in the regulation of body fluid levels in and out of cells. This movement affects blood volume as well, which is tied to the thirst mechanism and total body fluid levels. The blood proteins, such as albumin, that prevent the development of some types of edema also regulate blood volume.

Recommended Intake and Sources

The AI for sodium is 1500 mg/day for adults or about ¾ teaspoon of salt (sodium chloride). This dietary recommendation is based on the known adequate intake required for good health (Fig. 8.4). A UL for sodium has not been established as there is insufficient evidence to assess risk from high sodium intake, aside from the chronic disease risk. There is a CDRR (Chronic Disease Risk Reduction) intake set recommending for adults the reduction of sodium intake if the intake is above 2300 mg/day (National Academies of Sciences [NAS], 2019).

The average American adult consumes about 3300 mg of sodium a day, much higher than the AI for all ages (Institute of Medicine, 2013). Professional health organizations such as the American Medical Association, the American Public Health Association, and the American Heart Association, and other scientific groups support reduction of our dietary sodium intake. To achieve that public health goal, recommendations are to reduce daily intake to 2300 mg or lower based on the CDRR.

Most sodium enters our diet as sodium chloride (table salt). Sodium occurs naturally in many foods. It is also added to foods as salt during the cooking process and right before consumption (see the *Cultural Diversity and Nutrition* box A [Cooking] History of Salt). Processing of foods, particularly quick-serve foods, often adds substantial amounts of sodium, as listed in Table 8.2. Processed foods are carriers for other additives that often contain sodium. The sodium adds flavor that may be lost in processing.

Do you salt your food first, and then taste it? Some habits are hard to break but are worth the effort. However, breaking the salt-shaker habit will reduce sodium intake only 15% for most Americans; most of the sodium eaten comes from processed foods.

The more a foodstuff is processed, the higher the sodium content becomes (see Box 8.8). More nutrients are also lost along the way. Which is saltier, or to be more exact, which contains more sodium—a bowl of corn flakes or a large order of fast-food fries? The corn flakes win, containing 290 mg of sodium compared with 200 mg for the fries. Of course, the fries contain a lot more fat and calories.

Consider the potato. A plain baked potato contains only 16 mg of sodium. Prepared at a local fast-food restaurant, a baked potato with cheese sauce and broccoli skyrockets to

TABLE 8.2 Effects of Processing on the Sodium Content of Foods

Food Product	Total Sodium Content (mg)
Potatoes	
Baked potato (1)	16
French fried potatoes (10 strips)	108
Scalloped potatoes from dry mix (1 cup)	835
Chicken	
Baked chicken (3 oz)	64
Batter-fried chicken (3 oz)	231
Chicken nuggets (6 pieces)	542
Oats	
Oatmeal prepared with water (1 cup)	2
Oatmeal bread (1 slice)	124
Ready-to-eat cereal (1 cup)	307
Apples	
Apple (1)	Trace
Applesauce (1 cup)	8
Apple pie (1 slice)	476

(Data from US Department of Agriculture, Agricultural Research Service. 2016. *Nutrient Data Laboratory*. USDA National Nutrient Database for Standard Reference, Release 28 (Slightly revised). Version Current: May 2016. Accessed 24 December, 2020, from www.ars.usda.gov/nea/bhnrc/mafcl.)

CULTURAL DIVERSITY AND NUTRITION

A (Cooking) History of Salt

The course of history has been influenced by salt. Nations explored the world in search of salt because of its value in preserving foods. Bacterial and mold cells are inhibited from growing when placed in a concentrated salt solution, thus decreasing food spoilage. Although salt is no longer needed to preserve foods, we continue to value its ability to transform the taste of a dish from bland to sublime. Salt's importance to the human body cannot be denied because we have specialized taste buds to identify its consumption. Salt as a compound of sodium chloride contains two essential minerals without which the human body cannot survive.

Recognition of the importance of salt to human life began early. In the Old Testament of the Bible, salt was identified as an offering to God. Later on, Roman soldiers were given a stipend, called *salarium*, to buy salt. Today we can buy salt with our "salaries," a term that is derived from *salarium*. "Salt of the earth" was a phrase used by Jesus to describe his followers who were pure and of the earth.

Application to Nursing

Although salt has its virtues, it also has drawbacks. Health professionals continue to recommend moderate intakes of sodium to reduce the risk of hypertension. The amounts recommended for cooking vary because an amount that is pleasing to one person may vary for another. Amounts of salt listed in a recipe can usually be modified to suit the health and taste requirements of the cook and the eaters.

(Data from McGee H: *On food and cooking: The science and lore of the kitchen*, New York, 1997, Firestone; and O'Neill M: Let it pour, *New York Times Magazine*, 22 October, 1995, p. 77.)

having more than 400 mg of sodium and lots of fat. A cheese or sour cream mix prepared at home is even higher in sodium—close to 600 mg. The sodium in plain mashed potatoes from a mix (dehydrated and then reconstituted) jumps from 8 mg in its original whole form to more than 300 mg, and that's without butter or gravy. The point is that processing foods adds invisible sodium as sodium chloride; in fact, it's so invisible that we can no longer taste the saltiness.

Sodium enjoys widespread use in the American diet as a flavoring agent (sodium chloride, monosodium glutamate [MSG], sodium saccharin), dough conditioner (baking powder, baking soda), and preservative (sodium sulfite). Because of consumer demand, lower sodium versions of many products are available. Nutrition labeling information must include sodium content. This is powerful information that allows for the comparing of sodium contents of similar products.

Deficiency

Depletion of sodium can develop through dehydration or excessive diarrhea. Because of concern over the relationship between sodium and hypertension, some people may overly restrict sodium and thus be at risk for deficiency. Typical athletic activity or physical labor that produces excessive sweating may cause dehydration and sodium loss, but drinking fluids and consuming foods containing sodium soon restore body levels of sodium. Salt tablets, once a common remedy, are not recommended and may be dangerous.

Symptoms of sodium deficiency include headache, muscle cramps, weakness, reduced ability to concentrate, and loss of memory and appetite. For most people, sodium deficiency is unlikely to occur because we get enough sodium naturally from foods. These symptoms are similar to those of fluid volume deficit, which is more common.

Hyponatremia, or low blood sodium, may occur. The symptoms are the same as for sodium intake deficiency. Hyponatremia may be acute, as a one-time episode as a result of specific factors, or chronic—that is, a recurring condition. Acute hyponatremia is of concern for endurance athletes. Athletes completing endurance events or slower runners in marathon races who continually drink fluid without an equivalent loss of fluid through sweat or urination may so overhydrate as to experience hyponatremia. This condition is rare, but awareness is important, because medical treatments for FVD and acute hyponatremia are different even though the symptoms are the same. Blood testing determines the cause of the symptoms. Chronic hyponatremia may occur because of secondary disorders such as neurologic and kidney disorders that affect the fluid regulatory mechanisms of the body. Blood levels of sodium decrease as excess fluid is retained or too much sodium is excreted by the kidneys. Drug and dietary treatments may address chronic hyponatremia (Bailey et al., 2014).

Toxicity

Although there is no UL for sodium. an excessive intake is difficult for the body to handle. The kidneys have the primary responsibility to flush out the excess sodium. Some individuals are sodium sensitive and may experience hypertension and edema in response to high intakes of sodium. Levels consumed in diets based on highly processed foods and high-sodium foods may be enough to initiate hypertension in sodium-sensitive individuals. Although others may not experience negative ramifications of high-sodium intakes, there are no benefits either. This is one of the few nutrients that we can overdose on from foods we consume.

An occasional very salty meal may produce edema but not hypertension. The best remedy for occasional edema is simply to drink more water to equalize the sodium concentration of body fluids. The kidneys take care of the rest by filtering out the excess sodium.

Potassium

Function

Although sodium as a cation maintains the fluid levels extracellularly, potassium, as the primary intercellular cation, maintains fluid levels inside the cells. Potassium is also crucial for normal functioning of nerves and muscles, including the heart.

Recommended Intake and Sources

The AI for potassium ranges from 2600 mg/day to 3400 mg/day for women and men, respectively (NAS, 2019). The best sources for potassium for these purposes are the forms found naturally in fruits and vegetables.

Sources of potassium include whole unprocessed foods, white potatoes with skin, sweet potatoes, tomatoes, bananas, oranges, other fruits and vegetables, dairy products, and legumes.

Although evidence exists for potassium supplementation reducing high blood pressure, a CDRR has not been created, as the evidence does not clearly explain the relationship between potassium consumption and chronic disease criteria (NAS, 2019).

Deficiency

Like magnesium deficiency, potassium deficiency may be caused by dehydration from vomiting or diarrhea, diuretics, and misuse of laxatives. If long-term use of diuretics is warranted to reduce edema associated with hypertension, particular attention should be paid to consuming adequate levels of potassium from foods. Some diuretics are potassium wasting; some are potassium sparing. Potassium supplementation with use of a potassium-sparing diuretic could be dangerous. Clients ought to be informed when diuretics are prescribed as to whether the medication is potassium wasting or sparing. Potassium supplements should be taken only when prescribed by a primary health care provider.

Most often, bananas and oranges are suggested to patients at risk for potassium deficiency. These fruits may not be the best sources according to nutrient content, satiety, and economy. Whereas an edentulous (toothless) older person with congestive heart failure who is taking potassium-wasting diuretics and is on a low-income budget can make a meal out of a whole baked potato, they cannot be equivalently satisfied with a banana. A baked potato eaten with the skin contains 844 mg of potassium, whereas a whole banana contains 891 mg. A whole orange yields only 326 mg. A potato stores easily without refrigeration for much longer than a banana, and somewhat longer than an orange, and fits better into a tight budget. Yet foods like a simple potato may not be suggested to patients. Nurses can create patient education nutrient/food lists that consider factors such as satiety and economy to enhance compliance.

Symptoms associated with potassium deficiency include muscle weakness, confusion, decreased appetite, and, in severe cases, cardiac dysrhythmias.

Toxicity

In general, potassium toxicity occurs only from supplements, not from consuming excess from foods. Therefore, a UL has not been determined. Toxicity does not usually occur with foods as long as a person has properly functioning kidneys. For individuals with renal disease, high-potassium foods are toxic. Even clients undergoing dialysis may still be at risk for potassium toxicity. Symptoms of toxicity are similar to those of a deficiency. They include muscle weakness, vomiting, and at excessively high levels, cardiac arrest.

Chloride

Function

As the key anion of extracellular fluids, chloride assists in maintaining fluid balance inside and outside cells. In addition, chloride is a component of hydrochloric acid, an indispensable gastric juice produced by the stomach.

Recommended Intake and Sources

The AI for chloride is 2300 mg/day for adults. For adults more than 50 years old, the AI is 2000 mg, and for those older than 70 years, 1800 mg. These requirements are easily met by consumption of sodium chloride; foods containing sodium usually provide chloride as well.

Deficiency

Deficiency of chloride is rare; adequate amounts are easily consumed. Although chloride deficiency is possible, it would occur from the same circumstances as sodium deficiency or from excessive vomiting.

Toxicity

Chloride toxicity may occur because of dehydration, which can cause an imbalance of chloride with the other electrolytes. However, the other effects of dehydration are more severe than those of chloride toxicity.

Table 8.3 provides a summary of the major minerals.

TRACE MINERALS

Trace minerals as a group of nutrients function primarily as cofactors by performing metabolic and transport functions.

Iron

Function

Iron is responsible for distributing oxygen throughout our bodies. Oxygen depends on the iron in the hemoglobin (an oxygen-transporting protein) of red blood cells (erythrocytes) to bring

TABLE 8.3 Major Minerals

Mineral	Function	Clinical Issues Deficiency/ Toxicity	Recommended Daily Intakes[a]	Food Sources	Absorption Issues
Calcium (Ca)	Bone and tooth formation; blood clotting; muscle contraction/ relaxation; central nervous system; blood pressure	Deficiency: reduced bone density; osteoporosis Toxicity: constipation; urinary stones; reduced iron and zinc absorption	RDA: Adults: 1000–1200 mg Pregnancy/ lactation: 1000 mg UL: 2500 mg	Milk (whole, low-fat, skim), milk-based products, green leafy vegetables, legumes	Absorption based on need: increased by vitamin D; decreased by binders, inactivity, coffee/tea
Phosphorus (P)	Bone and tooth formation (component of hydroxyapatite); energy metabolism (enzymes); acid–base balance	Deficiency: rare Toxicity: increased calcium excretion	RDA: Adults: 700 mg Pregnancy/lactation: 700 mg UL: 4000 mg	Dairy foods, egg, meat, fish, poultry	Absorbed with calcium
Magnesium (Mg)	Structure/storage; cofactor; nerve and muscle function; blood clotting	Deficiency: secondary with muscle twitching, weakness, convulsions from FVD	RDA: Men: 420 mg Women: 320 mg Pregnancy/lactation: 320–360 mg UL: 350 mg	Whole grains, legumes, green leafy vegetables (broccoli), hard water	—
Sulfur (S)	Component of protein structures	Deficiency: only with protein malnutrition	Protein-adequate diets contain adequate levels	Protein-containing foods	—
Sodium (Na)	Major extracellular electrolyte for fluid regulation; body fluid levels; acid–base balance; nerve impulse and contraction; blood pressure/volume	Deficiency: FVD with headache; muscle cramps, weakness, decreased concentration, memory and appetite loss Toxicity: sodium-sensitive hypertension	AI: Adults: 1500 mg CDRR: Reduce intake if above 2300 mg	Table salt; natural in many foods; processed foods	—
Potassium (K)	Major intracellular electrolyte for fluid regulation; muscle function	Deficiency: muscle weakness, confusion, decreased appetite, cardiac dysrhythmias caused by FVD from vomiting/diarrhea or diuretics Toxicity: from diet or supplements if renal disease present	AI: Adults: Men: 3400 mg Women: 2600 mg	Unprocessed foods, fruits, vegetables, dairy products, meats, legumes	—
Chloride (Cl)	Acid–base balance; gastric hydrochloric acid for digestion	Deficiency: FVD caused by vomiting/ diarrhea	AI: Adults: 1800–2300 mg UL: 3600 mg	Table salt	—

AI, Adequate Intake; *CDRR*, Chronic Disease Risk Reduction; *FVD*, fluid volume deficit; *RDA*, recommended dietary allowance; *UL*, Tolerable Upper Intake Level.
[a]Ages 19–30 years.

oxygen to all cells. Myoglobin (an oxygen-transporting protein) holds oxygen in the muscle cells for quick use when needed. Because of its ability to change ionic charges, iron also assists enzymes in the use of oxygen by all cells of the body.

Iron is conserved and recycled by the body. When red blood cells are old or damaged, the spleen removes their iron component. Some iron is kept in the spleen for later use, and the rest is sent to the liver for processing. From the liver, iron is transported as transferrin to bone marrow and recycled for use in new red blood cells. Some iron is lost through the shedding of tissue cells in urine and sweat and when bleeding occurs; this lost iron must be replaced by dietary sources.

Recommended Intake and Sources

When red blood cells break down, the iron in the hemoglobin is recycled to the liver and used to form new red blood cells. Whenever blood is lost from the body, iron is lost as well and cannot be recycled. Internal bleeding, such as from acute ulcers, can be a deceptive cause of iron loss. More obvious is the loss of blood by women from menstruation. On the basis of this monthly loss and the greater iron demands of pregnancy, women's overall need for iron is higher than men's. The RDA for men is 8 mg, and that for women is 18 mg. During pregnancy the requirement is 27 mg; the blood supply of a pregnant woman is 1.5 times greater than her normal level.

The RDA allows for the unusual absorption rate of dietary iron. Only about 10% to 15% of dietary iron consumed is absorbed; this amount increases up to 20% if body levels are deficient. Higher percentages are absorbed during pregnancy and during periods of growth.

Intestinal mucosal cells contain two proteins that assist in absorption of dietary iron. One protein, mucosal transferrin,

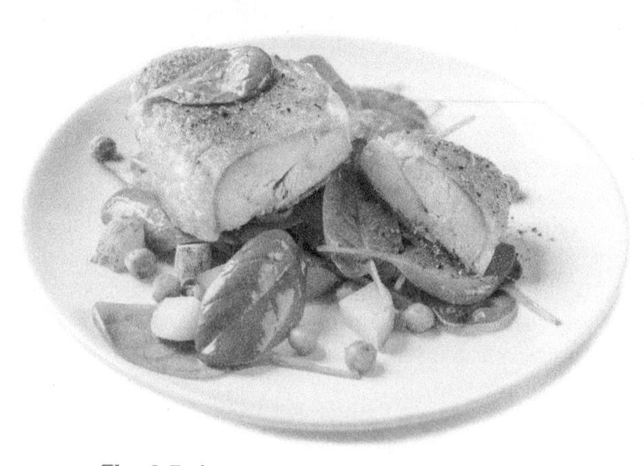

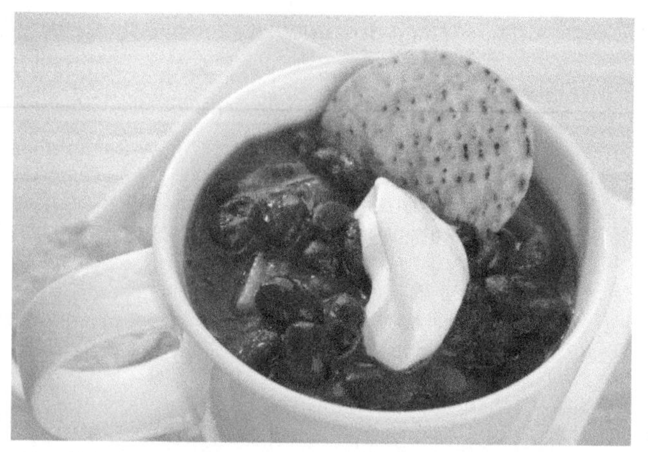

Fig. 8.5 An assortment of foods containing iron includes chicken, spinach, and beans in black bean soup.

moves iron to a protein carrier in blood transferrin. This allows for the movement of iron through blood to bone marrow and tissues as needed. The second, mucosal ferritin, stores iron in the mucosal cells as a reserve if iron is needed. If not used, mucosal cells are replaced every few days, so a continuous short-term supply of iron is available.

The RDA is also set to provide adequate storage levels of iron in the liver; iron is also stored in the spleen and bone marrow. In these organs, iron is contained in the protein's ferritin and hemosiderin. Ferritin is always being made and is easily available as an iron source. Hemosiderin is made when iron levels are high. Although it is a source of iron, hemosiderin must be moved from storage to be used by the body, so it is not as readily available as ferritin.

Iron is found in both plant and animal sources (Fig. 8.5). **Heme iron**, found in animal sources of meat, fish, and poultry, is more easily absorbed than nonheme iron found in plant foods. Animal sources of iron also contain nonheme iron in addition to heme iron. Although egg yolks contain iron, the iron in them is not absorbed as well as heme from other sources. **Nonheme iron** plant sources include vegetables, legumes, dried fruits, whole-grain cereals, and enriched grain products, especially iron-fortified dry cereals.

Increased absorption of iron occurs when dietary sources are consumed with foods containing ascorbic acid (vitamin C). For example, drinking orange juice or eating slices of cantaloupe with meals increases the amount of nonheme iron absorbed. Absorption of nonheme iron increases in the presence of heme iron. This means that consuming iron from several sources improves absorption of the total iron amounts of heme and nonheme iron.

Another way to increase dietary iron intake is to cook foods in cast-iron skillets. Iron in the skillet leaches into the foods, providing an easy means of boosting iron intake.

Factors that inhibit iron absorption include consumption of foods that contain binders (e.g., phytates and oxalates) that keep the dietary iron from separating from plant sources. Tannins in plants, most notably in teas and coffee, can also interfere with iron absorption. Continual use of antacids and excessive intake of other minerals competes with the absorption sites for iron. Pica, the consumption of nonnutritive substances, creates health problems. When the nonnutritive substances are excreted from the body, minerals are also excreted, decreasing mineral absorption. Pica is discussed in the next section.

Deficiency

Iron deficiency has been a public health problem for many years. Although the incidence has decreased in the United States, most likely because of greater fortification of foods with iron, it is still common for iron deficiency and iron-deficiency anemia to occur among young children, teenage girls, and women of childbearing age. These disorders are more common among women of color within lower socioeconomic status who have had many children. In other parts of the world, it is still the most widespread nutrient deficiency, primarily in the developing world. Children and women of childbearing age are most at risk. The effects of iron deficiency can be subtle and may be ascribed to other causes. A range of symptoms accompanies different degrees of deficiency. All levels of iron deficiency affect the availability of oxygen throughout the body.

Iron deficiency occurs when there is reduced supply of iron stores available in the liver. If neither the diet nor body stores can supply the iron needed for hemoglobin synthesis, the number of red blood cells in the bloodstream decreases. The blood hemoglobin concentration also falls. When both the percentage of red blood cells (called hematocrit) and the hemoglobin level fall, a health care provider should suspect iron deficiency.

In severe deficiency, the hemoglobin and hematocrit levels fall so low that the amount of oxygen carried in the blood is decreased and the person is pale, tired, and anemic. Iron-deficiency anemia is characterized by microcytes or small, pale red blood cells. Physical activity or work may be difficult to perform because not enough oxygen is available for use by the muscles. Cognitive functioning is compromised. In children, developmental delays and learning problems may develop; an iron-deficient child is easily distracted and unable to focus on learning tasks. A person may have a sensation of always feeling cold, as if body temperature cannot be regulated appropriately. The immune system is compromised as well, reflected in decreased wound-healing ability. During pregnancy, iron-deficiency anemia as a result of inadequate dietary intake is associated with greater risk of premature delivery and low birth weight.

Because infants receive more iron than in the past, a decline in iron-deficiency anemia among American children has occurred. However, prevalence has remained constant among women of childbearing age. The Centers for Disease Control and Prevention (CDC) has made guidelines for use by primary health care providers to prevent, detect, and treat iron deficiency. The guidelines focus on adequate iron nutrition for infants and young children, screening for anemia among women of childbearing age, and the value of low-dose iron supplements for pregnant women.

Deficiency of iron, even if not yet resulting in anemia, may also aggravate chronic inflammatory disease disorders such as chronic kidney disease, inflammatory bowel disease, and chronic heart failure. Treatment is dependent on disease-specific concerns but can lead to improvement of quality of life and clinical results (Cappellini et al., 2017).

A form of anemia called sports anemia occurs among endurance athletes. As the body adapts to aerobic development from intense exercise, the individual's volume of blood expands. This expansion lowers hemoglobin concentration, producing an appearance of anemia. This condition, however, is not an illness but a positive adaptation of the body.

To alleviate iron deficiency, the cause of the deficiency (either internal loss of blood or lack of dietary intake) needs to be addressed. Children may lack sufficient intake of iron foods. Iron-deficiency anemia may develop in toddlers from drinking too much milk, a poor source of iron, which fills them up and keeps them from eating other iron-containing foods. Women tend to be doubly at risk because of dieting habits and female physiology. Long-term dieting may affect the intake of iron-rich foods; loss of blood through menses and the high iron demands of pregnancy combine to greatly increase female iron requirements. The recent increased consumption of iced tea as a popular soft drink may also affect women's iron levels. The tannin in tea reduces iron absorption. For adults in the United States, iron deficiency is rarely caused by dietary deficiency; instead, it usually results from the blood loss of menstrual bleeding or internal bleeding in the GI tract, perhaps from bleeding ulcers or hemorrhoids.

An unusual behavior associated with iron deficiency is pica. Pica is characterized by a hunger and appetite for nonfood substances, including ice, cornstarch, clay, and even dirt. These substances contain no iron, and their consumption may even lead to loss of additional minerals because nonnutritive minerals may be absorbed, limiting iron absorption, particularly when clay and dirt are consumed. Pica may be missed as a factor for children diagnosed with iron deficiency, who may also be experiencing mental and/or emotional disabilities. The behaviors may lead to anemia and lead poisoning. Resolution of the behaviors occurs with education to recognize edible and inedible items while the child's emotional and physical health stressors are identified and addressed. In addition, support for the family's socioeconomic needs, if warranted, should be considered (Leung & Hon, 2019).

Pagophagia (excessive ice consumption) has been noted among all socioeconomic levels. Geophagia (pica of clay or dirt) and amylophagia (pica of cornstarch and laundry starch) are primarily recognized among women of rural and urban lower socioeconomic groups. There is a cultural history of the use of edible clays for medicinal and religious purposes since ancient times. The consumption of clays may precipitate iron deficiency (Gomes, 2018). Most at risk are pregnant women and preadolescent girls (Borgna-Pignatti & Zanella, 2016). Of particular concern is the practice of pica during pregnancy, when the risk and implications of iron-deficiency anemia are most severe. Among Hispanic women who are pregnant and are diagnosed with pica, there has been a strong association with food insecurity and iron deficiency (Aditi et al., 2018). Lead poisoning may also be present and related to pica behavior for immigrant pregnant women, particularly in urban areas (Thihalolipavan et al., 2013). A challenge to obstetric nurses is to elicit information about this type of dietary behavior when assessing clients.

If increases in dietary sources of iron-rich foods do not raise hematocrit levels, supplements may be prescribed. Determination of dose is based on physiologic requirements, as assessed by primary health care providers. Long-term compliance is necessary to adequately restore iron storage levels in the body. Client education and support from nurses are advantageous.

Strategies to enhance absorption of iron supplements are simple. Drinking a glass of orange juice when taking an iron supplement will maximize iron absorption. Avoid taking iron supplements with milk because the calcium in milk interferes with absorption. Use of iron supplements may cause stools to turn black and constipation to result.

Toxicity

Hemosiderosis, storing too much iron in the body, is a health concern. This condition may be caused either by hemochromatosis, a genetic iron overload disorder that allows more dietary iron to be absorbed than usual, or by consumption of very high levels of iron-containing foods, perhaps through iron fortification. The resulting iron overload can damage tissue cells when excess iron is stored. Bacterial microorganisms may thrive on the excessive amounts of iron circulating in the blood. These effects manifest as various symptoms, such as weakness and fatigue. More specific symptoms include liver and heart damage, diabetes, arthritis, and discoloration of skin (Kawabata, 2018).

Those at risk include men, people with chronic excessive alcohol consumption, and individuals who are genetically at risk for hemochromatosis. Because men lose no iron through menstruation or childbirth and may consume more foods fortified with iron, their bodies can potentially store more iron than needed. Excessive consumption of alcohol puts people at risk because their livers are affected by alcohol and may malfunction, absorbing too much iron. Iron overload may be a risk factor for diabetes (Simcox & McClain, 2013).

Hemochromatosis alters iron metabolism, allowing excess iron to be absorbed from food and supplements. Treatment for hemochromatosis is blood removal by giving blood regularly and by decreasing dietary intake of iron-containing foods. This disorder is sometimes misdiagnosed as diabetes or as liver disorders. Although both these disorders are caused by hemochromatosis, they are treated as individual ailments, and the underlying iron overload is not addressed. However, awareness of hemochromatosis is increasing among primary health care providers and other health professionals. Screening during regular checkups is recommended for those older than 30 years, particularly if they have diabetes. Screening is achieved with a blood test to assess transferrin saturation.

A final concern about iron toxicity is less a nutritional issue and more of a public health and safety issue. Accidental iron poisoning of a child who consumes iron supplements or vitamin or mineral supplements containing iron is a medical emergency. As few as 6 to 12 pills can be lethal, depending on the dose and the age of the child. All supplements, even the fruit-flavored shapes formulated for children, should be treated as medicinal drugs and be kept out of the reach of children.

Zinc

Function

More than 200 enzymes throughout the body depend on zinc. Zinc affects our growth process, taste and smell ability, healing process, immune system, and carbohydrate metabolism by assisting insulin function.

Recommended Intake and Sources

The zinc RDAs for men and women are 11 mg/day and 8 mg/day, respectively. During pregnancy and lactation, suggested levels for women increase to 11 to 12 mg.

Zinc-containing foods include meat, fish, poultry, whole grains, legumes, and eggs. In the United States, a variety of zinc sources are easily available. In parts of the world where animal foods are not regularly consumed and grains are a primary zinc source, deficiencies may develop because of the low bioavailability of zinc from fibrous whole-grain plant foods. Grains contain phytic acid, which remains bound to zinc in the intestinal tract; human digestive juices cannot break this bond. Use of leavening agents such as yeast to prepare whole-grain food products breaks this bond, making zinc available. Zinc deficiency still occurs in parts of the world where food sources may be limited and whole grains are consistently consumed as unleavened breads.

Deficiency

Deficiency symptoms are related to zinc's functions in the body. Symptoms include impaired growth, reduced appetite, and immunologic disorders. Severe zinc deficiency during the growth years may result in dwarfism and hypogonadism (reduced function of gonads), leading to delayed sexual development. Reduced appetite is most likely related to a diminished ability to taste (hypogeusia) and smell foods (hyposmia). The difficulty is that once appetite is reduced, fewer potential sources of zinc may be consumed, causing the zinc deficiency to worsen. Marginal deficiencies among children categorized as picky eaters have been noted to negatively affect height status. Among older adults, inadequate dietary intake resulting in reduced zinc intake appears to affect wound healing, taste and scent ability, and immune functions.

Toxicity

Zinc toxicity from inappropriate supplementation produces GI distress, leading to vomiting and diarrhea, fever, and exhaustion. The symptoms appear similar to those of the flu. Continual use of supplements decreases iron and copper levels in the body and reduces levels of high-density lipoprotein cholesterol, thereby increasing the risk of coronary artery disease. Intake should be no higher than the RDA unless directed by a primary health care provider; individuals should not self-medicate. Consequently, the UL of 40 mg should be observed.

Iodine

Function

Iodine is part of the hormone thyroxin produced by the thyroid gland. Thyroxin is involved with regulating growth and development, basal metabolic rate, and body temperature.

Recommended Intake and Sources

The RDA for iodine is 150 μg/day for both men and women. Many sources of iodine provide inconsistent amounts. Water may contain some iodine, but the amounts vary. Seafood is a good source, and dairy products and eggs may contain some iodine depending on the feed the animals consumed. Surprisingly, sea salt does not contain iodine; the iodine is lost in processing. The amount of iodine in plant foods depends on the amount in the soil in which the food is grown. Incidental sources of iodine are cleaning products whose residues adhere to cooking and baking equipment and dough conditioners. To ensure that the population receives adequate amounts of this nutrient, salt in the United States may be purchased fortified with iodine.

Deficiency

Iodine deficiency reduces the amount of thyroxine produced. Symptoms of iodine deficiency then reflect the effects of reduced thyroxine, including sluggishness and weight gain. Severe iodine deficiency during pregnancy causes cretinism of the fetus, resulting in permanent mental and physical retardation.

Goiter, enlargement of the thyroid gland, occurs during extended iodine deficiency (Fig. 8.6). The thyroid gland works to compensate for the low iodine levels and expands; the goiter often remains even after iodine intake is again sufficient.

The incidence of goiter in certain populations is endemic or regionally defined. In the past a goiter belt existed in the Midwestern states. Iodine was unavailable in the soil and water of the area because this region is untouched by oceans, which provide a natural source of iodine. Since then, fortification of salt with iodine and the wider availability of seafood because of improvements in refrigeration and transportation systems reduced this deficiency. Goiter, although extremely rare in North America, may still occur in parts of Europe, Africa, and South and Central America. To eliminate iodine deficiency globally,

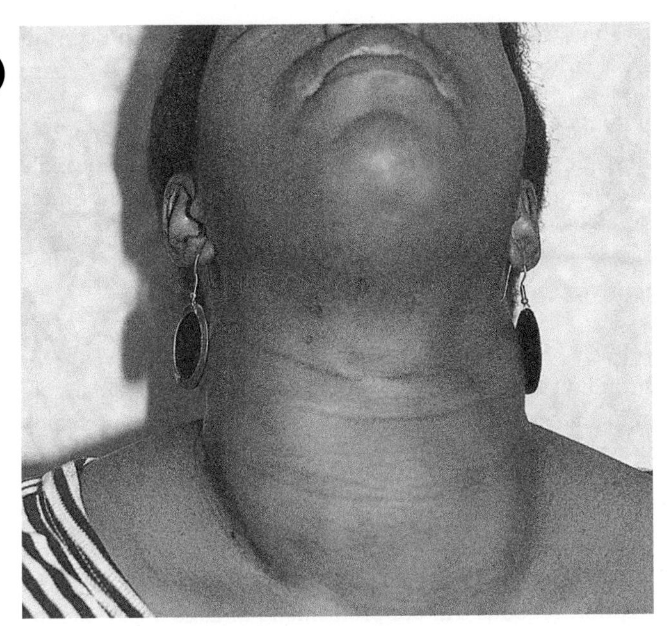

Fig. 8.6 Goiter caused by iodine deficiency. (From Swartz MH: *Textbook of physical diagnosis history and examination*, ed 3, Philadelphia, 1998, Saunders.)

the United Nations Joint Commission on Health Policy recommends universal salt iodization in countries in which iodine deficiency is a public health concern.

Goiter may also be caused by the action of goitrogens. When consumed as staple components of dietary intake, goitrogens (substances in the root vegetable cassava and in cabbage) suppress the actions of the thyroid gland. Although the thyroid gland swells as in iodine deficiency goiter, the iodine level is not the initiating agent; instead, substances in these vegetables suppress the actions of the thyroid gland. To control these iodine deficiency disorders (IDDs) in areas such as southern Ethiopia, programs are conducted to teach villagers how to use safer methods of preparing cassava.

Toxicity

Too much iodine can cause iodine-induced goiter called thyrotoxicosis; therefore, the UL is set at 1100 μg/day.

Fluoride

Function

Fluoride increases resistance to tooth decay and is part of tooth formation. Skeletal health also depends on fluoride for bone mineralization.

Recommended Intake and Sources

The AI for fluoride is 4 mg/day for men and 3 mg/day for women.

Sources of fluoride vary. The most consistent is fortified water to which fluoride has been added. Tea, seafood, and seaweed are other reliable sources. Unfortunately, these are not regularly consumed, particularly by children during tooth-formation years.

An inadvertent source of fluoride is toothpaste. Most toothpaste has fluoride added as a topical agent to strengthen tooth enamel. However, some fluoride is ingested during the rinsing process, providing a kind of dietary source of fluoride. Children can ingest a lethal dose of fluoride if a tube of toothpaste is consumed.

Deficiency

Low levels of fluoride raise the risk of dental caries. Factors such as hygiene, food choices, and possibly genetics also affect plaque and subsequent dental caries.

Toxicity

Too much fluoride causes fluorosis. Fluorosis consists of mottling or brown spotting of the tooth enamel; severe fluorosis may also cause pitting of the teeth. A UL of 10 mg/day reduces the risk of toxicity.

Selenium

Function

Selenium is part of an enzyme that acts as an antioxidant. Vitamin E and selenium work together to prevent cell and lipid membrane damage from oxidizing substances. Selenium is also associated with thyroid function. It is found extensively throughout the body.

Recommended Intake and Sources

The RDA for selenium is 55 μg/day. During pregnancy, the RDA is 60 μg/day, whereas during lactation the RDA goes up to 70 μg/day. Meats, fish, eggs, and whole grains are good sources of selenium. It is a nutrient for which the RDA is easily met.

Deficiency

Deficiency of selenium may predispose individuals to heart disease, particularly Keshan disease. Keshan disease was first noted in China, primarily in children and women of childbearing age. The symptoms of the disease include cardiomyopathy and other features common to selenium deficiency, including muscle pain and tenderness. It is difficult, however, to separate other environmental factors specific to China that may also affect long-term nutritional status. Deficiencies of nutrients other than selenium may have a role in the cause of Keshan disease. Keshan disease differs from the form of heart disease common in the United States because the myocardium of the heart is affected. In the United States, most heart disease is coronary artery disease. Therefore, selenium deficiency is probably not a factor affecting the American incidence of heart disease.

However, low dietary levels of selenium or reduced blood levels of selenium may be associated with an increased risk of cancer among Americans. The relationship of cancer to selenium consumption is probably caused by selenium's antioxidant functions, combined with those of other antioxidants in the body. This relationship continues to be explored.

Toxicity

The most common symptoms of chronic selenium toxicity are hair and nail brittleness and loss. Other effects are severe liver damage, vomiting, and diarrhea. Additional symptoms include metallic aftertaste, respiratory distress with lung edema and bronchopneumonia, and garlic-scented breath and sweat. Chronic toxicity is not likely to occur in the U.S. population because food is consumed from many regional areas, a pattern that dilutes consumption of food grown in naturally occurring high-selenium areas.

The toxicity of selenium highlights the delicate nature of the body's use of trace minerals. Although selenium is proposed as an antioxidant supplement, the amount suggested is that of the RDA for selenium (55 μg). To avoid toxicity, the UL for selenium is 400 μg/day.

Copper

Function

Although the body requires minute amounts of it, copper performs many functions. Some roles of copper are its actions as (1) a coenzyme involving antioxidant reactions and energy metabolism, (2) a component of wound healing, (3) a constituent of nerve fiber protection, and (4) a required element for iron use.

Recommended Intake and Sources

The RDA for copper is 900 μg/day for adults. Good sources include organ meats (liver), seafood, green leafy vegetables, legumes, whole grains, dried fruits, and water that flows through copper pipes.

Deficiency

Copper deficiency causes bone demineralization and anemia; this form of anemia can also be caused by zinc toxicity, which reduces body levels of copper. Copper deficiency does not occur in the United States.

Toxicity

Copper toxicity occurs from supplementation. A common toxic response consists of vomiting and diarrhea. Wilson's disease, an inherited disorder, results in the excessive accumulation of copper in the liver, brain, and cornea of the eye. Eventually the disorder can lead to cirrhosis, chronic hepatitis, liver failure, and neurologic disorders. Worldwide the incidence of copper toxicity appears tied to the use of brass and copper pots to prepare and store foods. Nutritional treatment for copper toxicity, whether caused by Wilson's disease or dietary sources, consists of dietary restrictions and chelation therapy that initiates excretion of excess copper from the body (Collins, 2014). In addition, 10 mg/day is the UL for copper.

Chromium

Function

Chromium has a role in carbohydrate metabolism as a constituent of the glucose tolerance factor that facilitates the reaction of insulin.

Recommended Intake and Sources

The AI of chromium is 35 μg/day for men and 25 μg/day for women. In adults older than 50 years, the AI is 30 μg/day for men and 20 μg/day for women. Found in animal-related foods, eggs, and whole grains, chromium is lost in food processing, particularly when wheat is refined to white flour.

Deficiency

Although chromium is lost through food processing, outright deficiencies of chromium are unusual. Inadequate chromium status may be responsible in part for some cases of impaired glucose tolerance, hyperglycemia, hypoglycemia, and unresponsiveness to insulin.

Toxicity

Chromium toxicity has been noted from environmental contaminants in industrial settings rather than from excessive dietary intake.

Other Trace Minerals

The amount needed of the following trace minerals is so low that it is easy to meet these amounts through ordinary consumption of foods. All are problematic in large doses; supplements are contraindicated.

Manganese is a component of enzymes involved in metabolic reactions. The AI for manganese is 2.3 mg/day for men and 1.8 mg/day for women. The mineral is found in whole grains, green vegetables, legumes, and other foods, and manganese deficiency in humans is unknown. The UL for manganese is 11 mg/day.

Molybdenum functions as a coenzyme. The RDA, 45 μg/day, is easily consumed through typical dietary selections. Deficiencies have not been recorded except under medical circumstances in which dietary intakes have been greatly altered. The UL for molybdenum is 2000 μg/day.

Other trace minerals found in our bodies that may have a role in human health are silicon, boron, nickel, vanadium, lithium, tin, and cadmium. The amounts required are so small that we naturally consume enough and are never deficient in these nutrients. Table 8.4 provides a quick reference to the trace minerals.

TOWARD A POSITIVE NUTRITION LIFESTYLE: PROJECTING

Projection is placing responsibility for our own unacceptable feelings or behaviors on others. In relation to health, we may attribute our poor eating patterns to hectic schedules and possibly to roommates or family members who do not want to shop for food or prepare meals. We project our unacceptable behaviors on others rather than take responsibility for our own health.

One mineral for which projection sometimes occurs is iron. Because iron deficiency often manifests as tiredness, paleness, and frequent infections, it is commonly self-diagnosed as the pathologic cause of poor health. Accurate diagnosis of iron deficiency is based on blood analysis, not on self-reporting. As an aspect of client education, we can help clients clarify the actual causes of their symptoms if they are not clinically iron deficient. Often these symptoms are caused by poor health habits: not enough sleep, irregular meals, and too little exercise. Rather than blaming ill health on the mineral iron, clients can take responsibility and modify their own health behaviors.

TABLE 8.4 **Trace Minerals**

Mineral	Function	Clinical Issues Deficient/Toxicity	Recommended Daily Intakes	Food Sources	Absorption Issues
Iron (Fe)	Distributes oxygen in hemoglobin and myoglobin; growth	Deficiency: microcytic anemia (children and women at risk) Toxicity: hemosiderosis; hemochromatosis	RDA: Men: 8 mg Women: 18 mg Pregnancy: 27 mg Lactation: 9 mg UL: 45 mg	Heme sources: meat, fish, poultry, egg yolks Nonheme sources: vegetables, legumes, whole grains, enriched grains	Conserved and recycled; only 10%–15% of dietary iron consumed is absorbed
Zinc (Zn)	Cofactor for more than 200 enzymes; carbohydrate metabolism (insulin function)	Deficiency: decreases wound healing; decreases taste and smell; impaired sexual and physical development; immune disorders Toxicity: similar to flu with vomiting/diarrhea/fever/exhaustion	RDA: Men: 11 mg Women: 8 mg UL: 40 mg	Meat, fish, poultry, whole grains, legumes, eggs	Binders may decrease absorption in whole grains
Iodine (I)	Thyroxine synthesis (thyroid hormone) regulates growth and development; regulation of basal metabolic rate	Deficiency: decreases thyroxine, causing sluggishness and weight gain, goiter, cretinism (if during pregnancy) Toxicity: thyrotoxicosis	RDA: Adults: 150 µg UL: 1100 µg	Iodized salt, seafood	—
Fluoride (Fl)	Bone and tooth formation; increases resistance to decay; increases mineralization	Deficiency: increases dental caries Toxicity: fluorosis	AI: Men: 4 mg Women: 3 mg UL: 10 mg	Fluoridated water, tea, seafood, seaweed	—
Selenium (Se)	Antioxidant cofactor with vitamin E; prevents cell and lipid membrane damage	Deficiency: possible Keshan disease/cancer Toxicity: liver damage, vomiting, diarrhea	RDA: Adults: 55 µg UL: 400 µg	Meat, fish, eggs, whole grains	—
Copper (C)	Coenzyme in antioxidant reactions and energy metabolism; wound healing; nerve fiber protection; iron use	Deficiency: bone demineralization and anemia (not in the United States) Toxicity: Wilson's disease or with supplements producing vomiting/diarrhea	RDA: Adults: 900 µg UL: 10,000 µg	Organ meats (liver), seafood, green leafy vegetables	—
Chromium (Cr)	Carbohydrate metabolism, part of glucose tolerance factor	Deficiency: possible link with cardiovascular disorders; hypoglycemia, hyperglycemia, and unresponsive insulin	AI: Men: 35 µg Women: 25 µg	Animal food, whole grains	—
Manganese (Mn)	Part of metabolic reaction enzymes	Deficiency: unknown	AI: Men: 2.3 mg Women: 1.8 mg UL: 11 mg	Whole grains, green leafy vegetables, legumes	—
Molybdenum (Mo)	Coenzyme	Deficiency: unknown	RDA: Adults: 45 µg UL: 2000 µg	Many foods	—

AI, Adequate Intake; *RDA*, recommended dietary allowance; *UL*, Tolerable Upper Intake Level.

SUMMARY

- Water and minerals are primary components of body fluids, and each performs other functions as well.
- Water supports a variety of functions: It is a structural component of the body, a temperature regulator, a lubricant, a fluid cushion, a transportation vehicle, a source of trace minerals, and a medium for and participant in biochemical reactions.
- Sources of water include beverages and foods with high water content; the best source is pure water.
- Minerals have diverse roles: provide structural rigidity and strength to teeth and skeleton, allow for proper muscle contraction and release, influence nerve function, assist enzymes, maintain proper acid-base balance of body fluids, and are required for blood clotting and wound healing.

- The 16 essential minerals are divided into two categories: major minerals (needed daily in amounts of ≥100 mg) and trace minerals (needed daily in amounts ≤20 mg).
  - Major minerals are calcium, phosphorus, magnesium, sulfur, and the electrolytes sodium, potassium, and chloride.
  - Trace minerals include iron, zinc, iodine, fluoride, selenium, copper, chromium, manganese, and molybdenum.
- Prime food sources of minerals include both plants and animals.
  - Plant sources include most fruits, vegetables, legumes, and whole grains.
  - Animal sources consist of beef, chicken, eggs, fish, and milk products.
- Minerals are stable when cooked.
- The bioavailability of some minerals may be limited, depending on the source.
  - Some plant minerals are not easily available to the human body because of binders inhibiting absorption.
  - Generally, minerals from animal foods can be absorbed more easily than those from plants.
- Dietary patterns consisting primarily of whole foods provide an adequate supply of minerals.

THE NURSING APPROACH

Clinical Judgment and Next-Generation NCLEX® Examination-Style Questions

Case Study 1

Deficient Fluid Volume

Ben, an 8-month-old infant, had a rectal temperature of 101.2° F. His mother suspected he had a viral infection and brought him to the emergency department (ED), worried he might be getting dehydrated.

It was November, and the nurse suspected Ben had rotavirus. After interviewing the infant's mother, the nurse did a physical examination, and Ben was admitted to the rapid treatment unit. The physician ordered laboratory tests, including blood and stool cultures, complete blood cell count (which includes white blood cell count and hematocrit), and comprehensive metabolic panel (which includes electrolytes). Prescriptions were written for acetaminophen given per rectum every 6 hours, Pedialyte by mouth as tolerated, and lactated Ringer's solution given intravenously.

Assessment/Recognize Cues

Subjective (From Mother's Statements)

- For 24 hours Ben vomited whenever his mother attempted to give him a bottle of formula.
- Ben had been crying and seemed weak.
- Ben had several loose brown stools in his diaper and probably urinated less than usual.
- One of his brothers also has had diarrhea and vomiting.

Objective (From Physical Examination)

- Dry skin and oral mucous membranes
- Sunken fontanelle
- Skin flushed and warm
- Temperature of 101.2° F (rectal)
- Rapid pulse and respirations
- Abdomen soft
- Bowel sounds hyperactive
- Urine concentrated

Diagnoses (Nursing)/Analyze Cues

1. Dehydration related to diarrhea and vomiting as evidenced by report from mother, dry mucous membranes, sunken fontanelle, and concentrated urine
2. Fever related to infection and dehydration as evidenced by temperature 101.2° F, skin flushed and warm

Planning/Prioritize Hypotheses

Patient Outcomes

Short term (within 24 hours):

- No further fluid loss, and fluid balance restored
- Temperature of 100° F or less

Nursing Interventions/Generate Solutions

- Carry out physician's orders.
- Monitor health status hourly.

Implementation/Take Action

1. Sent blood and stool cultures to the laboratory.
   Cultures can lead to identification of microorganisms, a correct diagnosis, and appropriate treatment.
2. Gave acetaminophen per rectum as ordered.
   Acetaminophen (Tylenol) can lower the temperature. Aspirin is not given to children because of its association with Reye's syndrome (an uncommon but potentially lethal complication).
3. Offered sips of Pedialyte in a baby bottle every hour.
   Pedialyte, containing glucose, water, and electrolytes, helps replace fluids and electrolytes lost through diarrhea and vomiting. Clear liquids minimize peristalsis and are better tolerated than formula when diarrhea and vomiting are present.
4. Administered intravenous fluids (IV), regulated by an IV pump.
   Intravenous fluids can immediately replace lost fluids. Rate must be carefully controlled to prevent fluid overload.
5. Checked vital signs hourly.
   Monitoring vital signs often aids early detection of complications and evaluation of health status.
6. Recorded intake and output and monitored for signs of dehydration.
   Once stabilized, intake (IV fluids and fluids by mouth) should be approximately equal to output (vomitus, diarrhea, urine). Diapers are weighed to determine amounts of urine.
7. Monitored laboratory reports.
   White blood cell count is commonly elevated by infections. Increased hematocrit can indicate a loss of fluids. Electrolyte levels are diminished by vomiting and diarrhea.

Evaluation/Evaluate Outcomes

Short term (within 24 hours):

- Blood and stool specimens were sent to the laboratory. Ben drank 2 ounces of Pedialyte but then vomited. Intravenous fluid was administered and urination increased. Oral mucous membranes were moist and fontanelle was flat.
  - Goal partially met. Plan: Continue to offer Pedialyte hourly. Continue IV fluids until Ben is taking fluids well by mouth.
- Temperature dropped to 100.8° F after acetaminophen was given. Pulse rate and respirations decreased.
  - Goal partially met.

Continued

THE NURSING APPROACH—cont'd

Discussion Questions

1. Why is it important to keep Ben hydrated?
2. How does Pedialyte help balance electrolytes as well as fluids? At what temperature should it be given?
3. What drinks and/or foods would be best for decreasing diarrhea in Ben's older brother?

Case Study 2

An elderly female who lives by herself has just been admitted to the emergency department (ED) complaining of nausea, vomiting, and diarrhea associated with the flu for a few days. She admits to taking a diuretic daily. Vital signs are temperature = 99.2° F, pulse = 96 beats per minute, respiration = 24 breaths per minute, blood pressure = 96/72 mm Hg. The client is alert and oriented. The weather has recently been hot and dry. The client complains of frequent urination, extreme thirst and weight loss. Upon examination by the nurse, the client has decreased skin elasticity, dry mucous membranes, and dry mouth.

Chose the **most likely** options for the information missing from the statement below by selecting from the list of options provided.

The assessment findings that require immediate follow-up include:

______________, ______________, ______________

______________, ______________ and ______________.

Options for 1	Options for 2	Options for 3
1. Alert and oriented	BP 96/72	Dry mouth
2. Decreased skin elasticity	RR 24	T 99.2 F
3. Orthostatic hypotension	Dry mucous membranes	Polyuria

APPLYING CONTENT KNOWLEDGE

Dorothy, a 77-year-old woman with a history of heart failure, presents to the hospital with shortness of breath. During your assessment you find that she has +3 edema on her lower extremities, bilateral lower lung crackles, and dyspnea on exertion, and she mentions she has gained 2 pounds since last week. The doctor orders a potassium-wasting diuretic to remove excess fluid. What are the signs and symptoms of potassium deficiency? What foods would you recommend Dorothy consume to prevent a potassium deficiency?

WEBSITES OF INTEREST

Centers for Disease Control and Prevention
www.cdc.gov/healthywater/
Offers many resources about water uses and safety.

Food and Nutrition Information Center
www.nal.usda.gov/fnic/food-composition
Provides resources on individual macronutrients, phytonutrients, vitamins and minerals. Created by U.S. Department of Agriculture, National Agriculture Library.

National Osteoporosis Foundation (NOF)
www.nof.org
Offers resources on causes, prevention, detection, and treatment of osteoporosis.

REFERENCES

Aditi, R., et al. (2018). Pica is prevalent and strongly associated with iron deficiency among Hispanic pregnant women living in the United States. *Appetite, 20*, 163–170.

Bailey, J. L., et al. (2014). Water, electrolyte, and acid-base metabolism. In A. C. Ross (Ed.), *Modern nutrition in health and disease* (11th ed.). Philadelphia: Lippincott Williams & Wilkins.

Bethel, M., et al 2017: Osteoporosis (Updated: 27 August, 2020), *eMedicine/Medscape*. From: emedicine.medscape.com/article/330598-overview#showall. (Accessed 24.12.20).

Borgna-Pignatti, C., & Zanella, S. (2016). Pica as a manifestation of iron deficiency. *Expert Review of Hematology, 9*(11), 1075–1080.

Cappellini, M. D., et al. (2017). Iron deficiency across chronic inflammatory conditions: international expert opinion on definition, diagnosis and management. *American Journal of Hematology, 92*(10), 1068–1078.

Collins, J. F. (2014). Copper. In A. C. Ross (Ed.), *Modern nutrition in health and disease* (11th ed.). Philadelphia: Lippincott Williams & Wilkins.

Coughlin, J. W., et al. (2014). Behavioral disorders affecting food intake: eating disorders and other psychiatric conditions. In A. C. Ross (Ed.), *Modern nutrition in health and disease* (11th ed.). Philadelphia: Lippincott Williams & Wilkins.

Fratianni, C.M. (2016). Osteoporosis in solid organ transplantation: Overview of treatment (updated: 2 November, 2016), eMedicine/Medscape. From: emedicine.medscape.com/article/128108-overview. (Accessed 01.01.18).

Gomes, C. F. (2018). Healing and edible clays: a review of basic concepts, benefits and risks. *Environmental Geochemistry and Health, 40*, 1739–1765.

Institute of Medicine. (2013). *Sodium intake in populations: Assessment of evidence (Report Brief)*. Washington, DC: The National Academies Press.

Kawabata, H. (2018). The mechanisms of systemic iron homeostasis and etiology, diagnosis, and treatment of hereditary hemochromatosis. *International Journal of Hematology, 107*(1), 31–43.

Leung, A. K., & Hon, K. L. (2019). Pica: a common condition that is commonly missed - an update review. *Current Pediatric Reviews, 15*(3), 164–169. https://doi.org/10.2174/1573396315666190313163530.

Meng, Y., et al. (2019). Dietary intakes of calcium, iron, magnesium, and potassium elements and the risk of colorectal cancer: a meta-analysis. *Biological Trace Element Research, 189*(2), 325–335.

National Academies of Sciences (NAS) (2019). *Consensus study report highlight: dietary reference intakes for sodium and potassium*, Washington, DC.

National Research Council. (2006). *Dietary reference intakes: The essential guide to nutrient requirements*. Washington, DC: The National Academies Press.

Simcox, J. A., & McClain, D. A. (2013). Iron and diabetes risk. *Cell Metabolism, 17*(3), 329–341.

Statista 2017: Sales volume of bottled water in the United States from 2010 to 2016 (in billion gallons). From: www.statista.com/statistics/237832/volume-of-bottled-water-in-the-us/. (Accessed 31 December, 2017).

Thihalolipavan, S., et al. (2013). Examining pica in NYC pregnant women with elevated blood lead levels. *Maternal and Child Health Journal*, *17*(1), 49–55.

Tucker, K. L., & Rosen, C. J. (2014). Prevention and management of osteoporosis. In A. C. Ross (Ed.), *Modern nutrition in health and disease* (11th ed.). Philadelphia: Lippincott Williams & Wilkins.

Weaver, C. M., & Heaney, R. P. (2014). Calcium. In A. C. Ross (Ed.), *Modern nutrition in health and disease* (11th ed.). Philadelphia: Lippincott Williams & Wilkins.

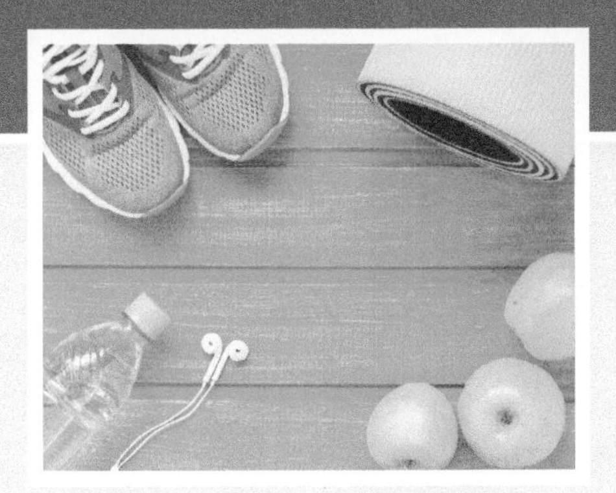

9

Energy, Weight, and Fitness

All people—the fat, the thin, and the in between—can benefit from adopting attitudes and behaviors that over time should promote the body composition appropriate to each individual's genetic makeup and contribute to true wellness.

http://evolve.elsevier.com/GRODNER/FOUNDATIONS

LEARNING OBJECTIVES

- Compare and contrast the two energy pathways.
- State the three major components of daily energy requirements.
- Define a healthy weight.
- List factors that influence body fat levels.
- Describe methods for assessing body fat composition and body weight.
- Discuss the nutritional needs of athletes.

ROLE IN WELLNESS

This chapter explores the issues of energy, weight, and fitness. Synergistic effects of energy intake and energy output are mediated by genetically defined physiology and behavioral options as influenced by environment. Body weight reflects factors within our control plus factors outside our control that are unable to be modified.

The meanings of weight and fatness in our contemporary culture and how they relate to wellness are considered. Because it is body fat that is really the issue, our focus is on fat rather than on weight. In addition, we use the approach management of body composition, specifically body fat levels, rather than achievement of ideal body fatness. In this context, management is defined as the use of available resources to achieve a predetermined goal. This definition recognizes that individuals differ in the resources available to them and in the goals they set.

Consideration of the physical, intellectual, emotional, social, spiritual, and environmental dimensions of health guides our understanding of the value of energy supply, fitness, and their potential impact on healthy body weight. Dietary intake and regular physical activity are essential to the achievement of optimal physical health and fitness. Exercise affects all muscles; even the muscles of our gastrointestinal tract function better when we exercise regularly. Managing body composition levels by decreasing or increasing body fat or lean body mass is, if appropriate, also an aspect of the physical dimension of health. Adequate levels of body fat allow the body to function most efficiently.

To strengthen our intellectual health dimension, the old saying "A sound body makes for a sound mind" still holds true. By being physically fit, we may be able to devote our full intellectual capacity to our work. The intellectual dimension of health also provides the skills to understand and critique the role of society in molding our attitudes to our levels of fitness and the shapes of our bodies.

The emotional health dimension may be supported by fitness because, for some people, depression seems to lift if they regularly engage in sustained aerobic activities. Even if we are not depressed, our general state of mind improves with daily physical exercise. Regardless of body size, our emotional health depends on our developing positive self-esteem.

Group sports provide an excellent opportunity for social activity while pursuing healthful goals that enhance social health. A sense of belonging and sharing occurs whether the group is a formal organization, such as a running club, or consists of friends who bike together. The social dimension of health may not be affected by body fat levels, although those at either extreme of body size may need to develop a circle of friends and family who accept their size differences.

Respecting and caring for our bodies by engaging in regular physical activity reflects the understanding of the unique nature of the human body, which in turn reflects spiritual health as tested as a belief in a higher being, providing support for some individuals who are struggling with behavior changes related to food consumption.

The environmental health dimension may be key to defusing the impact of obesogenic settings. Maintaining healthy levels of fitness and weight is significantly affected by the physical environments surrounding us. Are there safe areas in which to exercise outside? Are affordable gym memberships available, whether at a commercial facility or at the local community center? Are there supermarkets in the neighborhood that provide fresh produce and wholesome products at reasonable prices?

Obesogenic environments entice by limiting our need to be physical as well surrounding us with inexpensive food selections that are high in calories, fat, refined carbohydrates, and simple sugars. Considering ways to modify our environments to improve our individual and community health is a major contemporary health challenge (Box 9.1).

ENERGY

The abilities to perform work, produce change, and maintain life all require energy. Energy exists in many forms—mechanical, chemical, heat, electrical, light, and nuclear energies. The laws of thermodynamics tell us that each type of energy can be converted from one form to another. As our bodies function, chemical energy from food is converted to mechanical energy and heat.

The ultimate source of energy is the sun. Sunlight is used by plants to produce chemical energy in the form of carbohydrates, proteins, or fats. These foods possess stored energy. People are not capable of doing this. We must convert the chemical energy from the foods we eat into forms usable by the human body.

The energy released from food is measured in kcal (thousands of calories), or calories. Technically a calorie is the amount of heat necessary to raise the temperature of a gram of water by 1° C (0.8° F). As first noted in Chapter 1, to ensure accuracy, the term kilocalories is used throughout this text, abbreviated as kcal.

Two methods are used to determine the energy a food contains. One is using a bomb calorimeter (Fig. 9.1). This instrument is designed to burn a food while measuring the amount of heat or energy released. It provides an estimate of the energy available to humans. Because the bomb calorimeter method is more efficient than the human body, the kcal value assigned to a food item is adjusted to reflect the limitations of the human system. Amounts listed in food tables reflect this adjustment.

The other method of assessing food energy is proximate composition, which determines the grams of carbohydrates, proteins, and fats of a food item. The grams are then multiplied by the energy value of each (carbohydrates 4 kcal/g; proteins 4 kcal/g; fats 9 kcal/g). The sum of these calculations equals the total energy content of a specific food.

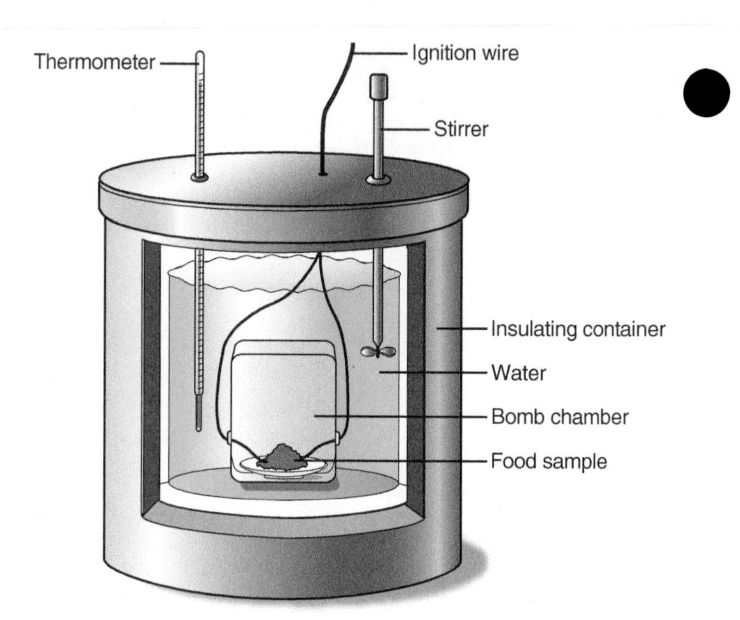

Fig. 9.1 Cross section of a bomb calorimeter. To determine energy, a dried portion of food is burned inside a chamber charged with oxygen that is surrounded by water. As the food is burned, it gives off heat. The heat raises the temperature of the water surrounding the chamber. The increase in water temperature indicates the number of kcal contained in the food. One kcal equals the amount of heat needed to raise the temperature of 1 kilogram of water by 1° C (0.8° F).

Energy Pathways

The processes of digestion, absorption, and metabolism for each of the three energy-supplying nutrients—carbohydrates, fats, and proteins—have been presented in previous chapters. (Alcohol also provides energy but is not considered a nutrient category.) Carbohydrate digests to glucose, triglycerides (fats) to fatty acids and glycerol, and protein to amino acids. Here we continue to follow their journey as they are used for energy in individual cells.

The nutrients release energy when they are catabolized (broken down), forming carbon dioxide and water. The released energy becomes caught within adenosine triphosphate (ATP), the fuel for all energy-requiring processes in the body (Fig. 9.2).

Carbohydrate as a Source of Energy

Glucose releases energy and is converted to carbon dioxide and water through three processes: glycolysis, tricarboxylic acid (TCA) cycle, and oxidative phosphorylation. These complicated processes are reviewed in general here; the intricate details are beyond the scope of this text.

Through glycolysis, which results in the conversion of glucose to carbon compounds, a glucose molecule produces pyruvic acid and ATP. Part of this process depends on niacin and other B-complex vitamins. Oxygen is not needed for glycolysis to occur, because it is an anaerobic pathway. The anaerobic pathway provides energy for sprint or speed-type exercise such as soccer, basketball, and football. We also depend on this energy source to run for the train, chase after toddlers, or bound across the room to answer the phone. This type of exertion is limited because oxygen is not available quickly enough to continue its support. Instead, the incomplete use of glucose causes the pyruvic acid to be converted to lactic acid. As lactic acid

BOX 9.1 Obesogenic Environments

Obesogenic environments refer to factors and conditions that increase the risk of development of obesity. Even if obesity does not occur, such environments may still have a negative impact on our health. During the past 50 years, so many aspects of life have changed, with many of those changes leading us to consume more dense foods in greater quantities while using the ever-evolving technologies that keep us "plugged in" with one another, without needing to leave our homes, our rooms, or our chairs, but also near the fridge! Add to this situation frenetic stressful work and/or school responsibilities leaving no time for physical activity, and we may find ourselves caught in lifestyle behaviors that keep us from achieving our personal health goals.

This is not just happening in the United States. Throughout the world, "globesity" is occurring in countries where a generation ago, hunger and malnutrition were of concern. Now overnutrition in the form of obesity is prevalent among children and adults as abundant, cheap, processed, high-calorie foods have replaced traditional sources of nourishment.

In the Social-Ecological Framework for Nutrition and Physical Activity Decisions model shown here, each circle can be considered "an environment" that, depending on the decisions made, could be an obesogenic environment. Consider for yourself or with your clients the influences of each of the social-ecological framework components on the risk that an environment is obesogenic.

A Social-Ecological Model for Food and Physical Activity Decisions

The Social-Ecological Model can help health professionals understand how layers of influence intersect to shape a person's food and physical activity choices. The model below shows how various factors influence food and beverage intake, physical activity patterns, and ultimately health outcomes.

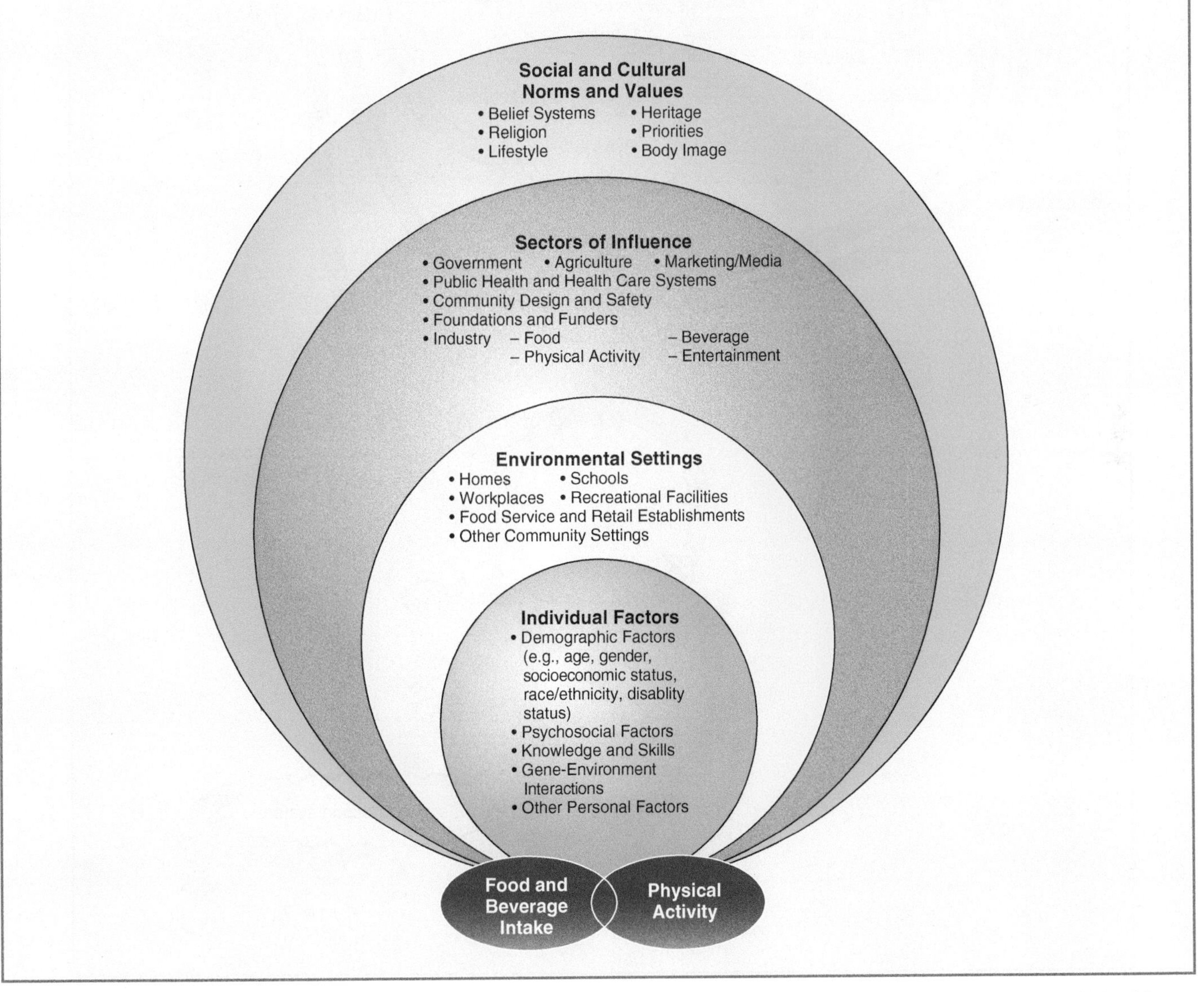

(From U.S. Department of Agriculture and U.S. Department of Health and Human Services: *Dietary guidelines for Americans, 2015–2020*, ed 8, Washington, DC, 2015, U.S. Government Printing Office. Accessed 8 January, 2018, from health.gov/dietaryguidelines/2015/resources/2015–2020_Dietary_Guidelines.pdf.)

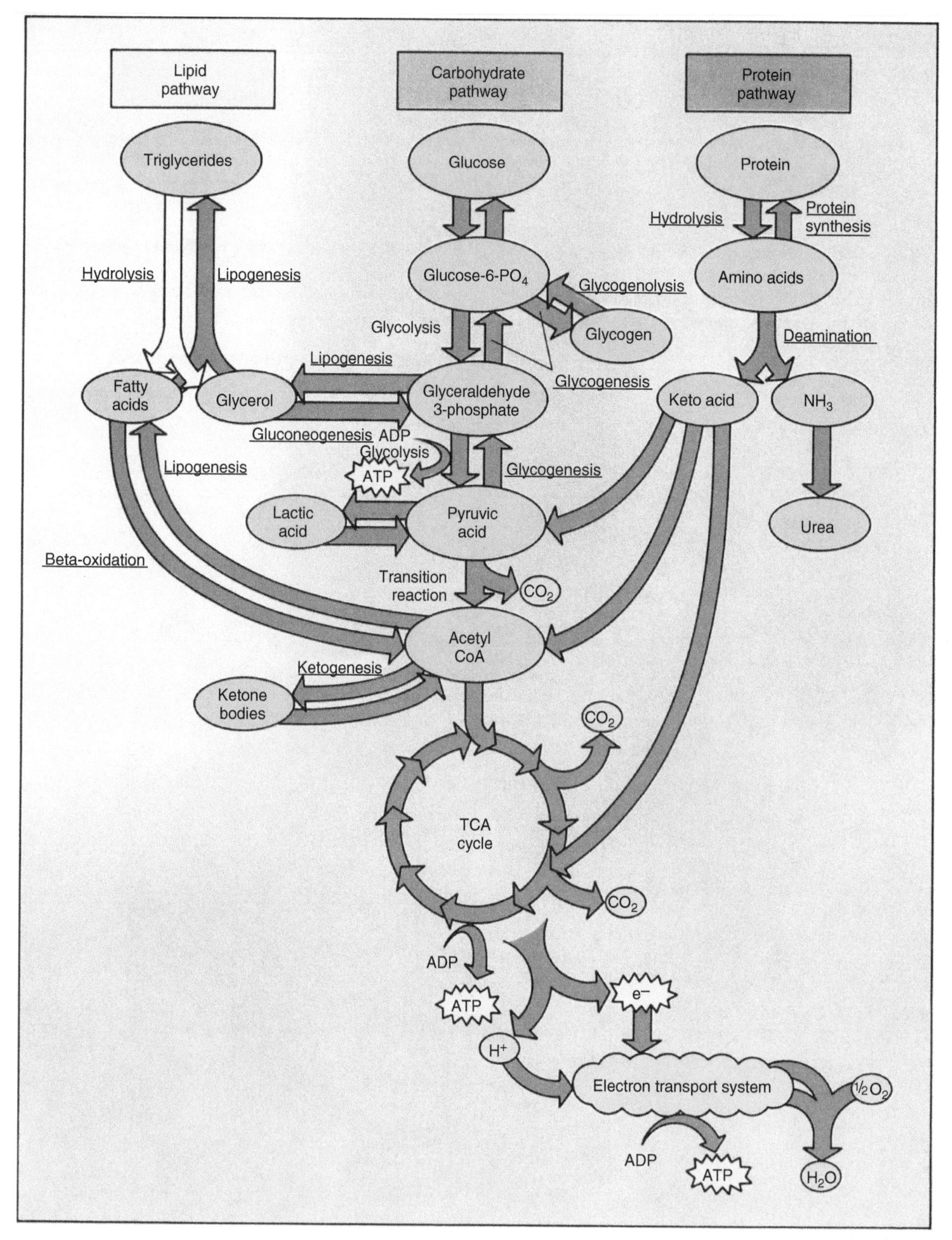

Fig. 9.2 Summary of key steps in the metabolism of glucose, fatty acids, glycerol, and amino acids. *ADP*, Adenosine diphosphate; *ATP*, Adenosine triphosphatase; *CoA*, coenzyme A; *TCA*, tricarboxylic acid cycle. (From Thibodeau GA, Patton KT: *Anatomy and physiology*, ed 4, St. Louis, 1999, Mosby.)

builds up, the muscles become sore and stiff. Consequently, the exertion ceases because of pain. Within a few minutes, enough oxygen is available to break down the lactic acid, relieving the physical discomfort. The effect is called oxygen debt.

Anaerobic glycolysis takes place in the cell cytoplasm, but oxygen-dependent aerobic glycolysis (the aerobic pathway) occurs in the mitochondria of the cell. In the mitochondria, pyruvic acid (made without oxygen) reacts with coenzyme A (CoA) to create acetyl CoA. The energy process continues as acetyl CoA reaches the TCA cycle. The reactions that are part of that cycle lead to the formation of additional ATP and carbon dioxide. The aerobic pathway is the primary energy source for exercises that are low enough in intensity to be carried on for at least 5 minutes. They include endurance-type exercise (e.g., swimming, bicycling, running), as well as walking and most of our daily activities.

The last process of glucose conversion to energy is oxidative phosphorylation. A number of actions lead to the release of hydrogens in the forms of water and additional energy that is captured in ATP. The term oxidative reflects the combination of hydrogen with oxygen to form water; phosphorylation is the creation of the phosphate bond to form ATP.

Fat as a Source of Energy

The first step in the use of fat for energy is the hydrolysis into glycerol and three fatty acids. Glycerol is changed into pyruvic acid and is used for energy. The fatty acids undergo an irreversible process known as beta-oxidation, which involves the breakdown of the fatty acids into acetyl CoA molecules, which then enter the TCA cycle and proceed like the acetyl CoA from carbohydrate (glucose).

Protein as a Source of Energy

Amino acids are first catabolized through deamination, as described in Chapter 6. Whereas the liver and kidneys process the nitrogen-containing amino acid groups, the other amino acid components enter the energy metabolism pathway, with each component entering at a different location. Some of the amino acid components are converted to pyruvic acid; others become intermediaries of the TCA cycle or part of the acetyl groups. If sufficient energy is available, amino acids are used for protein synthesis rather than for energy.

It is important to note that just as all three nutrients (carbohydrate, protein, and fat) can be used for energy when consumed in excess, they can also be stored as fat in the body. Likewise, when too little energy is consumed, these processes reverse. Energy that is consumed is used immediately, regardless of its source. The first stored energy used is glycogen, followed by the energy reserve of body fat in adipose cells. Bloodborne glucose must be available to the brain. Only a small portion of triglycerides (glycerol) can yield glucose, and continuous use of this source results in a buildup of ketones and the potential imbalance of the body pH (see Chapter 6). The body prefers to spare protein for its more important functions: building and repairing cells and tissues.

Anaerobic and Aerobic Pathways

How do anaerobic and aerobic energy pathways work together to supply energy? For the first minute or two of exertion, oxygen has not arrived at the muscles, and therefore energy must come from anaerobic sources. After several minutes the aerobic pathway takes over. However, as the exertion or exercise continues, there is a constant interchange or use of energy sources.

The energy source that muscles use during exercise depends on the intensity and length of exercise, the person's fitness level, and the foods eaten. Short-term, high-intensity activities such as sprinting rely mostly on the anaerobic pathway for energy, and only carbohydrates (primarily from muscle glycogen) can be used. On the other hand, exercise of low to moderate intensity is supported primarily by the aerobic system, and both carbohydrates and fats are used. Fats are an important energy source during exercise because, unlike carbohydrates, fatty acids are abundant in the body, and their use spares muscle glycogen.

The length of activity also determines what type of fuel the muscles will use during exercise. As the duration of exercise increases, glycogen stores become depleted, and fat becomes the primary source of energy (Fig. 9.3). A sedentary person breaks down glycogen faster and as a result accumulates more lactic acid in the tissues. The lactic acid causes muscle fatigue. A physically fit person has a higher aerobic capacity (the ability of the heart to supply oxygen) so that oxygen is available sooner and in greater quantity; this allows use of the aerobic pathway of energy, avoiding lactic acid buildup. This also means that more fat than glycogen can be used for fuel.

If we eat a diet high in carbohydrates, more glycogen can be stored as energy. The amount of carbohydrate stored in the body depends on how much carbohydrate we consume and our

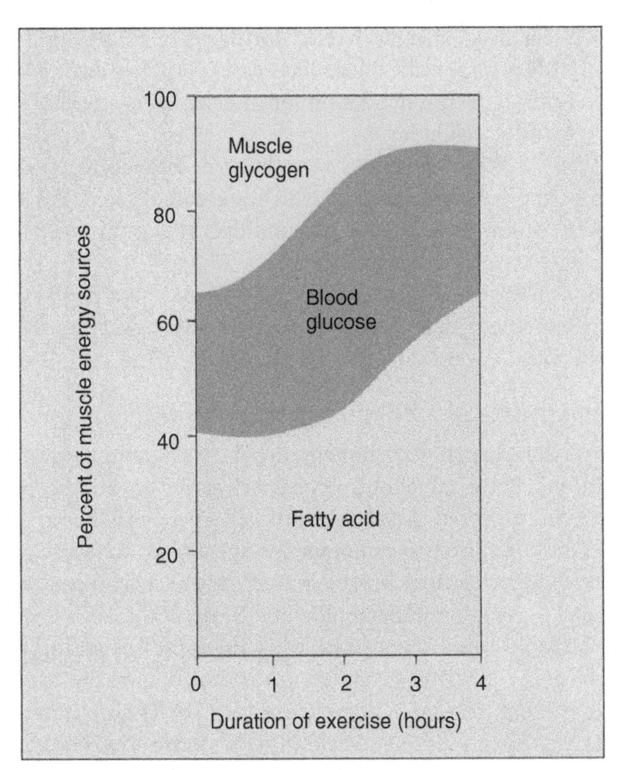

Fig. 9.3 Relative use made of energy sources in the body as exercise continues. (From Guthrie HA, Picciano MF: *Human nutrition*, New York, 1995, McGraw-Hill, with permission from Helen A. Guthrie.)

level of fitness. Endurance training increases the capacity of the muscles to store glycogen, but there is still a limit to the total amount of energy that can be stored. The more glycogen that we store, the more energy we have available for all kinds of everyday activities, not just for marathons.

ENERGY BALANCE

To maintain a healthy weight, we should consume only as much energy as we expend. Because of our sedentary lifestyles, some of us may need less energy than standard energy requirement charts recommend. In contrast, the serious competitive athlete's energy intake must support a training and competition schedule that allows the athlete to achieve their personal best.

Individuals who are acutely ill and hospitalized or are adapting to chronic disorders may require energy intake levels specifically calculated to meet their changing physiologic needs. Consultation with a registered dietitian/nutritionist may be warranted for patients, their family members, and other caregivers. Misconceptions about energy needs can be eliminated by nutrition counseling regardless of the nature of the health disorder.

Estimating Daily Energy Needs

The recommended energy allowances published by the National Research Council appear in Table 9.1. These energy values are based on individuals with a light to moderate activity level. The average daily energy intake for the referenced 19- to 24-year-old man is 2900 kcal, or 40 kcal/kg. It is 2200 kcal or 38 kcal/kg for the same age-referenced woman. If a person is more active or of a larger or smaller body size, further adjustments must be made. Most important, these levels are simply guidelines; the only accurate recommendation for individuals is one that supports healthy weight levels.

Many different formulas have been developed to estimate energy expenditure, some of which are complicated. An easy way to determine kcal need is to multiply weight by one of the numbers in Table 9.2. For example, a 77-kg (170-pound) man who participates in moderate exercise needs about 3060 kcal a day. Remember that these numbers represent averages. Some people need fewer kcal; others need more.

Components of Total Energy Expenditure

Our daily energy requirement depends on many variables, including basal metabolism, physical activity, and the thermic effect of food. **Basal metabolism** represents the amount of energy required to maintain life-sustaining activities (e.g., breathing, circulation, heartbeat, secretion of hormones) for a specific period. Basal metabolic rate (BMR) is the rate at which the body spends energy to keep all these life-sustaining processes going. BMR is measured in the morning on awakening, before any physical activity, and again at 12 to 18 hours after the last meal. Two methods are used. One consists of placement of the human subject in a chamber; the body heat the subject gives off changes the temperature of the chamber, reflecting the energy used by the body for the most basic functions. The second method, indirect calorimetry, uses a calorimeter. The calorimeter measures the respiratory quotient or exchanges of gases as a person breathes into the mouthpiece of the machine. This quotient determines the amount of oxygen used and carbon dioxide (CO_2) expired.

Several factors affect BMR, including age, body size, sex, body temperature, fasting/starvation, stress, menstruation, and thyroid function. BMR varies with the amount of lean tissue in the body; higher levels of lean body mass increase BMR. For example, men have higher BMRs than women because of larger body size and more lean body tissue. The BMR of adults slowly lowers after age 35 years because of decreases in lean body tissue associated with aging. The BMR of a physically fit person may not slow down as much with age as that of a physically unfit person. The process of sustaining fitness maintains the muscle mass of lean body tissue and slows the loss caused by aging. It is never too late to develop fitness; with the approval of a primary health care provider, exercise is appropriate at any age.

BMR also depends on thyroid function. The thyroid hormone thyroxine is a key BMR regulator; the more thyroxine produced in the body, the higher the BMR. Of course, production of too much thyroxine is not desirable either.

Many scientists, however, prefer to use a more practical measurement called resting energy expenditure (REE). REE is the energy a person expends in a normal life situation while at rest, and it includes some energy the body uses following meals and exercise. It accounts for approximately 60% to 75% of our total energy needs, similar percentages to those of BMR (Fig. 9.4).

Physical Activity

The second largest component of energy expenditure after REE (or BMR) is physical activity. **Physical activity** is any body movement produced by skeletal muscles that results in energy expenditure. It demands about 20% to 30% of our total energy needs. Of all the components, it varies the most among people. The amount of energy we expend depends on the intensity and duration of the activity. Walking requires more energy than sitting and walking for 60 minutes uses more energy than walking for 15 minutes. Thus, even a moderate activity can become one of high energy if it is carried on for a long time.

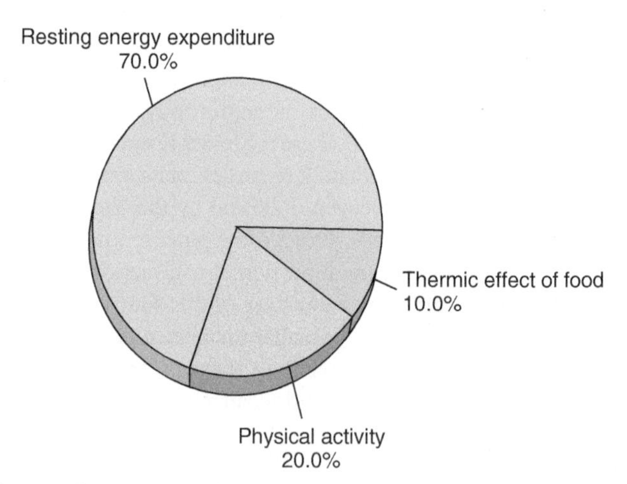

Fig. 9.4 Breakdown of human energy expenditure. (From Rolin Graphics.)

TABLE 9.1 **Estimated Calorie Needs per Day by Age, Gender, and Physical Activity Level**[a]

	MALE			FEMALE[b]		
Age (Years)	Sedentary[c]	Moderately Active[c]	Active[c]	Sedentary[c]	Moderately Active[c]	Active[c]
2	1000	1000	1000	1000	1000	1000
3	1200	1400	1400	1000	1200	1400
4	1200	1400	1600	1200	1400	1400
5	1200	1400	1600	1200	1400	1600
6	1400	1600	1800	1200	1400	1600
7	1400	1600	1800	1200	1600	1800
8	1400	1600	2000	1400	1600	1800
9	1600	1800	2000	1400	1600	1800
10	1600	1800	2200	1400	1800	2000
11	1800	2000	2200	1600	1800	2000
12	1800	2200	2400	1600	2000	2200
13	2000	2200	2600	1600	2000	2200
14	2000	2400	2800	1800	2000	2400
15	2200	2600	3000	1800	2000	2400
16	2400	2800	3200	1800	2000	2400
17	2400	2800	3200	1800	2000	2400
18	2400	2800	3200	1800	2000	2400
19–20	2600	2800	3000	2000	2200	2400
21–25	2400	2800	3000	2000	2200	2400
26–30	2400	2600	3000	1800	2000	2400
31–35	2400	2600	3000	1800	2000	2200
36–40	2400	2600	2800	1800	2000	2200
41–45	2200	2600	2800	1800	2000	2200
46–50	2200	2400	2800	1800	2000	2200
51–55	2200	2400	2800	1600	1800	2200
56–60	2200	2400	2600	1600	1800	2200
61–65	2000	2400	2600	1600	1800	2000
66–70	2000	2200	2600	1600	1800	2000
71–75	2000	2200	2600	1600	1800	2000
76+	2000	2200	2400	1600	1800	2000

(Data from U.S. Department of Agriculture: *Estimated calorie needs per day: Energy levels used for assignment of individuals to USDA food patterns.* Accessed 11 July, 2021, from https://fns-prod.azureedge.net/sites/default/files/EstimatedCalorieNeedsPerDay.pdf)
Estimated calorie needs are based on Estimated Energy Requirements (EER) equations, using reference heights (average) and reference weights (healthy) for each age-gender group. For children and adolescents, reference height and weight vary. For adults, the reference man is 5 feet 10 inches tall and weighs 154 pounds. The reference woman is 5 feet 4 inches tall and weighs 126 pounds.
[a]Estimated amounts of calories needed to maintain calorie balance for various gender and age groups at three different levels of physical activity. The estimates are rounded to the nearest 200 calories for assignment to a U.S. Department of Agriculture Food Pattern. An individual's calorie needs may be higher or lower than these average estimates.
[b]Estimates for females do not include women who are pregnant or breastfeeding.
[c]Sedentary means a lifestyle that includes only the light physical activity associated with typical day-to-day life. Moderately active means a lifestyle that includes physical activity equivalent to walking about 1.5 to 3 miles per day at 3 to 4 miles per hour, in addition to the light physical activity associated with typical day-to-day life. Active means a lifestyle that includes physical activity equivalent to walking more than 3 miles per day at 3 to 4 miles per hour, in addition to the light physical activity associated with typical day-to-day life.

Body size affects energy expenditure more than any other single factor. A heavier person uses more energy to perform a given task than a lighter person. Table 9.3 shows the number of kcal burned per hour for two individuals, one weighing 205 pounds and the other 125 pounds, as they engage in various activities.

Thermic Effect of Food

The third component of energy output is the energy required for our body to digest, absorb, metabolize, and store food. When we eat, the body's cells increase their activities. This increase in cellular activity is called the thermic effect of food (TEF), or diet-induced thermogenesis. The thermic effect is relatively small, accounting for approximately 7% to 10% of a person's total energy needs.

Adaptive Thermogenesis

Adaptive thermogenesis is the energy used by our bodies to adjust to changing physical and biologic environmental situations. This includes energy used to adapt to coldness, extreme changes in kcal intake (of several days' duration), and physical and emotional trauma. This category of energy need

TABLE 9.2 Factors for Estimating Daily Energy Allowances at Various Levels of Physical Activity for Men and Women (Ages 19–50)

Level of Activity	Activity Factor[a] (×REE)	Energy Expenditure[b] (kcal/kg per day)
Very Light		
Men	1.3	31
Women	1.3	30
Light		
Men	1.6	38
Women	1.5	35
Moderate		
Men	1.7	41
Women	1.6	37
Heavy		
Men	2.1	50
Women	1.9	44
Exceptional		
Men	2.4	58
Women	2.2	51

[a]Based on examples presented by World Health Organization (1985).
[b]Resting energy expenditure (REE) is the average of values for median weights of people ages 19 to 24 and 25 to 74 years: men, 24 kcal/kg; women, 23.2 kcal/kg.

incorporates additional demands from illness and the process of recovery. Because the expenditure depends on individualized variables, it is not calculated into average energy requirements.

Total energy expenditure has a direct impact on the maintenance of a healthy weight. Sustaining a healthy weight as influenced by energy input (consumption of food) and energy output (BMR/REE, voluntary physical activity, and TEF) is explored next.

HEALTHY WEIGHT

A healthy weight is a weight at which a person can physically move comfortably, maintain without undue restriction of food intake (but following healthy eating guidelines) or without excessive exercise, and live without experiencing any weight-related associative disorders such as diabetes, hypertension, coronary artery disease, or high blood lipid levels. If associative disorders do develop, lifestyle changes can be initiated to achieve a healthier weight. The definition of healthier weight involves a weight loss of 10 to 16 pounds accompanied by healthy lifestyle behaviors.

In response to increasing concerns about weight-related health disorders, similar concepts of healthier weight are being incorporated into many health promotion programs to change perspectives regarding healthy weight and management of body composition. These programs focus not on encouragement of dieting and weight loss but rather on prevention of obesity and promotion of healthy eating and exercise lifestyles. Thus, as more such programs are launched by government health departments, hospitals, and nonprofit health organizations, good prevention campaigns may lead to greater acceptance of individual differences in body size, shape, and fatness (see Box 9.1).

PERSONAL PERSPECTIVES

Who Wants to Be on a Diet? Not Me!

"Life in the post-diet age when you're not *supposed* to try to lose weight because there's not *supposed* to be any shame in not being skinny *unless* of course you're fat," wrote Taffy Brodesser-Akner in the *New York Times* Magazine article "LOSING IT" (Brodesser-Akner, 2017).

Everyone seems to know that weight-loss diets don't work; we are in the post-diet age. Instead, our efforts should be focused on following a wholesome way of life to maintain a healthy weight. This includes not only better food choices (for the healthier food patterns being followed, from omnivore to flexitarian to pescatarian to vegetarian to vegan) but also exercising regularly, whether running, yoga, strength-training, cycling, or high-intensity interval training (HIIT), in addition to a mindful lifestyle. And a person still needs to have a profession or at least a decent paying job!

My first introduction to shame in not being skinny was when I was 10 years old. I needed a fancy party dress for my brother's bar mitzvah celebration. My mother and I went to a fancy clothing store in Newark, New Jersey. (In 1960, this was equivalent to shopping on Fifth Avenue in New York City.) When my mother explained to the sales clerk what we needed, she looked me up and down and said, "Nothing in *this* department, we'll have to go to the *husky* department."

Since then, I have been on most every kind of weight loss diet for varying lengths of time. (To my credit, I never did the Cabbage Soup Diet!) I did limit "dieting" once I began studying nutrition and focused on eating well, which is another way of meaning healthier. I have developed a pattern of eating based on knowledge of nutrition and of what works well for my particular body to feel well and centered. My "body" weight goal is to fit into last year's seasonal clothes—that is, a stable weight within a range of about 5 pounds. I eat "clean," meaning few processed prepared foods, and although I've been doing so for decades now through years of vegan to omnivore dietary patterns and back again, I still crave ice cream, particularly hot fudge sundaes. Although I do occasionally indulge, I have proclaimed that once I turn 80, I will have a hot fudge sundae *every day*! Although I am about a bit more than a decade away from 80, I still won't be able to fulfill that proclamation because these days 80 is the new 70! Sigh!

The moral of this story is to experiment. Find a general eating pattern that works for you providing real food, containing valuable nutrients, emphasizing plant foods, and maintaining a stable healthy weight range.

Michele Grodner
Montclair, New Jersey

(From Brodesser-Akner T: LOSING IT, *The New York Times* Magazine, 6 August, 2017.)

Measuring Body Fatness

Body weight is the most common way to estimate fatness. Weight is used even though our bodies are made up not only of fat but also bone, muscle, and other nonfat tissue known as lean body mass. Weighing works fairly well as a means to determine fatness because usually the lean body mass changes slowly. Therefore, we assume if the scale shows we are a pound heavier this week than we were last week, the change is probably caused by a gain of fat.

TABLE 9.3 Approximate Calories Used per Hour in Various Athletic Activities

	CALORIES/HOUR	
Activity	By a 125-lb Person	By a 205-lb Person
Baseball:		
Infield or outfield	234	382
Pitching	299	488
Basketball:		
Moderate	352	575
Vigorous	495	807
Bicycling:		
On level ground, 5.5 miles per hour (mph)	251	409
13 mph	537	877
Dancing:		
Moderate	209	341
Vigorous	284	464
Football	416	678
Golf—twosome	271	443
Horseback riding:		
Walk	165	270
Trot	338	551
Mountain climbing	503	820
Rowing:		
Pleasure	251	409
Rowing machine or sculling 20 strokes/min	684	1116
Running:		
5.5 mph	537	887
7 mph	669	1141
9 mph level	777	1269
Skating:		
Moderate	285	465
Vigorous	513	837
Skiing:		
Skiing:		
Downhill	483	789
Level, 5 mph	586	956
Soccer	447	730
Swimming:		
Backstroke:		
20 yd/min	194	316
40 yd/min	418	682
Breaststroke:		
20 yd/min	241	392
40 yd/min	482	786
Butterfly	586	956
Crawl:		
20 yd/min	241	392
50 yd/min	532	869
Tennis:		
Moderate	347	565
Vigorous	488	797
Volleyball:		
Moderate	285	565
Vigorous	488	797
Walking:		
2 mph	176	286
4.5 mph	331	540
Wrestling, judo, or karate	643	1049

There are several situations in which weight is not a good measurement of fatness. One involves fluctuations in body fluid; fluid retention that occurs before menstruation or during hot weather may be interpreted as fat gain, and losses in a sauna may appear to be fat losses. In these circumstances, normalizing the fluid balance makes the apparent fat change promptly disappear. On the other hand, the scale is also misleading for anyone whose amount of lean body mass deviates from what is expected. A bodybuilder has a higher portion of lean body mass than the average person and thus will weigh more at the same height. Someone who suffers from a wasting disease has less lean tissue.

Because weighing is so convenient, it remains a useful assessment. However, to determine body composition (lean body mass plus body fat), other means, which generally involve other measurements of the size of the body (anthropometric measurements) or assessments that distinguish between fat and other body components on the basis of their physical differences, are used. Of the latter group, underwater weighing (densitometry) is the most widely accepted and is often used as a standard to assess the validity of other measures. Unfortunately, densitometry apparatus is bulky and expensive, and not everyone is willing or able to be submerged.

A practical alternative is bioelectric impedance analysis (BIA), a method often offered at health fairs and health and fitness centers. This method for better accuracy uses four electrodes placed at the wrists and ankles to monitor the ease of passage of a mild electrical current. (Two electrodes for foot-to-foot passage are not as accurate but are more available to consumers.) Fat is a poor conductor of electricity; the conductivity occurs through the nonfat parts of the body. BIA actually estimates the amount of lean body mass, and then the amount of fat is calculated from the difference between the lean body mass and the total weight. BIA is safe, inexpensive, easily performed, and reasonably accurate, but it is not considered sensitive enough to detect day-to-day changes experienced by someone trying to gain or lose fat. Hydration levels, though, may affect accuracy of the BIA readings. Other methods of assessing fat level are triceps skinfold and mid–upper arm circumference, but likewise these are unable to detect day-to-day changes.

Interpreting Weight

A convenient way to interpret weight is to determine body mass index (BMI). BMI is calculated by dividing the weight in kilograms by the square of the height in meters. This calculation

TABLE 9.4 Body Mass Index Table

Height (Inches)	Body Weight (Pounds)																
58	91	96	100	105	110	115	119	124	129	134	138	143	148	153	158	162	167
59	94	99	104	109	114	119	124	128	133	138	143	148	153	158	163	168	173
60	97	102	107	112	118	123	128	133	138	143	148	153	158	163	168	174	179
61	100	106	111	116	122	127	132	137	143	148	153	158	164	169	174	180	185
62	104	109	115	120	126	131	136	142	147	153	158	164	169	175	180	186	191
63	107	113	118	124	130	135	141	146	152	158	163	169	175	180	186	191	197
64	110	116	122	128	134	140	145	151	157	163	169	174	180	186	192	197	204
65	114	120	126	132	138	144	150	156	162	168	174	180	186	192	198	204	210
66	118	124	130	136	142	148	155	161	167	173	179	186	192	198	204	210	216
67	121	127	134	140	146	153	159	166	172	178	185	191	198	204	211	217	223
68	125	131	138	144	151	158	164	171	177	184	190	197	203	210	216	223	230
69	128	135	142	149	155	162	169	176	182	189	196	203	209	216	223	230	236
70	132	139	146	153	160	167	174	181	188	195	202	209	216	222	229	236	243
71	135	143	150	157	165	172	179	186	193	200	208	215	222	229	236	243	250
72	140	147	154	162	169	177	184	191	199	206	213	221	228	235	242	250	258
73	144	151	159	166	174	182	189	197	204	212	219	227	235	242	250	257	265
74	148	155	163	171	179	186	194	202	210	218	225	233	241	249	256	264	272
75	152	160	168	176	184	192	200	208	216	224	232	240	248	256	264	272	279
76	156	164	172	180	189	197	205	213	221	230	238	246	254	263	271	279	287
BMI	**19**	**20**	**21**	**22**	**23**	**24**	**25**	**26**	**27**	**28**	**29**	**30**	**31**	**32**	**33**	**34**	**35**
		NORMAL						**OVERWEIGHT**						**OBESE**			

(Modified from Aim for a Healthy Weight: Body Mass Index Table 1. Accessed 30 December, 2020, from www.nhlbi.nih.gov/health/educational/lose_wt/BMI/bmi_tbl.htm. *Note:* Additional BMI categories and BMI calculator may be accessed from this site.)
BMI, Body mass index.

yields a value that can be interpreted without further reference to height. BMI can be determined and related to the associated health risk by consulting the information shown in Table 9.4. BMI levels apply equally well to men and women without adjustment. BMIs in the normal to lower overweight category are associated with the fewest health risks (Thomas et al., 2016). Although some controversy exists as to whether the standards should be increased with age, health risk evidence supports relaxation of the recommended range for older adults. Mortality is higher for individuals at the lowest BMI and highest BMI levels, whereas those in the mid-range appear less at risk (Wellman & Kamp, 2017).

Bear in mind that although BMI is widely used and convenient, it is still a measure of weight and has all the shortcomings of using weight to estimate fat. When both weight and fat are measured on the same men and women, there are usually some individuals who have weight-to-height ratios considered normal but levels of body fat that are beyond what is recommended; they are normal weight for their height but obese. On the other hand, there are other individuals who are overweight but not "overfat"; this group is most likely to include very physically active persons.

HEALTHY BODY FAT

Functions of Fat

Body fat serves a number of vital functions. As discussed in Chapter 5, we could not live without some body fat. For most people, the major portion of body fat is storage fat. A layer of this fat under our skin provides protection from extremes of environmental temperatures, and cushions of fat defend many internal organs against physical trauma. Storing fat provides an efficient means of stockpiling energy so we can endure moderate fasts. In addition to this storage fat, there is a small amount of fat that serves vital functions such as membrane integrity; this minimal amount of fat is termed essential. Although there are individual differences, essential fat in men seems to be 3% to 8% of their body weight. When appropriate amounts of storage fat are added to essential fat for men, the recommended range for total fat is 15% to 20% of body weight. In women the concept of essential fat must be expanded to include gender-specific fat in their breasts, pelvic region, and buttocks, which is apparently an evolutionary feature providing energy during childbearing and lactation. Thus, for women the minimum levels of fatness compatible with health are based on the essential fat plus the gender-specific fat and are in the range of 12% to 14% of body weight; healthy levels of total fat range from 25% to 30% (Fig. 9.5).

Sometimes athletes and dancers may strive for body fat levels below these ranges. There is concern that low body fat levels may be responsible for the menstrual irregularities experienced by many athletic women. Amenorrhea (lack of menstruation) is associated with bone loss and increased risk of fractures. The fat level associated with the best athletic performance may not be the best level for all around long-term health. Working to achieve a lower level of body fat can be tempting; the desirability of doing this should be carefully assessed, with consideration of the effect on strength, general health, menstruation, and other individual factors.

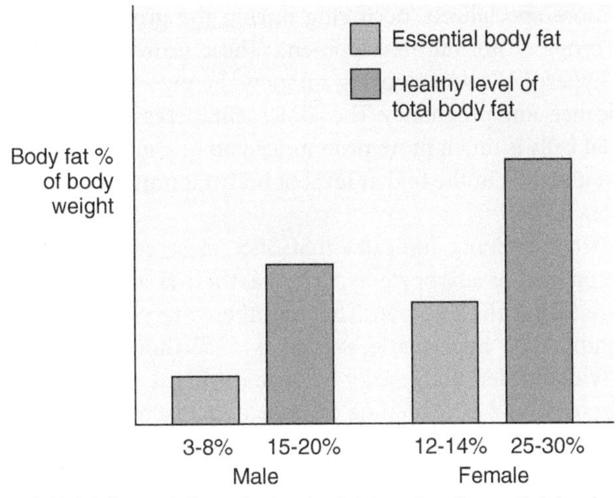

Fig. 9.5 Male and female body fat levels. Essential body fat, minimum level of body fat for biologic functions; total body fat, range of level of body fat that provides for biologic functions but that does not have the potential to negatively affect health. (From Rolin Graphics.)

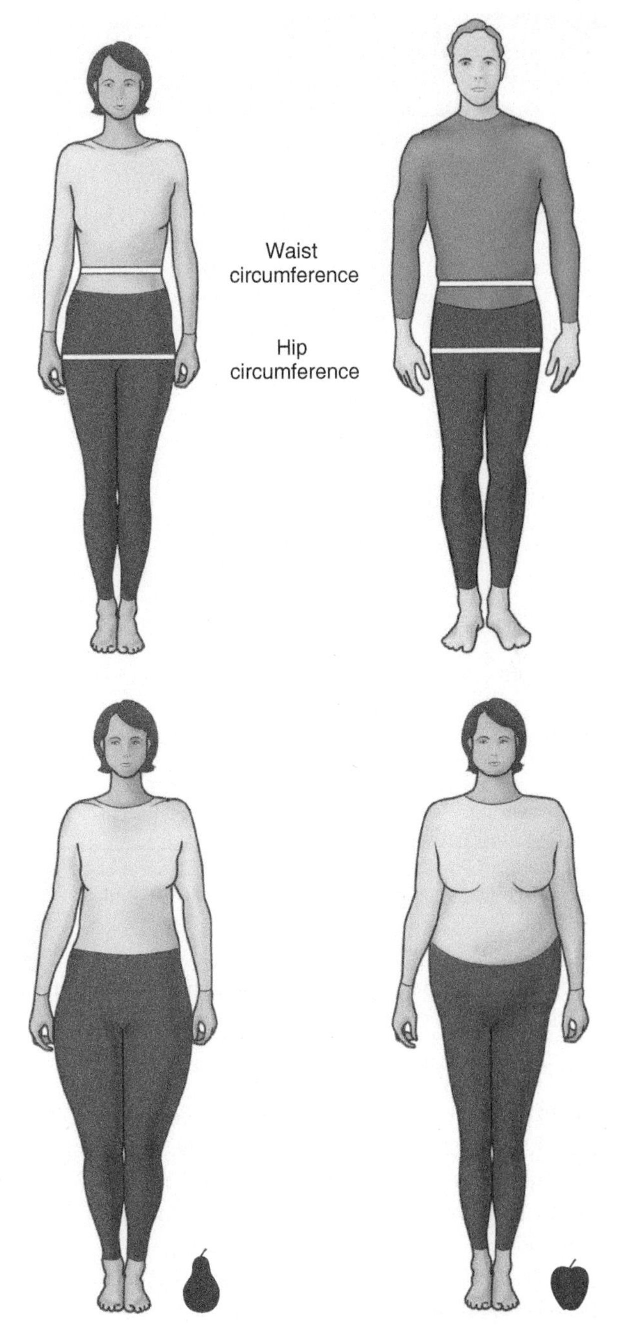

Fig. 9.6 Apple (android) and pear (gynoid) body shapes. To estimate your fat distribution, measure the circumferences of your waist and your hips. Divide your waist measurement by your hip measurement. You are an apple if you are a man, and your waist-to-hip ratio is greater than 0.95 to 1 or if you are a woman and your waist-to-hip ratio is greater than 0.8. You are a pear if you are a woman, and your waist-to-hip ratio is less than 0.8.

Body Fat Distribution

From both a health and an appearance perspective, it is not only the amount of fat but also its location that is important. Spend a few minutes at a popular swimming pool and notice the diverse patterns of fat distribution. Differences related to gender, age, and stage of development become apparent. Fat patterns may also vary among ethnic groups. These distinctions are genetically determined, and although the amount of exercise can affect the tone of the underlying muscle, it cannot change the pattern of distribution.

Imagine the various adult shapes seen at the swimming pool; try to classify them as either apples or pears. Apples (android body type) are biggest around the waist, and pears (gynoid type) are biggest in the hips, buttocks, and upper thighs. Although some evenly proportioned people will fit neither category, probably most of the pears are women and most of the apples are men and older women. Although this swimming pool visualization may seem frivolous, it focuses attention on the location of fat, which largely determines its effect on health. Fat that is visceral in the abdominal cavity seems to be much more dangerous than subcutaneous such as lower body fat or the fat under the skin in the abdominal area.

Although some sophisticated techniques accurately assess fat distribution patterns, a good estimate can be made by comparing waist circumference to hip circumference (Fig. 9.6). For men it is healthier to have a waist-to-hip ratio of less than 0.95 to 1, whereas women should have a ratio of 0.8 or less. The diameter of your waist alone provides a good estimate of the fat in your abdominal area; people with waist measurements more than 40 inches (102 cm) for men and more than 35 inches (88 cm) for women are at greater risk for the various chronic diseases associated with obesity (Thomas et al., 2016). (For those of Asian descent, higher risk is associated with waist measurements more than 36 inches [91 cm] for men and more than 32 inches [81 cm] for women.) When waist-to-hip measurements are combined with BMI ranges, the level of disease risk is further assessed (Table 9.5).

The two types of fat distribution also differ in their rate of turnover, with visceral fat being much more easily lost and also more quickly regained than subcutaneous abdominal fat or lower body fat. This is one of the factors contributing to men's apparent greater ease in losing and regaining fat. It is ironic that although the typical female fat pattern of lower body obesity is

TABLE 9.5 Potential Health Concerns Associated With or at Greater Risk in Obese Individuals

Cancer	Colon cancer
	Endometrial cancer
	Esophageal cancer
	Gallbladder cancer
	Kidney cancer
	Postmenopausal breast cancer
Metabolic disease	Cardiovascular disease
	Hyperlipidemia
	Hypertension
	Nonalcoholic fatty liver
	Stroke
	T2D
Reproductive disorders	Birth defects
	Cesarean section
	Fetal macrosomia
	Infertility
	Maternal death
	Miscarriage
	Preeclampsia
	Stillbirth
Other	Asthma
	Depression
	Osteoarthritis
	Sleep apnea

(Modified from Power ML, Schulkin J: The evolution of obesity, Baltimore, MD, 2009, The Johns Hopkins University Press.)

more benign, women tend to be more concerned with their fatness than men.

Body Fat Storage

Most of the fat in our bodies is stored in special cells called adipocytes. Each of these cells has a nucleus, mitochondria, and other organelles just as other cells do, but these features are usually squeezed over to the side to make room for the droplet of stored fat.

The fat in this droplet is in the form of triglycerides, the same type of molecule making up most of the fat we eat. These triglycerides are synthesized from glucose, glycerol, fatty acids, and some amino acids that are carried to the adipocyte by the bloodstream. The stored fat is in a constant state of flux, with some triglycerides breaking down while others are built. The net effect of this flux—that is, how much fat is in storage—is the result of our energy balance at that time. If we need energy, the balance shifts to favor breakdown and release of fatty acids and glycerol to be transported to various cells, where they are oxidized or converted to other needed molecules. When we have a ready supply of energy, especially shortly after a meal, the balance tilts toward storage.

At birth most of us have relatively small numbers of adipocytes, but during the next few years, these cells increase in number (a type of growth known as hyperplasia) and in size (hypertrophy). Hypertrophy occurs whenever we continue in positive energy balance for any time. Hyperplasia, however, is more specialized, occurring during the growth spurts that accompany normal development. These growth-related times of hyperplasia occur during infancy, the preschool years, adolescence, and pregnancy. The adolescent increase in the number of fat cells is much more pronounced among girls than in boys, and it results in the higher level of body fat normal for girls and women.

Most evidence indicates that once these cells form during the process of adipocyte hyperplasia, there is no natural means of reducing the number. Knowing there are predictable times of adipocyte hyperplasia, scientists once thought if we carefully controlled our energy balance during those critical periods, we would have lifetime insurance against becoming too fat. Unfortunately, we now know this is not true. If conditions are right, new adipocytes can form at any stage of life.

If more energy is consumed than expended, fat storage will go on until the fat droplet reaches its maximum size. If the positive energy balance continues, the body will make new adipocytes, thereby expanding the storage capacity. The stored fat is relatively equally divided, so all cells contain less than their maximum capacity. The body is then able to continue to expand our storage capacity as long as the positive energy balance persists.

When fat is lost, whether through reduced intake, increased physical activity, or illness, fat is mobilized from adipocytes to meet energy needs. This reduces the size of the droplet of stored fat, producing a smaller adipocyte.

If we have been obese and then lose a lot of fat, our adipocytes may become quite tiny—smaller than the cells of people who were never fat. Our bodies seem to monitor the size of adipocytes, interpreting the shrunken cells as evidence of imminent starvation. We may then feel compelled to eat more. Although the response mechanisms are not fully understood, the effects on metabolism and drive to eat clearly developed as a means to reverse the threat of further loss. This set of responses is a major part of the theory of set point, discussed later in this chapter.

REGULATION OF BODY FAT LEVEL

Our bodies form fat as a way of storing energy between eating episodes. When excess energy is available, we synthesize triglycerides and store them in adipose cells. When there is a shortage of energy, those stored triglycerides break down, and the stored energy is used. Thus, the bottom line in adjustment of body fat levels is the status of the body's energy balance: When energy intake exceeds expenditure, we gain fat; when it is less than expenditure, we lose fat. Sounds simple, doesn't it? But in fact, it is not simple at all. Our bodies are much more complex than the teeter-totter that is often used to illustrate energy balance. Many factors affect the rate of energy intake and expenditure. We all are familiar with the concept that some cars get good gas mileage and others don't. Humans have many systems regulating the mileage we get from our food energy.

Changes in Body Fatness

Levels of body fatness change when a disequilibrium in energy balance is established and maintained for a period. A pound of body fat is roughly equivalent to 3500 kcal. Thus, a cumulative positive balance of that magnitude should cause an estimated weight gain of 1 pound, whereas a negative balance of the same size should result in the loss of about a pound of fat. Recall that energy balance is determined by the relationship of the energy intake to the energy expenditure. The intake side of the equation is simple: It represents the kcal value of the food and drink consumed. The expenditure side is more complex, including the REE, the energy cost of physical activity and exercise, and the thermic effect of food. The levels of these expenditures are major factors in determining whether we will gain weight, lose weight, or stay the same weight with a given level of intake.

Earlier in this chapter we discussed how the effect of changes in one's physical activity alter the energy balance, an important factor when trying to achieve healthy levels of fatness. In addition to the effect of physical activity, the rate of energy expenditure is affected by a number of factors that cause individuals to vary significantly in the efficiency of their energy use. Although factors affecting BMR and TEF are of interest, there is no safe and practical way to alter them. Nevertheless, understanding these influences helps interpret the outcomes of the weight management efforts.

Influences on Body Size and Shape

Genetic effects on body weight are researched through family studies and investigations of specific genes and their mechanisms. The similarities of BMI values among first-degree family members are best explained by genetic similarity. This accounts for an increased risk of obesity for the first-degree relatives of obese individuals. Family studies reveal that obese children tend to be the offspring of obese parents. However, such studies cannot separate out the intermingled effects of natural genetic factors from those of the environment. Adoptive studies, though, favor the effects of genetics over environment. The adult weights of adoptive children mostly resemble the BMIs of their biologic parents rather than of their adoptive parents. This tendency negates or lessens the effects of environment on weight.

Genetic influences related to obesity include the endocrine influence of the hormones leptin and ghrelin. Leptin, produced by adipocytes, has a role in the complex system of the regulation of body weight and fat regulation. Leptin inhibits food intake and regulates long-term appetite. The size of adipose stores is regulated through messages transmitted by leptin between the brain and leptin receptors. Mutations in functions of leptin and leptin receptors may have a role in the development of obesity. This association is more theoretical than diagnosable (Polsky et al., 2014). In addition, leptin has a role in supporting functions of the body requiring substantial amounts of energy, such as reproduction and puberty. Leptin regulates these actions according to the adequacy of nutrient stores (Hussain et al., 2014).

Another hormone of interest is ghrelin, which is produced by the stomach and increases the appetite or food intake of humans (and rodents). When weight is lost, changes in appetite and energy use occur. Ghrelin, which circulates in plasma, makes up part of the adaptive response of the body to weight loss by leading the body to regain lost weight. As such, it acts as a long-term regulator of body weight. Consequently, depending on genetic predisposition, ghrelin may make maintaining weight loss harder—especially when the weight loss is accomplished through restrictive dieting. Its effect is less when weight loss occurs through the severe gastric bypass surgical intervention (see Chapter 13), probably because the stomach, under that circumstance, produces less ghrelin.

Studies of leptin and ghrelin are ongoing. Such studies significantly contribute to the understanding of the chemistry of appetite control and demonstrate that there are genetic factors associated with obesity. The work also serves to remind us that human fatness is complex, influenced by the interaction of many factors, both genetic and environmental.

The efforts of the scientists conducting these studies reveal that the role of genetics in fatness levels is complex. There is no single gene for human fatness or thinness. Therefore, fatness must be considered a multifactorial phenotype; that is, the displayed characteristic (phenotype) is the product of numerous genetic (DNA), epigenetic (potentially heritable traits that do not alter DNA), and environmental factors. The main genetic influences come from susceptibility genes—genes that do not in themselves produce a certain characteristic but rather affect the susceptibility to other factors (Fig. 9.7). Interactions between genes and gene-environmental influences, as well as nongenetic influences, complete the scheme of factors contributing to differences in body fatness levels.

Regardless of one's genetic makeup, one's fatness is also influenced by nutritional, psychologic, economic, and social factors. In addition, there are many different types of obesity and thinness. When a family is characterized by a marked degree of fatness or thinness, casual observations are unable to distinguish among the effects of a shared environment, those of shared genetics, and both. By extensive study of large numbers of people, geneticists have learned that a significant amount of the influence on one's fatness (and characteristics such as metabolic efficiency contributing to fatness) is genetic. Somewhat more influence comes from cultural or environmental influences shared by a family, and the remaining influence is related to factors beyond the shared genes and shared environment within a family (see Box 9.1 and the *Cultural Diversity and Nutrition* box Field Trips to Fast-Food Restaurants?).

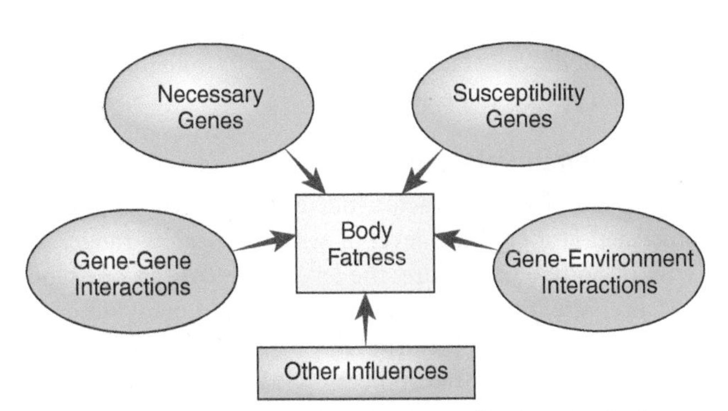

Fig. 9.7 Genetic factors and causes affecting body fatness levels. (Modified from Bouchard C: Genetic factors and body weight regulation. In Dalton S, editor: *Overweight and weight management*, Gaithersburg, MD, 1997, Aspen.)

CULTURAL DIVERSITY AND NUTRITION

Field Trips to Fast-Food Restaurants?

To initiate lifestyle behavior changes among high-risk, ethnically diverse, low-income adults, eight community nursing centers (CNCs) of the Midwest Nursing Centers Consortium conducted a 16-week course titled Wellness for a Lifetime for clients of the centers. The purpose of the course was to promote increased physical activity and to improve the quality of dietary intake of the participants.

Created by a multidisciplinary team, Wellness for a Lifetime was based on health behavior theory and included culturally appropriate content. Each CNC was provided with complete course content, including themes for support group discussions. Course topics were foods and nutrition, stretching and exercising basics, relationship between chronic diseases and diet and activity, and stress reduction strategies. The course was interactive; participants made trips to grocery stores and fast-food restaurants and explored walking routes.

Application to Nursing

CNCs provide services within neighborhood settings. By being "part of the neighborhood," each CNC was able to recruit clients for the course who might not have otherwise participated. The physical activity levels of the ethnically diverse populations served increased. Describing the need for exercise may not be enough; actually, leading clients through an exercise session or on a walking route models appropriate behaviors.

Although the Wellness for a Lifetime course was developed with culturally appropriate content, each site still needed to modify content to meet the specific needs of its population, such as offering the sessions in various languages (Spanish, Chinese, or Russian). When using other health education tools, we may need to modify aspects of the programs to meet the needs of our own target population.

(Data from Anderko L, et al: Wellness for a lifetime: Improving lifestyle behaviors of low-income, ethnically diverse populations, *Ann Fam Med* 3(Suppl 2): S35–S36, 2005.)

How would genes affect the amount and distribution of fat? Research suggests there is a strong genetic influence on certain components making up the energy balance equation: BMR or resting metabolic rate, TEF, and the energy cost of light exercise. Investigators also found genetic influences on the ability to use ingested fat for energy, on taste preferences, and on the ability to achieve a high level of physical conditioning. These findings help explain why people differ in the ease of gaining or losing weight. Nevertheless, for almost every component studied, there were not only genetic, but also environmental factors involved. Although genetics plays a part in the level of body fatness, it is not the only factor. The extent of its influence probably varies from person to person.

Set Point and Body Fatness

Many of our body characteristics are regulated so they are maintained at a constant level or within a narrow range. This is true of body temperature, the level of glucose in our blood, blood pressure, the acidity of body fluids, and many other features. Departure from the usual levels of these variables is usually a clear indication that something is wrong. Typically, when the problem is corrected, the characteristic returns to its usual level. This usual or natural level is called the set point. Actually, this term usually indicates not a single point but rather a narrow range defining the natural level for the characteristic. The adjustments our bodies make to return to the set point are called defending the set point. Thus, we can define set point as a natural level (of some characteristic) that the body regulates or defends.

Because energy is a high priority for the body, the level of energy stores is not left to chance or without regulation. Indeed, as described, the weight (and body fatness) of most adults is remarkably stable, returning to the usual level after minor gains and losses. Despite minor gains over the years, this is true of fat and thin people alike.

For the most part, our adult weights are pretty constant. Something regulates them. There is evidence that our bodies defend a set point. This regulation is skewed toward prevention of weight loss rather than avoidance of weight gain. Furthermore, it is clear that among adult humans there is quite a range of set points for body fatness.

Any theory describing set point mechanisms must be able to describe three components: (1) some characteristic that the body monitors, (2) some kind of messenger to carry the information to the central nervous system (CNS), and (3) some mechanism of response to exert the control. Evidence suggests that fatness, lean body mass, and body mass in general are all monitored.

Our attention is on the possible mechanisms of response, the actual regulation. The only options for exerting this control are (1) changing the amount of energy ingested, (2) changing the level of physical activity, or (3) changing the efficiency with which we use ingested and stored energy. These options are exercised through overlapping neural, endocrine, and metabolic mechanisms to exert both short- and long-term adjustments. Defending our bodies' fat stores is a matter of some complexity. Undoubtedly, this complex system, with lots of checks and balances and backup schemes, reflects the fact that energy is of prime importance to survival.

The concept of a set point for body weight or composition is controversial. Some of the controversy involves the question of set point versus set range. Other experts debate what characteristic (weight, fat, or lean body mass) is under regulation. Still others resist the concept because they feel it discourages individual responsibility for one's own health behaviors. The importance of these controversies is that they do not refute the basic concept.

Food Intake Adjustments

In the discussion of the regulation of food intake, one aspect of set point control was identified. When an individual's weight or fatness is less than what the body perceives as appropriate, the drive to eat is activated. Although the person experiences short-term satiety, this long-term hunger drive apparently is maintained as long as the lower weight exists. Although an individual may learn to ignore this drive, there is no evidence that it goes away. The individual is vulnerable to disinhibition, leading to potential excessive food intake or binge eating. It seems to take effort and attention to resist this hunger drive. People don't always have the psychologic energy to devote to such resistance.

Some people come back from a holiday or other situation during which they overate and gained weight, saying, "I ate so much then that I'm just not hungry now." Unfortunately, this type of hunger adjustment is rare. It is much more common for people to experience their usual degree of hunger and usual intake even after a period of overeating. The regulation system works poorly, if at all, in limiting food intake in this situation. Fortunately, the energy use efficiency part of regulation works somewhat better.

Adjustments in Energy Use

The body can adjust the efficiency of energy use in numerous ways; only a few are examined here. A fundamental mechanism of control is the rate of energy metabolism. This is implemented primarily in adjustments in the REE. The level of the TEF and the energy cost of a given amount of physical activity are probably affected as well. REE is a major component of total energy expenditure and usually accounts for at least half of total energy expenditure. Reducing food intake produces an immediate and significant depression in REE, which drops promptly and stays depressed throughout the period of lowered intake. If the reduction in intake is not too great, the drop in REE may be sufficient to prevent weight loss; this is a successful defense of set point. With greater dietary restriction, weight is lost, producing a departure from set point (at least temporarily). When weight is lost, there is less body to use energy; this change also depresses REE. Thus, these adjustments greatly slow the rate of weight loss. Most often the weight is then regained.

NUTRITION: WEIGHT ESSENTIALS

Gaining, Losing, or Maintaining: A Wellness Approach

Although it is untrue that we can mold our bodies to any size or shape we desire, we do have the power to change our attitudes and behaviors if needed so that we can achieve satisfaction and wellness at the body composition most natural for each of us. This section describes some guidelines that are equally applicable to nurses and to their patients who are fat, thin, or just right. This concept is commonly referred to as a nondiet approach. All of the behaviors recommended focus on long-term changes. Those who adopt these attitudes and implement these behaviors can expect to feel more comfortable with their bodies and probably better about themselves in general. If we eat well and are physically active, we will look and feel good. Body fatness may or may not change. Although this approach may seem discouraging, the harmful and disheartening effects of diets and other programs that promise a lot but deliver only worse problems will be avoided. Box 9.2 describes dietary procedures for those few people who have a serious health condition that justifies the risks of traditional weight-loss efforts (see also the *Health Debate* box Can "Commercial" Diet Programs Teach Healthy Eating Habits?)

HEALTH DEBATE

Can "Commercial" Diet Programs Teach Healthy Eating Habits?*

With the ever-advancing epidemic of obesity in the United States, health professionals are constantly telling the American population, "Don't gain weight! Lose weight!" But at the same time the health professionals are also saying, "Don't go on a diet! Stay away from those dangerous fad diets advertised on television!" So, what is the average person supposed to do? How can we expect nondietary experts to lose weight even while we health professionals struggle with our own weight control? Surely there must be some positive aspects of weight loss programs that we can use in our national "battle of the bulge."

This box presents discussion of healthy food aspects of programs like WW, formerly Weight Watchers—focusing on moderation and portion control and intake of fruits, vegetables, and fiber—and the Mediterranean Diet—emphasizing whole grains and fruits and vegetables—as helping individuals normalize eating patterns and food portions, *without* weeks of deprivation! Perhaps we need to change our approach to the use of commercial diet programs. Let's consider how to customize a program whether online or through books. This approach applies to men and women.

Portion Sizes

Programs that either provide premeasured food *or* have no limit on portion sizes do us a disservice. After years of eating out of control or even just eating our "usual" servings, we may consume portions that are just too large for our caloric needs. It is better to spend a few weeks with measuring cups, learning that your favorite cereal bowl actually holds three servings of cereal, not just one.

Cooking Skills

Eating out may be convenient, but it is more nutritious and economical to cook simple meals. Some programs include easy-to-follow recipes that taste good to both dieters and nondieters. Because more families consist of busy two-career parents and children have many extracurricular activities, children may grow up without learning basic cooking skills. As young adults they can easily teach themselves by following simple directions. Better healthy eating programs provide recipes for novice cooks.

Personal and Time Management

Goal-oriented individuals succeed. They plan and follow through. These skills are woven into the higher-quality weight-management programs. Planning ahead, shopping, and cooking for meals for the week involve time-management skills. Consider whether a particular week includes difficult social events involving food and how to cope with them; some programs are flexible enough to educate participants as to strategies for dealing with such situations.

Food Records

Keeping a food record or journaling has become an established means of tracking foods eaten. It is a diary of all that is consumed, including portion sizes and time of day. Studies indicate that more success occurs when someone attempting to normalize food consumption keeps written records of food intake. There are now "blogs" or personal diaries online of individuals' food struggles that all can read. A person's food record may be part of an online program of a commercial weight-loss program or may be a free program available on the Internet.

Food for Thought?

When a commercial weight-loss program advertises that if we do exactly as the program states, we will lose weight, run the other way! A healthy eating plan to manage body weight should be customized to our individual needs. To achieve this, we must take personal responsibility for creating our own strategy for healthy eating.

What is your opinion? Is there a role for commercial weight-loss programs? How would you advise your clients who need to manage their body weight?

*This discussion does not advocate the use of any named commercial diet program.

BOX 9.2 Restricted Dietary Patterns

The goal of weight management is weight stabilization through the adoption and maintenance of healthy lifestyle behaviors, including consistent eating patterns. Although these changes in behavior may result in minimal weight changes, health status may improve.

Certain chronic medical conditions are improved by weight loss. Consequently, although kcal-restricted diets are associated with physical and psychologic risks, the benefits outweigh them. Following is a guide for comparison of weight loss programs and brief reviews of the primary weight loss formats of these diets. Programs should be contacted directly to determine current fees. New programs may become available through the Internet and should be judged according to the criteria presented here.

Examples of weight loss programs follow:[a]

WW (Weight Watchers)	www.weightwatchers.com 800-651-6000
Jenny Craig	www.jennycraig.com 866-706-4042
Nutri/System	www.nutrisystem.com 800-435-4074
South Beach Diet	www.southbeachdiet.com 888-841-2620
Health Management Resources (HMR)	www.hmrprogram.com 800-418-1367
Registered dietitians/nutritionists (RDNs)	www.eatright.org 800–877-1600
Physicians practicing alone	Available but may not be trained to treat obesity
MyFitnessPal	www.myfitnesspal.com/
SparkAmerica	www.sparkAmerica.com

[a]This is not an endorsement of these programs or services.

Comparison of Weight Loss Programs

Moderate Restriction of Kilocalories

The kcal restriction should be at least 500 kcal less than the individual's daily requirement for energy; daily intake should not be lower than about 1200 kcal. Adults, depending on their gender, height, and weight, may lose weight at intakes between 1200 and 1500 kcal. Intake less than this level cannot provide sufficient amounts of nutrients unless supplements are prescribed. The diet should still follow general dietary guidelines, providing 45% to 65% kcal from carbohydrates, about 10% to 35% kcal from protein, and 20% to 35% kcal from fat.

Very-Low-Calorie Diets

Very-low-calorie diets (VLCDs) are intended for use by moderately or severely obese individuals (body mass index [BMI] >30) whose attempts with more traditional methods have been unsuccessful and for individuals with BMIs of 27 to 30 or higher whose medical conditions depend on weight loss for improvement. Containing only 200 to 800 kcal, a VLCD causes rapid weight loss but increases the risk of gout, gallstones, and other related symptoms, including cardiac complications. Individuals must be under the complete and regular supervision of a physician. The Academy of Nutrition and Dietetics (AND, 2016) has developed medical nutrition intervention procedures for the use of VLCDs. Maintenance of the weight loss is difficult and depends on nutritional counseling, exercise, and lifestyle changes. Regain of lost weight most often occurs after 5 years even with adjunct support from behavior therapy.

Formula Diets

Developed by pharmaceutical and food manufacturers, diet solutions are available in a variety of forms. Designed to replace meals, they may provide a daily total of about 900 kcal and often contain or may be supplemented by vitamins and minerals (AND, 2016). Although such diets are helpful for quick weight loss, the loss is rarely maintained because boredom with the solution and the lack of learning new eating approaches soon lead to regaining of the weight.

Pharmacotherapy

The criterion for pharmacotherapy is having a BMI greater than 30 or having comorbidities and a BMI of 27. The pharmacotherapy should be accompanied by medical nutrition therapy and exercise. Generally, starting weight loss is only 5% to 15% of original weight. Weight loss is regained when drug therapy is discontinued.

The use of pharmacologic drugs for obesity intervention is controversial among health professionals because of the lack of data on long-term effects and the possibility of abuse when prescribed to patients who do not meet the criterion for pharmacotherapy.

(Data from Raynor HA, Champagne CM: Interventions for the treatment of overweight and obesity in adults, *J Acad Nutr Diet* 116 (1):129–147, 2016.)

Establishing Realistic Goals

In setting goals, we should consider two almost opposing factors: (1) our unique and individual values, needs, and characteristics and (2) the limits to the extent of control we have over our bodies and our level of fatness. It is fashionable to deny any limits to this control, but objective observation will reveal the fallacy in that thinking. Aspiring to total control is neither realistic nor healthy for most of us. In goal setting, we need to consider what is practical and feasible.

Changing Behavior

The most important goals are those related to changes in behavior. By choosing appropriate behaviors for change, we can work toward establishing habits that will become almost self-sustaining. The behavioral goals should be related to each person's unique needs. For example, in examining their lifestyle, one person may discover that they are always out of food and running out to grab whatever they can find, usually pizza and convenience store items. They may try to establish a habit of planning and shopping for the next week every Sunday afternoon. For them, this behavior change automatically leads to better food choices. For a different person, this particular goal might be irrelevant.

The *Teaching Tool* box Principles of Behavior Change outlines basic principles of behavioral modification applicable to choosing appropriate changes. In recent decades it has become popular to make superficial use of the principles of behavioral change in weight loss programs. These techniques had limited success because they were presented as just a list of handy hints (e.g., eat on a smaller plate, put down the fork between bites) rather than the individualized system described in the box. Do not confuse these principles with those hints having little to do with the original concepts.

TEACHING TOOL

Principles of Behavior Change

Set a positive, specific, and achievable objective. It is helpful to frame a goal in terms of the exact behavior to be practiced. Objectives like "I want to eat better" or "I don't want to be so inactive" fail to give you any guidance about how to achieve them and what constitutes success. On the other hand, an objective such as eating vegetarian meals five times a week can orient you in a helpful direction right from the start. It is easier to replace a behavior with a new one than to just stop doing it. Break down major behaviors into smaller, less daunting parts, and try only a few changes at a time.

Establish a system for monitoring the behavior to be changed. This observation helps you assess success in changing the behavior and determine what contributes to and detracts from mastery of it.

Modify the environment so that it supports the change. If you were trying to eat more vegetarian meals, for instance, it would be helpful if the environment included vegetarian cookbooks and ingredients and opportunities to be with vegetarian friends.

Set up a plan for rewarding successes. Be sure to choose rewards that will be appreciated but are appropriate to the magnitude of the achievement. The reward should be as immediate as possible. You can make a long-range reward seem immediate by awarding points that build toward the reward.

Recruit support from friends and family. These people may want to be helpful but may not be skilled at it. Tell them of your objectives and how they can help, but do not make them responsible for your personal behaviors.

Allow enough time for a new behavior to become a habit. A simple new behavior like taking smaller bites, if practiced faithfully for 3 weeks, should be well on the way to becoming habit. More complex lifestyle behaviors take much longer to change, usually at least 4 months. Under stress, most of us revert to old habits, so have a plan for how to deal with this occurrence.

Normalizing Eating

The goal of normalizing eating is to reclaim eating as a comfortable and natural process. It involves being in tune with the needs of one's body and its signals about those needs.

Enjoying eating. Normal eating should be enjoyable. Eating is a very sensual process and has the potential to be highly pleasant. Unfortunately, the ubiquitous dieting mentality dictates a love-hate relationship with food. We tend to label the foods we most love sinful and off-limits. Then we long for them and feel dissatisfied with the more ordinary foods we allow ourselves.

In normalizing eating, we strive to retain the enjoyment of the process. This involves eating with awareness, relaxation, and without guilt, allowing ourselves to eat, in appropriate quantities, all the foods we enjoy. It may also involve expanding our pleasure by learning to enjoy a wider variety of foods.

Enjoyment can be enhanced by keeping meals and snacks simple enough that the true flavors of each item can be tasted. Not only do toppings, sauces, and the like usually involve the addition of extra sugars and fats, but they also obscure flavors.

Despite all this emphasis on enjoyment, normal eating does not mean depending on food as a major source of pleasure. Just as drinking a tall, cold glass of water is a joy when we are thirsty (but is without appeal when we're not thirsty), eating should be a natural source of pleasure and not a preoccupation. We are not advocating that we all live to eat (Box 9.3).

BOX 9.3 MyPlate: Weight Management

The MyPlate food guidance system can also be used for weight management. Several tools of MyPlate can be used to supervise our own energy in/out equations to maintain, lose, or gain weight depending on our individual health needs. These tools are available through www.ChooseMyPlate.gov.

Potential MyPlate Tools

MyPlate Plan: A customized food guide providing recommended number of daily food group serving amounts based on an individual's age, gender, and activity level. Users can opt for servings and caloric intakes to either achieve a healthy weight or maintain current weight. Access: www.myplate.gov/myplate-plan.

Start Simple with MyPlate App: The *Start Simple with MyPlate* App is an online dietary personal assessment tool that provides information on diet quality and food group consumption based on the assessment and goal setting features and links to related resources. Access: www.myplate.gov/resources/tools/startsimple-myplate-app.

Letting hunger and satiety guide eating. As discussed earlier, most of us guide our eating not only by physiologic cues to hunger and satiety but also by environmental and cognitive factors. Of these three sets of stimuli, only the physiologic cues are triggered by the body's needs. Therefore, normalizing eating involves letting hunger and satiety guide eating. It means eating when hungry even if it is not a traditional mealtime, and it means stopping with the first signs of satiety even if there is still food on the plate.

Although it would seem that eating this way would be easy, trying to implement this advice is actually challenging. A person may fear that if the cognitive control that tells us what we should be eating is relinquished, all control will be lost, and huge amounts eaten. A few people actually do go through such a period—a pretty scary experience. Nevertheless, when they trust that they can eat again as soon as hunger dictates, most find they are no longer driven to continue eating such large quantities.

A great many people have a different problem: They have ignored their hunger/satiety cues for so long that they no longer sense them. Reversing this lack of awareness involves relearning how to feel and identify the body's signals for satiety. An individual can start this process by carefully noting feelings when several hours pass without eating. Then the person should interrupt a meal midway through it and examine body sensations for satiety cues. A few minutes will be needed to perceive the satiety. If there are no cues to satiety, eating should continue but be stopped again to assess satiety after a few more bites.

Most people are less aware of their satiety signals than of hunger cues. Eating slowly may enhance awareness of satiety. Keeping meals and snacks simple may help, too. Some research indicates there is a component of satiety tied to specific tastes: The greater the variety, the more food is required to reach satiety because each component is activated by the array of sensations. This relationship may be responsible for eating behaviors at generous buffets.

Sensations of hunger are often confused for those of tiredness, anxiety, relief of anxiety, and other states. Distinguishing the difference may require work. It may be helpful to keep a journal of the various sensations observed.

Minimizing the Use of Food to Meet Emotional Needs

Probably all humans use food and eating to help them deal with emotions. We use food to express positive feelings, to celebrate good fortune, to reward hard work, and to create a sense of companionship. Eating as a means of handling negative emotions such as boredom, frustration, anger, or loneliness is especially problematic for many people. Compared with some other ways of responding to strong emotions, eating may be relatively benign, but when we rely on it as our main means of coping, our consumption patterns may have little or no relationship to our physiologic needs. This emotion-driven eating often is followed by feelings of guilt that may feed into the original negative feelings, creating a destructive cycle.

Minimizing emotional eating requires being aware of feelings and any eating associated with them. For personal understanding or as an adjunct to patient education, a journal or eating record can help achieve this awareness by monitoring feelings, hunger, and eating. Records kept for several weeks catch a range of moods. Examine the records from both the perspective of what triggered eating and of how the feelings were expressed or handled.

When we practice eating in response to hunger, we will probably use food less to meet emotional needs. However, if a pattern of eating in response to feelings rather than to hunger still occurs, or if we regularly use food to deal with certain emotions, we need to learn some alternative ways to respond to emotions. We can often be our own best resource for discovering alternative responses by using the records to identify coping behaviors that are already working and that can be used more often. Books are available that deal with making these kinds of changes. Counseling also can help.

Although we are probably never going to completely give up using food to meet emotional needs, it is worth considering how to do so effectively so that we may increase our awareness of how food consumption and emotions are connected. The following guidelines may help:

- Be aware of the reasons behind food use. Verbalize the intended function of the food. Eat food slowly and with concentration.
- Eat without guilt. If this type of eating occurs only rarely, there is nothing about which to feel guilty.
- Arrange a safe circumstance for eating. If some rich, creamy chocolate is just the thing needed, that's fine. Have some, but make sure there is no danger of overdoing it. Buy just one piece, eat in public, or do whatever is necessary to ensure that you can enjoy a reasonable amount without feeling at risk of bingeing.

Eating Regularly and Frequently

Our bodies have evolved so that we function best when we eat several times a day at times spaced throughout our waking hours. Unfortunately, our modern hurried lifestyle often makes eating balanced meals inconvenient. We tend to snack on what is handy early in the day and do most of our eating between 5 PM and bedtime. This pattern has several undesirable effects, as follows:

- It puts the greatest food intake at the least active time of day. This means that the energy ingested must be stored as fat to await use the next day. Because many individuals do not efficiently mobilize stored fat for energy, they probably feel sluggish and curtail their activity the next day.
- It may mean long stretches of time with little food. During these times we often find it too inconvenient to eat, and therefore we deny our hunger or stave it off with inadequate snacks. By late afternoon our hunger, now joined by tiredness and frustrations of school and work, overwhelms us, and we eat frantically, often far more than we need. Thus, this pattern runs counter to our goal of hunger-directed eating. Furthermore, with little or nothing to break the overnight fast, it's hard to get a good start in the morning.
- The quick meals or snacks we grab during the day usually are high in sodium and fat with little nutritive value.

There is nothing magical about eating three meals a day. Five may be better. Fewer than three results in long fasting times and may induce the problems described earlier. Whatever pattern works best, it should space food throughout active hours and should not produce overwhelming hunger or the drive to consume excessively. For most of us, how often we eat has to reflect the difficulties of providing ourselves with nourishing options throughout the day. Normalizing eating involves planning ahead to ensure that we don't get caught without any alternatives to chips and candy bars.

Adopting an Active Lifestyle

Does physical exercise help maintain a desirable body composition? The conclusions from research are contradictory and confusing. A lot of the confusion disappears when one distinguishes between what is possible in a controlled laboratory experiment and what is probable in the reality of most people's lives. Although exercise is not a panacea, it is one of the few factors consistently associated with success in maintaining a healthy body composition.

NUTRITION: FITNESS ESSENTIALS

Major advances in technology have made the lives of our clients and our own more comfortable and simpler. We drive instead of walk, take the elevator instead of the stairs, and ride the lawn mower instead of pushing it. The amount of physical activity performed at work and in the home has declined steadily. How important is physical activity to health, fitness, and total well-being? Let's take a closer look.

Physical activity is defined as any body movement produced by skeletal muscles that requires energy expenditure. It varies by day, time of year, and stage of life. Physical activity is similar to yet different from **physical fitness**. Physical activity describes the actions or movements that we make, whereas physical fitness describes the limits on the actions that we are capable of making.

Being physically fit is more than just being fast or strong. True physical fitness consists of three major components:

flexibility, muscular strength and endurance, and cardiovascular endurance. Flexibility is the ability to move the muscles to their full extent without injury. Muscular strength and endurance describe the ability of the muscles to perform hard or prolonged work. Cardiovascular endurance is the ability of the body to take in, deliver, and use oxygen for physical work. Although flexibility and muscular strength and endurance are important components of health and well-being, cardiovascular endurance is the best physiologic index of total body endurance. Life depends on the strength of the heart and lungs to deliver nutrients and oxygen to the cells.

Health Benefits of Physical Exercise

Much of what we do today will affect our future health. We have many choices to make regarding health behaviors. These choices have positive and negative consequences. The choices include using seat belts, smoking cigarettes, consuming alcohol, nutrition, and frequency of exercise. Our choices reflect our lifestyles; we are responsible for those choices.

Exercise is one of the many lifestyle factors that can be controlled. Increased physical activity leads to improved physical fitness and to other physiologic changes (Box 9.4). It is the combination of these changes that leads to better health. People who exercise regularly often adopt a healthier lifestyle; they may stop smoking, have more energy, handle stress better, and make wiser food choices—all of which improve the quality of life.

Most Americans have little or no physical activity in their daily lives. National surveys indicate that approximately one in four adults have sedentary lifestyles. Inactivity increases with age and is more common among women than men.

Persons with physically disabling conditions also benefit from moderate amounts of physical activity. Although this population tends not to perform regular exercise, it is still at risk for chronic diseases for which risk may be reduced by regular moderate exercise appropriate to the level of physical abilities. Other benefits are increased stamina and muscle strength and improvement of feelings of well-being through potential reduction of anxiety and depression (U.S. Department of Health and Human Services [USDHHS], 2008).

Currently, disparities in physical activity levels exist among American subgroups. Higher numbers of women than men, of Black and Hispanic Americans than White Americans, of older adults than younger, and of less affluent than more affluent Americans report no leisure time physical activity. This means that generally women, Black and Hispanic Americans, older adults, and the less affluent are not exercising sufficiently to gain the health benefits associated with physical activity (USDHHS, 2018). Health care providers can reduce these disparities by teaching patients about the benefits of exercise and providing information or referrals for exercise programs.

Physical activity need not be strenuous to achieve healthful benefits. Even people who are usually inactive can improve their health by becoming moderately active on a regular basis. As we counsel clients and patients in community and acute care settings, we can incorporate suggestions for simple fitness activities into care plans. The *2018 Physical Activity Guidelines for Americans* provides recommendations regarding the quantity, intensity, and type of exercise to promote health and reduce risk for major chronic diseases, psychological well-being, and a healthy body weight (USDHHS, 2018).

BOX 9.4 MyPlate: Why Is Physical Activity Important?

Regular physical activity can produce long-term health benefits. People of all ages, shapes, sizes, and abilities can benefit from being physically active. The more physical activity you do, the greater the health benefits.

Being Physically Active Can Help You

- Increase your chances of living longer
- Feel better about yourself
- Decrease your chances of becoming depressed
- Sleep well at night
- Move around more easily
- Have stronger muscles and bones
- Stay at or get to a healthy weight
- Be with friends or meet new people
- Enjoy yourself and have fun

When You Are Not Physically Active, You Are More Likely to

- Get heart disease
- Get T2D
- Have high blood pressure
- Have high blood cholesterol
- Have a stroke

Physical activity and nutrition work together for better health. Being active increases the number of calories burned. As people age their metabolism slows, so maintaining energy balance requires moving more and eating less.

Some Types of Physical Activities Are Especially Beneficial

- Aerobic activities make you breathe harder and make your heart beat faster. Aerobic activities can be moderate or vigorous in their intensity. Vigorous activities take more effort than moderate ones. For **moderate activities**, you can talk while you do them, but you can't sing. For **vigorous activities**, you can only say a few words without stopping to catch your breath.
- Muscle-strengthening activities make your muscles stronger. These include activities like pushups and lifting weights. It is important to work all the different parts of the body—your legs, hips, back, chest, stomach, shoulders, and arms.
- Bone-strengthening activities make your bones stronger. Bone-strengthening activities, like jumping, are especially important for children and adolescents. These activities produce a force on the bones that promotes bone growth and strength.
- Balance and stretching activities enhance physical stability and flexibility, which reduces risk of injuries. Examples are gentle stretching, dancing, yoga, martial arts, and t'ai chi.

FOOD AND ATHLETIC PERFORMANCE

Physical activity and nutrition have been associated with health since the time of ancient Greece. Hippocrates said, "All parts of the body which have a function, if used in moderation and exercised in labors in which each is accustomed, become thereby healthy, well-developed, and age more slowly, but if unused and left idle they become liable to disease, defective in growth and age quickly" (Simopoulos, 1989). More than 2000 years later, this advice is still consistent with our knowledge about nutrition, physical fitness, and health.

Physically active people of all ages and levels of competition are seeking information to enhance their training and achieve a competitive edge. They want to know what kinds of foods to eat and specific dietary regimens to follow. The nutritional needs of athletes are basically no different from those of nonathletes, with the exception of kcal and fluids. A diet that provides a variety of foods supplying 45% to 65% of kcal intake from carbohydrate, 20% to 35% of kcal intake from fat, and 10% to 35% of kcal intake from protein is recommended for health and performance (National Research Council, 2006). However, some forms of heavy training increase the requirement for certain nutrients. For example, carbohydrates are an important source of energy during endurance exercise, and therefore runners, cyclists, and swimmers may need more carbohydrates (60%–70% of their total kcal intake) than other individuals.

Nutrition can affect an athlete in many ways. At the most basic level, nutrition is essential for normal growth and development and for maintaining good health. By staying healthy, an athlete will feel better, train harder, and be in better condition. Among comparable athletes, good eating habits can be the factor that determines the winner. However, these good habits do not come from the pregame meal or even from what the athlete eats the week before competition. They are built daily over a long period.

A number of dietary patterns provide good nutrition. The MyPlate program can be a useful outline for athletes of what to eat every day. Each food group provides some—but not all—of the nutrients an athlete needs. Foods in each of the food categories of MyPlate provide kcal from different combinations of carbohydrate, protein, and fat (see www.chooseMyPlate.gov). For example, fruits provide kcal from carbohydrates, and grain products contain carbohydrate, protein, and varying amounts of fat.

Athletes should eat at least the minimum number of servings for each group daily to meet energy needs. Depending on their body size and level of training, some athletes may need more than the larger number of servings.

Nurses and other health professionals should have a basic understanding of the nutritional needs of athletes to provide fundamental information and to conduct a simple assessment or screening of nutritional status as influenced by athletic activities. Referrals to a registered dietitian with expertise in sports nutrition is appropriate for athletes and coaches with more specific concerns, such as the creation of individualized eating plans to support training and competitive needs (Thomas et al., 2016).

Kilocalorie Requirements

As noted earlier, kcal requirements vary greatly from person to person and are affected by activity level, body size, age, and climate. Body size affects kcal requirements more than any other single factor. The smaller the athlete, the lower the kcal requirement.

Some sports demand high-energy expenditure, whereas others do not. A commonly asked question is "How many kcal should I consume?" Athletes are consuming enough kcal if they are maintaining their best competitive yet healthy weight. Ideally, kcal intake should balance energy expended. If intake is consistently more or less than an athlete's requirement, weight gain or weight loss will occur, both of which can affect performance.

Many athletes are concerned about their appearance and thus eat less to keep their body weight and percentage of body fat low. However, restricting kcal can have a negative impact on health and performance. As kcal intake decreases, so does nutrient intake. A minimum requirement for college athletes is 1800 to 2000 kcal a day. Eating less than this amount can leave the athlete feeling weak and listless and may lead to iron deficiency, stress fractures, and, for women, amenorrhea and osteoporosis.

On the other hand, increasing kcal intake to gain weight may also be difficult for athletes. Too much food can cause discomfort, especially if a workout takes place soon after eating. Furthermore, for an athlete balancing school, work, and practice, little time is available to eat. Small meals and snacks become an important source of nutrients. How often to snack depends on body size and kcal needs.

Water: The Essential Ingredient

Water is the nutrient most critical to athletic performance. Without adequate water, performance can suffer in less than an hour. Water is necessary for the body's cooling system. It also transports nutrients throughout the tissues and maintains adequate blood volume.

During exercise there is always the risk of becoming dehydrated (fluid volume deficit), especially when the temperature is hot. When athletes sweat, they lose water. Although sweat rates vary among people, losing as little as 2% to 3% of weight via sweat can impair performance (Bardis et al., 2013). When the water lost via sweat is not replaced, blood volume falls and body temperature rises, causing confusion and loss of coordination. To replace the lost water, athletes must consume extra fluids.

The athlete's sense of thirst is not the best indicator that the body needs water; fluid needs may be greater than thirst can gauge. Adequate water intake before, during, and after an event or practice session is of utmost importance. Table 9.6 lists recommendations based on evidence statements from the American College of Sports Medicine (ACSM, 2007) to ensure adequate fluid replacement, which leads to optimal performance.

Stress the importance of adequate fluid intake. Clients should weigh themselves nude before and after exercise to determine fluid replacement needs. Sweat loss of 1 pound (2.2 kg) of body weight is equal to 2 cups (480 mL) of water. For every pound lost, an athlete needs to drink 2 cups of fluid. Another criterion of hydration is that urine should be basically clear in color throughout most of the day. (See Chapter 8 for the effects of a fluid volume deficit.)

Athletes completing endurance events or slower runners in races who continually drink fluid without an equivalent loss of fluid through sweat or urination may so overhydrate themselves as to experience **hyponatremia** (low blood sodium). Fluid volume deficit (dehydration) is much more common. Awareness of dehydration and hyponatremia is important because their medical treatments differ even though the symptoms appear similar.

TABLE 9.6 Recommendations for Adequate Fluid Replacement

	What to Do	What to Eat and Drink
Before exercise	Hydrating several hours before exercise allows for fluid absorption and urine output to normalize.	Beverages with sodium and/or salted snacks or small meals with beverages can help stimulate thirst and retain needed fluids.
During exercise	Weighing before and after exercise is useful for determining replacement fluid amounts.	Beverages containing electrolytes and carbohydrates are best.
After exercise	Consuming normal meals and beverages restores average hydration.	Beverages and snacks with sodium help speed recovery by stimulating thirst and fluid retention.

(Data from American College of Sports Medicine, et al: American College of Sports Medicine position stand: Exercise and fluid replacement, *Med Sci Sports Exerc* 39(2):377–390, 2007.)

Sports Drinks

Athletes often wonder which is better for replacing fluids during exercise—water or sports drinks. The number one goal is to remain well hydrated. Whether the athlete drinks water or a sports drink is their choice. Cool water is what the body really needs during activities lasting less than 1 hour. However, athletes participating in endurance events requiring more than 90 minutes of continuous moderate to heavy exercise, such as distance running or cycling, may benefit from sports drinks that contain carbohydrate and electrolytes (sodium and potassium). Sports drinks provide fluids to keep the athlete well hydrated and provide extra carbohydrates for energy.

A major consideration in fluid replacement is how quickly the fluid empties from the stomach. To hydrate the total body, the fluid needs to leave the stomach quickly to be distributed throughout the body. Although larger volumes of fluid empty more rapidly from the stomach, many athletes cannot exercise with a full stomach. Cool fluids empty faster from the stomach than warm fluids. Kcal content is also important. The greater the kcal content of a beverage, the slower the emptying rate. Fluid recovery choices are most effective if carbohydrates, protein, and water are provided as a 3:1 or 4:1 ratio of carbohydrate to protein (Clark, 2020). Table 9.7 lists commonly used recovery fluids and foods.

TABLE 9.7 Some Commonly Used Recovery Fluids and Foods After Exercise

Fluids	Foods
Chocolate milk	Cheerios with milk
Gatorade	Yogurt, flavored
Endurox	Pasta with meat sauce

(Data from Clark N: Nutrition and exercise workshop, New York, September 2013.)

Carbohydrate: The Energy Food

Carbohydrate stores in the body (glycogen) are limited. Low levels of muscle glycogen can impair performance. Consuming carbohydrates before and during exercise will delay the onset of fatigue and allow the athlete to compete longer.

How much carbohydrate should an athlete eat each day to replace muscle glycogen? The amount depends mostly on body size. An athlete with more muscle mass will require more carbohydrate. Carbohydrate requirements also depend on intensity and level of training. Athletes participating in high-energy sports that require short bursts of energy (e.g., basketball, tennis, football, soccer) need about 5 g of carbohydrate per kilogram of body weight daily to maintain muscle glycogen stores. Endurance athletes who train aerobically for more than 90 minutes daily may need a higher intake of carbohydrate per kilogram of body weight to replace glycogen. Individuals who exercise regularly to maintain conditioning do well with the general guidelines of high complex carbohydrate diets, as represented by MyPlate. The *Teaching Tool* box How Much Carbohydrate Do You Need? shows how to calculate carbohydrate requirements.

TEACHING TOOL

How Much Carbohydrate Do You Need?

1. Divide body weight in pounds by 2.2 (number of pounds in a kilogram) to determine body weight in kg. For example,
   154 lb ÷ 2.2 = 70 kg body weight
2. Multiply each kg of body weight by 5 g to determine the number of g of carbohydrate needed daily. For example,
   70 kg × 5 g = 350 g of carbohydrate daily

Both complex and simple carbohydrates are effective in replenishing glycogen in the muscles. However, complex carbohydrates provide vitamins, minerals, and fiber as well. Examples of complex carbohydrates are whole grains, bread, potatoes, pasta, cereal, fruits, and fruit juices. Simple sugars include maple syrup, molasses, honey, agave nectar, and table sugar.

Carbohydrate Loading

Carbohydrate loading is the process of changing the types of foods eaten and adjusting the amount of training to increase glycogen stores in the muscle. This concept first became of interest around 1939, when scientists studied the effects of dietary manipulation on the ability to perform prolonged hard work. They found that men consuming a high-carbohydrate diet for 3 days could perform heavy work twice as long as men fed a high-fat diet for the same 3 days (Christensen & Hansen, 1939). Since then, researchers have investigated several techniques for increasing glycogen levels in the muscles.

To achieve maximum muscle glycogen stores through carbohydrate loading, athletes should consume a high-carbohydrate diet as part of their regular training program. At least 60% (preferably 60%–70%) of their total kcal should come from carbohydrate. For the athlete eating 3000 kcal a day, this proportion represents a minimum of 450 g of carbohydrate daily. Three days before competition, exercise should taper off to allow muscles to rest. Dietary carbohydrates should be increased to 60% to 70% of total kcal. This technique of combining rest and increased carbohydrate intake encourages greater glycogen storage. Kcal intake may need to be reduced to compensate for less training.

Carbohydrate loading is usually recommended only for athletes engaged in continuous exercise lasting more than 90 minutes, although benefits may be gained for shorter events as well. It is not recommended for athletes participating in short-term events such as sprints or in sports such as football, baseball, and wrestling, nor should individuals with diabetes or hypoglycemia consider this dietary pattern, which affects carbohydrate metabolism. Furthermore, the degree of benefit from carbohydrate loading varies among individuals. Therefore, athletes should determine before competition the value of this regimen for themselves and should refer to specific resources for detailed recommendations. The potential negative side effects of carbohydrate loading include increased water retention and weight gain, stiffness, cramping, and digestive problems (Williams et al., 2016).

A more practical concern is whether athletes are eating enough carbohydrate on a daily basis to maintain adequate levels of muscle glycogen for training and workouts. The following organization websites may be helpful for determining adequate carbohydrate intake to maximize muscle glycogen stores: President's Council on Fitness, Sports & Nutrition: www.fitness.gov/index.html; American College of Sports Medicine (ACSM): www.acsm.org; and Healthy Weight, Nutrition, and Physical Activity: www.cdc.gov/healthyweight/tools.

Protein

The importance of protein for athletes has been a subject of controversy for many years. Many athletes and coaches believe that a high-protein diet supplies extra energy, enhances athletic performance, and increases muscle mass. There is no evidence, however, that eating more protein than needed improves athletic ability.

Although carbohydrate and fat are the major fuels used for energy, studies indicate that protein use increases during exercise, and under certain conditions, protein may contribute significantly to energy metabolism (Williams et al., 2016). Two factors that influence the use of protein as an energy source are the length of exercise and the carbohydrate content of the diet. The body may depend on protein for a greater percentage of energy in prolonged exercise (>90 minutes), particularly when carbohydrate intake is low.

The Dietary Reference Intake (DRI) for protein for sedentary adults is 0.8 g per kilogram of body weight per day. Research suggests that athletes need between 1.5 and 2 g of protein per kilogram of body weight per day. For a 150-pound (68-kg) athlete (runner), this amounts to 102 to 136 g of protein per day. Factors such as kcal intake, protein quality, and type and intensity of the sport are important considerations. The lower the kcal intake, the higher the protein requirements. This is one reason why protein intake is often a concern among female athletes, because many do not consume enough calories.

The type of protein eaten also affects the amount of protein needed. The 1.5 to 2 g of protein per kilogram of body weight recommendation is based on a diet containing animal foods. Athletes who eat meat, fish, poultry, eggs, milk, or cheese will have little problem meeting their protein needs. Strictly vegetarian athletes, however, will need to plan their diets more carefully to ensure that their protein needs are met. Protein bars may be used to supplement protein and energy intakes for athletes. Products should be carefully chosen to avoid excess intake of protein and simple sugars masked as dietary supplement bars.

Protein and Amino Acid Supplements

The use of protein and amino acid supplements is a common practice among athletes. Various combinations of individual amino acids are sold to athletes with the promise that the acids will stimulate the release of growth hormone and thus increase muscle mass. Promoters claim that amino acids can build muscle, aid fat loss, provide energy, speed up muscle repair, and improve endurance. Others claim that they are more readily digested and absorbed than the protein consumed in foods.

The question is: Do athletes need to take these supplements, or can they get the protein they need from food alone? Many athletes eat more than the recommended amount of protein (and thus amino acids) from food alone. Amino acids as building blocks of all proteins are found in a wide variety of foods, from pork chops to bread, from beans and peas to milk and tacos. Because the body cannot store extra protein, excess protein and amino acids are broken down and used for energy or stored as fat. If protein or amino acid supplements provide more nutrients than needed for protein functions, the body treats supplements the same as any excess source of protein.

It is safer and cheaper to take amino acids in a glass of milk, a turkey sandwich, or other protein-rich foods. Muscle size and strength increase only after weeks of work. If athletes want to gain muscle mass, they need to become involved in a resistive strength training program and consume a diet rich in carbohydrates.

Fat

In athletic performance, carbohydrate and fat are the major sources of energy. The amount of fat used during exercise depends on the duration and intensity of exercise, the level of prior training, and the composition of the diet. Exercise performed under aerobic conditions will promote fat use as a source of energy. There is a good reason to increase your body's ability to burn fat as fuel; using fat as a source of energy will spare muscle glycogen.

Athletes need a certain amount of fat in their diets and on their bodies for optimal health and performance. The challenge is eating a diet that provides the right amount. The position of the American Dietetic Association, Dietitians of Canada, and the American College of Sports Medicine recommends moderate energy intake of 20% to 25% energy from fat (Thomas et al., 2016). Because each athlete is different, some may eat less and some slightly more than the recommended range of kcal from fat. Many athletes cannot get the kcal they need without

TABLE 9.8 **Ergogenic Aids Marketed to Athletes**

Substance(s)	Description	Claims	Actual Effect
Arginine, lysine, ornithine	Amino acids	Stimulate release of human growth hormone	No proven effect
Antioxidant vitamins C, E, beta carotene	Compounds that may prevent free-radical damage	Prevent muscle damage from oxidation after high-intensity exercise	Some evidence of proven benefit
Caffeine[a]	Stimulant	Improves performance, increases fatty acid oxidation, spares glycogen	Some evidence of proven benefit
Carnitine	Facilitates the transfer of long-chain fatty acids into the mitochondria	Enhances energy levels, decreases body fat	No proven effect on body fat
Creatine	Protein/amino acids	Increases intramuscular creatine, increases power output, promotes increase in lean body mass	Some evidence of proven benefit
Dehydroepiandrosterone (DHEA)	Hormone	Increases energy, increases muscle mass, decreases body fat	More research is needed to confirm these observations
Ginseng	Extract of ginseng root	Reduces fatigue and improves endurance, strength, and recovery from exercise	No proven effect
β-hydroxy-β-methylbutyrate (HMB)	Metabolite of the amino acid leucine	Increases lean body mass, decreases body fat, increases strength	More research is needed to confirm these observations

[a]The use of caffeine is considered a form of doping by the International Olympic Committee (IOC). The IOC has set an upper limit of 12 μg/mL of caffeine content in urine.

eating a little extra fat. However, fat intakes greater than 35% of total kcal have been associated with increased risk of certain diet-related diseases (e.g., heart disease, obesity, cancer).

To lower fat intake, athletes should choose lean meats, fish, poultry, and low-fat dairy products. Fat and oils should be used sparingly in cooking, and fried foods and high-fat snacks should be eaten in moderation. (See Chapter 5 for strategies designed to lower dietary fat intake.)

Vitamins and Minerals

A balanced diet generally supplies enough vitamins and minerals to meet the needs of most athletes, and consuming more has not been shown to improve performance. Nevertheless, the use of supplements by high school and college athletes is common. Their use is even higher among elite athletes. Female athletes tend to use vitamin/mineral supplements more than men, and patterns exist among sport groups; for example, bodybuilders, cyclists, and runners are bigger supplement users than wrestlers and basketball players.

There are reportedly many reasons why athletes take vitamin and mineral supplements, such as for extra energy, to make up for a poor diet, to recover more quickly after exercise, and for general well-being. The problem is that athletes may view supplements as "good" and therefore harmless. Such beliefs can lead to excessive intakes. For many athletes, the level of nutrients consumed from food alone is greater than 200% of the DRI. With the addition of a supplement, combined food and nutrient intakes can exceed 1000% of the DRI. Toxicity and adverse health effects can occur from consumption of high doses of vitamins and minerals over a long period.

On the other hand, athletes in "thin-build" sports (e.g., gymnastics, figure skating, wrestling, and distance running) often consume low-calorie intakes and thus are at risk for vitamin and mineral deficiencies. For these athletes, supplementation with a multivitamin/mineral providing 100% of the DRI can be beneficial.

Ergogenic Aids

In athletics, the term ergogenic aids is used to describe drugs and dietary regimens believed by some to increase strength, power, and endurance (Table 9.8). Because winning is often a matter of a split second, it is easy to see why athletes are continuously looking for the competitive edge. The fact that more and more nutritional supplements are marketed to athletes presents a challenge to coaches, trainers, nutritionists, and health care providers to provide sound nutrition information.

The nutritional supplements used by athletes constantly change. Often, as athletes find that one doesn't work, they search for another. Today commonly used nutritional aids include creatine monohydrate (a protein), chromium picolinate, β-hydroxy-β-methylbutyrate (HMB), and dehydroepiandrosterone (DHEA). Although the use of DHEA is banned in some states, athletes still use it. With the exception of creatine, research has not found these supplements to have a significant effect on performance. Despite a lack of scientific basis for the claims associated with these products, their widespread use continues.

Nutritional supplements are a multimillion-dollar business. Athletes are prime targets for the marketers of these products. Athletes make good consumers because, like many Americans, they believe that if a little is good, a lot is better. It is not uncommon for an athlete to consume five or six different supplements a day and to not know what substances are in them. Many of the supplements athletes purchase from specialty nutrition stores and mail-order catalogs are not subject to the regulations established by the U.S. Food and Drug Administration (FDA), presenting another concern. Athletes have no way of knowing whether these nutritional supplements are safe.

Taking several different supplements at one time, or one containing a large amount of one nutrient, such as vitamin A, can be toxic. There is also the risk of nutrient–nutrient interactions, in which an excess of one nutrient can interfere with the body's ability to use another nutrient. Such a situation may occur when excessive amounts of one amino acid are consumed, possibly affecting the body's use of other amino acids.

ROLE OF NURSES

Approaches to weight, body composition management, and fitness are being reformulated. Recognition that traditional weight loss approaches to eat less and exercise more are not successful and are often counterproductive is growing and is forcing health professionals to consider alternative and adjunct approaches. Some of these approaches are presented in this chapter. Acceptance of genetic limitations and redefinition of weight management and fitness goals provide health professionals and their clients with potentially achievable objectives to achieve and maintain health.

Within these changes it is important for nurses to understand that the role of the dietitian is evolving from that of a counselor/educator who gives only dietary advice to that of a therapist who practices advanced counseling skills using psychodynamic models of therapy to assist and coach clients. This new view expands nutrition therapy and involves a shift from a short-term to a long-term approach. Weight management is a lifelong process and so incorporates broader lifestyle skills to achieve healthy weight and fitness goals. Dietitians can coach clients about the process of food choice, shifting the responsibility of decision making about food and portion control to the client, who is then armed with skills and support from dietetic counseling. The goal is to ensure enjoyment of eating while still maintaining a healthy lifestyle. Everyone should be able to enjoy their favorite foods but make conscious choices about where, when, and how much of the foods are eaten.

Dietitians are often part of multidisciplinary teams that incorporate primary health care providers, physicians, nurses, behavior therapists, exercise therapists, and psychologists. Nurses can provide support during the formal and informal interactions within the health care system. An important aspect of this support involves nurses' considering their attitudes about their own bodies and about clients who struggle with their weight, body image, and possible associated health concerns. In addition, nurses need to be knowledgeable about the lifestyle changes and food choices needed to achieve long-term body composition management to further support client success. This may require the nurse to further specialize as a member of a multidisciplinary health team.

TOWARD A POSITIVE NUTRITION LIFESTYLE: EXPLANATORY STYLE

In his book *Learned Optimism*, Dr. Martin Seligman, a psychologist and professor, explores applications of explanatory styles to everyday life situations (Seligman, 2006). As a component of personal control, explanatory style is the way in which a person regularly explains why events happen. An individual with a pessimistic explanatory style spreads learned helplessness by having a pervasive negative view that no matter what they do, nothing will change. In contrast, a person with an optimistic explanatory style feels able to stop the reaction of learned helplessness and understands events in a more positive way. An optimistic person feels competent in that they can change the course of events.

Explanatory style has been studied in relation to health and wellness. A person's approach to dealing with issues of physical health can be helped or hindered by cognitions about personal control over health conditions and maintenance. Seligman notes the following:

- The way we think, especially about health, changes our health.
- Optimists catch fewer infectious diseases than pessimists do.
- Optimists have better health habits than pessimists do.
- Our immune system may work better when we are optimistic.
- Evidence suggests that optimists live longer than pessimists.

How does this information apply to body fat management? Having an optimistic explanatory style may mean accepting one's body as it is and acting in ways to improve health by attempting to eat well and exercise regularly. A pessimistic explanatory style would judge one's body negatively and would not attempt behaviors to improve body composition because physical attributes would be understood to be permanent and thus unchangeable. Consider other ways that our patients' explanatory styles affect their approach to their illnesses and that our explanatory styles affect the strategies of nursing care.

SUMMARY

- The abilities to perform work, produce change, and maintain life all require energy, which is converted from food eaten into adenosine triphosphate (ATP) energy.
- The two energy pathways are the aerobic pathway (depends on oxygen) and the anaerobic pathway (functions without oxygen).
- Carbohydrate in the form of glucose is the only fuel to be used anaerobically, without oxygen, to produce ATP.
- During low- to moderate-intensity exercise, muscle cells mainly use fat for fuel.
- Daily energy requirement depends on three major components: basal metabolism, physical activity, and the thermic effect of food (TEF), or diet-induced thermogenesis.
- Each component is affected directly or indirectly by many factors, including age, gender, and body size.
- A healthy weight is a weight at which a person can physically move comfortably, maintain without undue restriction of food intake or without excessive exercise, and live without experiencing any weight-related associative disorders.
- Lifelong management of body fat levels provides a more holistic health approach to body size than does body weight.
- Goals for body fat levels account for an individual's genetic and family factors as well as those of society and health.
- Ways of measuring body fat composition include densitometry and bioelectric impedance analysis.

- Body mass index (BMI), which is calculated by dividing the weight in kilograms by the square of the height in meters, can relate to the associated health risk for men and women.
- Weight may be maintained by set point, through which the body regulates its most natural weight.
- Individuals at both extremes of fatness—those very thin and those very fat—are at increased risk for certain health-related disorders.
- Physical fitness consists of three major components: flexibility, muscular strength and endurance, and cardiovascular endurance.
- The nutritional needs of athletes are generally no different from those of nonathletes, with the exception of kcal and fluids.
- For athletes, a diet that provides a variety of foods supplying 45% to 65% of kcal intake from carbohydrate, 20% to 35% of kcal intake from fat, and 10% to 35% of kcal intake from protein is recommended for health and performance.
- Eating enough carbohydrates daily maintains adequate levels of muscle glycogen for training and workouts.
- Recommendations for protein intake for athletes, 1.5 to 2 g per kilogram of body weight, are greater than those for of sedentary individuals (0.8 g/kg).
- Ergogenic aids are drugs and dietary regimens believed to increase strength, power, and endurance.

THE NURSING APPROACH

Clinical Judgment and Next-Generation NCLEX® Examination-Style Questions

Case Study 1

Nutrition for an Athlete

Tom, an 18-year-old freshman student on the university track team, is preparing for a marathon running event. He has been given instructions about diet from his coach but wants to confirm the information with the nurse at the student health center. He has been training hard and is highly motivated to do his best in the race.

Assessment/Recognize Cues

Subjective (From Patient Statements)

- "I eat healthy and follow the MyPlate guidelines."
- "How do I carbohydrate load before the marathon?"
- "I would like to know what types of sports drinks I should drink and how much and when I should drink them."
- "Please tell me about protein powders."

Objective (From Physical Examination)

- Height 5′9″, weight 140 lb.
- Blood pressure 120/80. Temperature 98.4° F, pulse 60, respirations 16
- Lean with well-defined muscles.

Diagnoses (Nursing)/Analyze Cues

Need for health teaching as evidenced by desire to know about carbohydrate loading before a marathon race, sports drinks, and protein powders.

Planning/Prioritize Hypotheses

Patient Outcomes

Short term (at the end of this visit):

- Tom will state specific plans for carbohydrate loading, hydration, and protein supplements.
- He will discuss the rationale for each dietary plan.

Nursing Interventions/Generate Solutions

1. Assess Tom's knowledge of nutrition, and teach him about nutrition for athletes.
2. Caution Tom to avoid steroids and other banned or illegal substances.

Implementation/Take Action

1. Assessed Tom's knowledge of nutrition.
   It is important to know the beliefs of an individual so that his knowledge can be confirmed or corrected. Teaching should proceed from the familiar to new information. Teaching should be centered on the learning needs.
2. Taught him the correct procedure for carbohydrate loading.
   During endurance training, at least 60% of calories should come from carbohydrates. A few days before the endurance event, exercise is tapered down to allow muscles to rest, and carbohydrates are increased to help build glycogen stores in the muscles and liver. On the day of the event, a light carbohydrate meal is consumed before the race.
3. Taught him that hydration is important before the event. About 6 oz of sports drinks should be consumed every 15 to 20 minutes during an event lasting longer than 90 minutes.
   Water is needed to cool the body and prevent dehydration. Carbohydrate supplies energy, and sodium and potassium replace electrolytes lost through sweat.
4. Taught Tom that endurance athletes may have higher protein needs than the general population but probably do not need protein powders.
   Endurance and strength-trained athletes may need 1.5 to 2 g protein/kg body weight per day. These recommendations are usually met through diet alone because most Americans actually consume almost twice the recommended amount of protein. Female athletes, though, may need to be aware of their protein intake in relation to their overall caloric intake.
5. Cautioned him to avoid steroids and other banned or illegal substances.
   Even when not asked about steroids and other banned or illegal substances, the nurse should address the subject for health promotion. Steroids are synthetic hormones that are anabolic and androgenic, taken by some athletes to increase muscle size and strength. They are very dangerous and can cause premature closure of bone growth, liver injury, heart disease, high blood pressure, and sterility and many other physical effects. Other banned or illegal substances could disqualify him from participating in sporting events.
6. Referred Tom to a dietitian to discuss specific personal diet questions and concerns.
   Although a nurse is qualified to discuss general nutrition, specific individualized diets should be planned by a dietitian.

Evaluation/Evaluate Outcomes

Short term (at the end of the visit):

- Tom was able to state correct plans for consuming carbohydrates, sports drinks, and protein foods.
- He was able to explain valid rationales for his plans.
- He stated that he does not take steroids and other banned or illegal substances and will continue to avoid them.

Goals met.

Continued

THE NURSING APPROACH—cont'd

Discussion Questions

Tom went to a dietitian to work out a personalized meal plan, and he reported to the dietitian after the race. He was able to finish his marathon running event but was not among the fastest runners. He planned to do more training to improve his time.

1. Describe one prerace dinner meal that would provide high protein and about 60% carbohydrate.
2. Would the basic principles in this case study be the same for a young woman who planned to run a marathon? What might be different?

Case Study 2

The dietitian is evaluating a referral and is reviewing the client's medical record. The dietitian knows that adults are likely to get specific conditions if they have a lack of physical activity.

Highlight those conditions in the grid below. Select all that apply.

1. Heart disease
2. Diabetes
3. Celiac disease
4. High blood pressure
5. Rheumatoid arthritis
6. Melanoma
7. Stroke
8. High blood cholesterol
9. Hepatitis

APPLYING CONTENT KNOWLEDGE

Darren, a college student, just started an aerobic exercise plan to lose some fat. Because he feels tired, he stops by the college health center and chats with a nurse practitioner about his exercise program. He asks, "If my muscles use simple carbohydrates for energy, why isn't it okay for me to have a soda and a candy bar rather than a regular meal? It's all calories isn't it?" How might the nurse practitioner respond?

WEBSITES OF INTEREST

President's Council on Fitness, Sports & Nutrition

www.fitness.gov/index.html

Provides comprehensive information on physical activity, nutrition, and obesity and related programs in the United States.

American College of Sports Medicine (ACSM)

www.acsm.org

Encourages developing active lifestyles for people of all ages.

Healthy Weight, Nutrition, and Physical Activity:

www.cdc.gov/healthyweight/tools/

Offers strategies and tools for achieving and maintaining a healthy weight. Developed by the Centers for Disease Control and Prevention (CDC).

REFERENCES

American College of Sports Medicine (ACSM). (2007). American college of sports medicine position stand: exercise and fluid replacement. *Medicine and Science in Sports and Exercise, 39*(2), 377–390.

Bardis, C. N., et al. (2013). Mild hypohydration decreases cycling performance in the heat. *Medicine and Science in Sports and Exercise, 45*(9), 1782–1789.

Christensen, E., & Hansen, O. (1939). Arbeitsfahigkeit and ernahrung. *Skandinavisches Archiv fur Physiologie, 81*, 160–171.

Clark, N. (2020). *Nancy Clark's sports nutrition guidebook* (6th ed.). Champaign, IL: Human Kinetics.

Hussain, S. S., et al. (2014). Control of food intake and appetite. In A. C. Ross (Ed.), *Modern nutrition in health and disease* (11th ed.). Philadelphia: Lippincott Williams & Wilkins.

National Research Council (NRC). (2006). *Dietary reference intakes: The essential guide to nutrient requirements.* Washington, DC: The National Academies Press.

Polsky, S., et al. (2014). Obesity: epidemiology, etiology and prevention. In A. C. Ross (Ed.), *Modern nutrition in health and disease* (11th ed.). Philadelphia: Lippincott Williams & Wilkins.

Seligman, M. E. P. (2006). *Learned optimism.* New York: Alfred A. Knopf.

Simopoulos, A. P. (1989). Opening address: nutrition and fitness from the first Olympiad in 776 BC to 393 AD and the concept of positive health. *The American Journal of Clinical Nutrition, 49*(5 Suppl), 921–926.

Thomas, D. T., et al. (2016). Position of the academy of nutrition and dietetics, dietitians of canada, and the american college of sports medicine: nutrition and athletic performance. *Journal of the Academy of Nutrition and Dietetics, 116*(3), 501–528.

U.S. Department of Health and Human Services. (2018). *Physical activity guidelines for americans* (2nd ed.). Washington, DC: U.S. Department of Health and Human Services. From https://health.gov/our-work/physical-activity/current-guidelines. (Accessed 27 December, 2020).

Wellman, N. S., & Kamp, B. J. (2017). Nutrition in aging. In L. K. Mahan (Ed.), *Krause's food & the nutrition care process* (14th ed.). St. Louis, MO: Elsevier.

Williams, M. H., et al. (2016). *Nutrition for health, fitness and sport* (11th ed.). New York: McGraw-Hill Science.

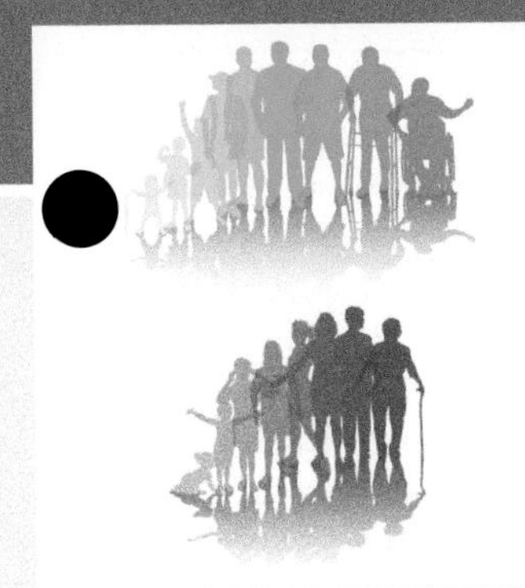

10 Nutrition Across the Life Span

Aging is a gradual process that reflects the influence of genetics, lifestyle, and environment over the course of the life span.

http://evolve.elsevier.com/GRODNER/FOUNDATIONS

LEARNING OBJECTIVES

- Discuss nutrient needs during pregnancy.
- Explain the process of lactation and the benefits of breastfeeding for mother and infant.
- Identify sound nutrition practices during the first year of life.
- Compare and contrast the nutrient requirements, eating styles, food choices, and community supports for childhood, adolescence, and adulthood.
- Describe approaches to prevent food asphyxiation, lead poisoning, overweight/diabetes, and iron deficiency during childhood and adolescence.
- Summarize nutrition strategies to reduce risk of the chronic disorders osteoporosis, cardiovascular disease, hypertension, and obesity.

ROLE IN WELLNESS

This chapter not only addresses the basic nutrition requirements of pregnancy, infancy, childhood, adolescence, and adulthood through older adulthood but also considers the factors that affect health promotion. As presented in Chapter 1, the goal of health promotion is to increase the level of health of individuals, families, and communities. Health promotion strategies often focus on lifestyle changes leading to new, positive health behaviors.

Development of these behaviors may depend on knowledge, techniques, and community supports. Knowledge is learning new information about the benefits or risks of health-related behaviors. Techniques are strategies used to apply new knowledge to everyday activities. By applying our knowledge, we modify lifestyle behaviors. Community supports (environmental or regulatory measures) are available that support new health-promoting behaviors within a social context.

Previous chapters have begun with a discussion of the relationship of the chapter topic to the six dimensions of health. Because this chapter covers the full range of the life span, a more fitting application of the dimensions is covered with the *Cultural Diversity and Nutrition* box, Live Long and Prosper … the Okinawa Way!

NUTRITION DURING PREGNANCY

Although the influence of nutrition on the course of pregnancy was assumed for some time, it was not until the twentieth century that research provided a scientific basis to substantiate such assumptions. Appropriate nutritional intake during pregnancy is integral to a successful pregnancy. Successful pregnancy outcomes include a viable infant of acceptable birth weight, an infant free of congenital defects, and a favorable long-term health outlook for both mother and infant.

Body Composition Changes During Pregnancy

After conception and continuing until parturition (childbirth), many metabolic, anatomic, hormonal, psychologic, and physiologic changes take place in the mother. This chapter focuses on those most affected by or affecting nutrient intake.

Hormones of Pregnancy

Numerous steroid hormones, peptide hormones, and prostaglandins influence the course of pregnancy. Some of them, such as the placental hormones human placental lactogen and human growth hormone, are produced only during pregnancy. Others, including insulin, glucagon, and thyroxine, are present in different amounts from those in the nonpregnant state and have profound influences on metabolism throughout gestation.

CULTURAL DIVERSITY AND NUTRITION

Live Long and Prosper ... the Okinawa Way!

Ageism, discrimination against the elderly, would cease to exist if we followed the lifestyles of the "successful-aging" elders of the Japanese island of Okinawa. According to the ongoing Okinawa Centenarian Study that began in 1976, the elders who follow Okinawa traditional ways experience lower levels of heart disease, stroke, and cancer; are generally healthier; and are more physically active for a greater number of years in comparison with other populations worldwide.

Because most of the present Okinawa centenarians are disabled, frail, and physically and/or cognitively impaired, the researchers decided to study the small number of successfully aging centenarians who are able to care for themselves by accomplishing activities of daily living (ADLs) and live independently in their villages. Although findings indicate genetic factors to be significant for their longevity and wellness, environmental factors may be even more important. The blend of these environmental factors of culture, attitude, and habits as an aspect of wellness may be understood through the definition of health as the blending of the six dimensions of health.

Okinawan Longevity and Wellness Through the Six Dimensions of Health

Physical health (efficient body functioning): *Nuchi gusui* and *hara hachi bu* address efficient body functioning through nourishing the body. *Nuchi gusui* means "let food be your medicine" by consuming a plant-based diet of fruits, vegetables, whole grains, sweet potatoes, legumes, fish, tofu, and other soy products. About 15 different foods, in small portions, are eaten every day. *Hara hachi bu* translates as eating in moderation until just about almost full. This approach allows the hypothalamus time to signal the brain that hunger has been satisfied, preventing overconsumption. The healthiest elders tend to be the most physically active, those who work, garden, and pursue interests.

Intellectual health (use of intellectual abilities): Rural Okinawan society views aging as a valuable achievement. Intellectual ability allows for acceptance of the aging process while maintaining one's active role in the community. Birthdays from ages 73 to 100 are observed with symbolic gestures such as elders patting family and friends to impart their good health and good fortunes.

Emotional health (ability to control emotions): *Taygay* represents a calm and relaxed approach to life. Traditional Okinawan society encourages being able to deal with stressors while maintaining appropriate control of one's emotions.

Social health (interactions and relationships with others): *Yuimaru* is the principle of mutual assistance on which Okinawan society is based. This concept applies to all ages as *moais* (groups of individuals who may be friends or work together) provide support for one another over many years. For the elders, their *moais* are important social links, providing daily interaction over shared pots of tea to discuss the news of the day.

Spiritual health (cultural beliefs about the purpose of life): "*Isha-hanbun, yuta-hanbun*" is a proverb meaning "To best understand your problem, see both a doctor and a shaman." This addresses the balance of life, to be aware of spiritual as well as physical well-being. Okinawan pursuits such as t'ai chi and karate provide both physical and spiritual benefits.

Environmental health (external factors that affect health and well-being): Life is organized around meeting the simple needs of community and personal well-being. The other five dimensions of health are supported within the natural setting of Okinawa.

Application to Nursing

Although we may not find ourselves in the semirural environment of the Okinawan villages in which these elders live, we can draw some strategies from their lifestyles to apply to our nursing practice.

We need to be mindful that elderly clients from diverse cultural backgrounds may have lost touch with their *moais*. Perhaps they have recently moved to live with their adult children, or have lost a spouse, or both. In addition to medical care, suggestions for seeking out a new *moai* may be most helpful. Art classes, card games, or discussion groups at a local senior center may be helpful in addition to medication for hypertension.

As we advocate for behavior change by our clients, particularly around food choices, consideration of the meaning of food is valuable. Asking an elder to make sweeping food changes is very unsettling. Perhaps introducing the traditional Okinawan concepts of *nuchi gusui* ("let food be your medicine") and *hara hachi bu* (eating in moderation until about almost full) may initiate a lively discussion about food choices and quantities consumed. Your client will remember "that interesting discussion I had with the friendly nurse."

(Data from Buettner D: The secrets of long life, *Nat Geogr* 208(5):2–27, 2005; Weil A: Longevity lessons from the Okinawans, *Dr. Andrew Weil's self-healing*, November 2005, p. 8; Suzuki M, et al: Successful aging: Secrets of Okinawan longevity, *Geriatr Gerontol Int* 4:S180, 2004; Willcox DC, et al: Healthy aging diets other than the Mediterranean: a focus on the Okinawan diet, *Mech Ageing Dev.* Mar–Apr;136–137:148–62, 2014.)

Progesterone and estrogen have a particularly strong influence on pregnancy. The action of progesterone promotes development of the endometrium (mucous membrane of the uterus) and relaxes the smooth muscle cells of the uterus. This relaxation serves to both help the uterus expand as the fetus grows and prevent any premature contractions of the uterus. The same effect also influences other smooth muscle cells, such as the gastrointestinal (GI) tract. The resulting slowing of the GI tract during pregnancy may increase the absorption of several nutrients, most notably iron and calcium. One perhaps annoying consequence of this decreased gut motility is the promotion of constipation. Progesterone causes increased renal sodium excretion during pregnancy. The body compensates for this sodium-losing mechanism by increasing aldosterone secretion from the adrenal gland and renin from the kidney. Sodium restriction during pregnancy, once thought to prevent hypertensive disorders of pregnancy, is actually harmful because it reduces plasma volume and cardiac output.

Estrogen promotes the growth of the uterus and breasts during pregnancy and renders the connective tissues in the pelvic region more flexible in preparation for birth.

Metabolic Changes

Profound changes in maternal metabolism occur during pregnancy, and successful adaptation to these changes is necessary for a favorable pregnancy outcome. The basal metabolic rate (BMR) rises during pregnancy by as much as 15% to 20% by term. This increase is caused by the greater oxygen needs of the fetus and the maternal support tissues. There are alterations in maternal metabolism of protein, carbohydrate, and fat. The fetus prefers to use glucose as its primary energy source. Changes occur in maternal metabolism to accommodate this need of the fetus. The adaptation allows the mother to use fat as the primary fuel source, thus permitting glucose to be available to the fetus (Turner, 2014). Increased macronutrient and micronutrient intake by the mother during pregnancy ensures that these higher metabolic needs are met.

TABLE 10.1 New Recommendations for Total and Rate of Weight Gain During Pregnancy, by Prepregnancy Body Mass Index

	TOTAL WEIGHT GAIN		RATES OF WEIGHT GAIN IN SECOND AND THIRD TRIMESTERS[a]	
Prepregnancy BMI	Range in kg	Range in lb	Mean (Range) in kg/week	Mean (Range) in lb/week
Underweight (<18.5 kg/m²)	12.5–18	28–40	0.51 (0.44–0.58)	1 (1–1.3)
Normal weight (18.5–24.9 kg/m²)	11.5–16	25–35	0.42 (0.35–0.50)	1 (0.8–1)
Overweight (25.0–29.9 kg/m²)	7–11.5	15–25	0.28 (0.23–0.33)	0.6 (0.5–0.7)
Obese (≥30.0 kg/m²)	5–9	11–20	0.22 (0.17–0.27)	0.5 (0.4–0.6)

[a]Calculations assume a 0.5- to 2-kg (1.1–4.4 lb) weight gain in the first trimester.
(Based on Siega-Riz AM, et al: Institute of Medicine maternal weight gain recommendations and pregnancy outcome in a predominantly Hispanic population, *Obstet Gynecol* 84[4]:565–573, 1994; Abrams B, et al: Factors associated with the pattern of maternal weight gain during pregnancy, *Obstet Gynecol* 86[2]:170–176, 1995; Carmichael S, et al: The pattern of maternal weight gain in women with good pregnancy outcomes, *Am J Public Health* 87[12]:1984–1988, 1997).

Anatomic and Physiologic Changes

Plasma volume doubles during pregnancy, beginning in the second trimester. Failure to achieve this plasma expansion may result in a spontaneous abortion, a stillbirth, or a low-birth-weight infant. One of the results of this increase in plasma volume is a hemodilution effect, or dilution of the blood. In other words, measured components in the plasma such as hemoglobin, serum proteins, and vitamins will appear to be at lower levels during pregnancy because there is a greater volume of solvent (the plasma) relative to concentrations of solute (the components). Cardiac hypertrophy occurs to accommodate this increased blood volume, accompanied by an increased ventilatory rate.

In the kidneys, the glomerular filtration rate (GFR) increases to accommodate the expanded maternal blood volume being filtered and to carry away fetal waste products. As a result of this increase in GFR, small quantities of glucose, amino acids, and water-soluble vitamins may appear in the urine. Although minor losses may be acceptable, a woman who excretes large amounts of protein may experience a more serious problem called preeclampsia, or pregnancy-induced hypertension, which needs strict medical monitoring. Preeclampsia is described in more detail later in the chapter.

As mentioned, progesterone may slow GI motility during pregnancy, leading to constipation, heartburn, and delayed gastric emptying. In late pregnancy, these problems may be exacerbated by the weight of the uterus and fetus as they compress the abdominal cavity.

Weight Gain in Pregnancy

There are three components to maternal weight gain: (1) maternal body composition changes, including increased blood and extracellular fluid volume; (2) the maternal support tissues, such as the greater size of the uterus and breasts; and (3) the products of conception, including the fetus and the placenta. Inadequate weight gain by the mother during pregnancy suggests that she may not have received the proper nutrients during pregnancy. Poor weight gain may then lead to intrauterine growth retardation in the infant. Infants born small for gestational age (SGA) or at low birth weight are more likely to require prolonged hospitalization after birth or to be ill or die during the first year of life. SGA is defined as an infant born at a lower birth weight than expected for the length of gestation, whereas low birth weight is a weight less than 5.5 pounds (2500 g) at birth. Additionally, infant mortality rate, which in part reflects maternal weight gain, is regarded as one measure of a country's health and well-being.

Between 2011 and 2016, rates of total infant, neonatal and post neonatal mortality rates were basically stable. During the same time span, rates of preterm and low birthweight newborn results were increasing. In the United States, maternal features such as the mother's age, race, and/or Hispanic origin vary in respect to total infant, neonatal, and postneonatal mortality occurrences. Infants born to non-Hispanic Black and Native American or Alaskan Native women have higher overall rates of mortality in addition to elevated rates of neonatal and postneonatal mortality compared with infants of women of other races and of Hispanic origin. Risk factors remain higher for infant deaths among younger (age <20 years) and older (age >40 years) women. Since 2007, the death rates have lowered for all groups. Nonetheless, there are notable differences between these groups (Ely et al., 2018).

There is strong evidence that the pattern of weight gain is just as important as the absolute recommended weight gains, as shown in Table 10.1. Failure to gain adequately during the second trimester of pregnancy is associated with poor infant birth weight, even if the net gain falls within the recommendations.

A balance must be struck regarding weight gain during pregnancy. Although women who are underweight or normal weight (as defined by body mass index [BMI]) are counseled to eat sufficiently to promote adequate gain, caution must be observed in counseling women who enter pregnancy while overweight or obese. Overweight and obese women should gain enough weight to support the fetus and maternal support tissues but without increasing total body fat. There are increased risks for operative delivery, increased maternal postpartum weight, gestational diabetes, and other long-term health consequences when maternal weight goes beyond the guidelines, particularly among women who are obese before pregnancy (Turner, 2014). In addition, there may be subpopulations, such as minorities and low-income women, who need special guidance regarding weight gain during pregnancy. Fig. 10.1 summarizes the possible determinants and the effects of gestational weight gain.

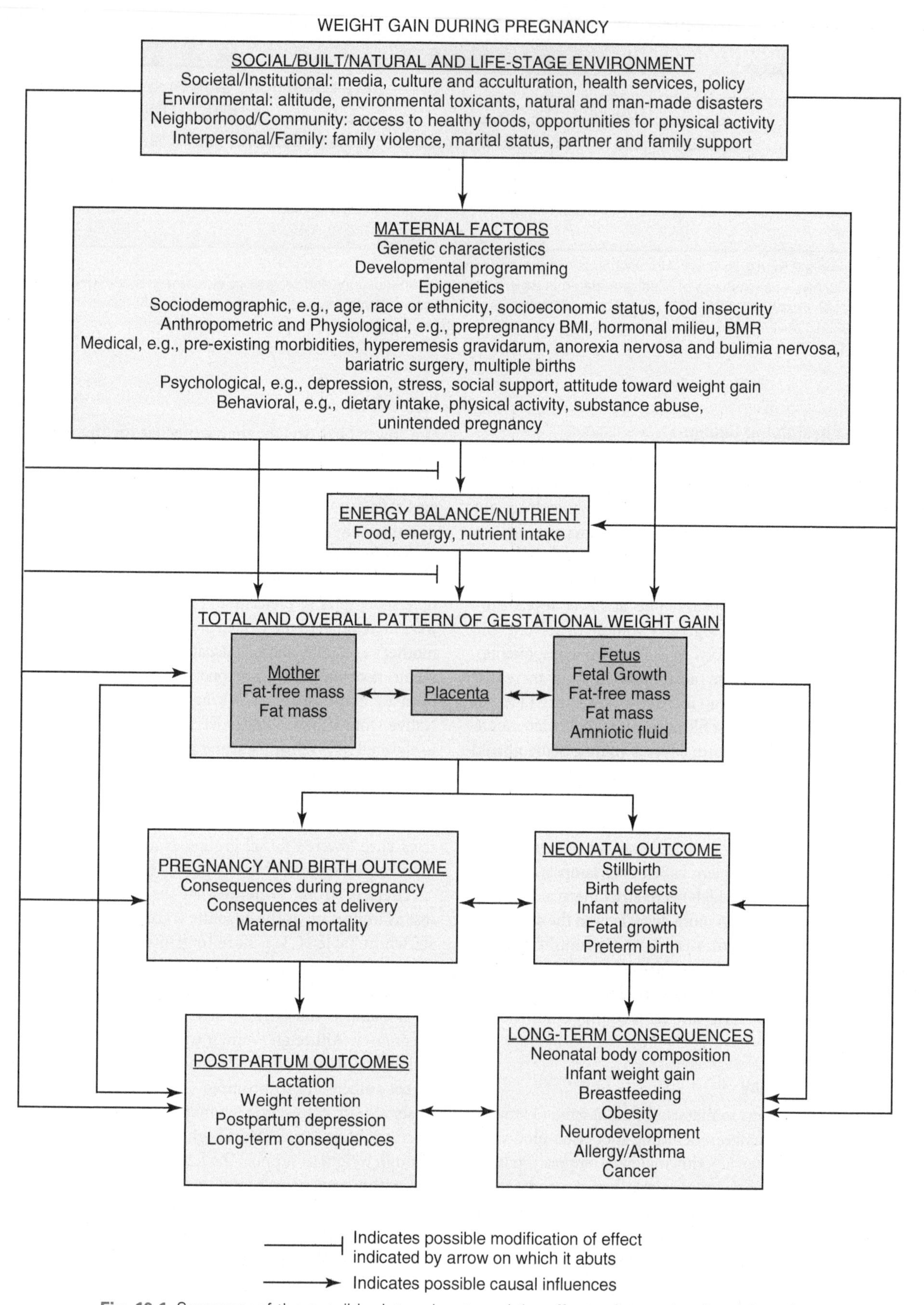

Fig. 10.1 Summary of the possible determinants and the effects of gestational weight gain. *BMI*, Body mass index; *BMR*, basal metabolic rate. (From the Institute of Medicine and the National Research Council: *Weight gain during pregnancy: Reexamining the guidelines*, Washington, DC, 2009, The National Academies Press.)

Additional issues arise when women who have undergone gastric bypass surgery become pregnant. Because of the smaller stomach size, less food is consumed, and intestinal absorption of nutrients may be compromised. Recommendations are to delay pregnancy until at least a year after bypass surgery and to seek nutrition services to support adequate nutrient absorption and energy intake.

Energy and Nutrient Needs During Pregnancy

The Dietary Reference Intakes (DRIs) recommend increases during pregnancy of all nutrients except vitamin D, vitamin E, vitamin K, phosphorus, fluoride, calcium, and biotin (Table 10.2). There are separate dietary recommendations for adolescents who are pregnant.

Energy

It is difficult to estimate the true energy cost of pregnancy, but the best estimates place the total energy cost somewhere between 68,000 and 80,000 kcal. The increase accommodates the rise in maternal BMR during pregnancy as well as the synthesis and support of the maternal and fetal tissues (Turner, 2014). The current recommendation is for a woman to consume an extra 340 kcal/day during the second trimester and 452 kcal/day during the third trimester of pregnancy. Although she appears to be eating for two, the expectant mother need not and should not double her food intake. An extra sandwich, fruit, and a glass of milk can easily provide the additional kcal per day, provided that she was eating well before pregnancy. Personal preference may guide particular food choices to provide the extra kcal, as long as the foods are nutritious.

What happens if a pregnant woman fails to increase her energy intake during pregnancy? The best-known example in the twentieth century occurred in Holland during World War II. Infants born during the famine of 1944 and 1945 had smaller birth weights and birth lengths than infants born either before or after the famine (Smith, 1947). Later research indicates that when women who begin pregnancy in energy deficit (e.g., those who are chronically undernourished in developing countries) are provided with energy supplementation throughout the course of pregnancy, there is a positive effect on maternal weight gain and infant birth weight (Bitler & Currie, 2005). On the other hand, some research suggests that women in the United States who are well nourished and do not increase their total energy intake by the recommended extra kcal per day can still have a positive pregnancy outcome. Most likely, in the third trimester, many women decrease their energy expenditure in pregnancy by reducing activity, thereby attaining a net increase in energy intake.

Pregnancy is not a time to restrict kcal or to lose weight, even if the mother begins the pregnancy as overweight. This issue may be particularly important to emphasize to the adolescent population. The mother should be encouraged to eat at least the minimum number of servings recommended during pregnancy from the MyPlate program. The interactive Daily Food Plan for Moms creates a personalized dietary food pattern based on height, weight, age, and other characteristics (www.myplate.gov/life-stages/pregnancy-and-breastfeeding). Sample menus can be helpful in showing the pregnant woman how MyPlate can be used (Box 10.1).

BOX 10.1 Sample Menu for Pregnant Women

Breakfast

Orange juice	½ cup
Whole-grain toast	1 slice
Banana	½ medium
Oatmeal	1 cup
Skim milk[b]	1 cup

Midmorning Snack[a]

Some examples are as follows:

- Cereal (ready to eat, ¾ cup) with skim milk (½ cup)
- Fresh or frozen berries (½ cup) with nonfat yogurt (½ cup)
- Apple/pear with cheese (1 oz) or peanut butter (1 tbsp)
- Fruit and yogurt shake
- Open-face peanut butter and apple sandwich

Lunch

Roast beef (2 oz lean) sandwich on whole-grain bread with lettuce and tomato

Green salad	1–1½ cups leafy greens, 1 tbsp balsamic vinegar dressing
Orange wedges	1 cup
Skim milk[b]	1 cup

Midafternoon Snack[a]

See list at Midmorning Snack.

Dinner

Sesame chicken (or fish)	4 oz
Broccoli	1½ cups
Sweet potato	1 medium
Mixed salad (carrots, tomato, 1½ cups spinach, romaine lettuce)	
Olive oil	2 tsp
Fresh lime juice or vinegar	2 tsp
Whole-grain bread	1 slice
Butter	1 tsp
Fresh fruit salad	½ cup
Skim milk	1 cup

Snack (Evening if Needed)[a]

See list at Midmorning Snack.

[a]Snacks are all interchangeable.

[b]Assumes water is consumed throughout the day as a beverage in addition to skim milk.

Protein

The recommended dietary allowance (RDA) for protein during pregnancy is 71 g/day for adolescent and adult women. Women can easily obtain this amount in the American diet; the use of special protein powder supplements is not recommended. Pregnant patients may be counseled to include appropriate sources of protein that provide vitamins, minerals, and moderate amounts of fat. Clients from low-income populations may need counseling or other assistance to ensure that their protein intake is sufficient; these clients may qualify for food vouchers through the Special Supplemental Nutrition Program for Women, Infants, and Children (WIC) of the U.S. Department of Agriculture (USDA) (see the *Social Issues* box Providing the Essentials).

SOCIAL ISSUES

Providing the Essentials

Nutrient-dense foods are the foundations for healthy expectant mothers and their offspring. Women at low socioeconomic levels may have difficulty affording these essentials. One way to ensure adequate nutrition is through a federal government program, such as the U.S. Department of Agriculture's Special Supplemental Nutrition Program for Women, Infants, and Children (WIC). More than 14.1 million women, infants, and children receive the benefits of WIC.

The WIC program began in 1974 and currently operates through approved clinics in all 50 states. Eligible participants must live in an area served by WIC, meet federal income guidelines (income no greater than 185% of U.S. poverty level), and have a nutritional risk factor such as anemia, poor weight gain during pregnancy, previous low-birth-weight infant, or inadequate diet. Pregnant and postpartum women (up to 12 months' postpartum if breastfeeding, 6 months if not) are eligible to participate, as well as infants and children up to 5 years of age.

WIC provides foods, including fresh fruits and vegetables high in protein, vitamin C, vitamin A, iron, and calcium—nutrients having been found to be lacking in this population. States issue either electronic benefit cards, paper checks or vouchers to participants to use at supermarkets, food convenience stores and other stores registered with the WIC program. Participants are also offered nutrition education or nutrition counseling, receive testing for anemia and routine anthropometric monitoring, and obtain referrals to other health care resources.

Community health care nurses can refer clients to local WIC programs for assistance. Contacting the city, county, or state health department can identify the closest WIC clinic.

(Data from U.S. Department of Agriculture (USDA) Food and Nutrition Service: WIC 2017 Eligibility and Coverage Rates, 2020. From: www.fns.usda.gov/wic-2017-eligibility-and-coverage-rates#:~:text=In%202017%2C%20an%20estimated%2014.1,WIC)%20in%20a%20given%20month. Accessed 1 January, 2021.)

The increase in protein intake over the nonpregnant state is necessary to build and maintain the variety of new tissues of pregnancy. A woman experiencing nausea and vomiting in the first trimester of pregnancy may find it difficult to increase sources of protein in her diet, particularly if meats (which have a strong cooking odor) aggravate the nausea. If this is the case, she should consume small amounts of high-quality protein as tolerated.

Vitamin and Mineral Supplementation

The DRIs are increased during pregnancy for most vitamins and minerals. Vitamins of concern are vitamins A and D. Although the RDA for vitamin A is 750 to 770 μg RAE (retinol activity equivalents) preformed vitamin A, the Tolerable Upper Intake Level (UL) is set at 2800 to 3000 μg RAE of preformed vitamin A per day because of the potential for birth defects from excessive intake (National Research Council [NRC], 2006). Similarly, excessive vitamin D during pregnancy may cause birth defects, so that the RDA (5 μg/day) and UL (50 μg/day) are the same for women regardless of physiologic state (NRC, 2006). Micronutrient needs may be met through a balanced diet, with a few notable exceptions, including folate and iron. All supplementation during pregnancy should be in the form of prenatal-type multivitamin-mineral supplements as recommended by primary health care providers or dietitians.

Folate. Substantial research has demonstrated that folate is important for the prevention of neural tube defects (NTDs) such as spina bifida and anencephaly, one of the most common congenital malformations in the United States. Approximately 2500 to 3000 infants are born with NTDs each year in this country, with an equal number likely lost to pregnancy termination and additional unknown numbers of spontaneous abortions. The U.S. Public Health Service and the American Academy of Pediatrics (AAP) now recommend that all women of childbearing age who are capable of becoming pregnant receive a daily intake of 400 μg of synthetic folic acid (from vitamin supplements, fortified grains, and other foods). Although fortification has been implemented, education continues to be needed to encourage awareness of folic acid intake by women of childbearing age. During pregnancy, the DRI increases to 600 μg dietary folate equivalents (DFE) per day (NRC, 2006).

Iron. The RDA for iron during pregnancy is 27 mg/day. This level may be difficult to achieve with a normal diet that maintains recommended fat and kcal guidelines. Therefore, all women should take a supplement with 30 mg ferrous iron daily beginning in the second trimester to prevent iron-deficiency anemia in pregnancy (Turner, 2014).

Iron-deficiency anemia is one of the most common complications of pregnancy. The iron requirement increases secondary to the expansion of the maternal red cell volume. Iron-deficiency anemia can impair oxygen delivery to the fetus, which may have severe consequences. In addition, during the last trimester, the fetus stores iron in its liver to use during the first 4 months of life.

As discussed in Chapter 8, an unusual behavior associated with iron deficiency is pica. Pica is characterized by a hunger and appetite for nonfood substances, including ice, cornstarch, clay, and even dirt. These substances contain no iron, and their ingestion may lead to loss of additional minerals, particularly when clay and dirt are consumed. Intestinal blockages caused by consumption of these substances may be life threatening. Of particular concern is the practice of pica during pregnancy, when the risk and implications of iron-deficiency anemia are most severe. Although more common among Black American women, pica has been diagnosed among all ethnic groups within all socioeconomic levels. A challenge to obstetric nurses is to elicit information about this type of dietary behavior when assessing clients.

Calcium. The RDA for calcium is 1000 mg/day for women and 1300 mg/day for adolescents, neither of which is an increase over the nonpregnant state. Although calcium needs are great during pregnancy, particularly for mineralization of the fetal skeleton, changes occur in maternal calcium homeostasis, which result in an increase in intestinal calcium absorption. Many women, particularly adolescents, may not consume the

BOX 10.2 Pregnancy in Special Needs Populations

Special considerations are needed during pregnancy for the following groups:
- Adolescents
- Vegetarians
- Women aged >35 years
- Women who are underweight
- Women who are overweight
- Women with phenylketonuria
- Women with multiple pregnancies
- Women who smoke or use drugs or alcohol
- Women with concurrent medical problems

RDA for calcium before pregnancy. Women who are unable to consume rich sources of calcium may need to seek advice from a dietitian/nutrition specialist to determine whether supplements are necessary.

Nutrition-Related Concerns

Some pregnant women require particular attention through the course of pregnancy because of exposure to potential nonnutritive substances that may act as teratogens, problematic lifestyle behaviors, or development of medical conditions unique to pregnancy. Box 10.2 lists special needs populations of pregnant women.

Other concerns affecting the course and outcome of pregnancy are maternal age and medical conditions requiring nutrition intervention, such as hypertension, diabetes, phenylketonuria (PKU), and human immunodeficiency virus (HIV) infection.

Alcohol

The use of alcohol during pregnancy may produce fetal alcohol syndrome (FAS) or fetal alcohol spectrum disorder (FASD) in the infant. Symptoms include central nervous system defects and specific anatomic defects such as a low nasal bridge, short nose, flat midface, and short palpebral fissures (separation between the upper and lower eyelids) (Fig. 10.2).

There is no safe level of alcohol intake during pregnancy. FAS is not confined to heavy drinkers; anyone who uses alcohol during pregnancy puts her infant at risk of this preventable syndrome. Therefore, all pregnant women should be urged to cease consumption of all alcoholic beverages. Because alcohol use by pregnant women has been increasing, health care providers should screen women for alcohol use and counsel clients appropriately.

Foodborne Illness

Foodborne illness is a concern during pregnancy. Pathogens such as *Listeria monocytogenes*, *Salmonella* species, and *Toxoplasma gondii* are high risks for a pregnant woman and her fetus. In addition, commonly consumed foods may contain pathogens, not usually viewed as high risk, that can be problematic during pregnancy. Food safety strategies take on greater importance when a woman's body has reduced immunity or protections against pathogens. Box 10.3 highlights these concerns.

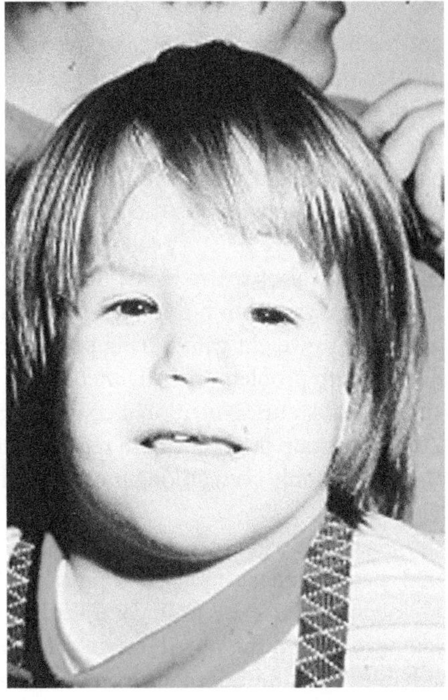

Fig. 10.2 A young child with fetal alcohol syndrome features. (From Streissguth AP, et al: Teratogenic effects of alcohol in humans and laboratory animals, *Science* 209(4454):353–361, 1980.)

BOX 10.3 Food Safety Risks for Pregnant Women and Newborns

During pregnancy, women and their unborn children are more likely to become very ill from food poisoning. Newborns and infants also are at risk because their immune systems are not fully developed. Infections from foodborne illness can be difficult to treat and can recur in these groups.

In addition to keeping good food-safety habits, there are certain foods that pregnant women should not eat, including the following:
- Rare, raw, or undercooked meats and poultry (rare hamburgers, carpaccio, and beef or steak tartare)
- Raw fish (including sushi, sashimi, ceviche, and carpaccio)
- Undercooked and raw shellfish (clams, oysters, mussels, and scallops)
- Fish containing high levels of mercury (swordfish, tilefish, king mackerel, and shark)
- Refrigerated smoked seafood
- Unpasteurized dairy products ("raw" milk and cheeses)
- Some fresh soft cheeses (Brie, Camembert, blue-veined varieties, and Mexican-style queso fresco) unless made with pasteurized milk
- Raw or undercooked eggs (soft-cooked, runny, or poached)
- Food items that contain undercooked eggs (unpasteurized eggnog, Monte Cristo sandwiches, French toast, homemade Caesar salad dressing, Hollandaise sauce, mayonnaise, some puddings and custards, chocolate mousse, tiramisu, and raw cookie dough or cake batter)
- Raw sprouts (alfalfa, clover, and radish)
- Deli salads
- Unpasteurized fruit and vegetable juices
- Refrigerated pâté or meat spreads

Some ready-to-eat foods require reheating before use. They include hot dogs, luncheon and deli meats, and fermented and dry sausages. Packaged items should be thrown away once their "use-by" dates have passed. If you think you have contracted a foodborne illness, contact your health care provider immediately.

(Modified from the Academy of Nutrition and Dietetics: Foodborne Illness and High-Risk Food, 2021. Accessed 12 July, 2021, from: www.eatright.org/homefoodsafety/safety-tips/food-poisoning/foodborne-illness-and-high-risk-foods.)

Maternal Age

Adolescents and women older than 35 years are at higher risk for poor pregnancy outcome. In any assessment of the nutritional status of the pregnant teen, there are several important factors to consider. These include the growth pattern of the mother, the psychologic maturity of the mother, possible lack of economic resources to provide for the infant, and potential delay in seeking medical care. Dietary factors to assess are the poor dietary habits typical of many teens, the frequency with which meals are eaten away from home each day, and the possible preoccupation with weight gain during pregnancy. This is still a major public health problem in the United States, affecting medical and nutritional status. Nutritional counseling targeted specifically to this age group is beneficial in reducing the risk of adverse outcomes commonly seen among pregnant adolescents (Wise, 2015) (Fig. 10.3).

Women who become pregnant after age 35 years have distinct nutritional needs, reflecting their longer medical history, potential long-term use of oral contraceptives (which may affect folate levels), and the possibility of a longer history of poor eating habits. In addition, older women are at risk for nutrition-related complications such as gestational diabetes. Careful nutritional evaluation of these patients can be useful in providing guidance to reduce the risk of nutritional imbalances that cause pregnancy complications.

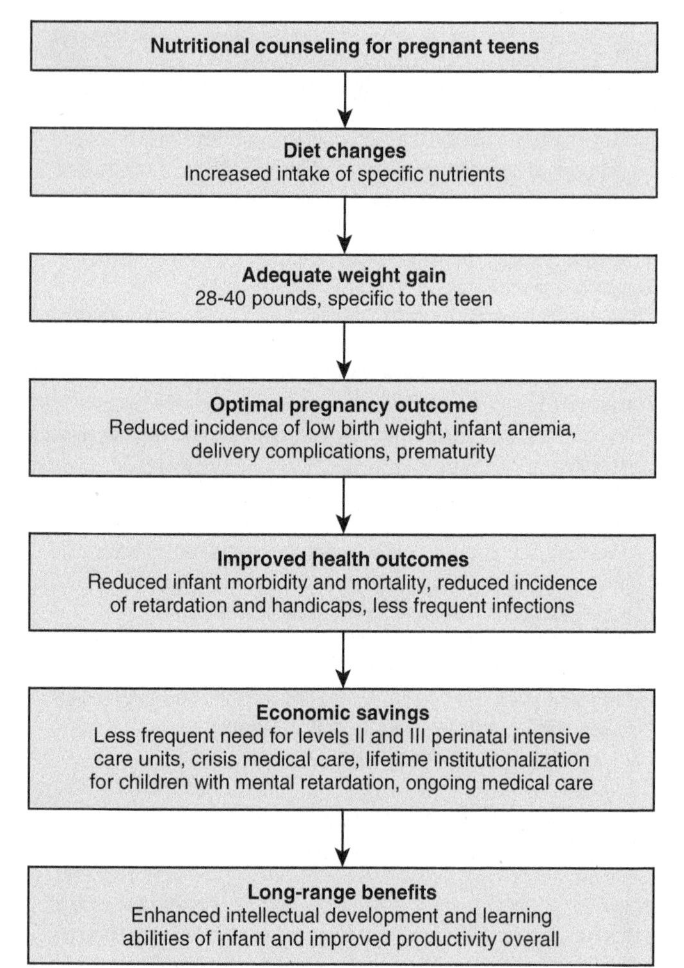

Fig. 10.3 Nutrition counseling during teen pregnancy. (From Mahan KL, Escott-Stump S: *Krause's food & nutrition therapy,* ed 12, Philadelphia, 2008, Saunders.)

Preeclampsia

Preeclampsia, also known as pregnancy-induced hypertension, is considered hypertension with proteinuria (excess protein in urine) after 20 weeks' gestation (Turner, 2014). Clinically, the mother experiences a sudden and severe rise in arterial blood pressure, rapid weight gain, and marked edema, often necessitating immediate delivery of the fetus to save the lives of both mother and infant.

Preeclampsia may occur in as many as 3% to 5% of pregnancies and is one of the leading causes of prematurity and maternal and fetal death. Risk factors for and symptoms of preeclampsia are listed in Box 10.4.

Preeclampsia may progress to eclampsia. This disorder may result in seizures that can be fatal to the mother and the infant. The cause of eclampsia is unknown, and no screening test is available for it (Turner, 2014).

BOX 10.4 Risk Factors for and Symptoms of Preeclampsia

Risk Factors

- First pregnancies
- Diabetes mellitus (type 1, type 2)
- Hypertension (for at least 4 years)
- Advanced maternal age
- African American heritage
- Multiple pregnancies
- Renal disease
- Age at conception:
  - 19 years or younger
  - 40 years or older
- Preeclampsia in earlier pregnancies:
  - Family history of mother or sister having preeclampsia
  - Family history of hypertension, vascular disease
  - Being researched: Inflammatory response, insulin resistance, and oxidative stress

Symptoms

- Headaches (continuous and severe)
- Hypertension (change from usual level)
- Edema of hands and face
- Sudden weight gain
- Excessive nausea and vomiting
- Vomiting blood
- Smaller amounts of urine or no urine
- Blood in urine
- Rapid heartbeat
- Dizziness and blurred or double vision
- Sudden blindness
- Ringing or buzzing sound in ears
- Drowsiness
- Fever
- Pain in the abdomen
- Slowed fetal growth
- Protein in urine (proteinuria)

Nutritional support during preeclampsia includes provision of a well-balanced diet with generous sources of protein to replace losses in proteinuria and with adequate vitamins and minerals. It should supply a sufficient amount of energy. Energy intake should not be limited in an attempt to restrict maternal weight gain.

Currently, low vitamin D status is being studied as an associative factor of preeclampsia. Lower levels have been reported in women with preeclampsia, particularly dark-skinned women from northern latitudes whose levels are lower than those of White women in the same area. Nonetheless, any women with preeclampsia may be experiencing hypovitaminosis D, and testing should be conducted. For those with low levels, dietary changes and/or supplementation may be appropriate (Erick, 2012).

Diabetes Mellitus

Women with preexisting diabetes mellitus (DM) (type 1 and type 2) require specialized care during pregnancy. Pregnancy significantly affects insulin requirements. Control of glucose levels and avoidance of ketosis by adjustment of nutrient intake and insulin dosage lend support for healthy birth outcomes. There is an increased risk of birth defects, especially of the heart and central nervous system (Turner, 2014). Other complications include macrosomia (larger body size), hypoglycemia, erythremia (abnormal increase of red blood cells), and hyperbilirubinemia. Hyperbilirubinemia is a neonatal condition in which excessively high levels of bilirubin (red bile pigment) lead to jaundice, in which bile is deposited in tissues throughout the body.

These infants may experience hypoglycemia after birth. The maternal source of glucose is no longer available, and because glucose readily crosses the placenta, levels of glucose in utero tend to be high, especially if the diabetes has been poorly controlled. Infants born to mothers with diabetes require immediate monitoring in the neonatal intensive care unit (NICU).

Fortunately, there may be a decreased prevalence of many of the maternal and fetal complications associated with DM when normal blood glucose level (normoglycemia) is achieved before conception and maintained throughout pregnancy. The current recommendation is for women to achieve tight glucose control before conception to maximize the likelihood of a healthy mother and infant while avoiding perinatal risks. Control involves prudent blood glucose monitoring, adherence to diet, moderate exercise, and strict adherence to the prescribed insulin regimen. Total energy intake and energy distribution will likely need modification during pregnancy because of the increased energy needs of pregnancy. Insulin dosages will require adjustment because many of the hormones of pregnancy, such as estrogen, progesterone, human chorionic gonadotropin (HCG), somatotropin, and maternal cortisol, act in an antagonistic fashion with insulin. All women with diabetes should discuss drug treatment options with their physicians before conception.

Gestational diabetes mellitus (GDM) is a form of diabetes occurring during pregnancy, most commonly after the twentieth week of gestation. Pregnancy affects glucose control and insulin needs. For nondiabetic women, insulin sensitivity is decreased by placental and ovarian hormones. In response, more insulin is secreted to ensure appropriate glucose levels. The pancreatic reserves of approximately 5% to 10% of women are unable to compensate and do not secrete adequate insulin, and gestational diabetes develops. Patients experience abnormal carbohydrate metabolism, much like other persons with diabetes. Of all forms of diabetes during pregnancy, GDM is the most common, affecting 4% of all pregnancies (Turner, 2014). All women should undergo screening for GDM during the second trimester, with repeat testing for women whose results are borderline.

Treatment of GDM consists primarily of dietary control combined with moderate exercise leading to an appropriate weight gain. Insulin may be required if glycemic control is not achieved through dietary control and exercise. Risk factors for GDM include delivery of a previous large infant, prepregnancy weight, family history of diabetes, ethnicity, a prior perinatal death, glycosuria, and maternal age greater than 30 years (Box 10.5). The majority of women with GDM have normal glucose tolerance after delivery, but they may remain at risk for T2D mellitus (T2DM) later in life.

BOX 10.5 Risk Factors for and Symptoms of Gestational Diabetes Mellitus

Risk Factors

- Obesity
- Advanced maternal age
- African or Hispanic heritage
- Recurrent infections
- Gestational diabetes in previous pregnancy
- In a previous pregnancy, child having a congenital malformation or birth defect and/or unexplained death of fetus or newborn
- Previous newborn weighing more than 9 pounds

Symptoms

Often there are no symptoms, but the following may occur:

- Increased thirst
- Increased urination
- Weight loss with increased appetite
- Fatigue
- Blurred vision
- Frequent infections, including those of the bladder, vagina, and skin
- Nausea and vomiting

Maternal Phenylketonuria

PKU is an inborn error of metabolism characterized by extremely low levels of the enzyme phenylalanine hydroxylase, which catalyzes the conversion of phenylalanine to tyrosine. Absence of this crucial enzyme causes a failure in the metabolism of the amino acid phenylalanine and low levels of tyrosine. Successful treatment of this disorder occurs through adherence to a strict diet low in phenylalanine and supplemented with tyrosine, beginning in the first week of life. Failure to detect the disease or a lack of compliance with the dietary therapy results in irreversible mental retardation.

Forty years ago most patients with PKU did not conceive and bear children. Most likely, they were disabled before they were diagnosed or able to properly adjust their diets. However, with the advent of neonatal PKU testing in all 50 states, diagnosis and treatment of the disorder allow many young women to lead normal, productive lives, including having children. Women with PKU require specialized nutrition care during pregnancy. Maternal PKU, particularly if not well controlled at the time of conception, poses a great risk to the unborn offspring. Mothers with untreated PKU have a high likelihood of experiencing spontaneous abortion or having an infant born with microcephaly, mental retardation, congenital heart defects, or intrauterine growth retardation, even if the infant does not have the genetic defect. Conscientious adherence to a low-phenylalanine diet may lessen, but not completely eliminate, the risk of an adverse pregnancy outcome (Elsas & Acosta, 2014). Total nutrient intake and maternal weight gain should be monitored throughout pregnancy.

All young women with PKU should continue their low-phenylalanine diets throughout the childbearing years. Family planning is strongly encouraged to establish safe phenylalanine levels before conception and to educate women regarding the high risk of poor pregnancy outcome, even with good dietary control.

Human Immunodeficiency Virus Infection

In the United States, most of the female cases of HIV infection are among women of childbearing age. Pregnancy may put an additional strain on the already fragile immune system of a woman with HIV, because the hormones and proteins of pregnancy (including estrogen, progesterone, HCG, alpha fetoprotein, corticosteroids, prolactin, and α-globulin) have immunosuppressive effects.

The HIV-infected woman experiencing an opportunistic infection during pregnancy has increased needs for kcal, protein, vitamins, and minerals. Weight gain must be strictly monitored, although there are no specialized weight gain recommendations for this population. Other issues pertaining to HIV are presented in Chapter 20.

Common Nutrition-Related Discomforts of Pregnancy

The following sections discuss the common discomforts of pregnancy and methods of relief.

Nausea and vomiting. Nausea and vomiting, often referred to as "morning sickness," during the first trimester of pregnancy can be annoying, but they generally begin to subside by the beginning of the second trimester. Symptoms of morning sickness may actually occur at any time throughout the day, although vomiting tends to be more common between 6 AM and noon. Although the etiology of nausea and vomiting during pregnancy is unknown, it may be caused by hormonal factors such as a rise in estrogen or the placental hormone HCG. Stress or fatigue may exacerbate the condition. There is no cause for alarm unless the mother begins to lose weight or becomes severely dehydrated. If she cannot retain either foods or fluid for 6 hours or longer, a physician should be contacted.

If nausea or vomiting persists into the second trimester or severely interferes with the mother's life, it may be a more serious condition. Hyperemesis gravidarum is severe and unrelenting vomiting and usually requires intravenous replacement of nutrients and fluids. If the mother receives total parenteral nutrition or nasogastric tube feedings for the treatment of hyperemesis gravidarum, appropriate levels of vitamins and minerals should be included, with careful monitoring and follow-up.

There are no specific foods to avoid, but many women find it is helpful to eat small, frequent meals, to drink liquids between rather than with meals, and to avoid fried and greasy foods. Some women find it helpful to reduce coffee intake and to prepare meals near an open window to avoid cooking odors. If nausea upon getting out of bed in the morning is a problem, dry toast or crackers eaten before getting out of bed may provide relief. Snacks to keep handy while working or traveling include dried fruit, crackers, and small cans of juice.

Heartburn. In late pregnancy, when the fetus rapidly grows in size, the uterus pushes up against the stomach, possibly causing a feeling of fullness in the mother. Additionally, because of the action of progesterone (which can cause relaxation of smooth muscles), a relaxation of the gastroesophageal sphincter may occur, resulting in some reflux of gastric contents into the lower esophagus. This is the cause of the heartburn so common during the final weeks of pregnancy. The best dietary remedies are eating small, frequent meals, avoiding foods high in fat, drinking fluids between rather than with meals, limiting spicy foods, and avoiding lying down for 1 to 2 hours after eating. Many women find relief by wearing clothing that is loose-fitting around the abdomen. Expectant mothers should not take antacids without approval of a primary care provider. Heartburn generally disappears after delivery of the infant.

Constipation. Constipation is common during the first and third trimesters of pregnancy. During the first trimester, progesterone (which slows GI motility) may be responsible. In the third trimester, the growing fetus crowds the other internal organs, again possibly slowing GI motility. Although bothersome, constipation responds well to dietary treatment. A generous intake of fiber, such as whole-grain cereals, fresh fruit, and raw vegetables, as well as inclusion of plenty of fluids should alleviate constipation. Moderate exercise such as a daily walk may also help. The recommendations for alleviating constipation also help prevent hemorrhoids. Over-the-counter laxatives or enemas should not be used by a pregnant woman unless prescribed by a physician.

NUTRITION DURING LACTATION

All sexually mature female mammals possess milk-producing mammary glands and are able to produce milk specifically formulated to provide optimum growth and development for their offspring. Although there are historical accounts of wet nurses and even artificial feeding implements dating back to Greek and Roman times, breastfeeding (lactation) was the primary mode of infant feeding until the previous century in the United States and around the world.

Since World War II there has been a dramatic decline in the incidence and duration of breastfeeding worldwide. Currently 80% of mothers in the United States initiate breastfeeding at hospital discharge, but by 6 months after birth, only about 22% of American infants are breastfed (Patnode et al., 2016). In many developed countries, such as Sweden, all women initiate breastfeeding and continue for most of the infant's first year of life. Although there is not one isolated cause for lower breastfeeding rates in the United States, it can be attributed to a multitude of causes. These include the advertising of breast milk substitutes, lack of support for the breastfeeding mother, lack of health care

BOX 10.6 Benefits of Breastfeeding

- Provides immunologic protection to the infant against many infections and diseases (especially respiratory and gastrointestinal)
- Offers uniquely suited nutrient composition with high bioavailability
- Reduces risk of food allergy in the infant
- Promotes infant oral motor development
- Offers convenience: always fresh, available, and at the right temperature
- Is generally less expensive than formula feeding
- May protect infant against some chronic diseases such as T1D and childhood leukemia
- Promotes mother-infant bonding
- Facilitates uterine contractions and controls postpartum bleeding
- Promotes return to prepregnancy weight

professional knowledge about lactation, short postpartum hospital stays, and the rise in maternal employment without appropriate facilities to nurse infants or pump and store breast milk (Lessen & Kavanagh, 2015).

The Academy of Nutrition and Dietetics and the American Academy of Pediatrics have policy statements advocating exclusive use of human milk as the preferred feeding choice for infants for at least the first 6 months of life (AAP, 2012; Lessen & Kavanagh, 2015). Ideally, breastfeeding should occur for the entire first 12 months, accompanied by appropriate weaning foods. Although primary nourishment is provided by breast milk for the first 6 months, introduction of complementary foods may first occur from 4 to 8 months of age, depending on individual feeding behaviors and needs. Breastfeeding offers advantages for both infant and mother (Box 10.6).

Anatomy and Physiology of Lactation

The human breast begins development in utero and goes through two further stages of change after birth: at puberty and during pregnancy. The mature human breast consists of a system of alveoli and ducts. Myoepithelial cells surround the milk-producing glands, located in the alveoli. The ductules emerge from the alveoli to carry the milk to the lactiferous ducts, which eventually empty into the lactiferous sinuses. The lactiferous sinuses are located behind the areola, or the darkened area of the nipple where the infant latches on during nursing (Fig. 10.4).

Throughout the course of pregnancy, the breast tissue undergoes considerable development. Under the influence of progesterone, the lobules or alveoli increase in size and number, and estrogen stimulates proliferation of the ductal system. Together these changes render the breast completely capable of milk production after delivery. An uncommon occurrence is a failure of the breasts to undergo development during pregnancy. A woman who does not notice any changes in her breasts during pregnancy, particularly if she is pregnant for the first time, should receive postnatal assistance to determine her ability to fully lactate. Most women are able to fully lactate with no problems. Actual size of breast has no bearing on the ability to breastfeed.

Lactation is a normal process beginning when various hormones interact after delivery of the infant. Before the onset of labor, there is a rise in serum levels of oxytocin. This hormone is instrumental in initiating the uterine contractions of labor that bring about birth. Oxytocin and another hormone, prolactin, set off the lactation process. Prolactin is primarily responsible for milk synthesis; oxytocin is involved with milk ejection from the breast.

When an infant is allowed to suckle after birth, a nerve impulse is sent to the mother's hypothalamus. This stimulates the anterior pituitary to secrete prolactin, which then stimulates milk production in the alveolar cells (Fig. 10.5). The infant sucking stimulus initiates the release of oxytocin from the posterior pituitary. The flood of oxytocin into the breast tissue causes the myoepithelial

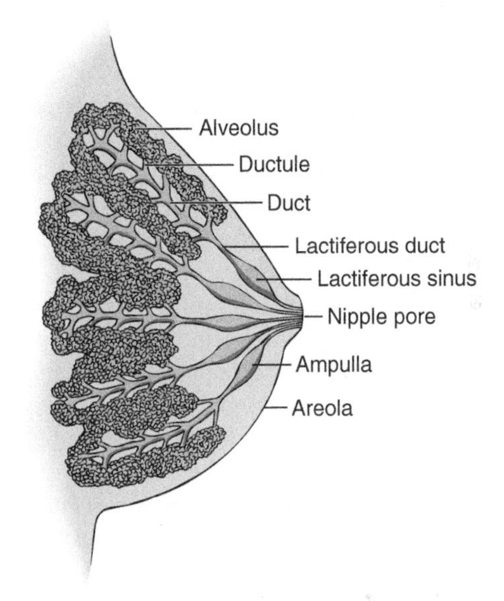

Fig. 10.4 Detailed structural features of the human mammary gland. (From Rolin Graphics.)

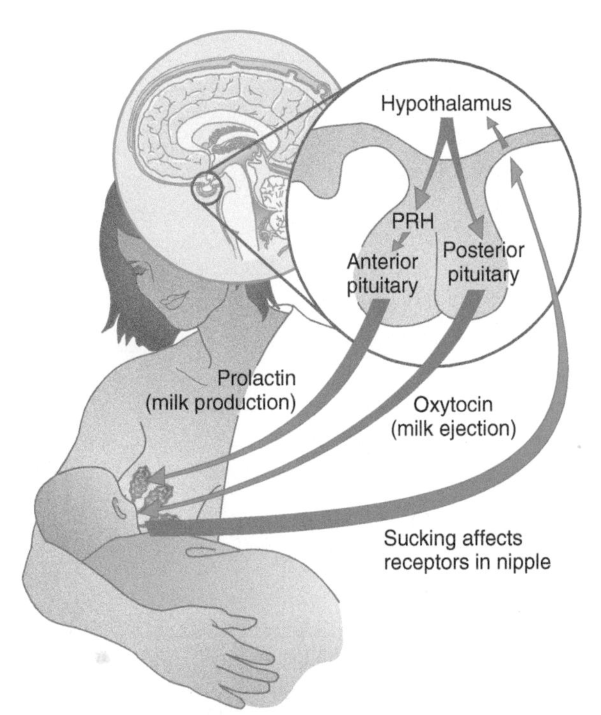

Fig. 10.5 Maternal breastfeeding reflexes. (From Mahan KL, Escott-Stump S: *Krause's food & nutrition therapy*, ed 12, Philadelphia, 2008, Saunders.)

cells around the glands to contract, thereby ejecting the milk into the infant's mouth. This is called the let-down reflex, or the milk-ejection reflex. Many women report feeling a tingling sensation in their breasts when the let-down occurs. Additionally, if a mother hears her infant's cry or sees another infant, she may experience a let-down accompanied by a rush of milk ejecting from her breasts. Deterrents to the let-down reflex include fatigue, stress, alcohol, smoking, and some prescription medications.

An important point to note is that milk production is a supply-and-demand mechanism. The more an infant is allowed to nurse, the more nerve stimulation there will be, resulting in a rise in prolactin levels followed by increased milk production. No restrictions should be placed on the number of times an infant, particularly a newborn, nurses per day (Lesson & Kavanagh, 2015).

Of particular value is colostrum, the fluid secreted from the breast during late pregnancy and the first few days postpartum. When consumed by a newborn, colostrum provides immunologically active substances (maternal antibodies) and essential nutrients.

Promoting Breastfeeding

To increase the incidence and duration of breastfeeding in the United States and around the world, health care professionals can take measures ensuring that appropriate breastfeeding policies are adopted and practiced in hospitals providing maternity care. In 1991, the World Health Organization and UNICEF (United Nations International Children's Emergency Fund) launched the Baby Friendly Hospital Initiative (Ebrahim, 1993). The initiative includes "Ten Steps to Successful Breastfeeding" that the hospital must be willing to take to become infant friendly. Among the steps is breastfeeding education for all mothers, no separation of mother and infant following birth, except for medical reasons, and no supplemental feedings unless medically indicated. Nurses play a key role in prenatal counseling and in postpartum support to help mothers successfully establish and maintain lactation. Obstetric nurses should consult a lactation specialist if an infant or mother has difficulties initiating breastfeeding.

Another influence on successful lactation is acceptability of lactation within the cultural and ethnic communities of which the mother is a part. Cultures in which breastfeeding is common are Chinese, Finnish, Indian, Saudi Arabian, Muslim, South African, and Swedish. In the following cultures, breastfeeding is common, but infants are not given colostrum because it is considered bad or unclean: Cambodian, Filipino, Haitian, Japanese, Korean, Laotian, Mexican, and Vietnamese. Socioeconomic and education levels are influences that help or hinder a mother's attempt at lactation. Organizations such as the La Leche League and community-based mothers' groups may provide invaluable support to nursing mothers, particularly those nursing for the first time.

Energy and Nutrient Needs During Lactation

A large proportion of the energy stores laid down as adipose tissue during pregnancy are mobilized in lactation. Both BMR and maternal activity return to their prepregnant levels. The energy cost of milk production is approximately 500 to 800 kcal/day, depending on the volume of milk production. The RDA recommends increases for protein (71 g/day) and for most of the vitamins and minerals over the normal adult levels. The mother can meet most of these increases by consuming a well-balanced diet (see Table 10.2).

TABLE 10.2 Dietary Reference Intakes to Meet Needs of Pregnancy and Lactation

	Adult Women 19–50 Years of Age	Pregnant Women Third Trimester	Lactating Mothers[a]
Energy (kcal)	2200	2652	2530
Protein (g)	46	71	71
Vitamin A (retinol equivalent, μg)	700	770	1300
Vitamin D (μg)[†]	15	15	15
Vitamin E (alpha-tocopherol equivalent, mg)	15	15	19
Vitamin C (mg)	75	85	120
Thiamin (mg)	1.1	1.4	1.4
Riboflavin (mg)	1.1	1.4	1.6
Niacin (niacin equivalent, mg)	14	18	17
Vitamin B_6 (mg)	1.3	1.9	2
Folate (μg)	400	600	500
Vitamin B_{12} (μg)	2.4	2.6	2.8
Calcium (mg)[b]	1000	1000	1000
Phosphorus (mg)	700	700	700
Iron (mg)[c]	18	27	9
Zinc (mg)	8	11	12
Iodine (μg)	150	220	290
Selenium (μg)	55	65	75

[a]During the first 6 months of lactation.
[b]Adequate intake.
[c]The increased iron requirement for pregnancy cannot be met by the usual American diet or from body stores; thus a supplement of 30 to 60 mg of elemental iron is recommended.
Data from Institute of Medicine, Food and Nutrition Board: *Dietary DRI references: The essential guide to nutrient requirements*, Washington, DC, 2006, The National Academies Press.

A woman need not avoid certain foods while breastfeeding unless a problem occurs. For example, some infants are fussy after the mother's consumption of gas-producing vegetables such as cabbage, onions, and broccoli.

Adequate fluid intake is important during lactation. The average woman produces 750 to 1000 mL of milk per day. She can replace this fluid through consumption of water or juice. Coffee or cola drinks should be avoided or used on a minimal basis. They may act as diuretics in the mother's body, and caffeine, a stimulant, passes into breast milk in small amounts. The old myth stating that alcohol helps a mother relax and enhances milk production should not be followed. Alcohol not only passes into milk, thus becoming available to the infant, but also may inhibit oxytocin, consequently reducing the let-down reflex.

Despite the desire of most women to return to their prepregnancy weight quickly, rapid weight loss should not be encouraged during breastfeeding; reduction in milk production may result. Research indicates that women may achieve weight loss without compromising their nutritional intake or the infant's if they breastfeed without the use of supplementary formula for at least 6 months. Sufficient milk may be provided with a modest caloric reduction for healthy lactating women with a 1-lb per week loss. An energy intake of at least 1800 kcal/day should be maintained for adequate lactation regardless of maternal fat stores (Erick, 2012).

Nutrition-Related Concerns

Common colds, the flu, and even most illnesses requiring short-term antibiotic therapy do not require cessation of breastfeeding. A number of maternal illnesses or conditions, however, are contraindications to breastfeeding:

- Active tuberculosis
- Human immunodeficiency virus/acquired immunodeficiency syndrome (HIV/AIDS)
- Herpes simplex lesions on the maternal breast
- Maternal alcoholism
- Maternal drug addiction
- Malaria
- Maternal chickenpox (first 3 weeks postpartum only)
- Maternal breast cancer requiring treatment
- Maternal hepatitis C

Most medications for mild illnesses are safe for the mother to take while breastfeeding. If the need for a medication arises, the mother should always remind her health care provider that she is nursing an infant. The American Academy of Pediatrics has classified medications into five categories based on safety considerations. For mild illnesses, as well as for chronic diseases, a medication compatible with breastfeeding can usually be found and substituted for one that is contraindicated. The amount of the maternal dose of drug actually secreted into the milk depends on the route of administration, the size of the molecule, ionization, the pH of the medication, solubility, and protein binding (AAP, 2012). Health care providers might keep this information in mind as they consider prescription medications for nursing mothers.

The Centers for Disease Control and Prevention (CDC) and the Academy of Pediatrics recommend that all women in the United States infected with HIV not breastfeed their infants (CDC, 2020). In contrast, the World Health Organization (WHO) advises that HIV positive mothers who are exclusively breastfeeding while adhering to antiretroviral treatment by breastfeeding their babies greatly reducing the risk of transmitting HIV to their babies while providing high quality nutrition. In some parts of the world, the cost and availability of infant formula and safe drinking water supplies for bottle feeding may be beyond the reach of many mothers. Therefore, WHO recommends exclusive breastfeeding for the first six months, then continue breastfeeding for 12 months with the addition of complementary foods (CDC, 2020; WHO, 2010).

Because of the advent of hepatitis B vaccinations given at birth, hepatitis B is no longer a contraindication to breastfeeding. However, there is mother-to-infant transmission of hepatitis C, and therefore mothers with hepatitis C should not breastfeed.

NUTRITION DURING INFANCY

Energy and Nutrient Needs During Infancy

Dramatic changes in growth and development occur during the first 12 months of life. In the first year, a human infant is expected to triple their birth weight and increase length by 50%. In addition, after birth, organs such as the kidney and brain continue to develop and mature. In no other period of life do growth and development occur so rapidly. To support this rapid growth and development, the appropriate balance of all nutrients is essential. At the same time, parents, caregivers, and health care professionals must realize that infants have specialized nutrient needs. Advice that is appropriate for adults, and even older children, is inappropriate for infants, particularly with regard to fat and fiber intake and weight-gain patterns.

Energy

Adequate energy intake will be reflected in satisfactory gains in length and weight as plotted on a National Center for Health Statistics growth chart (www.cdc.gov/growthcharts/clinical_charts.htm). Infants' fat intake should not be restricted. Well-meaning parents should not put their infants on low-fat diets. Human milk, in fact, is high in cholesterol and fat content. Omega-3 fatty acids are plentiful in human milk, particularly if the mother includes fish in her diet on a regular basis. These fatty acids have been found to be essential for proper brain and nervous system development.

Protein

Protein needs of infants have been hard to determine because of the difficulty of performing nitrogen balance studies on this population. Requirements are estimated on the basis of the intake and growth rates of normal, healthy breastfed infants. Protein requirement is highest during the first 4 months of life, when growth is the most rapid. It is suggested that infants receive 9 g/day from birth to 6 months of age and 11 g/day for the second half of the first year. An excess of protein in an infant's diet can be problematic. Protein has a significant influence on renal solute load. The infant kidney is immature and unable to handle the large renal solute loads of an adult's. Therefore, increasing a normal infant's protein intake above the recommended amount should be avoided.

VITAMIN AND MINERAL SUPPLEMENTATION

The DRIs may be consulted for appropriate levels of vitamins and minerals for infants. Breast milk or commercial formula should provide infants with all the vitamins and minerals needed for proper growth and development (Table 10.3).

During the third trimester of pregnancy, the fetus stores iron in its liver to be used during the postnatal period. By 4 months of age, this supply of iron is usually depleted. The iron in breast milk, although lower in absolute amounts, is more bioavailable than iron from commercial formula. Many breastfed infants do not need an iron supplement. However, their iron levels should be assessed periodically. Infants who consume commercial formula should be given the iron-fortified variety to prevent iron-deficiency anemia.

Humans can manufacture vitamin D through exposure to the sun; many young infants may not receive enough sun exposure for adequate synthesis. Breast milk contains vitamin D, but it may not be present in levels sufficient to prevent vitamin D-related rickets. In the United States, there have been several documented cases of vitamin D-related rickets, particularly among fully breastfed infants who receive little or no sunlight exposure. Therefore, it is recommended that all breastfed infants receive a daily oral supplement of vitamin D, unless they receive substantial sunlight exposure. Vitamin D can be toxic, so the recommended dosage should not be exceeded. Because vitamin D is present in commercial infant formula, formula-fed infants need not receive a supplement. Use of milk alternatives such as "milks" made from rice, soybeans, almonds, or coconut have also resulted in rickets. These alternatives, which are low in protein, calcium, and vitamin D, are not nutrient dense compared with breast milk, formula, or cow's milk. Health care providers need to emphasize to caregivers that although the term milk is used in reference to these beverages, they are not nutritionally equal to milk produced by humans or animals.

The water supply of most major cities in the United States contains fluoride as a preventive measure against tooth decay. The availability of fluoride may be particularly important for infants and young children whose teeth are developing. Routine fluoride supplementation is not recommended for infants younger than 6 months. Older infants may need to receive fluoride if their local water supply is not fluoridated, but an assessment of total exposure to fluoride (via water, or juice prepared from local water source) should be made before systemic fluoride is prescribed. For example, many rural families who rely on well water should have their water supplies assessed for fluoride content. Excess fluoride can result in fluorosis, or mottling of tooth enamel, so precise dosing of this mineral is critical.

Newborns are vulnerable to vitamin K deficiency (and thus hemorrhaging) in part because they lack intestinal bacteria to synthesize the vitamin. As a preventive measure, U.S. hospitals routinely give infants 0.5 to 1 mg of vitamin K by injection, or 1 to 2 mg orally, once shortly after birth.

Food for Infants

The ideal food for the first 4 to 6 months of life is exclusive use of breast milk, which has the correct balance of all the essential nutrients as well as immunologic factors that protect the infant from acute and chronic diseases. The breast should be offered at least 10 to 12 times per 24 hours in the first several weeks. As the infant develops a stronger suck, more milk will be extracted with each nursing session, and the frequency of feeding may decline. Although there is no specified time the infant should stay on the breast, between 10 and 15 minutes per breast (offering both breasts per session) is a good recommendation. It is important to realize this is a general guideline because all infants have different nursing styles. It may in fact be more appropriate to watch the infant—not the clock—in an effort to allow the infant to dictate when satiety is reached. The *Teaching Tool* box Guidelines for Successful Breastfeeding offers some suggestions to facilitate breastfeeding.

TEACHING TOOL

Guidelines for Successful Breastfeeding

Although breastfeeding is the most natural and easiest way to feed infants, mothers who decide to breastfeed will welcome the following suggestions:

- Offer both breasts at each nursing session.
- Open infant's mouth wide to latch on correctly.
- Place at least ½ to ¾ inch of the areola in the infant's mouth, not just the nipple.
- Check that the infant's lips make a tight seal around the breast.
- Sore nipples are usually caused by incorrect positioning; position the infant correctly in a tummy-to-tummy fashion or in a "football hold." Support the newborn's head and back with extra pillows on your lap or with your arm cradling infant.
- Do not limit nursing time in the first several days. Doing so does not prevent sore nipples and may hinder milk production.
- Remember that milk is produced by supply and demand—the more often the infant nurses, the more milk produced.
- Expect growth spurts at approximately 10 days, 2 weeks, 6 weeks, and 3 months. At these times, expect a fussy infant who wants to nurse frequently.
- Offer no bottles of formula or water while the milk supply is being established. The artificial nipple may confuse the infant, and substitute feedings that replace breast stimulation may diminish milk production.
- Once milk supply is established, breast milk may be expressed manually or by a pump and saved in a bottle in the refrigerator (up to 48 hours) or in the freezer (several months).
- Learn your infant's cues for satiety.

TABLE 10.3 Recommended Supplementation of Infant Diets

Type of Feeding	Iron	Vitamin D	Fluoride	Vitamin K
Human milk	1 mg/kg/day[a]	10 µg/day	0.25 mg/day	Single intramuscular dose of 0.5 to 1 mg or oral dose of 1 to 2 mg
Formula	Iron-fortified formula	—	0.25 mg/day[b]	Single intramuscular dose of 0.5 to 1 mg or oral dose of 1 to 2 mg

[a]May be provided through iron-containing foods after 6 months of age.
[b]If fluoride content of water is less than 0.3 part per million.
Modified from American Academy of Pediatrics Committee on Nutrition: *Pediatric nutrition*, ed 8, Itasca, IL, 2019, American Academy of Pediatrics.

If a mother chooses not to breastfeed or if she has a medical condition contraindicating breastfeeding, a variety of formulas made from either cow's milk or soy are available. In addition, a number of specialty formulas, such as protein hydrolysate formulas, are available for infants with medical problems. The parents should consult their primary health care provider or nutrition care specialist to identify the most appropriate formula for their infant.

Formulas are supplied either as ready-to-feed, with no mixing required, or as a powder or liquid concentrate to be mixed with water (Box 10.7). In older homes and buildings, old pipes, joints, or faucets may contain lead. To reduce the chance of lead leaching into water, tap water should be run for 15 to 30 seconds before using for drinking, cooking, or formula preparation. Only cold water should be used for formula preparation. The formula should be mixed exactly as stated on the package unless otherwise directed by a primary health care provider. Adding insufficient water can result in a high renal solute load, putting strain on the immature infant kidneys; overdiluting will precipitate undernutrition.

For parents or caregivers who may be non-English speaking or may have low literacy skills, pictorial mixing instructions may be useful. Alternatively, asking the caregiver to demonstrate appropriate formula mixing may be suitable. Formula should never be heated in a microwave oven because microwaves heat food unevenly. Contents of a bottle appearing to be cool on testing may actually have portions that could scald an infant. All unused formula at the end of a feeding should be discarded if not used within 2 hours because of contamination by enzymes and bacteria in the infant's saliva. Home-prepared formulas made from evaporated milk, popular in some cultures, are likely to be low in iron, vitamin C, and other essential nutrients and should be avoided.

Before 1 year of age, cow's milk, regardless of fat content or form (evaporated, liquid, or dried), should not be fed to infants. The fat in cow's milk is less digestible than the fat in breast milk or formula and contains less iron and more sodium and protein. These higher levels of solutes may lead to dehydration caused by the increase in urine volume that occurs to reduce solute levels in the body. Deficiencies of other nutrients, such as vitamin C, essential fatty acids, zinc, and possibly other trace minerals, develop because cow's milk is a poor source of these nutrients.

Cow's milk may be introduced after 1 year of age, when at least two-thirds of energy needs are fulfilled by foods other than milk. The delay in cow's milk consumption reduces the risk for development of a milk allergy. Reduced-fat milk and nonfat milk are not recommended until age 2 years.

BOX 10.7 Formula Preparation

1. Clean all necessary equipment and wash hands before preparing formula.
2. Read formula label, and dilute formula exactly as recommended by the manufacturer.
3. Use cold tap water for preparation of concentrated or powdered formula, unless directed otherwise by physician or nurse.
4. Never heat formula in a microwave oven.
5. Discard unused prepared formula after 2 hours.

Introduction of Solid Foods

Solid foods may be added to the infant's diet between the ages of 4 and 6 months. Infants who are introduced to solid foods before this time may be at risk for excessive kcal intake, food allergies, and GI upset. Many parents and even some health care professionals believe that offering an infant cereal in the evening will promote sleeping through the night. This belief, however, is not supported by research.

Two basic issues when one is considering the introduction of solid foods to the infant's diet are how to introduce them and what foods to introduce.

How to introduce solid foods. Parents and other caregivers may be anxious to introduce foods other than breast milk or formula to their infant's diet. Health professionals can assure them that it is best for the infant to be developmentally ready for solid foods. The infant should be able to sit with some support; move the jaw, lips, and tongue independently; be able to roll the tongue to the back of the mouth to facilitate a food bolus entering the esophagus; and show interest in what the rest of the family is eating. For example, the infant may try to reach and grab an item off of a family member's plate at mealtime. Likewise, parents should become familiar with satiety cues so as not to overfeed the infant. To indicate fullness, the infant may turn the head to the side, refuse to open the mouth, or grimace when the spoon comes close to the mouth. The caregiver should respect these cues. The infant should never be force fed. If the infant is overtired or is not interested in food, they ought to be removed from the highchair and the foods offered again later.

At age 9 to 12 months, an infant may enjoy self-feeding. Although this may be a messy process, caregivers should encourage the development of these skills through food exploration (Fig. 10.6).

Appropriate solid foods during the first year of life. The second half of the first year of life should be thought of as a transitional period; breast milk or formula is still the primary food, and the solid foods are complementary. Solid foods should be

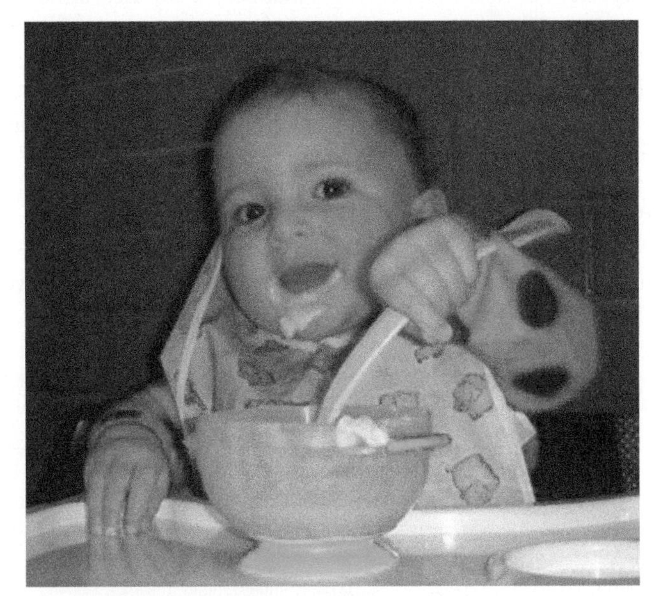

Fig. 10.6 A messy experience as an 11-month-old infant strives to feed herself with a spoon.

introduced gradually and one at a time with a 4- to 5-day interval between new foods. This timing is suggested because if the infant has any type of allergic reaction, such as GI upset, upper respiratory distress, or skin reactions (e.g., eczema, hives), the offending food can be easily identified. Families with a documented history of allergies should delay introduction of solid foods until the infant is about 6 months old. If solid foods are introduced too early, the large protein molecules of the offending food may cross the intestinal barrier and elicit an immunologic response in the infant. As the gut matures, it is less likely to allow large unhydrolyzed proteins to cross the mucosa.

Solid foods offered to the infant need not be commercial. Home-prepared foods are good, practical alternatives. Strict attention should be paid to sanitary food preparation procedures. Although infants should not be offered excessive sweets, naturally sweet fruits such as peaches offer them a taste satisfaction. Although salt should not be added to an infant's food, complete elimination of sodium from foods in the diet is neither practical nor recommended.

A variety of textures, colors, and tastes is important for infants, whether they receive home-prepared or commercial infant foods. General guidelines for infant feeding are listed in Table 10.4.

BOX 10.8 Baby Bottle Tooth Decay

Baby bottle tooth decay (BBTD), also known as early childhood caries (ECC), nursing bottle caries, nursing bottle mouth, and nursing bottle syndrome, is a distinctive pattern of tooth decay in infants and young children. It most commonly affects the maxillary incisors, although other teeth may be affected as well. For BBTD to develop, the mouth requires the presence of fermentable carbohydrate and a pathogenic organism.

BBTD commonly occurs in infants who are allowed to sleep with a bottle of milk, juice, or other sweetened liquid. As the infant falls asleep, the vigorous suck-swallow pattern that normally occurs during feeding diminishes. Moreover, saliva production decreases, resulting in a loss of saliva's buffering action in the mouth. Liquid pools in the infant's mouth, particularly behind the central incisors, becoming a ready source of fermentable carbohydrate for the bacteria colonizing the oral cavity. The acid produced by bacterial metabolism then destroys tooth enamel and initiates caries.

Prevention of BBTD is important for long-term dental health. Infants should never be put to bed with a bottle of milk, formula, juice, or other sweetened liquid. If a bottle is needed at bedtime, it should be plain water only. Oral hygiene may begin as soon as teeth erupt, as a daily gentle cleaning of the tooth surfaces with gauze or a washcloth. Finally, sharing of food and utensils between adults and infants should be discouraged because of transmission of bacteria from the adult to the infant. Weaning from the bottle should occur as soon as the child can drink from a cup.

Beverages During the First Year of Life

Fruit juice, particularly apple juice, is offered to many infants. Fruit juice can make an important contribution to the diet as a source of vitamin C, water, and possibly calcium (if fortified). Its use, though, needs to be monitored. From age 6 to 12 months, no more than 4 to 6 fluid ounces per day should be offered. Excess fruit juice (>12 fluid ounces per day) may lead to diarrhea from carbohydrate malabsorption, growth failure, or, in some children, obesity caused by excess calories. Juices can be diluted with water, providing a beverage with less sweetness. All fruit juices given to infants (and children) should be pasteurized. As discussed earlier in the chapter, it is important to note that beverages made from soy, rice, almond, or coconut do not contain the level of nutrients found in breast milk or infant formula unless they are specifically fortified as infant formulas.

An additional issue is the dental health effects when infants fall asleep with fluids in their mouths (Box 10.8).

Nutrition-Related Concerns

The nutrition requirements of children with congenital or acquired health problems deserve special attention. These infants often have higher nutrient requirements, increased losses, or malabsorption. Significant drug-nutrient interaction often takes place as well. Although it is beyond the scope of this chapter to describe all of such children's special needs one might encounter in practice, a few of the major disorders are outlined. In all of these cases, a registered dietitian/nutritionist should be a part of the medical team.

The Premature Infant and the Low-Birth-Weight Infant

An infant is considered premature if born before 37 weeks' gestation. Low birth weight infants may be full term or premature but weigh 2500 g or less at birth. As medical technology becomes increasingly sophisticated, infants are surviving at younger ages and lower weights. However, their developmental outlook may still be tenuous. Nutrition support of these infants plays a crucial role in successful long-term outcome. The major issues of concern in the premature infant are low birth weight, immature lung development, poor immune function, immature GI and neurologic function, insufficient production of digestive enzymes, inadequate bone mineralization, and minimal energy and mineral reserves.

TABLE 10.4 Solid Foods During the First Year of Life

Age	Food	Foods to Avoid in the First Year of Life
4–5 months	Iron-fortified infant cereal	Honey (may cause infantile *Clostridium botulinum* poisoning); hot dogs, grapes, hard candies, raw carrots, popcorn, nuts, peanut butter (choking hazards); skim milk (insufficient calories); cow's milk (potential allergen, may replace breast milk or formula); egg whites (potential allergen)
5–6 months	Strained fruits and vegetables	
6–8 months	Mashed or chopped fruits and vegetables Juice from a cup	
9–12 months	Crackers, toast, cottage cheese, plain meats, egg yolk, finger foods	

Because the coordinated suck-swallow reflex is not fully developed until an infant reaches 34 weeks' gestation, initial feeding of the premature infant may need to be via total parenteral nutrition, tube feeding, or gavage feeding. Many criteria influence the route of nutrient delivery, and thus each infant should receive an individualized nutrition assessment by a registered dietitian who specializes in high-risk pediatric patients.

Premature infants have increased needs for protein, kcal, calcium, phosphorus, sodium, iron, zinc, vitamin E, and fluids. The best feeding choice for a premature infant is mother's milk with the addition of "human milk fortifier," which contains additional minerals and protein needed by the premature infant. Although the infant may not suckle well or may tire easily at the breast, the nurse can play a key role in helping the mother pump and store her milk in the neonatal nursery. The milk may then be given by gavage even when the mother is not present. If the mother chooses not to breastfeed, a variety of specialized infant formulas are available to meet the special nutritional requirements of the infant.

Research suggests these formulas should be fortified with long-chain fatty acids to mimic what would be delivered via the placenta. Long-chain fatty acids are essential for proper retinal and neurologic development. Premature and low-birth-weight infants require continual nutritional follow-up after discharge for at least the first year of life because they are at risk for feeding problems, developmental delays, and growth retardation.

Failure to Thrive

Failure to thrive (FTT) is defined as a drop of two standard deviations in weight gain over an interval of 2 months or longer for infants younger than 6 months of age or over an interval of 3 months or longer for infants older than 6 months of age. An alternative definition is a weight-for-length measurement less than the fifth percentile or weight for age less than the third percentile.

FTT may have organic causes, such as an underlying metabolic disorder. Congenital heart disease or HIV infection may cause such an increased energy requirement that oral intake is not able to keep up with metabolic need.

Nonorganic FTT may be diagnosed when no medical reason for poor growth can be recognized. There may be psychosocial causes for FTT, such as either extreme of parental attention (neglect or excessive attentiveness). Neglect may include inadequate maternal-infant bonding, poverty, child abuse, or neglect. Treatment for nonorganic FTT must include nutrition intervention to promote weight gain and therapy to correct developmental delays and any psychosocial problems in the home environment (Krugman & Dubowitz, 2003).

Inborn Errors of Metabolism

PKU and galactosemia are described next. Other inborn errors of metabolism that require nutrition therapy that are not discussed further include urea cycle disorders, maple syrup urine disease, and homocystinuria.

Phenylketonuria. All 50 states have newborn screening programs to detect PKU. When it is discovered early, dietary therapy can begin immediately, and long-term prognosis is good. Without treatment, phenylalanine and its metabolites reach toxic levels in the blood, resulting in damage to the central nervous system, including mental retardation. Likewise, because phenylalanine cannot be converted to tyrosine, low levels or absence of tyrosine may contribute to the mental retardation.

Treatment consists of a low-phenylalanine diet to be followed throughout the individual's life. In infancy the use of a special formula such as Lofenalac is recommended. Partial breastfeeding is permitted, but phenylalanine levels in the infant's blood must be monitored carefully (Elsas & Acosta, 2014). As children with PKU are introduced to solid foods and make the transition to table foods, meals require careful planning. The use of low-protein breads and pastas is advised. This condition requires close monitoring of dietary intake by specialized dietitians.

Galactosemia. Galactosemia is another rare, autosomal recessive disorder caused by an enzyme deficiency and is part of the newborn screening panel. Absence of the enzyme galactose-1-phosphate uridylyltransferase results in an inability to metabolize galactose. Because the milk sugar lactose is a disaccharide of glucose and galactose, infants without this enzyme are unable to tolerate any milk products containing lactose. Manifestations include diarrhea, growth retardation, and mental retardation. Treatment is dietary therapy that excludes all milk products, including human milk. Soy formulas and casein hydrolysate formulas are acceptable. Even with lifelong diet therapy, there may be long-term health consequences, such as nervous system or ovarian dysfunction (Elsas & Acosta, 2014). Specialized pediatric dietitians closely monitor the diet of infants and children who have this disorder.

NUTRITION HEALTH PROMOTION: PREGNANCY, LACTATION, AND INFANCY

Knowledge

The metabolic, hormonal, anatomic, psychologic, and physiologic changes that occur during pregnancy can be bewildering for the mother and for those around her. Understanding the process can ease adaptation to these changes. Focusing on the nutrient needs of the mother assures appropriate weight gain to support the growth of the fetus. Knowledge of the anatomic and physiologic changes that occur after childbirth prepares the mother's body for lactation. Nutrient requirements of the mother remain elevated during lactation to produce nourishment for the infant. Recommendations for the specific nutrient needs of the first year of life are important for parents and caregivers to provide.

Techniques

There are numerous resources to assist with pregnancy, lactation, and infancy. Whether in printed form or on the Internet, strategies for dealing with challenges abound. Care needs to be taken to assess the credibility of the source of information. Government sites (.gov) are trustworthy, and applicable sites are available for each of the areas of concern. For example, the MyPlate site (MyPlate.gov) includes specific categories for pregnancy and lactation. In addition, sites from professional medical associations also provide potential solutions to the challenges of this life span category.

Community Supports

Community supports may be government sponsored, such as the WIC program discussed in the *Social Issues* box Providing the Essentials. Health care providers can be familiar with such programs and recommend patients to take advantage of the services. In addition, interest groups have a strong presence either locally or through the Internet. Notable is the La Leche League (www.llli.org), which provides mother-to-mother support of breastfeeding women, ranging from local chapter meetings through a larger mission as an international nonprofit organization. Within individual communities, mothers (and fathers) may organize to assist one another with the trials and tribulations of pregnancy and the first year of life issues of their babies. This interaction may occur through a group blog or on a dedicated website.

NUTRITION DURING CHILDHOOD

Once we pass the specific nutrition and health necessities of pregnancy and infancy, the rest of the life span categories share more similarities than differences regarding nutrient intake and dietary patterns.

Stages of Development

The life span stages reflect psychologic and physiologic maturation. Approaches to health promotion take into account these stages and their impact on nutrient requirements, eating styles, and food choices.

Childhood (1–12 Years)

The accelerated growth of infancy slows down by about age 1 year, marking the transition to childhood. Growth then occurs unevenly until puberty heralds the onset of adolescence. This growth deceleration during childhood results in varying hunger levels, reflecting physiologic need. Parent and caregiver awareness of these fluctuations allows children to stay in tune with their internal hunger cues.

Nurses sensitive to normal growth patterns as affected by genetics and environmental influences can help families to understand the growth curves of their children. Height, weight, and head circumferences are used with the standard growth charts from the National Center for Health Statistics to monitor growth (available at www.cdc.gov/growthcharts). See Chapter 11 for a detailed description of clinical nutrition assessment procedures.

Childhood categories are based on a combination of psychosocial and physiologic developmental stages. Physiologic requirements are the basis of the age and gender divisions of the DRIs. This discussion highlights the nutrients of concern—protein, iron, calcium, and zinc. For other specific age-related nutrient recommendations, refer to the DRI tables.

Children depend on adults for the provision of food. A discussion of the nutrient needs of the growing body is not complete without a consideration of the role of adults in nourishing children. Children are influenced by adults and model the behaviors of adults. Adults control the quantity and quality of foods prepared, as well as the environment within which foods are presented for consumption. Serving sizes should represent appropriate quantities for the ages of the children. The children themselves, however, control the actual amount consumed. Easily distracted children may need gentle coaxing to try new foods or to ingest sufficient amounts to meet energy and nutrient needs.

Adults are responsible for not only what meals are offered but also when meals are offered. Regularity of mealtimes at home—breakfast and dinner—helps support success at school. Breakfast supplies energy in the morning for school learning (see the *Teaching Tool* box What's the Best Breakfast?); dinner supports the ability to complete homework, study, and relax before bedtime. Most children eat lunch away from home and either bring a prepared lunch from home or purchase meals through a school lunch program. (School lunches are discussed later in this chapter, under the heading "Community Supports.")

TEACHING TOOL

What's the Best Breakfast?

Foods considered best for breakfast have changed. Although traditional breakfasts consist of eggs, bacon, white toast, and whole milk, this combination is now recognized as being too high in fat and protein. In addition, in the rush of morning preparation, few of us have the time to prepare this type of meal. Nonetheless, breakfast, which breaks our fast, is an important contributor of nutrients and energy.

As we teach clients and their families about nutrition and optimum dietary intake patterns, we can assure them that breakfast can be simple yet still provide appropriate levels of nutrients. Following are some ideas for parents to use to ignite their children's breakfast appetites:

- For children (and adults) who eat and run, have quick foods available such as fruit, granola bars (low fat/low sugar), muffins (low fat/low sugar), and raisins/nuts.
- For older children, offer to prepare a simple breakfast. Although they are able to prepare their own meal, the extra nurturing—and time saved—will be appreciated.
- To create appetite, toast bread while family members are dressing. The enticing scent will spark their taste buds.
- For picky eaters, create small smorgasbord plates with several choices such as a small container of yogurt, crackers with cheese, and some pear slices.
- Be a role model by also eating breakfast yourself.

Snacks boost daily nutrient intake; for children whose energy and general dietary intake are adequate, snacks may sometimes include sweets, such as cookies and even an occasional candy bar. A common myth is that sugar makes children hyperactive; studies have found no convincing evidence that consumption of sugar causes attention-deficit/hyperactivity disorder. High-sugar-containing foods, however, can displace more nutritious foods and contribute to nutrient deficiencies (such as of calcium and dietary fiber) or excessive caloric and dietary fat intake. Of significant concern is childhood excess adiposity or overweight bodies. No food should be forbidden; frequency and quantity should be the guides.

Children too young for school may attend daycare programs if their parents work. The impact on their nutrition may be positive or negative, depending on the quality and attitude of the programs to nutrition and mealtimes. Most young children, regardless of parental employment, attend some form of preschool; for many, the food and social experiences broaden acceptance of a variety of foods and eating styles.

Although adults may have predominant influence over the eating behaviors of children, another primary influence for some children is television. The influence of TV commercials has been studied extensively and is most often condemned as negatively influencing children's food choices. In addition, watching television while family meals are eaten appears to affect the types of foods served, resulting in consumption of foods higher in fat and lower in fiber—possibly reflecting the categories of foods most often advertised on television. Parents and caregivers can watch television with their children to assess the type of products advertised and then discuss their nutritional value. As more healthful products are marketed, even if targeted at adults, acceptance by children may increase. Occasional treats of advertised products may lessen their appeal if children are accustomed to high-quality snacks and meals.

The acceptable macronutrient distribution range (AMDR) for daily dietary fat intake recommends about 30% kcal intake. This level of dietary fat intake may also assist with obesity prevention and emphasizes fruits, vegetables, and complex carbohydrates. It is easier to enjoy whole foods that are naturally low in fat throughout childhood than to convert one's eating style as an adult. Other AMDRs include for carbohydrates 45% to 65% kcal; for protein 5% to 20% kcal for young children and 10% to 30% kcal for older children; and adequate intake dietary fiber of 19 g/day for children 1 to 3 years, 25 g/day for those 4 to 8 years, 31 g/day for boys 9 to 13 years, and 26 g/day for girls 9 to 13 years (Ogata & Hayes, 2014). *Dietary Guidelines 2020–2025* recommends that added sugar comprise less than 10% of caloric intake regardless of age.

Despite national dietary recommendations, trends in children's total energy intake have indicated an increase. Although calories increased, total intake of milk, vegetable, soups, breads, grains, and eggs decreased, and intake of fruits, fruit juices, sweetened beverages, poultry, and cheese increased. When food groups were considered, about 16% of U.S. children did not meet any food group recommendations, whereas only 1% consumed recommended amounts for all food groups. Approximately two-thirds of U.S. children do not consume suggested servings of fruits and vegetables. Consumption of whole grains is extremely low, with consumption of two or more servings of whole grains daily by less than 13% of children. Those who did meet dietary recommendations had intakes that were high in fat (CDC, 2019; Krebs-Smith et al., 2010). Consider that for some children the principal vegetable is French fries. These findings indicate that nutrition education is still needed for parents and their children. (The *Cultural Diversity and Nutrition* box Child Health Education for Foreign-Born Parents offers suggestions for educating foreign-born parents about their child's health.)

CULTURAL DIVERSITY AND NUTRITION

Child Health Education for Foreign-Born Parents

Providing child health education for foreign-born parents for whom English is not their primary language presents special concerns related to language and culture. An innovative, culturally relevant approach should be used to present basic child health information in English, with translators present as facilitators. Foreign-born parents who need a partial or complete language interpretation then have readily available access to translation support. Parents can ask questions, provide comments and suggestions, and evaluate the presentation through the translator. Because participants can be grouped with an appropriate translator, each presentation can accommodate more than one language.

The presentation, conducted in English, is paced to allow for discussions. Child care is provided in a nearby setting, allowing parents to focus on the presentation without the concern of child care. Vocabulary relative to health care is developed from English into the parents' primary language with the support of the translator.

Application to Nursing

This is an example of one culture-specific strategy used to meet minority and ethnic health needs. Nurses are also encouraged to provide translated health education materials for the populations with whom they teach.

(Data from Baker R: Child health education for the foreign-born parent, *Issues Compr Pediatr Nurs* 24:45–55, 2001.)

Stage I: Children 1 to 3 Years Old

Usually referred to as "toddlerhood," the age span of 1 to 3 years old is a busy time for young children. They are dealing with issues of autonomy. Often food and eating create an arena for asserting newly discovered independence. The eating relationship between parent (or caregiver) and child is forming, and adult reaction to autonomy sets the stage for future encounters. Consistency of mealtimes is important. Meals are best accepted when hunger, tiredness, and emotions are still controllable; an overly tired child just cannot eat. Equally important is fostering self-reliance by allowing young children to feed themselves in a manner most appropriate for their psychomotor abilities. Regardless of the messy results, children's attempts to self-feed provide the roots of self-empowerment crucial to overall physical and psychologic development.

Hunger, rather than adult meal schedules, guides the child's perception of time to eat. Meals for toddlers are based on the same design and food selections as adults, only in smaller portions. (Of course, overly spicy foods may not be acceptable to young taste buds.) Snacks are a necessity in addition to meals. Toddlers are able to eat only small amounts at each meal or food encounter. Planned snacks provide required additional nourishment between meals to ensure an adequate dietary intake.

Nutrition requirements. Growth, BMR, and endless activity require an energy supply of 1300 kcal/day for children aged 1 to 3 years. Protein needs increase to 16 g to meet the demands of growing muscles. For children aged 1 through 6 years, a general guideline is one fruit or vegetable serving equals one level-measuring tablespoon of fruit or vegetable per year of age. A serving of bread or cereal is equal to about one fourth of an adult's serving. Up to age 3 years, children should consume two or three 8-ounce cups of milk per day or about 16 to 24 ounces per day, and meats or meat substitutes can be offered at least twice per day (Heird, 2014). Caregivers should be advised that alternative milk products such as rice milk and soymilk, unless sufficiently fortified, may not provide the same quality of nutrients as animal-derived foods.

When children are between 1 and 3 years old, they should be introduced to lower-fat versions of commonly eaten foods. Fat-containing foods should not be obsessively restricted; however, high-fat foods are often filling and may displace other nutrient-containing foods.

This is also a prime time to introduce toddlers to a variety of foods. Toddlers imitate the adults around them; therefore, adults can model behavior by eating a variety of foods themselves. Clever introductions to foods are always helpful to catch the attention and appetite of toddlers. Broccoli is more than just a vegetable; cut up, it looks like little trees. Peas steamed in their pods are not just peas but green pearls waiting to be discovered.

Although breast milk or formula is the milk of choice until age 1, toddlers should drink breast milk, whole milk, or formula until age 2, after which low-fat or skim milk is best. Sometimes toddlers consume too much milk or juice, particularly if they are given an unlimited number of servings. Perhaps drinking from feeding bottles throughout the day simply becomes a habit. Unfortunately, the child fills up on milk or juice, both low sources of iron, and then does not have an appetite for iron-containing foods such as meat, fish, poultry, eggs, or legumes. Iron-deficiency anemia may develop. Additionally, apple juice is sweet tasting and has few nutrients beyond carbohydrate kcal. Its frequent consumption may habituate young children to sweet drinks. Later, apple juice may be replaced with sugar-laden sodas or beverages, which displace more nutrient-dense beverages. One possible solution is to dilute juices with water. Milk can be served with meals and diluted juices drunk between meals. Parents and caregivers can view bottles as cups or glassware. Few of us drink from a cup continually while watching television, reading, or playing games. Similarly, once past infancy, young children's use of feeding bottles and/or lidded cups or "sippy" cups should be viewed as beverages that are part of a meal or snack. Healthful snacks can provide energy for playing.

Stage II: Children 4 to 6 Years Old

Stage II is characterized by independent eating styles, although modeling of adults still occurs. Children of this age clearly understand the time frame of meals and can save their appetite for meals. Snacks are still an integral part of the children's nutrient intake. Far from the messy eating styles of toddlers, these children accept foods more easily if presented separately, not mixed in a casserole style. Variations in hunger and appetite levels may confuse parents and caregivers. The most practical approach is to be respectful of these variations of hunger; this approach diffuses power plays over food consumption.

New foods can continue to be introduced. Children may require repeated exposures, as many as 8 to 10 attempts, before they accept a food. For some families, backup meal plans can encourage trying new foods. For instance, if a child does not accept a new dish after a reasonable attempt, the child may be allowed to prepare a peanut butter sandwich or cereal and fruit. By establishing backup meals in advance, parents avoid becoming short-order cooks preparing three or more individualized meals for dinner.

Another approach is to have at least one meal (eaten at home) include new foods along with favorite foods. In addition to the new foods, the child will recognize some familiar foods on his or her plate. A meal can consist of a sampling of food items; several will probably be acceptable.

At this stage, children can develop a sense of responsibility for healthful food selections. They can understand that although all foods are okay, some foods, such as fruits, vegetables, and low-fat foods, can be eaten more often than others.

Sometimes a child develops a food jag, wanting to eat only a narrow range of foods. Parents and teachers can educate the child that each food contains a different assortment of nutrients and offer substitute choices that contain additional nutrients, with the child making the final selections. Eventually food jags diminish, and the child consumes a broader selection of foods.

Nutrition requirements. Energy requirements jump to 1800 kcal/day at 4 to 6 years of age, reflecting continued growth and activity levels. Protein intake needs increase to 24 g.

Stage III: Children 7 to 12 Years Old

The years from 7 to 12 are tumultuous. Although actual growth may slow down, the body is preparing and seemingly storing up for the puberty growth spurt. Puberty may begin for girls from around age 9 years; boys may reach puberty in the early teen years. This prepuberty time may be reflected by weight buildup; an increase in chubbiness is not alarming if moderate eating and physical activities are maintained. Adults must be careful not to overreact, or they may plant the seeds of eating disorders. To rule out overeating, children can be asked whether they are really hungry for food or only tired or thirsty. These are different sensations. A child can be reminded to "stop eating when you are full" (Fig. 10.7). If hunger returns, a snack of fruit can be provided. By taking time to consider these sensations, children can stay in touch with internal cues of true hunger.

Exposure to other dietary patterns takes place as children spend more time away from home at school and in socializing

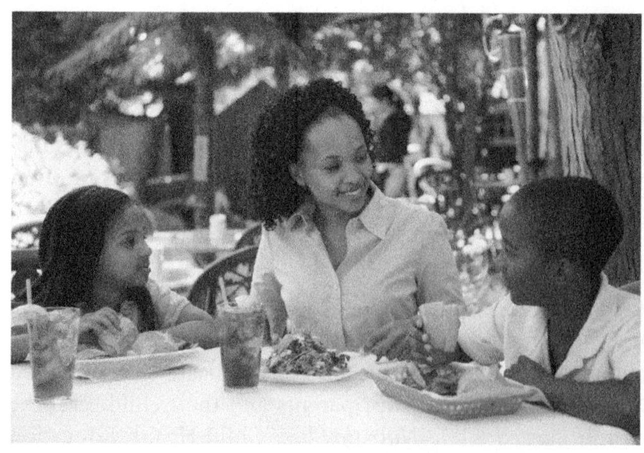

Fig. 10.7 A child can be reminded to "stop eating when you are full." (From www.thinkstockphotos.com)

with friends. Peer influence at school lunchtime increases; having the right kind of lunch may be as important as wearing the right kind of clothes. Adults need to be sensitive to these issues. As long as a basic lunch of some protein, complex carbohydrates, and a beverage (preferably milk, juice, or water) is consumed, missing nutrients can be adjusted for later in the day, especially through after-school snacks.

It is at this age—when midmorning school snacks disappear and school lunch scheduling has more to do with numbers of students than with actual lunchtime appetites—that after-school hunger may intensify. This is the time to provide healthful snacks or at least stock the kitchen shelves with an assortment of nutrient-dense treats (Box 10.9). If children purchase snacks away from home, adults can develop guidelines with children this age to maintain positive eating styles.

The intent is to supplement the nutrients received during meals with nutrient-dense snacks so the total caloric and nutrient intake is adequate to meet the needs of growth at each childhood stage. Snacking, though, seems to have changed in definition and frequency. A study of 31,337 children and adolescents assessed snacking and meal intake trends from 1977 to 2006 (Piernas & Popkin, 2010). On average, the numbers of both calories and eating events (a total of snacks and meals) increased substantially over time. Compared with the 1970s, about half of American children in the twenty-first century average 4 snacks a day, whereas others consume snacks and meals as many as 10 times a day, or basically eat nonstop. This means that an excessive number of calories, most likely less nutrient-dense snack foods, are being consumed and that the consumption of nutrient-dense mealtime foods is decreasing. Although the increase in snack calories is only 168 kcal, this number represents an average, signaling that for many children the excess intake is higher. With increased eating episodes, there can be a concern that eating is due not to physiologic hunger but to a habit from needing a constant state of satiation.

Nutrition requirements. Energy needs for 7- to 12-year-olds increase to 2000 to 2200 kcal/day. Protein requirements rise to between 28 and 46 g, depending on sexual maturity. Sexual maturity leads to an increase in lean body mass, particularly for boys, which requires more dietary protein for growth and maintenance.

Mineral needs rise as well. Because of greater bone growth and mineralization, calcium RDA recommendations jump from 800 mg/day at age 8 years to 1300 mg/day throughout adolescence. Iron and zinc allowances increase as well. Well-chosen dietary intakes will provide sufficient amounts of these nutrients. Marginal intakes of zinc have been noted among schoolchildren who are finicky eaters; low zinc intakes can affect growth rates (Willoughby & Bowen, 2014).

BOX 10.9 Healthy Snacks

Snacks are a way to bridge energy levels between meals. They are not meant to be so energy dense that intakes during meals are compromised or that daily total caloric intakes are significantly increased. Frequent snacking (or nonstop eating) throughout the day has been associated with increased body weight in children (and adults!).

Here are some suggestions for healthy snacks:

- Ready-to-eat cereals: reserve presweetened cereals as special snack treats or mix a sweet cereal with a less sweet cereal—the best of both worlds
- Snack smorgasbord: cut-up apples and oranges, popcorn, cheese, crackers, and cookies
- Fruit juice pack
- Low-fat chocolate milk pack
- Open-face peanut butter sandwich (child-made) with cut fruit, jelly, coconut, and raisins
- Sliced apple or pear with thin spread of nut butter (peanut, almond, or cashew)
- Fresh or canned fruit (in fruit juice) with cottage cheese (in 4-ounce size)
- English muffin (oat bran, raisin, or sourdough) with a small amount of fruit spread
- Healthier Danish: a slice of toasted bread with low-fat ricotta cheese and preserves
- Bagel with a spread of whipped cream cheese, margarine/butter, or nut butter (peanut, almond, or cashew); freeze a variety of bagels
- Smoothie or fruit shakes made with skim milk or fruit juice, plain or fruit-flavored yogurt, fresh or frozen fruit—just mix in a blender
- Leftovers from lunch or dinner; a bowl of soup with bread for dipping instead of a prepackaged snack

NUTRITION HEALTH PROMOTION: CHILDHOOD (1–12 YEARS)

Knowledge

The growth cycle of this age span is important for both parents and children to understand. Attention to issues related to weight, appropriate appetite, and meal patterning is crucial for positive eating relationships and may prevent the development of eating disorders. By understanding the relationship of nutrients and kcal to their growth needs, children possess sufficient information to take responsibility for certain aspects of their food choices and dietary patterns. Children with special needs who are challenged by physical and/or mental limitations may require additional support to achieve nutritional adequacy (Box 10.10). Ultimately, however, adults must provide nourishment for children and guidance as to positive health behaviors.

Techniques

Several techniques can be used with children this age. MyPlate for Kids is similar to the adult version but presents games and other creative approaches for children to visualize and understand the serving sizes and types of foods that result in a balanced nutrient intake. It can be found at www.myplate.gov/life-stages/kids. Another source for appropriate techniques is the Produce for Better Health Foundation website, which offers resources for parents and children (www.fruitsandveggies.org).

Community Supports

Community supports for children are currently divided into two categories based on location and services or education offered: (1) school food service and (2) classroom nutrition education.

School food service. The National School Lunch Program (NSLP) was established to protect the health and wellness of American children. Formalized in 1946, the program provides

BOX 10.10 Nutrition Requirements of Children With Special Needs

Although the basic nutrition needs of all children are the same, some children may be challenged by the limitations of physical and mental differences and the physical and pharmacologic consequences of chronic disease treatment. The ability to self-feed may be highly related to life expectancy. Enhancing feeding skills to the greatest extent possible is an involved procedure. Nutrition education has valuable skills and experiences to offer. Keep the following issues in mind:

- All children can enjoy working together to prepare foods. The process of measuring, mixing, arranging, and eating food that they helped to prepare enhances self-esteem and provides the acquisition of other skill competencies such as math and science and the interpersonal skills of cooperation.
- Positioning of children with physical handicaps may require adaptive equipment and alternative eating strategies for special conditions. Oral stimulation before eating may be required for children with low muscle tone, and certain textures of foods may be better received than others. If chewing and swallowing are problematic, textures of foods may need adjustment. Low muscle tone may also affect functioning of the large intestine and require adequate fiber and water to reduce the risk of constipation.
- Medications may increase or decrease appetite. Caregivers and teachers should be aware of these effects, and meals and snacks should be offered when hunger is the strongest.
- Children with sensory integration difficulties may be sensitive to textures, temperature, and even colors of foods. Preferences should be accommodated when possible to ensure adequate nutrition and to provide the children a sense of control over food choices.
- Children experiencing growth retardation or malnutrition should be reassessed by a registered dietitian/nutritionist (RDN) to determine whether alternative feeding strategies can improve their nutritional status. Parents should regularly receive assessments of nutritional status to fully understand their children's conditions.
- Periodic nutritional assessments of children with special needs should be conducted by RDNs who have the expertise to evaluate nutritional status and offer practical strategies for everyday eating situations.

(Data from Fung EB, et al: Feeding dysfunction is associated with poor growth and health status in children with cerebral palsy, *J Am Diet Assoc* 102(3):361, 373, 2002; and correspondence on Society for Nutrition Education (SNE) listserv 19 February, 1998, from Susan Piscopo, associate professor, University of Malta; Sharon Davis, education director, Home Baking Association; Collette Janson-Sand, associate professor, University of New Hampshire; and others.)

lunches at varying cost, depending on family income, to all schoolchildren at public and nonprofit private schools and residential child care institutions. At the federal level, the program is administered by the Food and Nutrition Service (FNS) of the USDA, at the state level by various agencies, and locally by school boards. As an entitlement program, the NSLP provides funds to all schools that apply and meet the criteria of eligibility. Approximately 95% of all school districts participate in this program. Every school district is required to implement a local school wellness policy to focus on obesity prevention and, through modification of school environments, to support healthy eating habits and physical activity (Food Research & Action Center [FRAC], 2019).

At participating schools, there are two types of eligibility to qualify for free or reduced-price meals; both usually require the family to complete and return application forms. Categorical eligibility is based on the child's household receiving the Supplemental Nutrition Assistance Program (SNAP) or Temporary Assistance for Needy Families (TANF) or participating in the Food District Program on Indian Reservations (FDPIR), and free meals for the homeless, runaways, and children of migrant workers. Income-based eligibility offers reduced-price meals to children whose household income is less than 185% of the federal poverty level; free meals are available to those with incomes less than 130% of the poverty level. Through the process of direct certification, school districts qualify children without requiring submission of family applications. School districts work with state or local SNAP, TANF, and FDPIR agencies to certify children in households.

During the 2018–2019 school year, NSLP served meals daily to about 30 million children in almost 97,000 schools and residential childcare institutions. More than 70% of these children received free or reduced-price lunches (FRAC, 2019).

New standards were issued by USDA in January 2012 as required by the Healthy, Hunger-Free Kids Act to provide school meal nutrition standards that implement the U.S. Department of Health and Human Services *Dietary Guidelines for Americans*. The new standards include increasing the amount of fruits and vegetables served, with a focus on whole-grain-rich foods. Only lower-fat or nonfat milk is to be served, and other reductions in saturated fat, sodium, and calories are required. Also included are increasing cultural food options to meet the needs of local communities.

Basically, lunch must provide approximately one-third or more of the recommended levels for key nutrients, providing no more than 30% kcal from fat and less than 10% of kcal from saturated fat. For low-income children participating in the program, this lunch provides one-third to one-half of their daily intake.

The School Breakfast Program, created in 1966, has reduced tardiness and improved school attendance, while increasing test scores and improving student health through reducing food insecurity. During the 2018–2019 school year, about 90,000 schools and institutions participated in the School Breakfast Program, serving 14.6 million children. Over 80% of the participants qualify for free or reduced-priced meals. More than 58% of the children from low-income families receive both school lunch and school breakfast (FRAC, 2020).

The breakfast can comprise an assortment of foods, but the program requires milk (either as a beverage or with cereal), a serving of fruit (either whole or as juice), and two servings of a bread/cereal product or meat/meat alternative or a combination of bread and meat servings. The breakfast is designed to provide one fourth or more of the daily recommended level for key nutrients and limits fat to no more than 30% kcal with less than 10% kcal of saturated fat.

During summer, the Summer Food Service Program for Children (SFSP) functions through a range of eligible organizations including schools, summer camps, and community agencies, as well as various federal, state, and local government departments. The purpose is to serve meals to school-age children when schools are not in session in communities where children depend on school meals as an essential component of their daily nourishment.

School nurses and community health nurses should be aware of these programs as valuable sources of nutrition. Sometimes children do not participate because school payment policies create a stigma associated with participation. Intervention by a health professional may be required to ensure that children's health needs are met in a socially sensitive manner. As health advocates, nurses may be able to highlight the importance of school lunch and breakfast programs to educational administrators and the community at large.

Classroom nutrition education. Health has been taught for many years in most school systems. What varies are the depth of school health curricula and the qualifications of the instructors. Both may affect the quality of the nutrition education. Although basic nutrition facts can be taught within a short-term health course, lifestyle changes that affect dietary patterns take longer to achieve. Unless they have special preparation, instructors may not feel comfortable teaching the intricate and ever-changing discipline of nutrition. This may lead to either poor-quality teaching or the imparting of negative attitudes to nutrition and food selections.

NUTRITION DURING ADOLESCENCE

The adolescent years (13–19 years) are marked by change. Not only does puberty initiate growth acceleration, but emotional and social developmental struggles also occur as academic and personal responsibilities escalate. Adults often assume that teenagers can take care of themselves. Although teens need to take responsibility for their behavior and overall health status, they still need the guidance and nurturing of caring adults. There is a fine line between allowing adolescents to be responsible and neglecting their needs. Adult involvement is still necessary to provide physical and emotional support during the stressful years of adolescence.

Part of the physical and emotional support includes creating guidelines for dietary patterns and providing food for consumption. Creating guidelines means maintaining a household in which meals are available, even if family members may not be able to eat together. Knowing that dinner just needs to be reheated means someone was thinking of the welfare of all family members. Of course, shared responsibility for meal preparation may be an appropriate component of family duties. A kitchen stocked with nourishing snack foods and ingredients for simple meals helps make stressful, chaotic teenage schedules more manageable.

Older teens may be adjusting to the new demands of the college environment, including adapting to dining hall meals. Some campuses provide flexible meal plans with several locations for meal acquisition around campus. Others offer salad bars and food "stations" to provide a variety of selections. Individuals requiring special dietary requirements such as kosher meals or lactose-reduced meals should discuss these issues with food service staff or with student service personnel.

As their sense of social awareness develops, some teens may adopt a vegetarian dietary pattern. Creative planning on the part of the teen and the family meal planner results in meals that meet everyone's nutritional needs without compromising personal convictions.

Discussions of the eating habits of teens tend to be critical of their fast-food consumption. Fortunately, most teens can afford the extra kcal that typically higher-fat foods such as hamburgers, fries, and pizza may contain. If teens have grown up accustomed to well-balanced meals, they will more than likely still prefer those meals to high-fat delights. Eating in fast-food restaurants, where prices tend to be low, may have more to do with socializing among peers than with nutrient values.

When fast foods become the mainstay of an individual's diet, regardless of age, some nutrients, such as vitamins A and C, may be lacking, and overconsumption of dietary fats and kcal may occur. Although teens may be seen at such restaurants, most other customers are families with young children as well as older adults. Fast foods affect the nutrient intake of all ages.

Nutrition Requirements

Because of the natural physiologic differences between adolescent boys and girls, nutrient requirements from age 9 years and older are divided by gender. Girls need about 2200 kcal and 45 g of protein daily. Recommendations for boys are 2500 to 2900 kcal and 45 to 59 g of protein daily. These values for kcal and protein reflect the greater lean body mass developing in males. They do, however, only represent suggested amounts; physical activity, either work or athletic endeavors, affects the actual nutrient needs for both boys and girls.

Calcium RDA recommendations are the same for the two genders, 1300 mg/day, to allow for skeletal growth (particularly for boys) and for bone mineralization, a prime physiologic function during adolescence. Bone mineralization for girls is a concern because teenage girls often do not consume enough calcium-rich foods.

Teenage girls and sometimes teenage boys are at risk for dieting-related disorders and eating disorders. By regularly under consuming nutrients during a time when the human body is completing maturation, girls are at risk for various deficiencies as they progress to adulthood and the nutrient requirements of potential pregnancies. In addition to calcium, iron allowances are important to fulfill, particularly for girls who begin menstruation; iron is also needed by boys, whose accelerated growth necessitates an increased blood volume and lean body mass.

NUTRITION HEALTH PROMOTION: ADOLESCENCE

Knowledge

The adolescent body benefits from a dietary intake most similar to an adult's; however, some nutrient needs are greater. Energy requirements are higher than at any other time of life, especially for adolescents involved in competitive athletics. Calcium recommendations increase to ensure adequate mineralization of bones. Parental tolerance for alternative food styles enhances overall dietary intake and allows for the acceptance of dietary suggestions to maintain appropriate nutrient consumption.

Teenagers can comprehend the body's physiology and nutrient needs. Ideally, this information should be taught within family life, health, or science curricula in schools. This knowledge provides a rationale for consumption of nutrient-dense foods, especially as preparation for sports activities. Although adults may supply provisions for meals and snacks, especially those that can be reheated, ultimately, most adolescents take responsibility for their own nutrient intake. Teens can help shop for and plan meals that meet the family's nutritional needs while incorporating alternative food styles.

Awareness of the risk factors for and symptoms of disordered eating and drug/alcohol abuse can be provided through health classes or interactions with health and educational professionals and parents. (See Chapter 19.) Even mild substance abuse in the face of the increased nutritional needs of adolescence can compromise nutritional status. For example, alcohol adversely affects absorption of folate and zinc, two nutrients required for normal growth. Nurses need to be aware of the indicators of substance abuse so they can guide adolescents into treatment. Nutrition assessment, intervention, and support are part of comprehensive physical and psychologic rehabilitation of all substance abusers.

Techniques

As they do for children, the concepts found at the MyPlate and Fruits & Veggies—More Matters websites provide a basis for adolescent food choices (adolescents use MyPlate for adults). Often the forces overriding good food choices are lack of time and scheduling demands. One strategy accommodating both is to ensure the availability of simple meals that are easily eaten and reheatable. Scheduling of meals in a home or institutional setting (e.g., school cafeterias, dining halls) can take into account school, sports, work, and recreational agendas. To improve the quality of food choices, adolescents should be included in meal planning and food preparation.

Community Supports

Except for federal government programs serving children and adults, no food programs are specifically targeted at adolescents. At a time when teens are developmentally ready to be empowered to take care of themselves, society provides few supports. In fact, school, sports, and work schedules often hinder adolescents from taking responsibility for their health behaviors. Television, radio, Internet, and social media rarely promote healthy behaviors. Although the increased interest in physical pursuits of basketball, soccer, biking, skateboarding, weightlifting, and other recreational sports enhances fitness, the nutrition component is often overlooked or cloaked in misinformation. This is an area to which all health professionals should be sensitive.

One of the few community supports is a comprehensive school health program. The depth of health issues covered varies and may not include sufficient nutrition guidance, but at the least these programs highlight basic concerns of nutrition and health.

NUTRITION-RELATED CONCERNS OF CHILDHOOD AND ADOLESCENCE

Food Asphyxiation

Asphyxiation from food is possible at any point in the life span, but toddlers and older adults tend to be more at risk. (Older adults are discussed in the next section of this chapter.) As toddlers first become accustomed to a variety of food textures and substances, they sometimes misjudge the size of food being chewed or may be too active while eating and accidentally swallow before sufficiently chewing. Some foods that are potential problems are peanut butter (large clumps can stick in the throat), peanuts, popcorn, hot dogs, potato chips, hard candies, gum, grapes, and foods containing bones (e.g., beef, poultry, fish). Efforts by parents and caregivers to serve appropriate foods to young children can prevent choking incidents (Box 10.11); adults with responsibility for caring for children should know how to perform the Heimlich maneuver. Children can be reminded to chew food well and sit quietly while eating.

Lead Poisoning

Lead poisoning can be an invisible health hazard. Found in old paint dust or chips, enameled porcelain fixtures (bathtubs), soil, and water or air from industrial and transportation pollution, lead can be absorbed into the body in excessive amounts. (See Chapter 8 *Personal Perspectives* box Do Not Take Water for Granted.) Children are most at risk; they naturally absorb greater amounts of minerals than adults. Nutritional deficiencies of iron, calcium, and zinc tend to increase the absorption of lead. Lead poisoning and iron-deficiency anemia are sometimes diagnosed concurrently. Excessive exposure to lead can permanently affect cognitive and perceptual abilities. These reduced functions affect learning ability (Wessling-Resnick, 2014).

Role of Nurses

School and community nurses in higher-risk areas should be sensitive to this risk to both physical and intellectual health. Higher-risk areas for children include lower socioeconomic areas with poor housing conditions. Once lead poisoning is determined through blood testing, local health departments work with families to ascertain the sources of contamination in the home or school environment while physicians implement lead-reduction therapy.

Overall levels of lead in the environment are lower than in the past because of standards established and enforced by the Environmental Protection Agency. Levels of lead in some communities, however, are still high enough by CDC standards that primary prevention activities to further reduce lead poisoning should remain a community-wide goal.

Obesity

During childhood and adolescence, weight and height continually change. This affects the standard measurements used to assess body composition of fat and lean mass. Therefore, direct application of standards used to evaluate obesity in adults to children is inappropriate. Gender and age also affect body composition during growth. For example, during adolescence, fat redistributes differently for boys and girls. Boys gather body fat centrally around the waist, whereas girls tend to collect body fat gluteally on the lower body. Overweight may be determined as a BMI of 30 or greater and/or through skinfold measurements.

The prevalence of obesity or excessive body fat composition among American children and adolescents has grown substantially over the past 30 years. Among children aged 6 to 18 years,

BOX 10.11 Choking Prevention

Choking prevention for young children can be approached through the following measures:

1. Appropriate selection of foods based on size, shape, and texture
2. Application of prevention strategies.
3. Knowledge of the Heimlich maneuver procedures for use with children

Food Selection for Choking Prevention

Size

Both small and large pieces of food can cause choking. Small, hard pieces of food may get caught in the airway if they are swallowed before being chewed well. Larger pieces, those that are more difficult to chew, are more likely to completely block the throat. Examples include the following:

- Nuts
- Raw carrots, broccoli, and cauliflower
- Hard fruit, especially with peels, such as crisp apples

Shape

Food items shaped like a tube may cause choking because they are more likely than other shapes to completely block the throat. Examples include the following:

- Hot dogs
- Link sausage
- Whole carrots
- Grapes
- Frozen banana pieces

Texture

Foods that are firm, smooth, or slick may slide down the throat into the airway. Examples include the following:

- Hard candy
- Whole-kernel corn
- Peanuts, especially Spanish peanuts

Dry, hard foods may be hard to chew but easy to swallow whole. Examples include the following:

- Hard pretzels
- Tortilla chips
- Popcorn

Sticky foods can stick to the back or roof of the mouth and block the throat and are difficult to remove. Examples include the following:

- Nut butters alone
- Processed cheese chunks or slices
- Gummy bears
- Marshmallows
- Fruit roll-ups

Hard-to-chew foods that are fibrous and tough can present hazards. Examples include the following:

- Bagels
- Steak, roast, or other fibrous meats
- Meat jerky
- Toddler biter biscuits

Applying Prevention Strategies

Always supervise eating: Children do best when sitting to eat. It lets them concentrate on chewing and swallowing. Join the children at the table. Eating or drinking while running or playing is a distraction and can cause choking problems.

Decrease outside distractions: Reduce activities such as television, games, pets, and so on during meals and at snack times.

Cut food into bite-sized pieces or thin slices: Grind or mash tough food.

Cook food until soft, especially beans, pasta, and rice: These foods are favorites but need to be soft enough to chew easily.

Steam vegetables, such as carrots and broccoli.

Eating in cars/buses may also cause problems: It is hard for the driver to safely pull over fast enough if a child is choking.

Serve small amounts of food at a time: Keep portion sizes small. With babies, be sure the mouth is clear before giving the child another spoonful of food.

Heimlich Maneuver

Choking is fairly common. Choking deaths occur most commonly in children younger than 3 years old and in senior citizens, but they can occur at any age. The Heimlich maneuver has been valuable in saving lives and can be administered by anyone who has learned the technique.

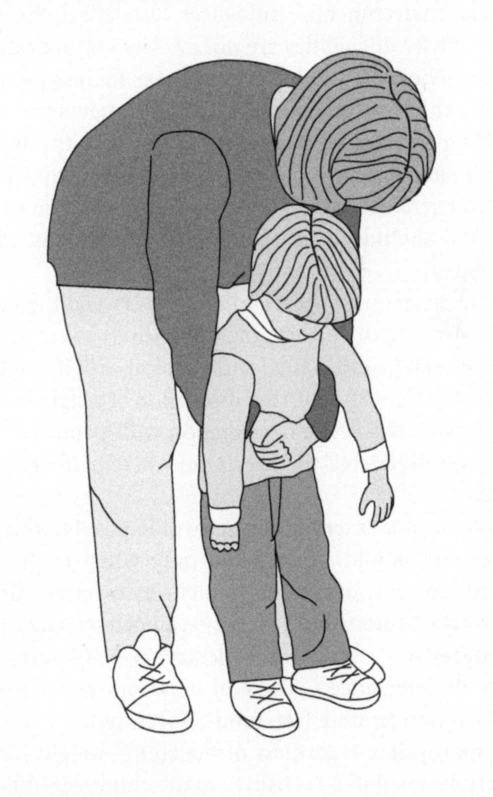

(Modified from New York State, Department of Health: *Choking Prevention for Children* New York State, Department of Health, revised 2017, Author. Accessed 4 August, 2018, from https://www.health.ny.gov/prevention/injury_prevention/choking_prevention_for_children.htm).

the proportions who were obese rose from 6% in 1980 to 17% by 2010 to about 20% in 2019. (CDC, 2019; Polsky et al., 2014). Racial, ethnic, and gender differences reveal that Black non-Hispanic American girls and Mexican American boys have been at greater risk of being overweight than other American children. Severe overweight or obesity has increased more quickly than even the increases of moderate overweight.

The etiology of these changes is not obvious but may be considered multifactorial. Eating more food as snacks and meals away from home may be a subtle factor for children and adults. These food portions are larger and higher in calories and dietary fat than those eaten at home. Another factor may be the increase in sedentary lifestyles. Physical activity has decreased, with a related decline of fitness. Although TV watching has not

TABLE 10.5 Recent Societal Changes That Affect Children's Diet and Activity Patterns

Change	Consequences
More families with working parents	Parents unable to supervise children's meals and active play
Neighborhoods and parks perceived as increasingly unsafe	Children unable to play outside without supervision
Reduced tax revenues for schools	Introduction of soft drink contracts, vending machines, fast food, and food advertising in schools
Limits on school physical education	Less play during and after school
Increased agricultural production	Increased competition for market share; promotion of more junk food directly to children
Increased demands for convenience foods	More eating occasions; more calories consumed
Greater consumption of food prepared outside the home	Larger portions; more calories consumed
Business deregulation	Unrestricted marketing to children
Television deregulation	More commercials for junk foods during children's programming
Increased use of computers	Food marketing on the Internet; more sedentary behavior
Increased media consolidation	Alliances with food companies to market to children
Increased Wall Street expectations for corporate growth	Expansion of fast-food chains, food products, and marketing to children

From Nestle M: Preventing childhood diabetes: The need for public health intervention, *Am J Public Health* 95(9):1497–1499, 2005.

increased substantially over the years, children may be more sedentary than in the past because they play video games, surf the Internet, and scroll through social media. Physical and behavioral environmental influences also affect the level of physical activity. If facilities are not available or not safe to use, physical activity is limited. Concerns over increasing numbers of latchkey children (grade-school children arriving home without adult supervision until the evening) focus on the use of food for emotional comfort and security. All these factors affect the influence of genetics, which may predispose children to heavier weights and should be considered as interventions are being contemplated.

Clinical assessment of childhood overweight consists of completing a health history, including the pattern of weight gain, emotional health status, and physical activity patterns. If BMI is greater than 30, a further discussion of weight issues may be appropriate, but first a consultation with parents or guardians may be preferable to determine whether intervention is warranted.

As with adults, intervention regarding weight with a child or adolescent should be initiated only when the patient is motivated or is experiencing weight-associative disorders. Conducting a 24-hour food intake recall provides an opportunity to engage in a discussion of dietary intake patterns such as excessive or imbalanced intake of non–nutrient-dense foods like sodas, sweets, and fast foods. (This type of discussion may be appropriate regardless of the child's weight.) Physical examinations need to be sensitive to the child regarding his or her weight and body issues. If weight is excessive, the assessment can determine whether the weight is causing physical symptoms such as sleep apnea. Morbidly obese adolescents may require a more comprehensive physical examination and intervention approaches.

T2D Mellitus

Obesity during childhood, when combined with lack of physical activity, is of significant concern as a risk factor for T2DM. Until recently, T2DM was a concern just of older adults, but with the significant increase in childhood overweight combined with lack of physical activity and poor-quality dietary intakes, the age of risk has gotten progressively younger. Risk is multidimensional because genetics and race also predispose individuals to T2DM. Asian people experience diabetes at lower body weights than people of other races; Hispanic and Black Americans appear to have diabetes in greater numbers than other ethnic groups. Increased risk is also tied to the everyday lifestyle habits often set in childhood; such habits as sedentary activities (Internet/video games/TV) and excessive fat/sweet snacking have a lasting impact on diabetes risk. As the incidence of T2DM rises among the American adult population, the behaviors that put these adults at risk are being adopted by their children (Nestle, 2005).

T2DM is almost completely preventable by a balance of energy intake with energy output. This may sound like a simple solution, but as the rates of obesity and T2DM increase among children, particularly Hispanic and African American children, societal changes seem to fuel the risk factors, creating much more complex situations. Societal changes affect family structures, educational system, communities, consumer demands, food production, and business practices, all of which affect behaviors associated with overweight and diabetes risk for all ages (Nestle, 2005). Table 10.5 lists the consequences of these changes.

Prevention efforts focus on the responsibility of the individual to reduce their risk factors for overweight and diabetes. Instead, a public health approach would be more effective. A public health approach provides community supports to ease the transition to positive health-promoting behaviors. For example, local governments could create and provide funds for after-school programs for different types of physical activities suitable for children of varying sizes and ages.

Treatment

Treatment of obesity, if warranted, must include the family. The goal is to maintain the current weight of the child while growth continues. Children should not be "dieting," but guidance can be provided to the child and caregivers as to healthier eating patterns. Education about dietary patterns such as those on the

MyPlate site and food choices to restructure dietary intake patterns may be sufficient and should be conducted by a dietitian who has the expertise to work with children and their families. The goal of treatment should not be to reach an "ideal weight" but to develop and maintain a healthy lifestyle that includes acceptance of diverse body sizes. Additional T2DM treatment concerns are discussed in Chapter 15.

Role of Nurses

Nurses support the goals of health promotion for overweight children by being sensitive to the emotional, social, and physical dimensions associated with weight and body composition. As allies, nurses create an affirming medical environment for large children through awareness of their own behavior when they conduct physical examinations, such as quietly recording weight rather than announcing weight aloud in a medical office or school setting. Pediatric offices should also have examining gowns large enough for larger pediatric patients.

Iron-Deficiency Anemia

For children, poverty is a significant risk factor for iron-deficiency anemia. Economically deprived children of inner cities are most at risk because of the dual risks of lead poisoning, which reduces the amount of iron absorbed by the body, and of chronic hunger, which limits the intake of adequate nutrients. Lead poisoning and iron deficiency each contribute to learning failure. The ability to learn is decreased because cognitive and motor abilities are altered, limiting the ability to explore, focus on, and benefit from the education environment. Poor Americans of any group are at risk, but Black American, Hispanic American, and Native American children are most likely to have inadequate intakes of iron.

Malnourished children may be developmentally delayed and unable to benefit from educational experiences. The effects of iron-deficiency anemia may begin in childhood and carry through adolescence and into adulthood, limiting the productivity and potential accomplishments of individuals.

Although iron deficiency has been recognized as a public health issue for many years, it is still a concern. It is possible that federal government programs to improve nutrition status among Americans experiencing poverty may actually work against decreasing iron deficiency. For example, the U.S. Federal Commodity Food Program releases cheese and butter to the poor. Not only are these foods high in fat, but they also are particularly poor sources of iron and may contribute to the continuing prevalence of iron deficiencies. Another contributing factor may be that in 1997 the USDA began to allow the School Lunch Program to substitute yogurt for meat/protein requirements. For the general population, the effect on iron intake may be minimal, but for economically disadvantaged children, the amount of iron consumed through school lunch servings of meat, poultry, fish, and beans is significant. The effects of chronic poverty and malnutrition are so intertwined that simple nutritional intervention will not overcome the deficits of social deprivation (Perez-Escamilla, 2014).

Role of Nurses

Nurses, particularly school nurses, can educate teaching staff about the relationship between iron deficiency and learning ability. Children may be labeled as slow learners and as having "behavior problems" in whom iron deficiency may be the true cause of learning difficulties.

NUTRITION DURING ADULTHOOD

Aging is a gradual process that reflects the influence of genetics, lifestyle, and environment over the course of the life span. The purpose of cell creation begins changing around age 30 years. No longer supplying new cells for growth and development, cell metabolism slows down and instead creates new cells to replace old cells. At older ages this process of cell replication slows even more, and the effects of aging on body organs begin to appear. Some body systems are more affected than others, and the changes may begin to affect nutritional status. Other organ functions that may be altered include taste and smell, saliva secretions, swallowing difficulties, liver function, and intestinal function. For example, the GI tract functions are diminished by reduced production of gastric juices such as hydrochloric acid, which results in decreased absorption of nutrients. The systems and the effects of aging are listed in Table 10.6.

TABLE 10.6 Effects of Aging

Effect on Nutritional Status	Cause	Organ(s) Involved
↓ Ability to taste salt and sweets	↓ Taste buds	Tongue and nose
↓ Palatability of food	↓ Taste and olfactory nerve endings	
↓ Food intake		
↓ Taste and smell		
↓ Sense of thirst/dry mouth	↓ Saliva production	Salivary glands
Minor effects on swallowing (but may progress to dysphagia)	Muscle contractions may malfunction	Esophagus (and swallowing process)
↓ Bioavailability of vitamins, minerals, proteins	↓ Hydrochloric acid (HCl) secretion and intrinsic factor	Stomach
↓ Absorption of vitamin B_{12} and folate	↓ Pepsin	Stomach
↓ Drug doses (adjustments possible to prevent overdosing)	↓ Production of drug-metabolizing enzymes	Liver

↓, Reduction in.
Data from Rosenberg, I.H. et al: Aging and the digestive system. In Munro, H.N., editors: *Nutrition, aging, and the elderly*, New York, 1989, Plenum Press.

How an individual body responds to these changes reflects health status across the life span. Consequently, everyone ages differently. The role of nutrition during the life span categories of adolescence through the middle years (40s and 50s) provides a foundation to adequately support body processes to effectively deal with the effects of lifestyle and environmental factors. Nutrient intake and dietary patterns directly influence the risk of developing the chronic disorders of osteoporosis, coronary artery disease (CAD), diabetes, hypertension, and obesity. The effect of nutrient intake, though, is mediated by lifestyle behaviors, including physical activity, stress, smoking, alcohol consumption, and exposure to environmental factors. For example, how a young woman eats and the amount of exercise she performs affects the density of her bones and the level of lean body mass of her body. If her nutrient intake is adequate and the exercise is weight bearing, she may reduce her risk of osteoporosis (as well as the risk of the other chronic disorders) decades later when she is in her 60s or 70s.

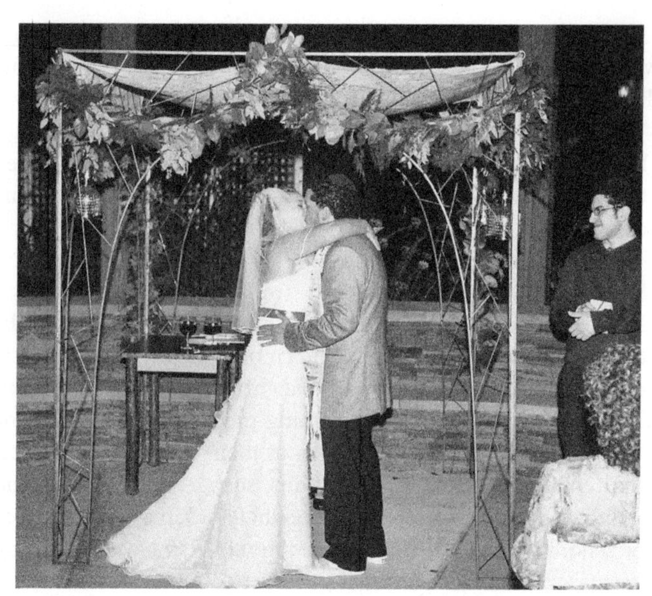

Fig. 10.8 The early years of adulthood often include the forming of long-term relationships. Copyright Jean Kallina, 2005.

Stages of Adulthood

The Early Years (20s and 30s)

Students tend to imagine that once they finish high school or college and enter the working world, they will then be able to eat better, sleep more, and generally take better care of themselves than they do during their hectic school years. Unfortunately, that is rarely the experience of young adults. Many find that their lifestyles may be even more time restricted, and positive health behaviors such as regular meal patterns and exercise may fall by the wayside.

These years mark a transition from one stage of the life span to another; young adults separate from their family of origin, focus on personal and career goals, and often face reproductive decisions (Fig. 10.8). As such, it is a prime time to either refine or establish an eating style that promotes health, possibly preventing future development of diet-related diseases. National surveys, though, continue to report that few adults consume the health-promoting recommended intakes of fruits and vegetables. A self-review or assessment by a nutrition professional can assist in creating a personal schedule that allows time for planning and preparation of simple yet high-quality meals.

Many women bear children during these years. The nutrition and health requirements of pregnancy are detailed earlier in this chapter. Layered on these needs during this life span stage are often employment and other family commitments, all of which affect nutritional and health behaviors. Physically caring for young children, although eminently rewarding, may be exhausting. Throughout the mother's pregnancy and during childbearing, the father's role in terms of health issues is often ignored. Although the woman's body is nourishing fetal development, the father is under stress as he prepares to support additional responsibilities. Fathers also need to be at optimum health, especially during the first few years of childrearing when physical stamina is put to the test.

Nutrition requirements. Growth tends to be completed by the late teens for women and early 20s for men, as reflected by the DRI. For women, the RDA for energy is 2200 kcal daily; for men, it is 2900 kcal. This reflects the typical differences in body weight and lean body mass of men and women. When this stage includes a departure from high school or college sports training, energy intake should be reduced to meet actual need, or weight gain could occur. A teenage boy's serious athletic training may require as much as 5000 to 6000 kcal/day to maintain weight. Switching to a desk job and exercising for 1 hour per day do not equal previous energy requirements.

The RDA for protein increases for women from 46 to 50 g and for men from 58 to 63 g daily; these ranges reflect lean body mass growth that may occur in both men and women through about age 24 years. Vitamin and mineral needs do not significantly change. Calcium and phosphorus needs for men and women decline after age 18 because skeletal growth is almost complete. Daily RDA recommended calcium levels up to age 18 are 1300 mg, dropping to 1000 mg from 19 years on. For phosphorus, RDA levels up to age 18 are 1250 mg/day, dropping to 700 mg from 19 years on. Maintaining calcium and iron intake continues to be a concern for women because of their often-restricted intake of food during dieting. (See also Box 7.1 or Box 8.3 regarding nutrients and their functions.)

The Middle Years (40s and 50s)

The years from 40 to 50 are marked by a continuation of family demands and career involvement. Some middle-year adults may be faced with caring for aging parents; this increased stress and responsibility may be offset by the seemingly reduced parenting of their own children. As older children leave for college or move into their own residences, the resultant "empty nest" necessitates rediscovering preparation of dinners for two or, for single parents, dinners for one. With family meals no longer a requirement, many middle-year adults often have the finances and time for restaurant dining. However, making the transition to food preparation styles and dietary patterns that maintain healthful dietary patterns is crucial.

The impact of continued positive dietary patterns coupled with regular exercise provides continued prevention or delay of diet-related diseases such as T2DM and CAD. Increased stamina is an additional benefit of such behaviors.

Nutrition requirements. During the middle years, cell loss rather than replication occurs. Kcal needs decline as lean body mass is lost and replaced by body fat, which is less metabolically active. Women in particular experience an increase in body fat composition. Body fat increases can be slowed by exercise and strength training to continue maintenance of lean body mass. After age 50 years, daily energy needs drop from 2200 to 1920 kcal for women and from 2900 to 2300 kcal for men. It is a challenge to meet the same nutrient needs with reduced kcal intake. Protein needs remain constant for both genders. Iron requirements for women drop from 18 to 8 mg, which reflects reduced iron loss because of menopause. (See also Box 7.1 or Box 8.3 regarding nutrients and their functions.)

Overall, dietary patterns that are nutrient dense and feature lower-fat protein foods coupled with fiber-containing fruits, vegetables, and grains best meet the nutrient needs of middle-year adults.

The Older Years (60 s, 70 s, and 80 s)

The United States has never had a population with as high a percentage of older adults as it has now. As our life span increases in years, senescence (older adulthood) is for many people a time of life for continued professional or career advancement and recreational enjoyment. Others are in transition, adjusting to retirement and settling into new patterns of activities. Gerontology, the study of aging, has provided insights into the emotional, physical, and social aspects of the later years of life. Preparation for the social and physical transitions of aging actually begins many years earlier, as individual approaches to lifestyle health behaviors, career fulfillment, and leisurely pursuits evolve.

Overall, quality of life for older adults depends on factors that influence daily experiences. These factors include health status; nutritional well-being; spirituality; living arrangements; physical activity; social interactions; physical, mental, and emotional functioning; disease management; and level of financial and physical independence. The level of wellness experienced during this stage of life often reflects the quality of life resulting from health behaviors through the several life span stages.

Physical activity. A lifetime of physical fitness and good nutrition allows an individual to enter these years with more stamina, cardiovascular conditioning, and solid health-promoting habits, which enable them to overcome the inevitable slowing down or physical limitation of the later years. Even those who were not always active have been found to benefit from regular exercise. Strength training has improved the muscle tone and stamina of older men and women.

Physical, mental, and emotional functioning. During these later years, individuals may struggle with the deaths of family members and friends and adjustment to retirement. Although some delight in retirement, others view it as a loss of social status. This combination of death and loss of status may lead to isolation and depression, resulting in loss of appetite (anorexia) or other forms of malnutrition. The economic realities of retirement without a solid financial base may thrust some older adults into unexpected poverty, because Social Security and Medicare payments may not be sufficient to cover living and medical expenses. Resources for food purchases may be limited and may negatively affect nutritional status. Unless social networking and family supports are strong, these conditions may persist. Older adults may abuse alcohol as a way to deal with these perceived difficult events.

BOX 10.12 Signs of Dehydration in Older Adults

Confusion
Weakness
A hot, dry body
Furrowed tongue
Decreased skin turgor (may not be valid finding in older adults)
Rapid pulse
Elevated urinary sodium

Disorientation or senility often associated with aging may be caused by improper use of medications, marginal nutrient deficiencies (e.g., vitamin B_{12}), or simple dehydration. Older clients may intentionally restrict fluid intake because of incontinence, nocturia (excessive urination at night), or the inability to get to the toilet on their own. Some older adults lose their sense of thirst and forget to consume enough fluids. Fluid requirements in older adults remain the same as in younger adults (about 8 cups daily is sufficient) unless a medical condition or medication prescribes otherwise. The signs of dehydration are listed in Box 10.12. Medical diagnosis should be sought to determine the specific etiology of these signs.

Nutritional well-being. Nutritional status of older adults may be affected by restrictions in access to food and ability to prepare meals. Shopping may be difficult without transportation, and mobility to walk through stores may be limited. Funds for food may be constrained, and often food quantities available are beyond the amounts that can be used by individuals living alone (Fig. 10.9). Once foods are purchased, preparation may be affected by physical limitations caused by progressive chronic illnesses such as arthritis. Some older adults may no longer have an interest in cooking. Others have become so frightened about foods containing too much fat or cholesterol that they become malnourished. For individuals in this age bracket, there is not sufficient evidence to warrant restrictive dietary intake; in actuality, malnutrition and underweight are more detrimental than excess dietary fat and cholesterol intake. Box 10.13 lists risks factors for malnutrition in older adults.

Dietary management for older adults may be more complicated than for other stages of adulthood. For younger adults, reducing BMI decreases health risks. For older adults, decreased BMI may be associated with increased risk of strokes. Having an average BMI provides healthful weight reserves during times of illness (Chapman, 2010). Studies of weight reduction strategies seldom include older participants, so their complex physiologic, behavioral, and social needs are not considered.

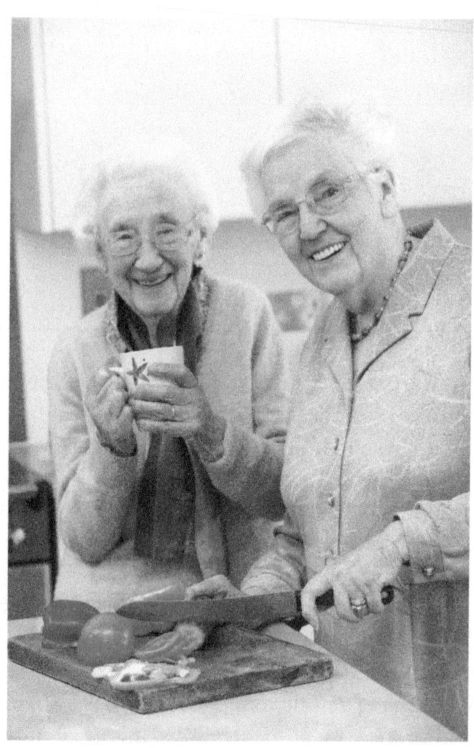

Fig. 10.9 Socializing around food preparation assists with the adjustments of the older years. (From www.thinkstockphotos.com)

BOX 10.13 Risk Factors for Malnutrition in Older Adults

- Alcoholism
- Anorexia
- Chewing and swallowing problems (dysphagia)
- Consuming only one meal a day
- Dental difficulties
- Depression or dementia
- Diabetes
- Diminished physical functioning
- Feeding problems
- Food purchasing/preparation difficulties
- Impaired acuity of taste and smell
- Living in long-term care institution
- Loss of spouse
- Taking multiple medications
- Nerve disorders
- Poverty
- Pulmonary disease
- Surgery

Data from Chernoff, R. Nutrition and health promotion in older adults, *J Gerontol A Biol Sci Med Sci* 56(Spec 2[2]):47–53, 2001; copyright the Gerontological Society of America.

Additionally, such strategies may overly limit intake of essential nutrients, further worsening malnutrition.

Another aspect of older adult dietary management is protein adequacy. Total body protein decreases as aging progresses. Although the loss of skeletal muscle is the most noticeable body protein lost, organ tissue, blood components, and immune bodies are also affected, leading to compromised wound healing, loss of skin elasticity, reduced ability to battle infection, and longer recuperation from illness and surgeries (Chernoff, 2004). Dietary intake may be further altered when these physical factors combine with social factors, leading to reduced protein intake. Consumption of micronutrients found in protein foods also may be limited, leading to deficiencies of vitamins B_{12}, A, C, and D, calcium, iron, zinc, and others. Frail elderly women are most at risk for these micronutrient deficiencies. This need, combined with the greater turnover of whole-body protein in aging bodies, results in a need for greater dietary protein intake in older adults. Protein consumption may be improved by consumption of 30 g of protein per meal (Paddon-Jones & Leidy, 2014).

Living arrangements. Living arrangements also affect nutritional status. A variety of living arrangements exists for older adults. Although many continue to live in their own homes or with family members, some opt for retirement communities, and others, because of health conditions, may reside in long-term care facilities or nursing homes. Living in one's own home provides the freedom to prepare and eat foods whenever desired; illness, however, may make shopping for and preparing food difficult. Retirement communities may provide transportation to food stores and more social events involving meals (see Fig. 10.10), although residents may still be responsible for their own food preparation. Long-term care facilities usually provide prepared meals, but the style of cooking may not be as appealing or comforting as home-prepared meals.

A challenge for meeting the nutritional needs of institutionalized older adults is that the DRIs used to guide nutrient levels are intended to meet the needs of healthy older adults. Adjustments are necessary for individual circumstances of acute or chronic illness to achieve rehabilitation, recuperation, or maintenance to reduce the risk of further complications. Consequently, it is now recommended that diets in long-term care facilities be liberalized to improve dietary intake of this age group (Kuczmarski et al., 2005).

Dietary patterns and preferences of older adults are the result of long-established habits. When they are ill, lonely, or under stress, older adults may strongly prefer foods they associate with pleasant memories. Ethnic favorites may provide security and comfort. The psychologic and social meanings of foods can play an important part in helping an older client recover from illness or adjust to changed circumstances.

Demographic and lifestyle characteristics may, as noted, put older adults at nutritional risk. Factors may include gender, smoking, alcohol abuse, dietary patterns, educational level, dental health, chronic illnesses, and living situations. Interventions to assist older adults must account for these influences and should view support services through a continuum of care. Continuum of care provides continuity of care while the older individual moves through different living situations, and services such as health, medical, and supportive services are provided in suitable care environments. Care settings may range from acute medical settings to community and daycare, from assisted-living retirement housing to traditional nursing home facilities and hospices.

PERSONAL PERSPECTIVES

Settling into a New Home

When 80-year-old Yetta Kaemmer moved to an adult independent living community after living in her own home, she made some adjustments, including eating meals with others every day in the congregate dining room, no longer needing to even cook for herself.

It's like living in a hotel. I don't have to cook, and I always have someone to eat with. Every morning I go to the dining room for breakfast. It's good to be dressed and have a schedule to follow. By the time breakfast is over, you forget about the aches and pains you woke up with. For lunch I have something in my refrigerator to eat, or I may go out. Before dinner I relax by watching television. Then I always freshen my makeup and go to the dining room to eat at my assigned table with three others. When new people arrive, they sometimes feel awkward until they get to know others, especially when entering the dining room for dinner, because everyone seems to know each other. After dinner, there is often a program to attend.

Although we are served balanced meals, we actually eat more food than before, because we have full dinners every night. There are always choices of appetizers, main dishes, and desserts. You get to choose. And so most of us have put on a few pounds! I don't really miss cooking. Sometimes, though, I will feel a twinge in the supermarket when I see the ingredients of favorite meals I used to prepare. I made a really good meatloaf and, for company, Cornish hens each with a pineapple ring and cherry. Oh, they would look so nice!

Yetta Kaemmer
Teaneck, NJ

Nutrition requirements. The DRIs remain constant from age 51 years and older for men and women, except for vitamin D. What does change is the ability of the body to either process or synthesize certain nutrients. Synthesis of vitamin D is reduced; the RDA for vitamin D for individuals older than age 70 increases to 20 μg/day, up from 15 μg/day for those aged 51 to 70 years. Older adults either need more exposure to sunlight to produce required amounts of vitamin D or require a supplement if so diagnosed by a physician, qualified nutritionist, or dietitian. Because of decreased production of gastric juices and intestinal enzymes, digestion and absorption may be reduced, further highlighting the need for optimum nutrient intake. The production of the intrinsic factor required for vitamin B_{12} absorption also may be reduced, increasing the risk of pernicious anemia. New recommendations suggest the use of vitamin B_{12} supplements or consumption of foods fortified with vitamin B_{12} to meet the RDA of 2.4 μg/day. (See also Box 7.1 or Box 8.3 regarding the functions of nutrients.)

Other factors may affect nutritional status. A marginal deficiency of zinc can alter the sensitivity of taste receptors. This deficiency heightens the ability to taste bitter and sour flavors and reduces sweet and salty sensations; excessive use of sugars and salt to make foods taste appealing may result.

Overconsumption of simple sugars and sodium may exacerbate other diet-related disorders, such as diabetes and hypertension. As the muscularity of the digestive system weakens, constipation may be a problem, especially after a lifetime of low-fiber foods. Constipation may be alleviated by slowly increasing consumption of whole-wheat products, fruits, vegetables, and fluids as well as increasing exercise.

Dental health may also affect the ability of older adults to be well nourished. Loss of teeth caused by periodontal disease limits the ability to chew foods such as meats, a prime source of zinc. For some, chewing ability may still be compromised after dentures have been fitted to replace missing teeth. Dentures may need to be periodically refitted. When dentures do not fit properly, some people do not use them. Instead, they tend to eat foods that can be gummed rather than chewed.

The Oldest Years (80s and 90s)

As life expectancy increases in years, the number of those in the most golden years rises. Although nutrient needs remain basically stable after age 80 years, the effects of aging may continue to reduce the ability of the body to absorb and synthesize nutrients. Optimum nutrition continues to be critical. The healthiest of the oldest develop individual patterns of dietary intake that most meet their physical and social needs.

Nutrition requirements. Malnutrition and being underweight become a concern during this stage (see Box 10.13). As food preparation becomes more physically difficult to accomplish, kcal intake may diminish. Illness and accompanying medications may reduce appetite; malnutrition is associated with increased complications. Relatives, friends, and health care professionals can assist in ensuring that adequate meals are available and consumed (Box 10.14). Those in the oldest years may be most at risk for dehydration. Particularly at risk are Black Americans and men. Risk rises because of decreased ability of the kidneys to concentrate urine, limited movement, drug interactions, and malfunctioning thirst sensation. Limited ability to move may increase fears of incontinence that lead to decreased fluid intake. Nearly half of older adults hospitalized as Medicare patients experience dehydration (Kuczmarski et al., 2005). (See also Box 7.1 or Box 8.3 regarding functions of nutrients.)

Older adults may be at risk for asphyxiation of food because of reduced chewing ability from loss of teeth or poorly fitting dentures. Neurologic conditions such as Parkinson's disease and effects of stroke may result in chewing and swallowing difficulties (dysphagia) that may cause asphyxiation (see Chapter 19). Counseling older adults about problematic foods may avert asphyxiation. Referrals to a registered dietitian/nutritionist with expertise in these disorders should be considered.

Although assessment is the responsibility of all health care professionals, home health nurses are particularly able to conduct routine nutrition screening and implement appropriate interventions to prevent or halt malnutrition among this population. Government and community meal programs help fill this need and are discussed later in the section on community supports.

NUTRITION HEALTH PROMOTION: ADULTHOOD

Knowledge

Health promotion integrates nutrition education and focuses on three areas of knowledge: (1) adequate intake of nutrients found in foods (rather than supplements), (2) the relationship between diet and disease, and (3) moderate kcal intake

BOX 10.14 Strategies for Overcoming Barriers to Good Nutrition

Counteract Decreased Senses of Taste and Smell

Recommend that smokers refrain from smoking at least 1 hour before meals.
Suggest sipping water before and during the meal to moisten a dry mouth.
Amplify flavors with the use of seasonings other than salt.
Recommend chewing food thoroughly to fully release flavor and aroma.
Vary food textures and flavors.

Encourage Social Interaction

Find others who are willing to share food preparation and mealtimes.
Investigate congregate meal programs available through senior citizen centers, religious organizations, and hospital community outreach programs.
Avoid noisy dining areas for people with hearing aids.

Present Food Attractively

Use colorful foods and table settings.
Provide enough lighting to see food clearly.

Provide Outside Support

Arrange for Meals on Wheels for homebound adults.
Refer eligible clients to the Supplemental Nutrition Assistance Program (SNAP), Emergency Food Assistance Program, Child and Adult Care Program, or community food banks or soup kitchens.
Locate grocery stores with delivery service.
Refer to the Expanded Food and Nutrition Education Program (EFNEP) of the Cooperative Extension Service for recipes, meal suggestions, and budgeting assistance.
Refer clients to home health nurse for routine nutrition screening and appropriate interventions.

coupled with regular exercise for physical fitness and obesity prevention.

Techniques

Many strategies can be used for adult health promotion:

1. To reduce risk of diet-related disorders such as coronary heart disease, some cancers, T2DM, and obesity, consider:
   - Scheduling routine food shopping so staples such as fruits, vegetables, and grains are available for meal preparation.
   - When shopping, occasionally comparing fat content of commonly purchased foods with that of similar products and purchasing the lower-fat product.
   - Aiming to limit foods that contain visible fat.
   - Reorganizing work and personal priorities if necessary to allow time for meal preparation and consumption; for example, get up earlier for breakfast, pack a lunch or afternoon snack, preplan easy-to-prepare dinner menus.
   - Keeping track of dietary intake using MyPlate resources (www.myplate.gov) such as the Start Simple with MyPlate App (www.myplate.gov/resources/tools/start-simple-myplate-app). Utilize the resources of Have a Plant (https://fruitsandveggies.org/) from the Produce for Better Health Foundation. Review Chapter 5 for other dietary fat–lowering techniques and Chapter 4 for approaches that increase the use of complex carbohydrates and fiber-containing foods.
2. To reduce osteoporosis risk and strengthen bone health, consider:
   - Focusing on routine dietary habits—for example, drink a glass of milk at lunch each day. A food pattern assessment can assist in creating a practical calcium consumption plan.
   - Reviewing Chapter 8 for other approaches to increasing calcium consumption.
3. To decrease the risk of sodium-sensitive hypertension and CAD, consider:
   - Adopting the DASH (Dietary Approach to Stop Hypertension) eating plan, which focuses on increasing intake of fruits and vegetables. See Chapter 17 for more details.
   - Learning the food categories that are generally salty, and either consume them only occasionally or, if available, purchase low-sodium versions. See Chapter 17 for other sodium-reducing strategies.
   - Reducing overall intake of fat, particularly saturated fat, while increasing consumption of health-promoting "good" fats such as monounsaturated and polyunsaturated fats found naturally in whole foods.
4. To achieve a healthy body weight and decrease the possibility of diet- and lifestyle-related obesity, consider:
   - Responding to actual hunger with low-fat, high-fiber foods (with occasional splurges) rather than focusing on dietary restrictions.
   - Exercising regularly to increase stamina, strength, and a sense of wellness. Depending on conditioning, incorporate exercise gradually. A 10-minute walk may be comfortable for some, but others can begin with more strenuous endeavors.
   - Consulting Chapter 9 for related strategies. (See also the *Cultural Diversity and Nutrition* box Live Long and Prosper … the Okinawa Way!)

Community Supports

Government, corporate, and social institutions create the environments and structures that can support lifestyle health promotion behaviors. Although the actions of these institutions affect particular groups of the public, employees, or communities, it is the individual who can choose to reap the rewards.

Government agencies such as the U.S. Food and Drug Administration (FDA) create regulations that either provide consumer information for decision making (e.g., nutrition labeling) or control the quality of foods, which in turn affects the nutrient viability of manufactured products.

In New York City, an ordinance was passed that requires restaurants and food chains with 10 or more locations to post the nutrient content of foods served. This information may be posted on signs, as in fast-food restaurants, or on menus in traditional restaurants. Whether this requirement will influence consumer choices is yet to be determined, but at least it makes the possibility of informed decision making available. A similar requirement is to be implemented nationally but the date of implementation is still under consideration. Ordinances banning the use of artificial *trans* fats in the preparation of foods for direct consumption by consumers in restaurants and other food outlets have been implemented in several cities in the United States. The FDA has removed artificial *trans* fat from the generally recognized as safe (GRAS) list of ingredients because of its effect on blood cholesterol levels. Any use of *trans* fat would then be as a food additive requiring specific regulations to allow for its use.

Corporations can support health promotion activities by offering comprehensive employee health promotion programs to their employees. This can be accomplished through wellness centers providing programs about healthy lifestyles. Although most corporations may not be able to provide on-site gyms or similar facilities, some have arranged for corporate discounts at local gym facilities.

Government agencies and community groups provide socioeconomic support within the community. Government programs include SNAP, The Emergency Food Assistance Program (TEFAP), and community food banks and meals. Boosting people's food purchasing power improves their overall nutrient intake. SNAP is administered nationally by the USDA and on the state and local levels by welfare or human services agencies. The federal government pays the actual food assistance costs; administration costs are divided among the other agencies.

As an entitlement program, SNAP is available to all who are eligible without restriction of age or family size. Financial and nonfinancial factors of households are considered to determine eligibility. Financial factors include income and economic resources, such as savings and vehicles; nonfinancial considerations consist of a variety of factors, such as social security eligibility, citizenship, and work requirements. Gross incomes must meet certain percentages of the poverty level on the basis of overall factors; the level of support varies according to family membership and net income (USDA, 2021).

The Food and Nutrition Service of the USDA administers TEFAP. Various local agencies may administer the program. State agencies determine their own criteria for eligibility based on household income. The program serves two functions: to reduce government-held surplus dairy commodities and to supplement the dietary intake of low-income households through the distribution of basic commodities. The types of foods distributed vary between actual surplus foods and foods purchased especially for this program. In addition to dairy products such as nonfat dry milk and cheese, TEFAP has distributed canned meat, peanut butter, citrus juices, legumes, dried potatoes, and canned and dried fruit. Some of this program's funds are used by states to fund emergency feeding programs such as soup kitchens and food banks (USDA, 2021).

Community food banks and emergency feeding programs may be partially funded by TEFAP in addition to support from foundations and other charitable organizations (Fig. 10.10). Some programs also collect food from the surrounding community and surplus donations from supermarkets and restaurants. Personnel at these facilities are usually volunteers from youth groups, religious organizations, and civic associations. Food banks often provide a bag of food staples to help bridge the gap that may occur when food stamps and monthly welfare support are exhausted before the beginning of the next month. Emergency feeding programs such as soup kitchens may provide hot meals as a safety net to help individuals of lower socioeconomic populations avoid malnutrition.

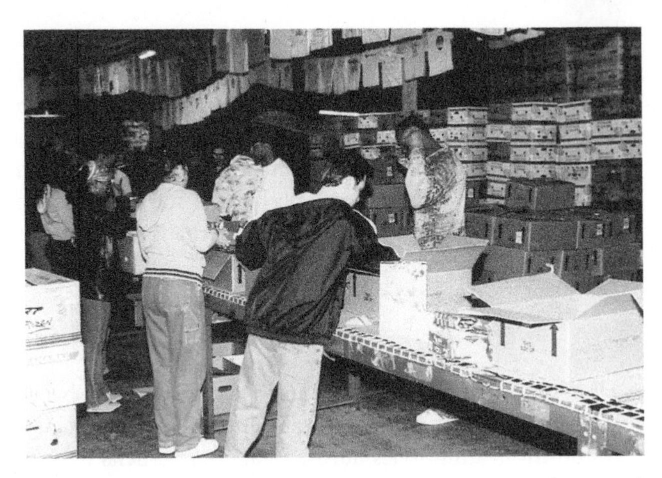

Fig. 10.10 Food bank volunteers sorting foods. (Courtesy Community Food Bank of New Jersey, Hillside, NJ.)

Other USDA supports specifically for older adults are the Child and Adult Care Food Program and the Senior Nutrition Program. Community groups may sponsor some of the government programs or may develop their own local programs.

The Child and Adult Care Food Program provides meals and snacks for children up to age 12 years and to senior citizens and specific categories of handicapped people participating in daycare programs that are nonprofit, licensed, or receive agency approval. Reimbursement rates differ for programs that serve children and adults. Family income of the participants may be considered. Like other programs, it is administered on the federal level by the Food and Nutrition Service of the USDA and on the state level by human services or education departments. Adult daycare programs may be administered locally by a variety of community sponsors. For children, eligible programs include Head Start, after-school programs, and family daycare (USDA, 2021).

The Senior Nutrition Program serves only older adults and was created to offer inexpensive meals, education, and socialization. The Congregate Meals Program and Home-Delivered Meals Program are both part of the Senior Nutrition Program. This program provides for those in financial need as well as those in social need. Eligibility is open to everyone 60 years or older; spouses of participants may also be served regardless of their age. To participate in the Home-Delivered Meals Program, individuals must reside in the program service area and be unable to prepare their own meals. Meals are generally provided Monday through Friday. Those receiving meals at home may also be given frozen meals for weekend consumption (USDA, 2021). Distribution of meals varies among programs.

TOWARD A POSITIVE NUTRITION LIFESTYLE: RATIONALIZING

Rationalization is one of the psychologic defense mechanisms used to protect our sense of self when we are under stress. When our behaviors, feelings, or perceptions are irrational or unreasonable, we may use rationalization to assign reasonable explanations to ourselves as to why we behaved as we did.

For example, from adolescence on through the older years, some individuals rationalize their poor eating habits. The list of reasonable explanations may include not enough time to prepare better meals, lack of knowledge about nutrition, and lack of cooking skills. Although these may be reasonable explanations, they do not help improve nutritional status. Often these types of rationalizations make it harder to change unproductive behaviors.

Consider the same explanations in a more positive way:

- Not enough time to prepare better meals but can reorganize schedule to create time.
- Lack of knowledge about nutrition or of cooking skills but can take a nutrition or cooking course or read books on nutrition and use simple cookbooks to learn basic skills.
- Instead of continuing negative rationalization, positive rationalization may provide the means to change.

SUMMARY

- The importance of nutrition during pregnancy, the benefits of breastfeeding, and the establishment and maintenance of positive eating styles during infancy are crucial to overall health goals.
- Lactation is a natural, physiologic process beginning shortly after delivery and completing the cycle of the female body from pregnancy through motherhood.
  - Human milk is the best health promoter for the neonate.
  - Breastfeeding should begin immediately after birth and continue every 2 to 3 hours during the initial postpartum weeks.
  - Lactating women should continue to consume a diet with adequate sources of protein, energy, vitamins, and minerals.
- Sound nutrition practices during the first year of life lay the foundation for good health.
  - The ideal food for the first 4 to 6 months of life is breast milk.
  - Supplemental foods may be introduced one at a time at 4 to 6 months of age.
  - Feeding of breast milk (or formula) should continue until the infant reaches 1 year of age.
- Children with medical problems may require specialized nutrition support.
- Psychologic and physiologic maturation reflect life span stages: childhood (ages 1 through 12), adolescence (ages 13 through 19), and adulthood.
- Health promotion depends on knowledge, techniques, and community supports.
  - Approaches to health promotion take into account these stages and their effect on nutrient requirements, eating styles, food choices, and supports from the larger community.
- Barriers to health promotion during childhood and adolescence may include food asphyxiation, lead poisoning, overweight/diabetes, and iron-deficiency anemia.
- The role of nutrition in each of the adult life span categories reflects the value of adequate nutrient intake to reduce the risk of chronic disorders of such as osteoporosis, coronary artery disease, diabetes mellitus, hypertension, and obesity.
- During the early years (20 s and 30 s), establishment of positive health behaviors is desirable because these years are the childbearing and childrearing years, with health implications for both women and men.
- The middle years (40 s and 50 s) are years of career and family demands. Chronic diet-related diseases, such as T2D mellitus and cerebrovascular disease, may occur during these years. Positive dietary and exercise behaviors may provide protection. Nutrient needs for women change as menopause occurs. In particular, adequate calcium consumption is recommended to offset loss of bone density.
- The older years (60 s, 70 s, and 80 s) are most reflective of lifestyle behaviors practiced over many years, although psychosocial issues may affect adequacy of nutrient intake.
- During the oldest years (80 s and 90 s), malnutrition and underweight bodies are of concern.

THE NURSING APPROACH: CLINICAL JUDGMENT AND NEXT-GENERATION NCLEX® EXAMINATION-STYLE QUESTIONS

Case Study 1

Breastfeeding

Rebecca, aged 24 years, delivered her first child 2 days before meeting with the nurse practitioner. She said she and the baby boy, Bobby, were doing well, but she had some questions about breastfeeding.

Assessment/Recognize Cues

Subjective (From Patient Statements)

- "He nurses OK and seems happy, although he wants to eat every 2 hours."
- "My nipples are not sore, but I feel really tired."
- "I plan to keep breastfeeding until Bobby is about 6 months old. I like the closeness I feel to him."
- "I'm wondering what to do about feeding when I need to leave the baby with my husband for a few hours."
- "How do I know if Bobby is getting enough to eat?"

Objective (From Physical Examination)

- Birth weight 7 pounds 10 ounces and length 19.7 inches
- Newborn at fiftieth percentile for weight and length
- Loose yellow stool and light-yellow urine in diaper

Diagnoses (Nursing)/Analyze Cues

1. Effective breastfeeding as evidenced by the mother's statement that the newborn infant "nurses OK and seems happy," the fact that the newborn is at fiftieth percentile for weight and height, and the loose yellow stool and light-yellow urine in infant's diaper.
2. Need for health teaching as evidenced by questions about saving milk and evaluating adequacy of milk intake.

Continued

THE NURSING APPROACH: CLINICAL JUDGMENT AND NEXT-GENERATION NCLEX® EXAMINATION-STYLE QUESTIONS—cont'd

Planning/Prioritize Cues

Patient Outcomes

Short term (at the end of this visit):

- Rebecca will state how to determine whether the infant is eating enough.
- She will demonstrate how to express milk and state how to save milk for the infant for times when she cannot breastfeed.
- She will identify resources for continued success with breastfeeding.

Long term (follow-up visit after 4 weeks):

- The infant will continue to gain weight to stay in the fiftieth percentile for weight and length.
- Rebecca will say she is satisfied with breastfeeding.

Nursing Interventions/Generate Outcomes

1. Assess Rebecca's feelings about breastfeeding.
2. Discuss nutrition requirements for breastfeeding and promote a healthy lifestyle.
3. Educate Rebecca on the benefits of breastfeeding, how to express and store breast milk, and how to determine whether the infant is getting enough milk.
4. Provide resources for Rebecca.

Implementation/Take Action

1. Assessed Rebecca's feelings and attitudes about breastfeeding.
   The nurse can accept and support a woman's decision to breastfeed or bottle feed. If the mother is not successful with breastfeeding, the nurse can try to help her. If the mother is not happy with breastfeeding, the nurse should present her with the alternate choice of using formula in bottles.
2. Encouraged drinking at least 3000 mL of water, milk, and juices per day, and eating a well-balanced diet per recommendations from ChooseMyPlate.gov.
   Adequate hydration, adequate nutrients, and extra kcal (~500 kcal more than usual) are needed to support lactation and the health of the mother. Alcohol and caffeine should be avoided because they can be secreted in the breast milk.
3. Reviewed benefits of breastfeeding.
   It is rewarding for the mother to know that the infant may have fewer infections, fewer allergies, and easier digestion with breast milk. In addition, it is usually more convenient and economical to breastfeed rather than bottle feed.
4. Discussed how to express breast milk and save it in a bottle.
   Milk may be expressed manually or with a pump. It needs to be saved in a bottle in the refrigerator (up to 48 hours) or in the freezer (several months). Cleanliness and good hand washing are essential to preventing infection.
5. Discussed how to determine whether the infant is getting enough milk.
   Breastfeeding should be done on a demand schedule, and the infant should generally be content after eating. At least six wet diapers and one bowel movement per day indicate adequate hydration and milk. Weight gain should follow a standard growth chart.
6. Provided literature about breastfeeding and La Leche League support groups, and wrote down a contact number for the clinic.
   Written materials reinforce learning. Contacts and support personnel are helpful when questions arise about breastfeeding.

Evaluation/Evaluate Outcomes

Short term (at the end of the first visit):

- Rebecca identified how to determine whether the infant is getting enough milk.
- She demonstrated how to express milk and stated how she can save milk.
- She said she might contact someone from La Leche support group.

Goals met.

Long term (in 1 month):

- Infant gained weight and remained in fiftieth percentile for height and weight.
- Rebecca reported her satisfaction and infant's contentment after breastfeeding.
- She reported that infant has a bowel movement with each feeding and urinates several times a day.
- Rebecca said she rented a breast pump and was able to save enough milk to go on a date with her husband while the grandmother cared for the infant.

Goals met.

Discussion Questions

At the follow-up visit, Rebecca said she was drinking a lot of diet cola to increase her fluid intake and production of breast milk. She was restricting her calorie intake so that she could quickly lose the 25 pounds she needed to lose to get back to prepregnancy weight. She would like to begin introducing solid foods into the infant's diet but is not sure what foods to start with or whether Bobby is ready.

1. Role-play a conversation the nurse could have with Rebecca about her fluid intake and her restriction of calories.
2. How soon should Rebecca add solid food to the infant's diet? What food may be tolerated best?

Case Study 2

A nurse is caring for a pregnant client in the gynecologist's office. The client has been diagnosed with gestational diabetes mellitus. She is normally in good health and lives with her husband. The client is very concerned about this condition. She asks the nurse, "How did I get this?"

What are some of the risk factors the nurse shares with the client?

Highlight the correct risk factors for gestational diabetes mellitus. Select all that apply.

1. Obesity
2. Younger than 25 years of age
3. European heritage
4. Young maternal age
5. Recurrent infections
6. No history of gestational diabetes in previous pregnancies
7. Previous newborn weighed less than 9 pounds
8. In previous pregnancy, child having a congenital malformation or birth defect and/or unexplained death of fetus

APPLYING CONTENT KNOWLEDGE

Elena, age 18 years, is a client at the city Special Supplemental Nutrition Program for Women, Infants, and Children (WIC); she is beginning her third trimester of pregnancy. She attended nutrition education classes taught by the WIC nutritionist. The nutritionist, though, is concerned because Elena has not been gaining sufficient weight to support her pregnancy although she is otherwise healthy. The nutritionist suspects that Elena does not understand the relationship between her dietary intake and the health of her fetus. The nutritionist asks you as a WIC nurse to reinforce these concepts when Elena comes in for her monthly checkups. What will you discuss with Elena?

WEBSITES OF INTEREST

Black Mothers' Breastfeeding Association
blackmothersbreastfeeding.org/
Advocates breastfeeding success for black families through creation of foundational networks of direct service and education, leading to reduction of racial inequities and multigenerational breastfeeding support and encouragement.

KidsHealth
www.kidshealth.org
Provides information for children, teens, and parents on health, food, and fitness, including games and colorful animations.

Office of Minority Health and Health Disparities (OMHD)
www.cdc.gov/omhd
Aims to eradicate health disparities for vulnerable and at-risk populations and to maximize the health impact of the Centers for Disease Control and Prevention (CDC) on the U.S. population.

National Women's Health Information Center
www.womenshealth.gov
Functions as a single point of entry for federal and private sector sources on women's health issues; created by the Office on Women's Health, U.S. Department of Health and Human Services.

REFERENCES

American Academy of Pediatrics (AAP). (2012). Policy statement on breastfeeding and the use of human milk. *Pediatrics, 129*(3), e827–e841.

Bitler, P. M., & Currie, J. (2005). Does WIC work? The effects of WIC on pregnancy and birth outcomes. *Journal of Policy Analysis and Management: [the Journal of the Association for Public Policy Analysis and Management], 24*(1), 73–91.

Centers for Disease Control and Prevention (CDC). (2019) Childhood Nutrition Facts, rev 29 May. From: www.cdc.gov/healthyschools/nutrition/facts.htm#:~:text=Americans%20do%20not%20meet%20federal%20dietary%20recommendations. (Accessed 5 January, 2021).

Centers for Disease Control and Prevention (CDC). (2019) Childhood Obesity Facts, rev 24 June. From Childhood Obesity Facts. Overweight & Obesity. CDC. (Accessed 5 January, 2021).

Centers for Disease Control and Prevention (CDC). (2020). *Breastfeeding: Human Immunodeficiency*, rev 4 February. From Human Immunodeficiency Virus (HIV), Breastfeeding, CDC. Accessed (1 January, 2021).

Chapman, I. M. (2010). Obesity paradox during aging. *Interdisciplinary Topics in Gerontology, 37*, 20–36.

Chernoff, R. (2004). Protein and older adults. *Journal of the American College of Nutrition, 23*(6 Suppl), 627S–630S.

Ebrahim, G. J. (1993). The baby-friendly hospital initiative. *Journal of Tropical Pediatrics, 39*, 2.

Elsas, L. J., II, & Acosta, P. B. (2014). Inherited metabolic diseases: Amino acids, organic acids, and galactose. In A. C. Ross (Ed.), *Modern nutrition in health and disease* (11th ed.). Philadelphia: Lippincott Williams & Wilkins.

Ely, D.M., et al. (2018). Infant mortality by age at death in the United States, 2016, NCHS Data Brief No.326.

Erick, M. (2012). Nutrition during pregnancy and lactation. In L. K. Mahan (Ed.), *Krause's food & the nutrition care process* (13th ed.). Philadelphia: Saunders.

Food Research & Action Center (FRAC). (2019) School Meals are Essential for Student Health and Learning. From: School-Meals-are-Essential-Health-and-Learning_FNL.pdf (frac.org). (Accessed 3 January, 2021).

Food Research & Action Center (FRAC). (2020). School breakfast scorecard school year 2018–2019. From: Breakfast-Scorecard-2018-2019_FNL.pdf (frac.org). (Accessed 3 January, 2021).

Heird, W. C. (2014). Nutritional requirements of infants and children. In A. C. Ross (Ed.), *Modern nutrition in health and disease* (11th ed.). Philadelphia: Lippincott Williams & Wilkins.

Krebs-Smith, S. M., et al. (2010). Americans do not meet federal dietary recommendations. *The Journal of Nutrition, 140*, 1832–1838.

Krugman, S. D., & Dubowitz, H. (2003). Failure to thrive. *American Family Physician, 68*(5), 879–884.

Kuczmarski, M. F., et al. (2005). Position paper of the American Dietetic Association: Nutrition across the spectrum of aging. *Journal of the American Dietetic Association, 105*(4), 616–633.

Lessen, R., & Kavanagh, K. (2015). Position of the Academy of Nutrition and Dietetics: Promoting and supporting breastfeeding. *Journal of the Academy of Nutrition and Dietetics, 115*, 444–449.

National Research Council (NRC). (2006). *Dietary reference intakes: The essential guide to nutrient requirements*. Washington, DC: The National Academies Press.

Nestle, M. (2005). Preventing childhood diabetes: The need for public health intervention. *American Journal of Public Health, 95*(9), 1497–1499.

Ogata, B. N., & Hayes, D. (2014). Position of the Academy of Nutrition and Dietetic: Nutrition guidance for healthy children ages 2 to 11 years. *Journal of the Academy of Nutrition and Dietetics, 114*(8), 1257–1276.

Paddon-Jones, D., & Leidy, H. (2014). Dietary protein and muscle in older persons. *Current Opinion in Clinical Nutrition and Metabolic Care, 17*(1), 5–11.

Patnode, C. D., et al. (2016). Primary care interventions to support breastfeeding: updated evidence report and systematic review for the US preventive services task force. *JAMA: the Journal of the American Medical Association, 316*(16), 1694–1705.

Perez-Escamilla, R. (2014). Food insecurity in children: Impact on physical, psychoemotional, and social development. In A. C. Ross (Ed.), *Modern nutrition in health and disease* (11th ed.). Philadelphia: Lippincott Williams & Wilkins.

Piernas, C., & Popkin, B. M. (2010). Trends in snacking among U.S. children. *Health Affairs, 29*(3), 398–404.

Polsky, S., et al. (2014). Obesity: Epidemiology, etiology, and prevention. In A. C. Ross (Ed.), *Modern nutrition in health and disease* (11th ed.). Philadelphia: Lippincott Williams & Wilkins.

Smith, C. (1947). The effect of wartime starvation in Holland upon pregnancy and its product. *American Journal of Obstetrics and Gynecology*, *53*, 599–608.

Turner, R. E. (2014). Nutrition during pregnancy. In A. C. Ross (Ed.), *Modern nutrition in health and disease* (11th ed.). Philadelphia: Lippincott Williams & Wilkins.

U.S. Department of Agriculture. (USDA). Food and Nutrition Services (FNS) 2021: Programs and services. From: www.fns.usda.gov/programs-and-services. (Accessed 6 January, 2021).

Wessling-Resnick, M. (2014). Iron. In A. C. Ross (Ed.), *Modern nutrition in health and disease* (11th ed.). Philadelphia: Lippincott Williams & Wilkins.

Willoughby, J. L., & Bowen, C. N. (2014). Zinc deficiency and toxicity in pediatric practice. *Current Opinion in Pediatrics*, *26*(5), 579–584.

Wise, N. J. (2015). Pregnant adolescents, beliefs about healthy eating, factors that influence food choices, and nutrition education preferences. *Journal of Midwifery & Women's Health*, *60*, 410–418. https://doi.org/10.1111/jmwh.12275.

World Health Organization (WHO). (2010). Guidelines on HIV and infant feeding: *Principles and recommendations for infant feeding in the context of HIV and a summary of evidence*. Geneva, Switzerland: WHO Press. 2010.

11

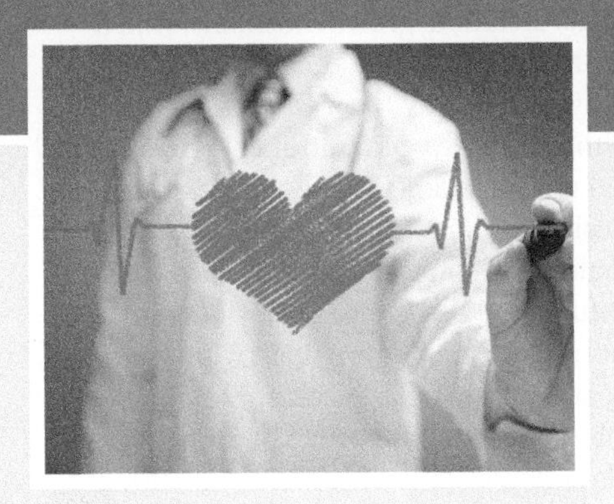

Nutrition Assessment and Patient Care

Hippocrates made the link between nutrition and disease almost 3000 years ago, but the modern medical community has just rediscovered its importance. The tremendous advances of medical technology are meaningless if the individual is at nutritional risk or already malnourished.

http://evolve.elsevier.com/GRODNER/FOUNDATIONS

LEARNING OBJECTIVES

- Discuss the basic nutrition status assessment performed by nurses.
- Explain how the nutrition status of patients may be compromised by illness and the impact of nutrition status on recovery.
- Describe the role of the registered dietitian (RD/RDN).
- Outline the process and data collection of a comprehensive nutrition assessment conducted by a dietitian.
- Compare and contrast the Nutrition Care Process (NCP), the Nursing Process and the National Council of State Boards of Nursing (NBSBN) Model of Clinical Judgment.
- Summarize the types of potential interactions among food or nutrients and drugs.

NUTRITION IN DISEASE MANAGEMENT

The first half of this text discusses nutrition as it relates to health and wellness. The second half provides information for nursing professionals on how nutrition pertains to the physiologic stresses of disease states. The Quality and Safety Education (QSEN) nursing competencies (patient-centered care, teamwork and collaboration, quality improvement, safety, and informatics) are basic and serve as the underlying theme.

Role of Genetics on Disease Onset

Knowing how genes affect nutrient metabolism and how nutrients affect gene expression affirms the old adage "We are what we eat." In fact, a woman's prenatal diet affects the long-term health of her children (referred to as the fetal origins of adult disease). Placental insufficiency, maternal malnutrition, and intrauterine growth restriction (IUGR) can impair infant growth and eventually lead to hypertension, cardiovascular disease, and T2D in adults (Simeoni et al., 2018). Not only is it important to eat well during pregnancy, but we now realize that the lifelong adequacy of a person's diet affects the onset and severity of acute and chronic illnesses. Accumulation of errors in the genome and damage to biomolecules cause functional tissue changes, even aging. With exciting research in the field of nutritional genomics, more will become known about the role of specific nutrients and genes in health and wellness. A DNA analysis may become part of the routine nursing assessment!

THE NUTRITION TEAM

Doctors are generally responsible for writing admission orders, including diet. However, nurses are often the first health professionals with whom the hospitalized patient comes into contact. By using information gathered during assessments, they are in a good position to identify patients in need of nutrition services. Furthermore, nursing staff often perform basic nutrition screening and provide nutrition education.

On admission, key issues include decreased appetite and unintentional weight loss, which are red flags for nutritional decline. A patient's age, medical history, hydration status, and illness severity are also important to share with the nutrition team. When more in-depth nutrition assessment/recognize cues and interventions/generate solutions are needed, care is provided by registered dietitians-nutritionists (RDNs). This text will refer to the "RD" or "RDN" for simplification, but both credentials require the minimum Bachelor of Science degree from an accredited university, 1200 hours of supervised practice (often a dietetic internship), and passing the national examination. Most states also require licensure to practice.

The RD is specially qualified to conduct the Nutrition Care Process (NCP) and serve as a valuable partner with the nursing team. The NCP encompasses detailed nutrition assessments, establishment of a nutrition diagnosis, provision of nutrition therapies, monitoring, and evaluation of outcomes. Nutrition therapy is often needed to treat an illness, injury, or related condition. Dietetic technicians, registered (DTRs) can assist the RD by taking diet histories, collecting information for nutrition screening and assessment, and working directly with patients who are having problems with their meals. A DTR may provide basic nutrition education but should not be asked to counsel patients about complex disease modifications.

Medical nutrition therapy (MNT) is a legal term that applies to patients with prerenal failure and diabetes who receive nutrition treatments under Medicare. To avoid confusion, this text will use the term nutrition therapy to discuss the provision of food and nutrients, nutrition education, nutrition counseling, and coordination of care.

NUTRITION RISK AND MALNUTRITION

An important relationship exists between dietary intake and a healthy population. The capacity for recovery from illness or disease depends on good nutrition status. Poor nutrition status delays recovery and decreases quality of life (QOL). It is important, therefore, to determine the current nutrition status of those undergoing medical treatment or cure. A return to wellness is the goal.

Nutrition Risk From Hunger

Many people have inadequate access to food. Hunger and food insecurity are prevalent in both developed and developing countries. According to the Food and Agriculture Organization (FAO, 2020), people experience food insecurity when they lack access to enough safe and nutritious food for normal growth and development or to have an active, healthy life. With more hunger and food insecurity because of the COVID-19 pandemic and economic recession, it is unlikely that there will be "Zero Hunger" by 2030 (World Health Organization, 2020).

Undernutrition and chronic micronutrient deficiencies are forms of "hidden hunger" (Amoroso, 2016). Older adults (>65 years) are at high risk for nutrition-related chronic diseases (heart disease, diabetes) as well as infections (pneumonia, influenza, COVID-19), thus requiring strategies, policies, and interventions to address hidden hunger (Eggersdorfer et al., 2018). When admitted to hospitals or nursing homes, many are already "at nutritional risk" and may experience poor wound healing, longer lengths of stay, and a decline in overall health. In addition, both frail elderly and sick people may experience loss of appetite, depression, or alterations of taste and smell perception.

A diet with low-quality protein and amino acids is especially detrimental for growing children, and stunting may result. Achieving one's genetically programmed height is controlled by nutrient-sensitive hormones, including growth hormone, which is enhanced during sleep (Millward, 2017). The master growth regulation pathway (rapamycin complex 1 [mTORC1] pathway) integrates nutrients, growth factors, oxygen, and energy to regulate growth of bone, skeletal muscle, nervous system, gastrointestinal (GI) tract, blood cells, immune effector cells, organ size, and whole-body energy balance (Semba et al., 2016). Infections can lead to intestinal dysfunction and endogenous inflammation; micronutrient replacement must be combined with access to clean water, sanitation, and high-quality protein.

In the United States, "food deserts" are urban or rural locations where individuals lack access to healthy, affordable food at local grocery stores (U.S. Department of Agriculture [USDA], 2020). The problem became more widespread during the COVID-19 pandemic, when people had to line up to receive items from food banks or soup kitchens already stretched to their limit. Thankfully, more women and minorities are growing produce for personal consumption through gardening or farming (Barnes & Bendixsen, 2017).

Although adults do not need nutrients for growth, they do require high-quality protein for general health and tissue repair. Nurses and RDs have a responsibility to help patients achieve their optimal nutrition status (Xu et al., 2017).

Challenges of the Hospital Setting

Imagine you have been taken to a place where, after answering a multitude of questions about your condition, insurance, financial status, and durable power of attorney (a legal document in which a competent adult authorizes another competent adult to make decisions for themselves in the event of incapacitation), you are whisked off to a sterile-looking room that you must share with a stranger. In this room, your clothes are replaced with a thin, flimsy gown that won't close in the back. You answer more questions about your medical history from the nurse who admits you. Once they finish, a resident or intern comes into your room to ask many of the same questions and conduct a physical examination (Fig. 11.1).

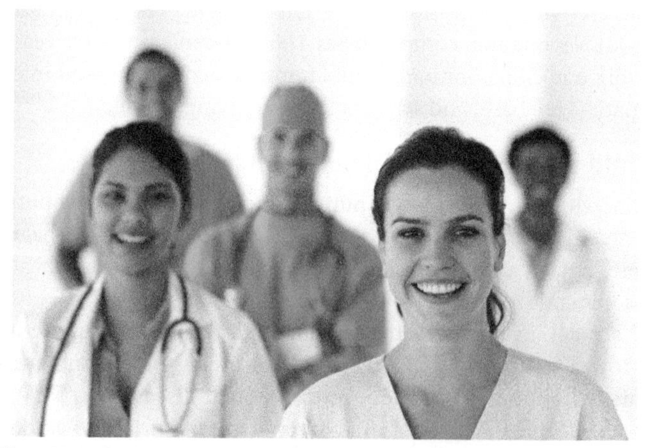

Fig. 11.1 Patients are interviewed by many members of the health care team. From www.thinkstockphotos.com.

During a hospital stay, eating habits are open to scrutiny and change. You are away from your own kitchen, and meals are served on a schedule that may or may not coincide with your personal preferences. Depending on your medical diagnosis, the food may be modified in texture, consistency, nutrients, or energy. While you're in the hospital, different staff routinely enter your room to ask questions, ranging from what you ate yesterday to your elimination habits, to draw blood, and to take you elsewhere in the hospital for tests that may or may not be invasive. Although no harm is intended, little privacy is afforded while you undergo tests and examinations that may provide critical information about your prognosis. During these trying times, food becomes very important, physiologically and psychologically. Food is one of the few familiar experiences encountered in a hospital setting (see the *Personal Perspectives* box Sharing an Orange).

PERSONAL PERSPECTIVES

Sharing an Orange

Machines were whirling as I entered the cardiac intensive care unit to visit my husband Lenny's grandmother. I didn't know what to expect. Grandma Ethel was the most energetic older adult I ever knew. She was 86 years old, still running her own gift shop, and always ready to go out with Lenny and me, until she had this heart attack.

Grandma Ethel was sitting upright in a chair with all kinds of wires attached to her body. She was pale, but immediately her radiant smile spread across her face. She said, "Come and sit, have lunch with me," as she invited me to share the hospital lunch that was on a tray in front of her. Now I certainly wasn't going to eat any of her lunch, especially hospital food. But I was definitely needed. She wanted the soup but, with the wires and being somewhat weak, couldn't get the lid off the Styrofoam cup. So, I came to the rescue. Uncover the lid from the plate of soft chicken and mashed potatoes? Again, I was handy. Open the juice container and decaffeinated coffee cup? Who knew I was so competent?

"Michele, here, have the orange." The orange was in a bowl surrounded by plastic wrap. I gently suggested she should have it because it was good for her. "No, I'm too full. Take it home ... take it home for the boys [my sons; her great-grandsons] and take the brownie too!" I then realized that the real issue was not to feed Grandma Ethel's body, but to let her soul feed us. Her soul needed to nourish us with her gift of a sweet orange and a rich brownie. And we were nourished.

Michele Grodner
Montclair, NJ

Particularly for hospitalized toddlers and adolescents, food can become a battleground because of its emotional connotations (Fig. 11.2). The same is true for elderly patients when they receive meals that contain unfamiliar or disliked foods. A temper tantrum is possible—at any age!

Food or an alternative method of nourishment can mean the difference between a good and a poor prognosis. Part of the initial assessment should include questions related to cultural, ethnic, or religious food preferences (see the *Cultural Diversity and Nutrition* box Asking the Right Questions and Improving Cultural Competency).

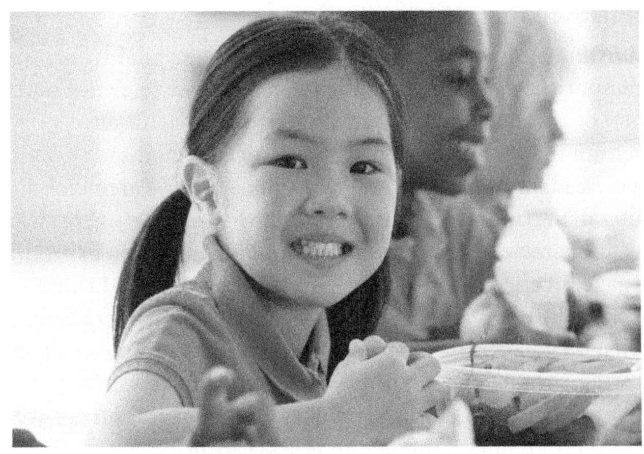

Fig. 11.2 Food provides emotional comfort as well as nutrition, especially for children. From www.thinkstockphotos.com

CULTURAL DIVERSITY AND NUTRITION

Asking Right Questions and Improving Cultural Competency

Health care professionals serve patients from a variety of diverse backgrounds in hospitals, nursing homes, the community, and sometimes patients' homes. When providing care, nurses must be sensitive to the cultural needs and expectations of their patients and family members. To be culturally competent, nurses need to understand the knowledge and attitudes of each cultural group in relation to food, especially those with symbolic or religious connotations.

It is impossible to know all the specific cultural food practices of diverse groups around the world, so asking the right questions is important. Use of a Cultural Nutritional Assessment Guide, modified here from Andrews and Boyle (2020), helps obtain information for a patient's health history. Information obtained from the patient or family member can improve the patient's satisfaction, the nurse's cultural competency, and the patient's nutrition outcome.

Cultural Nursing Assessment Guide: Nutrition

- What nutritional factors are influenced by the client's cultural background? What is the meaning of food and eating to the client?
- With whom does the client usually eat? What types of foods are eaten? What is the usual timing and sequencing of meals?
- What does the client define as food? What does the client believe comprises a "healthy" versus an "unhealthy" diet?
- Who shops for food? Where are groceries purchased (e.g., special markets or ethnic grocery stores)? Who prepares the client's meals?
- How are foods prepared at home—preparation methods, cooking oils used, length of time foods are cooked (especially vegetables), amount and type of seasonings added to various foods during preparation?
- Has the client chosen a particular practice such as vegetarianism or abstinence from alcohol or fermented beverages?
- Describe how the client's religious beliefs and practices influence the type, amount, preparation, or delineation of acceptable food combinations (e.g., kosher diets, fasting). Does the client fast or abstain from certain foods at regular intervals, on specific days of the week, or on certain dates determined by the religious calendar?
- If the client's religion mandates or encourages fasting, what does the term fast mean (e.g., refraining from certain types or quantities of foods, eating only during certain times of the day)? For what length of time is the client expected to fast?
- During fasting, does the client refrain from liquids/beverages? Does the religion allow exemption from fasting during illness? If so, does the client believe that an exemption applies to them?

(Modified from Andrews M, Boyle J, Collins JW: *Transcultural concepts in nursing care*, ed 8, Philadelphia, 2020, Wolters Kluwer Health.)

Nutrition Risk Assessment

Nutrition risk assessment focuses on the potential to become malnourished because of primary (inadequate intake of nutrients) or secondary (caused by disease or iatrogenic affects) factors. For the past decade, the Academy of Nutrition and Dietetics (the Academy) and the American Society for Parenteral and Enteral Nutrition (ASPEN) have standardized the use of diagnostic characteristics to document adult malnutrition in routine clinical practice (Mueller et al., 2011; White et al., 2012).

Stays in acute care hospitals play havoc with patients' nutritional intake. During hospitalization, patients admitted in good nutrition status encounter psychological and physiologic factors that put them at nutrition risk. Tests, surgical procedures, interruptions, medications, and illness can all cause a decline in nutrition status. If patients are admitted in compromised nutrition status, as nearly half are, risks are even greater and of more consequence. Moderate to severe nutritional depletion is associated with longer lengths of stay and can contribute to high readmission rates or even death (Whitley et al., 2017).

An interdisciplinary approach to addressing malnutrition both in the hospital and in the acute posthospital phase is a reasonable request (Reber et al., 2019). Nursing personnel can help prevent malnutrition by paying attention to inadequate diet orders. Risk is high when patients have had nothing to eat, liquid diets for more than 24 hours, or intravenous feedings that contain only glucose and saline. Those are the times to contact the RD for a more complete evaluation of the patient's nutrition status.

Effects of Bed Rest on Nutrition

Occasionally, complete bed rest is prescribed as part of patients' medical care. Some patients may be unable to ambulate because of the severity of their illnesses or because they are "hooked up" to a multitude of necessary lifesaving equipment at bedside. Although it is often necessary or unavoidable, complete immobilization because of bed rest can have injurious effects on a patient's body. Short-term bed rest or disuse accelerates the loss of muscle mass, function, and glucose tolerance (Galvan et al., 2016). It is especially detrimental in older adults. Emerging evidence suggests that low-intensity exercise and leucine-supplemented meals may partially and temporarily protect skeletal muscle (English et al., 2016; Galvan et al., 2016). Leucine-rich foods include whey protein, milk, beef, chicken, yogurt, peanuts, and soy foods.

Skin integrity may be compromised after just 24 hours of immobilization. Nursing personnel can prevent or delay some injurious effects by frequently turning and repositioning patients. Good nutrition, hygiene, and skin care are essential during this time.

Malnutrition

Nearly 40% of patients admitted to hospitals are malnourished on admission or demonstrate malnutrition during their hospitalization (Jensen et al., 2010). In chronically ill patients with complex needs, the percentages are even higher (Burgos et al., 2020). Patients may experience physiologic stress from injury or illness, which increases nutritional demands. Nutrition needs may be further compromised because of periodic fasting needed before laboratory testing or diagnostic procedures. Highly restricted, nutritionally inadequate diets, meals missed because of procedures and tests, and unmonitored dietary intakes can lead to malnutrition; see Chapter 12 for details on managing diet orders.

Adult forms of malnutrition are classified as starvation-related malnutrition when there is chronic starvation without inflammation, chronic disease-related malnutrition when inflammation is chronic and of mild to moderate degree, and acute disease- or injury-related malnutrition when inflammation is acute and severe (Jensen et al., 2010). The indicators are used to assess individuals. Examples include starvation-related malnutrition in a patient with anorexia nervosa, chronic malnutrition in a patient with cancer, and acute disease-related malnutrition for the febrile patient with burns.

NUTRITION CARE PROCESS

Most patients entering the health care system have special nutrition needs, depending on their injury or illness. Patients at nutrition risk need to be identified so that high-quality nutrition interventions can be provided. Poor nutrition status may lead to complications such as increased morbidity and mortality, longer lengths of stay, and higher cost of care (Reber et al., 2019). For nutrition intervention to be efficacious and successful, a systematic, logical methodology is necessary. The Nutrition Care Process serves this purpose (Box 11.1).

Screening

It is not possible, or necessary, to complete a full nutrition assessment on every patient. It is necessary, however, to have a system in place to quickly identify patients at risk for nutrition problems such as malnutrition (The Joint Commission [TJC], 2020). Nutrition screening is the process of identifying patients, clients, or groups who may have a nutrition diagnosis and benefit from nutrition assessment and intervention by an RDN; the process should apply valid, reliable tools that can be quickly performed (Academy of Nutrition and Dietetics, 2020).

The Joint Commission (TJC) requires that all patients admitted to a hospital be screened for nutritional concerns. Screening is performed when warranted by the patient's needs or condition, with written criteria identifying when more in-depth assessments are required; screenings must be completed within 24 hours after inpatient admission (TJC, 2020). In long-term care facilities, screening and assessments must be completed on all residents within 14 days of admission.

Nutrition screening can be executed by nurses, RDs, DTRs, dietary managers, physicians, or other trained personnel. Whether the RDs directly perform the nutrition screening or not, they are responsible for establishing suitable screening parameters. The nutrition screening process facilitates completion of early intervention goals, includes collection and interpretation of relevant data, helps determine the need for a nutrition assessment, is cost effective, and may be completed in any setting.

BOX 11.1 Academy of Nutrition and Dietetics: Nutrition Care Process

Definition of Nutrition Care Process

Providing nutrition care starts when a patient is recognized as being at nutritional risk and requiring additional support to attain or maintain positive nutritional status. The Nutrition Care Process (NCP) is defined "as a systematic problem-solving method that dietetics professionals use to critically think and make decisions to address nutrition-related problems and provide safe and effective quality nutrition care." It is composed of the following four separate but interrelated and associated steps:

1. Nutrition assessment
2. Nutrition diagnosis
3. Nutrition intervention
4. Nutrition monitoring and evaluation

Each stage builds on the preceding one, but the process is not necessarily linear. Fig. 11.3 provides a visual illustration of the model.

Step 1: Nutrition Assessment

Techniques such as those outlined previously in the chapter are used to systematically obtain information necessary to determine or reassess whether a nutrition problem (or diagnosis) exists. If so, the problem is diagnosed using the PES (problem, etiology, signs/symptoms) statement described in Step 2.

Step 2: Nutrition Diagnosis

Before nutrition intervention can take place, the nutrition problem(s) must be identified. This identification is accomplished with the nutrition diagnosis. Standardized language has been developed to make the nutrition diagnosis clear to other nutrition and health care professionals. When the nutrition problem has been identified, it is labeled with a specific, standardized diagnostic term. The nutrition diagnosis statement, or PES statement, is organized in three distinct parts: the problem (P), etiology of the problem (E), and signs and symptoms associated with the problem (S). Typically, nutrition diagnoses fall into one of three categories or domains: intake, clinical, and behavioral-environmental.

Here is an example of how a nutrition diagnosis is written:

"Disordered eating pattern related to harmful belief about food and nutrition as evidenced by reported use of laxatives after meals and statements that calories are not absorbed when laxatives are used."

Step 3: Nutrition Intervention

Intervention begins once the nutritional diagnosis is identified. It is generally aimed at the etiology (E) of the nutrition diagnosis and is directed at reducing or eradicating the effects of the signs and symptoms (S). Nutrition interventions are intended to modify a nutrition-related problem and comprise two interconnected

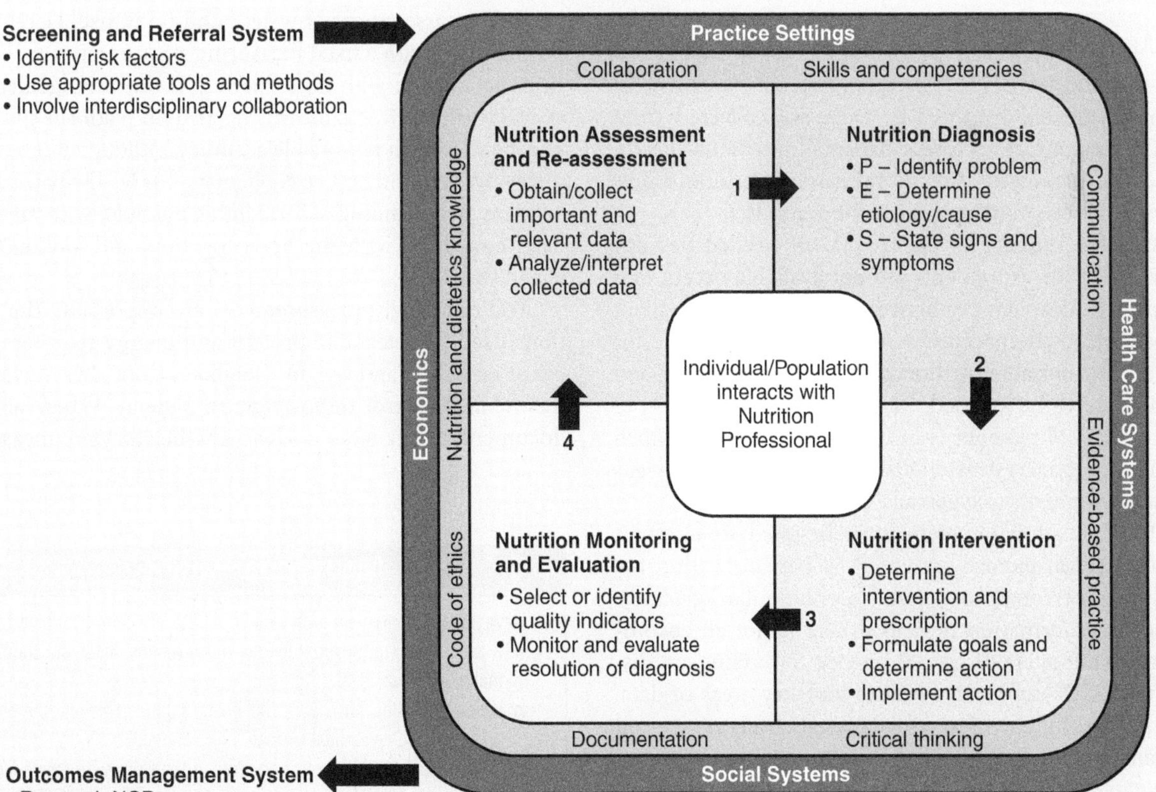

Fig. 11.3 Nutrition Care Process and model. PE. (Modified from https://www.eatrightpro.org/-/media/eatrightpro-files/practice/nutrition-care-process/ncp/nutritioncareprocessandmodelupdate.pdf?la=en&hash=4280DC4E03C6084FCA44CED6EE0A1E2904635F2D; with permission from the Academy of Nutrition and Dietetics.)

Continued

BOX 11.1 Academy of Nutrition and Dietetics: Nutrition Care Process—cont'd

components: planning and implementation. Nutrition diagnoses are prioritized in the planning component, whereby implementation is the "action phase." The plan is communicated and carried out, data continue to be collected, and the nutrition intervention is revised as necessary. Four categories or domains of nutrition intervention have been identified:

- Food and/or nutrient delivery
- Nutrition education
- Nutrition counseling
- Coordination of care

Step 4: Nutrition Monitoring and Evaluation

The point of the nutrition monitoring and evaluation step in the NCP is to measure improvement made by the patient in meeting nutrition care goals. The patient's progress is examined by determining whether the nutrition intervention is being executed and by providing evidence that the intervention is or is not altering the patients' nutrition status. Nutrition monitoring and evaluation terms are organized into four categories or domains:

- Food/nutrition-related history
- Biochemical data, medical tests, and procedures
- Anthropometric measurements
- Nutrition-focused physical findings

Summary

The NCP allows for continuous monitoring and evaluation of the patient. As the condition of the patient changes, plans or interventions change, as do diagnoses and/or interventions. If the patient shows no response to interventions, new interventions can be developed. Additionally, any or all nutrition interventions should be planned along with patients and/or their caregivers or significant others.

From Academy of Nutrition and Dietetics: *International dietetics and nutrition terminology (IDNT) reference manual: Standardized language for the nutrition care process*, ed 4, Chicago, 2012, Author; The Writing Group: Nutrition Care Process and model: Part 1: The 2008 update, *J Am Diet Assoc* 108:1113–1117, 2008.

A referral to an RD is necessary when a patient shows signs of nutrition risk, especially unintended weight loss or poor appetite. The RD is responsible for conducting the nutrition assessment, selecting relevant nutrition diagnoses, and providing appropriate nutrition care.

Nutrition Assessment

The first step of the formal NCP is a comprehensive nutritional assessment conducted by the RD. Data are collected from several different sources to assess patients' nutritional needs, because no one parameter directly measures nutrition status, determines nutrition problems, or identifies needs.

Estimating the number of calories (kcal) needed per day is not easy. Direct measurements are not available except in a research setting. Although predictive equations are convenient and inexpensive, their inaccuracy makes them unreliable for designing an appropriate nutrition plan. Both overfeeding and underfeeding are to be avoided. The best method used, especially for critically ill patients, is indirect calorimetry, in which the type and rate of energy metabolism are determined from gas exchange measurements (oxygen and carbon dioxide).

A combination of parameters must be used to interpret the overall nutrition picture presented by patients within the context of their personal, social, and economic backgrounds. The assessment information described here is not all encompassing; only parameters of special interest to nursing are discussed. An "ABCD" approach includes four key areas of data: **A**nthropometrics, **B**iochemical tests, **C**linical observations, and **D**ietary evaluation.

Anthropometric assessment. Anthropometric measurements are simple, noninvasive techniques that measure height and weight, head circumference, and skinfold thickness. Effectiveness of single anthropometric measurements is limited, but certain serial measurements can be useful to assess body composition changes or growth over time. Standardized techniques must be used to obtain valid and reliable measurements. Evaluation of anthropometric data involves a comparison of data collected with predetermined reference limits or cutoff points that allow classification into one or more risk categories. Discussion of various anthropometric measurements follows.

Height. Stature (height/length) is important in evaluating growth and nutrition status in children. In adults, height is needed for assessment of weight and body size. Height should be measured with a fixed measuring stick or tape on a true vertical, flat surface with no carpeting. If this arrangement is not available, the movable measuring arm on platform clinic scales may be used with reasonable accuracy, although it tends to produce lower measures (Lee & Nieman, 2013). The patient should be measured standing as straight as possible, without shoes or head coverings, with the heels together, and looking straight ahead (Box 11.2).

Accurate height measurements are important. The calculations used to determine protein and energy requirements are based on height and weight. Heights are not always available in the medical records of hospitalized patients. When heights are documented, it is often unclear whether they are measured, or

BOX 11.2 Measuring Height

1. Have patient stand erect with weight equally distributed on both feet.
   a. If the legs are of unequal length, place boards under the short limb to make the pelvis level.
   b. When possible, make sure the head, shoulder blades, buttocks, and heels all touch a vertical surface.
   c. Instruct patient to let arms hang free at the sides with palms facing the thighs.
2. Have patient look straight ahead (so the line of vision is perpendicular to the body), take a deep breath, and hold that position while the horizontal headboard is brought down firmly on top of the head. (Measurer's eyes should be level with the headboard to read the measurement.)
3. Read the measurement to the nearest 0.1 cm or ⅛ inch.

From Lee RD, Nieman DC: *Nutritional assessment*, ed 6, New York, 2013, McGraw-Hill.

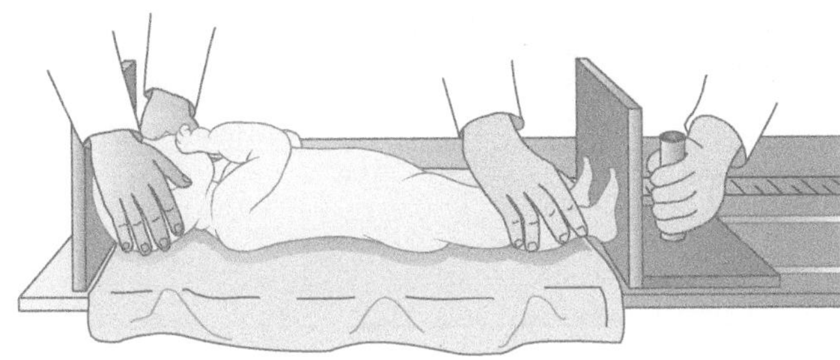

Fig. 11.4 A recumbent length board used to take height measurements horizontally. (From Mahan LK, Escott-Stump S, Raymond JL: *Krause's food & nutrition therapy*, ed 13, St. Louis, 2012, Elsevier.)

just reported by the patient. As people age, their height tends to decline, so a current height is valuable information.

Asking patients about their height does not usually produce accurate information. On average when asked, people report being slightly taller than they are. Men overstate height more often than women, and the extent of overstating height increases as people age (Lee & Nieman, 2013). If the height of a patient recorded in the medical record is not a measured height, it should be documented as a stated height.

When measuring an infant or child (age >2–3 years) who cannot stand or another patient unable to stand erect without assistance, a **recumbent measure** can be taken while the subject is lying down or reclining. A recumbent length table can be used. A recumbent length table or board has a fixed headboard, a movable footboard, and a permanent measuring scale along the side (Fig. 11.4). To measure a patient, they should be placed supine on the board or table with shoulders and legs flat against the measuring board (table) and arms at the sides. The head should firmly touch the headboard while the line of vision is perpendicular to the board or table. Soles of the feet should be vertical, and the footboard should touch the bottoms of the feet so that the soft tissue is compressed. Length can be recorded from the measure at the footboard. Two people may be needed to take an accurate measurement.

When the patient is comatose, critically ill, or unable to be moved for other reasons, taking a recumbent bed height may be possible (Box 11.3). Note that compared with standing height, bed height is significantly greater by at least 2% (Gray, 1985). A more accurate measurement for patients who cannot stand is knee height, which is minimally affected by aging but requires the use of special calipers. Other possible

BOX 11.3 Measuring Recumbent Bed Height

1. Remove pillows and make the bed level.
2. Straighten the patient out in the bed but with the feet flexed.
3. With a clipboard or ruler, extend perpendicular lines from the top of the head and the bottom of the feet out to the side of the bed.
4. Mark the two positions on the bed sheet, and measure the distance between them to the nearest ½ inch.

Data from Gray D: Accuracy of recumbent height measurement, *J Parenter Enteral Nutr* 9:712–715, 1985.

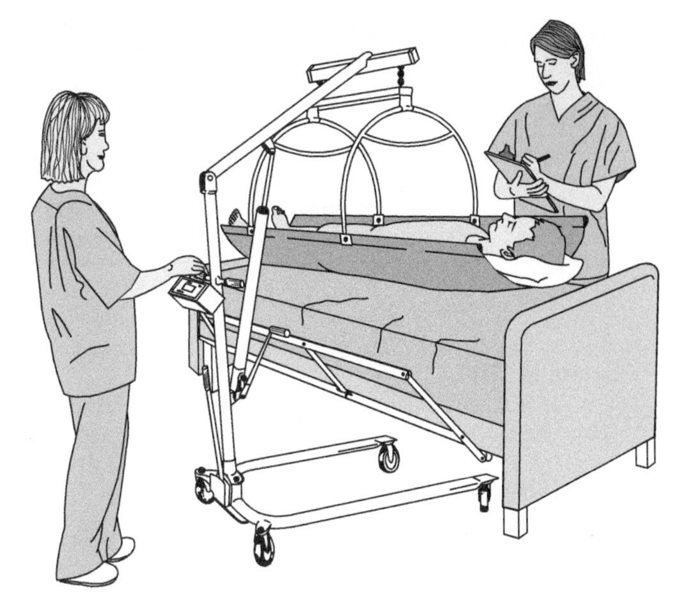

Fig. 11.5 If a patient is nonambulatory, a bed scale can be used to measure patient weight.

measurements are forearm length (useful for patients with contractures) and demi-span (useful for patients with lower limb dysfunction); details on measuring heights in bedridden patients can be found at the following website: http://www.rxkinetics.com/height_estimate.html.

Weight. When accurately measured, body weight is a simple, gross estimate of body composition. In fact, body weight is one of the most important measurements in assessing nutrition status and is used to predict energy expenditure (Psota & Chen, 2013).

Beam scales with movable but nondetachable weights or accurate electronic scales are recommended to obtain accurate results. Spring scales are not recommended. If the patient is not ambulatory, wheelchair or bed scales should be used (Fig. 11.5). Scales should be checked for accuracy periodically and recalibrated when necessary.

Like heights, actual measured weights are more accurate than self-reported weights. Studies suggest that concurrent self-reports of height and weight may be more useful than previously thought (Cui et al., 2016).

For accurate weights, the patients should be clothed in underwear or a hospital gown. Weight should be measured at the same time of day and after voiding. The patient should stand still with the weight evenly distributed on both feet while weight is recorded to the nearest 0.1 kg, or 0.25 pound (Lee & Nieman, 2013).

As a nutrition screening tool, weights can be used to detect changes that may represent or suggest serious health problems. Magnitude and direction of weight change are more meaningful when dealing with sick or debilitated patients than standardized desirable weight references (Table 11.1). Percent weight change is a useful nutrition index and may be computed as follows:

$$\% \text{ Weight change} = (\text{Usual weight} - \text{Actual weight}) \div \text{Usual weight} \times 100)$$

TABLE 11.1 Weight Change as an Indicator of Nutrition Status

% Weight Change	Time	Nutrition Status
1–2	1 week	Moderate weight loss
>2	1 week	Severe weight loss
5	1 month	Moderate weight loss
>5	1 month	Severe weight loss

TABLE 11.2 Classifications of Overweight and Obesity by Body Mass Index

	Body Mass Index (kg/m²)
Underweight	<18.5
Normal	18.5–24.9
Overweight	25.0–29.9
Obesity	≥30

Example 11.1

Mrs. Welch is admitted to your unit. Her weight on admission is 120 pounds. During the admissions interview, she indicates that 3 months ago she weighed 135 pounds. Her percent weight change from usual weight is calculated with the formula:

$$\%\text{ Weight change from admission weight} = (\text{Usual weight} - \text{Actual weight}) \div \text{Admission weight} \times 100$$

as follows:

$$(135 - 120) \div 135 \times 100 = 15 \div 135 \times 100 = 0.11 \times 100, \text{ or an } 11\% \text{ Weight change}$$

Mrs. Welch's (actual) weight is 11% less than her usual weight.

Example 11.2

Mr. Tucker is a patient in the long-term care facility where you work. When he was admitted more than a year ago, he weighed 180 pounds. He has weighed 170 pounds for the past 6 months, but today you weigh Mr. Tucker and he weighs 165 pounds. His percent weight change from admission weight is calculated as follows:

$$\text{Admission weight minus current weight} = 180 - 165 \text{ (15 lbs)}$$
$$15/180 = 8\% \text{ loss}$$

$$\text{Recent weight} - \text{current weight} = 170 - 165 \text{ (5 lbs)}$$
$$5/170 = 3\% \text{ loss}$$

Mr. Tucker's actual weight is 3% less than his admission weight. His percent weight change since a nutrition intervention is as follows:

$$(\text{Usual weight} - \text{Actual weight}) \div \text{Preintervention weight} \times 100$$

Example 11.3

Mrs. Bussard was started on a feeding tube because her weight has decreased from her usual weight of 130 pounds to 115 pounds. She has been on the feeding tube for 1 week, and when you weigh her today, she weighs 122 pounds. Her percent weight change since nutrition intervention is calculated as follows:

$$(130 - 122) \div 115 \times 100 = 8 \div 115 \times 100 = 0.067 \times 100 = 6.96\%, \text{ or a } 7\% \text{ Weight change}$$

Mrs. Bussard's weight has increased 7% since the tube feedings were initiated.

Special care should be taken to identify patients with ascites, edema, or dehydration. Their weight changes may be fluid shifts rather than actual changes in body composition. A gain of more than 1 pound in 1 day may signify excess fluid. It is also important to examine any unplanned weight loss the patient might experience (Table 11.2). Reported or measured percent weight losses of these magnitudes could be cause for alarm.

For older adult patients who cannot be weighed because of the severity of their medical condition, or if bed or chair scales are not available, gender-specific equations are available to predict body weight in people 60 to 90 years of age (Chumlea et al., 1988). These estimated weights are based on recumbent measures of arm circumference (AC), calf circumference (CC), subscapular skinfold (SSF), and knee height (KH).

The equation for women is as follows:

$$\text{Weight (cm)} = [0.98 \times \text{AC (in cm)}] + [1.27 \times \text{CC (in cm)}] + [0.4 \times \text{SSF (in mm)}] + [0.87 \times \times \text{KH (in cm)}] \; 62.35$$

The equation for men is as follows:

$$\text{Weight (cm)} = [1.73 \times \text{AC (in cm)}] + [0.98 \times \text{CC (in cm)}] + [0.37 \times \text{SSF (in mm)}] + [1.16 \times \text{KH (in cm)}] \; 81.69$$

Another challenge in obtaining weights occurs in patients who have missing body parts because of accidents or amputation. Fig. 11.6 shows the approximate percentages of body weight contributed by individual body segments; using this information allows a patient's desirable weight to be calculated.

Body mass index. Body mass index (BMI) is a ratio of weight to height and has been associated with overall mortality and nutrition risk (Aune et al., 2016). BMI does not determine body composition (lean body mass or adipose tissue) but is a gauge of total body fat (National Heart, Lung, and Blood Institute [NHLBI], n.d.). Some genetic makers have correlated high body fat percentages with death from cardiovascular disease (Schnurr et al., 2016). Although BMI measurements are useful, they also have limits (Lefton & Malone, 2015; McCauley & Beavers, 2014):

- BMI has not been validated in acutely ill patients.
- BMI may underestimate body fat in the elderly and others who have lost muscle mass.
- BMI may overestimate body fat in individuals who have a muscular build.
- Cardiorespiratory fitness (CRF) is a potential modifier because the risk of all-cause mortality is lowest in the overweight category.

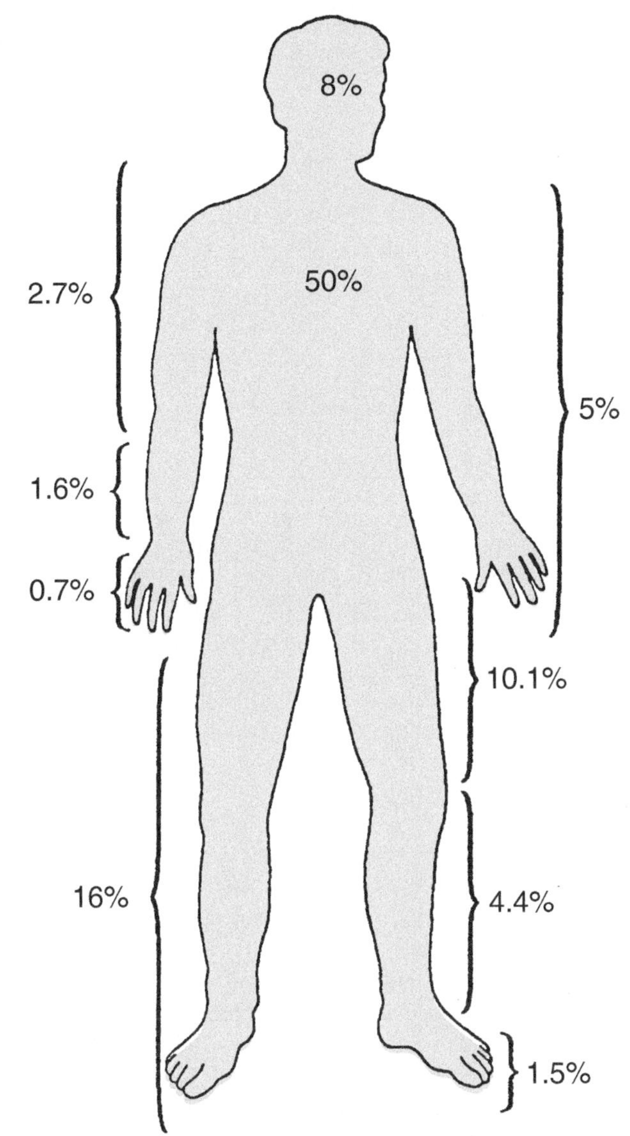

Fig. 11.6 Approximate body weight percentages. (Modified from Brunnstrom S: *Clinical kinesiology*, Philadelphia, 1962, FA Davis.)

You can determine BMI by dividing weight in kilograms by height in squared meters—(BMI = Weight [kg] ÷ Height [m]^2)—using the following three steps:

1. Divide weight in pounds by 2.2 to convert it into kilograms.
2. Multiply height in inches by 2.54, and divide the result by 100 to convert height to meters; then multiply height in meters by itself (i.e., square it).
3. Divide weight in kilograms (result of step 1) by the square of height in meters (result of step 2). The result is BMI.

The desired BMI range for healthy adults is 18.5 to 24.9 kg/m^2, which reflects a healthy weight for height; see Table 11.2. Although at low risk for health problems, people with BMI values between 25 and 29.9 kg/m^2 are approximately 20% above desirable levels. A patient with a BMI less than 18.5 kg/m^2 is classified as underweight; this status is associated with risk factors such as respiratory disease, tuberculosis, digestive disease, and some cancers (NHLBI, 1998).

Waist measurements. Waist circumference (WC) is an economical and straightforward measure that can be used to assess abdominal (visceral) fat content. A circumference greater than 40 inches in men and 35 inches in women indicates risk for disease. Note that visceral adiposity may vary among racial and ethnic groups; more research is needed for making targeted recommendations (Heymsfield et al., 2016).

Waist-to-hip ratio (WHR) is sometimes used for patients with human immunodeficiency virus–acquired immunodeficiency syndrome (HIV-AIDS). For WHR, measure waist circumference and divide by hip circumference.

Waist-to-height ratio (WHtR) has greater predictive capacity than either BMI or WC for diabetes, hypertension, and cardiovascular risks and outcomes in both men and women (Ashwell et al., 2012). For WHtR, measure waist circumference and divide by height. A simple goal here is to keep WC to less than half of height (<0.5).

Nutrition-Focused Physical Examination and Functional Assessments

A nutrition-focused physical examination includes fluid assessment, functional status, wound status, and clinical signs of malnutrition, overnutrition, or nutrient deficiencies (Esper, 2015). Involuntary weight loss should be addressed by an interdisciplinary team. Obesity is another condition that warrants a team effort; see Fig. 11.7.

Poor muscle quality is often a predictor of mortality, especially in the elderly. Manual muscle testing (MMT) and handgrip strength (HGS) dynamometry assessments have been used to evaluate muscle weakness in patients. Further study is needed to verify whether these tests are valid as part of a nutrition screening or assessment.

Biochemical assessment. Many routine blood and urine laboratory test results recorded in patient charts are useful for objective assessment of nutrition status. However, care should be taken in interpreting test results for several reasons. First, no single test is available for evaluating short-term response to nutrition therapy. Laboratory values should be used in conjunction with anthropometric data, clinical data, and results of dietary intake assessments. Second, some tests may be inappropriate for certain patients; for example, serum albumin might not be useful in the evaluation of protein status in patients with liver failure because this test assumes normal liver function. Third, laboratory tests conducted serially will give more accurate information than a single test.

Although serial measures can be obtained in long-term care settings, patients in acute care facilities are rarely hospitalized long enough for serial measures to be obtained. Therefore, it is often appropriate to compare test results with known standards. Biochemical parameters can be used to evaluate visceral proteins and immune function, which may reflect nutrition status.

Visceral proteins are proteins found in internal organs and blood rather than in muscle. Visceral protein status is estimated through tests of serum albumin and prealbumin. Interpretation of albumin values must be cautious, however, because inflammation, infection, hydration, and illness affect these values. Low values do not necessarily indicate poor dietary intake.

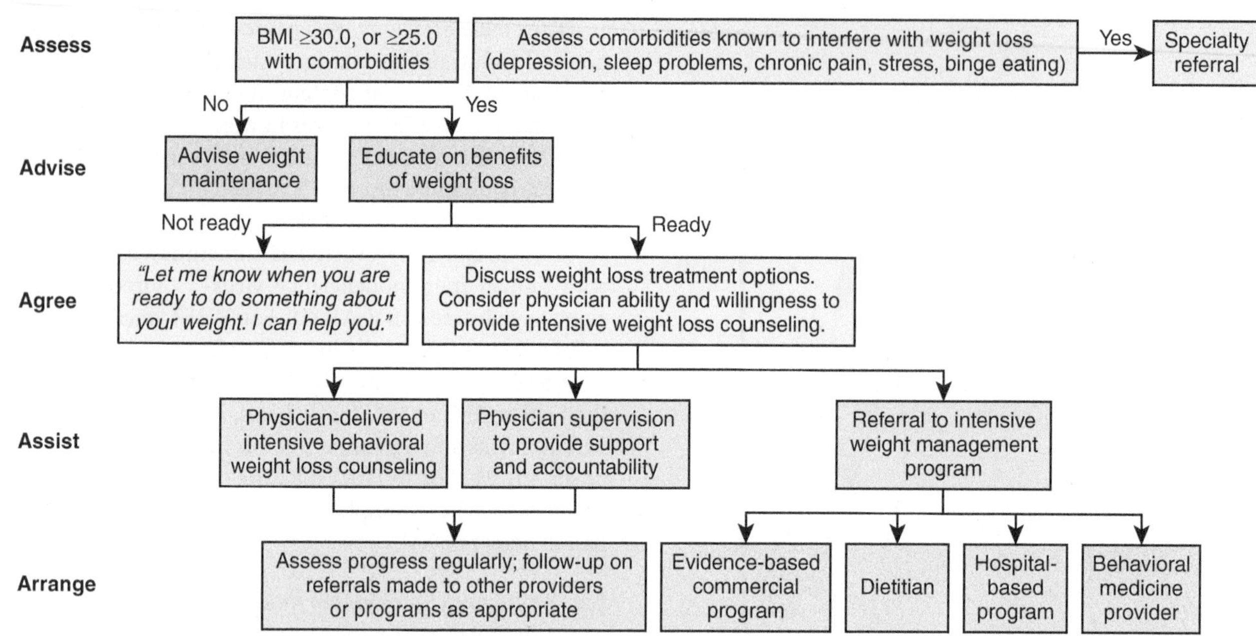

Fig. 11.7 Interdisciplinary care plan for involuntary weight loss. Flow chart for a model of obesity management in primary care. The flow chart allows for the categorization of patients according to their readiness to lose weight. *BMI*, Body mass index. (Modified from Fitzpatrick SL, Wischenka MA, Appelhans BM, et al. An evidence-based guide for obesity treatment in primary care. *Am J Med* 129: 115.e1–115.e7, 2016.)

Normal serum albumin values are within 3.5 to 5 g/dL. For nutritional analysis, values between 2.8 and 3.5 g/dL indicate compromised protein status; values less than 2.4 g/dL may precede pressure ulcer development. If patients are experiencing dehydration or have received infusions of albumin, fresh frozen plasma, or whole-blood serum albumin, serum levels may appear normal. Abnormally low values may be caused by various conditions, including nephrotic syndrome, heart failure, hepatic cirrhosis, and protein malnutrition; however, most cases of hypoalbuminemia are caused by acute and chronic inflammatory responses (Peralta, 2020). Low serum albumin levels are an important predictor of morbidity and mortality, especially for burns or severe sepsis. Low serum albumin concentration (<3.5 g/dL) worsens the prognosis of patients with stable cardiovascular disease (Chien et al., 2017). At best, albumin reflects long-term changes in nutritional intake because the half-life is 14 to 20 days. Serum levels usually only rise when the inflammatory insult is resolved.

Prealbumin (transthyretin) is ordered for monitoring short-term changes in visceral protein status because of its short half-life of 2 days. Normal values range from 16 to 40 mg/dL. Compromised protein status is indicated when levels are between 10 and 15 g/dL. It is wise to remember that changes in prealbumin may reflect conditions such as inflammation, infection, or trauma; it is more of a prognostic tool than a valid indicator of nutritional status.

Serum hemoglobin measurement is a useful test. This oxygen-carrying protein molecule is especially important for children; iron-deficiency anemia affects their health and their cognitive development (Berglund et al., 2017). In adults, iron-deficiency anemia leads to fatigue, pale skin, weakness, and cold extremities. Indeed, many biochemical assessments provide useful information to determine the effects of nutrition or of medical conditions on the health status of patients. Table 11.3 provides more content.

Immune function may be evaluated with serum levels of several nutrients. Zinc, vitamin A, and omega-3 fatty acids play a role. Of greater prominence is vitamin D because it affects hundreds of genes in the body (National Institutes of Health [NIH], 2020). Vitamin D receptors (VDRs) have been found in bone, skin, placenta, and cancer cells. Adequate serum levels may help with immunity, pregnancy, and aging as well as possibly preventing autoimmune diseases, cancer, obesity, cardiovascular and respiratory disorders, erythropoiesis, diabetes, and muscle dysfunction (Wilson et al., 2017).

Vitamin D is produced by the body when sunlight strikes the skin; then two metabolic steps are required in the liver and the kidney to convert to the active form, vitamin D_3 (calcitriol). Dietary sources of this vitamin are few, and the rate of conversion to the active form is lower with aging. Thus, individuals who avoid the sun, have darker skin, are older, consume no vitamin D–rich foods, or habitually use sunscreens with high sun-protective factors may not acquire sufficient amounts. Serum vitamin D levels should be 50 to 125 nmol/L; a level between 30 and 50 nmol/L is mildly inadequate, and levels less than 30 nmol/L are detrimental for bone and health.

Clinical assessment. Clinical assessment includes data from several sources: medical history, social history, and physical examination. Environmental, social, family history, and past and present medical factors can alter nutrition status. Information can be found by reviewing the patient's medical record, as well as through direct interview. Many physical signs and symptoms

TABLE 11.3 Serum Biochemical Parameters[a]

Serum Analyte Normal Value/Range	Function	Comments
Albumin Normal: 3.5–5.0 g/dL Depletion: Mild: 3.0–3.4 g/dL Moderate: 2.4–2.9 g/dL Severe: <2.4 g/dL Half-life: ~14–20 days	Maintains plasma oncotic pressure; carrier for small molecules	Not sensitive or specific for acute protein malnutrition or response to nutrition therapy; affected by hydration status, disease state, clinical condition Often low because of inflammation Can be used as prognostic indicator of morbidity, mortality, and severity of illness
Prealbumin (transthyretin, thyroxin-binding prealbumin) Normal: 16–40 mg/dL Depletion: Mild: 10–15 mg/dL Moderate: 5–9 mg/dL Severe: <5 mg/dL Half-life: ~2–3 days	Carrier protein for thyroxin Combined with retinol-binding protein, transports vitamin A	Influenced less than albumin by intravascular fluid volume Not affected as early or as significantly with liver disease (compared with albumin) More likely to be a reflection of recent dietary intake than an accurate indicator of nutrition status
Hemoglobin Normal: Males: 13.8–17.2 g/dL Females: 12.1–15.1 g/dL Depletion: Males: <13.5 g/dL Females: <12 g/dL In general: Mild anemia = 10–12 g/dL Moderate anemia = 8–10 g/dL Severe anemia = <8 g/dL	Carries oxygen to cells; gives blood cells red color	Hemoglobin estimation is a useful index of the overall state of nutrition; in addition to anemia, it also suggests protein and trace element status High levels may be indicative of dehydration but not necessarily a high dietary iron intake The hemoglobin finding interpretation must be made in concert with that of other values before iron-deficiency anemia can be diagnosed Low serum levels may occur from blood loss, hidden gastrointestinal bleeding, or absorption problems (celiac disease, inflammatory bowel disease, etc.) Patients may exhibit shortness of breath, pale skin and gums, fast heartbeat, and extreme fatigue
Glucose (70–99 mg/dL [fasting])	Used for monitoring diabetes mellitus (DM) and other conditions such as hypoglycemia and ketoacidosis	Fasting glucose >125 mg/dL indicates DM (oral glucose tolerance tests are not needed for diagnosis); fasting glucose >100 mg/dL is indicator of insulin resistance
Creatinine (Males: 0.6–1.2 mg/dL; 53–106 µmol/L Females: 0.5–1.1 mg/dL; 44–97 µmol/L)	Muscle breakdown molecule	Increased in renal disease and decreased in malnutrition (i.e., blood urea nitrogen [BUN]/creatinine ratio >15:1)
BUN (5–20 mg urea nitrogen/dL; 1.8–7 mmol/L)	Protein in the bloodstream	Increased in renal disease and excessive protein catabolism Decreased in liver failure, negative nitrogen balance, and pregnancy
Total bilirubin (0.3–1.0 mg/dL; 5.1–17.0 µmol/L)	Important value in liver disorders	Increased in gallstones, biliary duct diseases, hepatic immaturity
Serum electrolytes Na$^+$ (135–145 mEq/L)[b] K$^+$ (3.6–5 mEq/L)[b] Cl^{2-} (101–111 mEq/L)[b]	Used to monitor most patients, especially those with cardiac, pulmonary, renal, or liver problems	Sodium levels are altered by hydration status Hypokalemia associated with diarrhea, vomiting, and licorice ingestion, and with diuretics and some other drugs Hyperkalemia occurs in renal diseases, crush injuries, and infection Chloride levels may be low with prolonged episodes of vomiting
Total calcium (8.5–10.5 mg/dL)	Transported bound to albumin; level may be altered by albumin level Important in bone and blood health	Hypercalcemia associated with endocrine disorders, malignancy, and hypervitaminosis D Hypocalcemia associated with vitamin D deficiency and inadequate hepatic or renal activation of vitamin D, hypoparathyroidism, magnesium deficiency, renal failure, and nephrotic syndrome
Phosphorus (phosphate) (3–4.5 mg/dL)	Important part of energy metabolism (forms adenosine triphosphate molecules)	Hyperphosphatemia associated with hypoparathyroidism and decreased intake Hypophosphatemia associated with hyperparathyroidism, chronic antacid ingestion, and renal failure
Total cholesterol (<200 mg/dL)	Cholesterol is an important precursor of steroid hormones and vitamin D	Decreased in patients with some forms of malnutrition, liver diseases, and hyperthyroidism
Triglycerides (40–160 mg/dL)	Levels vary by age and sex	Increased in patients with glucose intolerance and in some alcoholics

[a]Biochemical assessment for nutrition starts from a general overview but will then be targeted according to medical diagnosis. Reference ranges may vary slightly among laboratories.

[b]mEq/L = 1 mmol/L.

Modified from Lab Tests Online. Accessed from http://labtestsonline.org/map/sindex; Lee RD, Nieman DC: *Nutritional assessment*, ed 6, New York, 2013, McGraw-Hill; and Thompson CW: Laboratory assessment. In Charney P, Malone AM, editors: *Academy of Nutrition and Dietetics pocket guide to nutrition assessment*, ed 3, Chicago, 2015, Academy of Nutrition and Dietetics.

associated with malnutrition are also sought as an integral part of assessing health status.

Features associated with nutrition deficiency may be identified through histories and clinical categories. Acquiring historical data includes asking about poverty, avoidance of specific food groups (e.g., dairy, meat, fruits or vegetables), weight changes, nicotine use, drug or alcohol use, family medical history, and use of dietary supplements. Clinical factors include recent surgery or wounds, blood loss, skin and hair changes, and many other indicators. Findings may be organized according to symptoms of the eyes, face, skin, muscles, tongue, and central nervous system (Table 11.4). Although these signs are taught thoroughly to dietitians, nurses may overlook them. For example, in a patient with spoon-shaped nails, an assessment for iron-deficiency anemia may be an appropriate request for the physician to review.

Dietary intake assessment. There are several methods for collecting information regarding actual and habitual dietary intake. Most commonly, data are collected using dietary recall methods (historical/retrospective) or documented food records (current/prospective). Each method has its pros and cons, so it is important to choose a method suitable for the type of information needed.

TABLE 11.4 Physical Signs That Suggest Nutrient Imbalance

Area of Concern	Possible Deficiency	Possible Excess
Hair		
Dull, dry, brittle	Pro	
Easily plucked (with no pain)	Pro	
Hair loss	Pro, Zn, biotin	Vitamin A
Flag sign (loss of hair pigment in strips around head)	Pro, Cu	
Head and Neck		
Bulging fontanel (infants)		Vitamin A
Headache		Vitamin A, D
Epistaxis (nosebleed)	Vitamin K	
Thyroid enlargement	Iodine	
Eyes		
Conjunctival and corneal xerosis (dryness)	Vitamin A	
Pale conjunctiva	Fe	
Blue sclerae	Fe	
Corneal vascularization	Vitamin B_2	
Mouth		
Cheilosis or angular stomatitis (lesions at corners of mouth)	Vitamin B_2	
Glossitis (red, sore tongue)	Niacin, folate, vitamin B_{12}, and other B vitamins	
Gingivitis (inflamed gums)	Vitamin C	
Hypogeusia, dysgeusia (poor sense of taste, distorted taste)	Zn	
Dental caries	Fluoride	
Mottling of teeth		Fluoride
Atrophy of papillae on tongue	Fe, B vitamin	
Skin		
Dry, scaly	Vitamin A, Zn, EFAs	Vitamin A
Follicular hyperkeratosis (resembles gooseflesh)	Vitamin A, EFAs, B vitamin	
Eczematous lesions	Zn	
Petechiae, ecchymoses	Vitamin C, K	
Nasolabial seborrhea (greasy, scaly areas between nose and lip)	Niacin, vitamin B_{12}, B_6	
Darkening and peeling of skin in areas exposed to sun	Niacin	
Poor wound healing	Pro, Zn, vitamin C	
Nails		
Spoon-shaped nails	Fe	
Brittle, fragile	Pro	
Heart		
Enlargement, tachycardia, failure	Vitamin B_1	
Small heart	Energy	
Sudden failure, death	Se	
Arrhythmia	Mg, K, Se	
Hypertension	Ca, K	

Continued

TABLE 11.4 Physical Signs That Suggest Nutrient Imbalance—cont'd

Area of Concern	Possible Deficiency	Possible Excess
Abdomen		
Hepatomegaly	Pro	Vitamin A
Ascites	Pro	
Musculoskeletal and Extremities		
Muscle wasting (especially temporal area)	Energy	
Edema	Pro, vitamin B_1	
Calf tenderness	Vitamin B_1 or C, biotin, Se	
Beading of ribs, or "rachitic rosary" (child)	Vitamin C, D	
Bone and joint tenderness	Vitamin C, D, Ca, P	
Knock-knee, bowed legs, fragile bones	Vitamin D, Ca, P, Cu	
Neurologic		
Paresthesia (pain and tingling or altered sensation in the extremities)	Vitamin B_1, B_6, B_{12}, biotin	
Weakness	Vitamin C, B_1, B_6, B_{12}, energy	
Ataxia, decreased position and vibratory senses	Vitamin B_1, B_{12}	
Tremor	Mg	
Decreased tendon reflexes	Vitamin B_1	
Confabulation, disorientation	Vitamin B_1, B_{12}	
Drowsiness, lethargy	Vitamin B_1	Vitamin A, D
Depression	Vitamin B_1, biotin, B_{12}	

Ca, Calcium; *Cu*, copper; *EFAs*, essential fatty acids; *Fe*, iron; *K*, potassium; *Mg*, magnesium; *Na*, sodium; *P*, phosphorus; *Pro*, protein; *Se*, selenium; *Zn*, zinc.

The intake records provide information about calories (kcal), protein, carbohydrate, fat, vitamins, minerals, and fluid. Results can be calculated manually with food composition tables or analyzed by computer software. More than 100 computer programs are available to analyze dietary intake.

24-hour diet recall. In 24-hour diet recall, the patient is asked by a trained interviewer to report all foods and beverages consumed during the past 24 hours. Detailed descriptions of all foods, beverages, cooking methods, brand names, condiments, and supplements, along with portion sizes in common household measures, are included. Food models, measuring cups, life-size pictures, or abstract shapes (squares, circles, and rectangles) are used to assist the patient in estimating correct portion sizes of foods consumed. This method is useful in screening or during follow-up to evaluate adaptation of or compliance with dietary recommendations. The advantages of this method are that it is quick (only 15 to 20 minutes is needed) and that it can be used with most age groups. Because it is retrospective, the patient does not modify their actual intake. The information can be obtained by face-to-face interview, telephone interview, or patient self-reporting. Some of the drawbacks of this method are that it relies on the memory, motivation, and awareness of the patient. Also, because it records only a single day's intake, the results may not be representative of the patient's actual diet.

Food records. Estimated or measured food records can provide a more realistic picture of a patient's usual intake. For this method of dietary data collection, the patient must be literate, numerate, and well-motivated (Lee & Nieman, 2013). All foods, beverages, snacks, and supplements are recorded by the patient, usually over 1 to 7 days using household measures. The patient must be trained with food models, measuring cups, or other measuring devices that will help ensure recording of proper or actual portion sizes. Cooking methods, recipe ingredients, and descriptions should be recorded as completely and accurately as possible. If information is needed to identify behavioral as well as nutritional patterns, the recorder is also asked to record locations, times, events, and feelings in addition to foods eaten. A 7-day food record is considered optimal for gathering this kind of information, but it does tend to be tedious. Shorter periods are less representative of usual intake, but a 3-day record (2 weekdays and 1 weekend day) is most common.

Calorie counts. In an acute- or a long-term care setting, one of the most common forms of food records is a calorie count. In actual practice, all nutrients can be assessed, but energy and protein intakes are most often quantified. Information gathered in this manner is used to determine the adequacy of patients' daily oral intake or to document need for **nutrition support** (any nutrition intervention used to minimize patient morbidity, mortality, and complications).

Nursing observations are essential for early identification of malnutrition and prevention of weight loss during the hospital stay. Staff responsible for recording calorie intake must be accurate in their recordings. It is important to record foods and beverages consumed in measurable amounts (e.g., cups, ounces, teaspoons, tablespoons, milliliters) or in percentage of amount eaten (50% baked chicken, 75% bread, 25% green beans). Subjective terms such as "two bites, ate well," and "three swallows" are not useful and cannot provide objective information needed to calculate protein and kcal intake. See the *Teaching Tool* box Conducting an Effective Calorie Count.

TEACHING TOOL

Conducting an Effective Calorie Count

Policy

Residents and patients will receive a Calorie Count/Nutrient Intake Analysis, as ordered by the physician.

Procedure

A Calorie Count/Nutrient Intake Analysis is the calculation of a resident's food and beverage intake for calories and protein for 72 hours. In addition, the analysis of other nutrients sometimes is ordered.

1. A physician's order is obtained for a calorie count, which is conducted for 72 hours (3 days). Extensions sometimes are ordered.
2. Nutrient intake analysis begins with the first breakfast meal after the order is written and received by the Nutrition Department.
3. Nursing staff must contact the nutrition professional and give the name, room number, and current diet order. The diet sheet must indicate that a calorie count has been ordered.
4. Nursing staff will initiate the 72-hour (3-day) calorie count.
5. Nursing staff will record the resident's food and beverage intake for each meal on the actual menu and attach it to the calorie count form (shown here). It is also necessary to record all between-meal snacks, nourishments or nutrition supplements on the calorie count form.
6. The nutrition designee picks up the completed calorie count form.
7. The nutrition professional records a summary of analysis in the resident's medical record.
8. The nutrition professional makes recommendations in the medical record and communicates these recommendations to the physician, as per policy, if findings indicate a need for further assessment or interventions.
9. References to help calculate nutrient intake may include the following:
   - Nutrient analysis of menu items
   - *Food Values of Portions Commonly Used*, ed 19, 2009, Lippincott Williams & Wilkins.
   - *USDA Agriculture Handbook 8: Composition of Foods—Raw, Processed, Prepared*, and its revisions, and/or supplements
   - Exchange lists

Modified with permission from https://drnancycollins.com/personnel/dr-nancy-collins/.

Managing Nutrition Risk

The nutrition care process involves assessing patients' nutritional status, estimating nutrition needs, determining whether there is a problem (nutrition diagnosis) to treat, and planning nutrition intervention. If done appropriately, early intervention works as treatment of established malnutrition or prevention of malnutrition among those at high nutrition risk. Areas to consider for nutrition risk are age, weight, laboratory test results, body systems, and feeding modalities (Table 11.5), as follows (Rasmussen et al., 2010):

Age: Age-related high risk is possible for patients aged 75 years or older. For children, high risk most often occurs for those younger than 5 years.

Disorder severity: Conditions affecting various body systems can pose either moderate or high nutrition risk. Moderate nutrition risk may be experienced when a patient undergoes chemotherapy because of its effects on dietary intake. High risk is incurred among individuals with eating disorders or pregnant women with diabetes.

Feeding mode: Risk is high with modified diets that have the potential to cause nutrient deficiencies. Patients may be at high risk if they receive parenteral feeding or tube feeding, are nil per os (NPO—i.e., nothing by mouth), or are consuming only clear liquids for more than 3 days.

Laboratory test results: Biochemical tests provide a cursory assessment of nutrition risk.

Weight: Weight loss is a potential nutrition risk factor, depending on its cause.

Remember that there is no single index for measuring nutrition status. Accurate and meaningful assessment can be made only by incorporating anthropometric, biochemical, clinical, and dietary data.

Screening and Assessment Tools

A variety of tools have been established to evaluate nutrition screening and assessment factors, especially in relation to length

TABLE 11.5 Nutrition Risk Categories

Data Source	Moderate Risk	High Risk
Age	65–75 years Children >5 years of age	≥75 years Children <5 years of age
Weight	Evaluation of loss (i.e., self-induced)	5% weight loss in 1 month 10% loss in 6 months Length/height for age <5th percentile Weight/height <5th percentile or <80th percentile of standard
Laboratory	Albumin 3–3.5 g/dL[a]	Albumin ≤3 g/dL
Systems (risk depends on the individual population)	Heart, antepartum, pain, orthopedics, selected oncology, short hospital stay, chemotherapy	Renal, pancreas, gastrointestinal, liver, diabetes with pregnancy, eating disorders, oncology, transplants, any condition in children associated with development of protein-calorie malnutrition
Feeding modalities	Transitional (stable) Some selected modified diets with education component	Parenteral nutrition, tube feeding, nothing per mouth (NPO), or clear liquids >3 days

[a]A *Nutrition Risk Score* (NRI), developed originally for populations with acquired immunodeficiency syndrome (AIDS) or cancer, was derived from the serum albumin concentration and the ratio of actual to usual weight, as follows: NRI = (1.519 × serum albumin, g/dL) + (41.7 × present weight [kg]/ideal body weight [kg]) (Aziz EF, Javed F, Pratap B, et al: Malnutrition as assessed by nutritional risk index is associated with worse outcome in patients admitted with acute decompensated heart failure: An ACAP-HF data analysis, *Heart Int* 6:e2, 2011.)

Data from Grant A, DeHoog S: *Nutritional assessment and support*, ed 5, Seattle, 1999, Anne Grant/Susan DeHoog.

of hospital stay and morbidity. It is important to determine how the tools were validated, how reliable they are, and for which population and care setting they were developed (Rasmussen et al., 2010). Of the many tools, six are mentioned here: Nutrition Risk Screening 2002 (NRS-2002), Malnutrition Universal Screening Tool (MUST), Mini Nutritional Assessment (MNA), Short Nutritional Assessment Questionnaire (SNAQ65+), Subjective Global Assessment (SGA), and Malnutrition Screening Tool (MST).

The NRS-2002 can be used in the community, in the hospital, or for the elderly. Some tools have been designed by groups, such as the MUST from the British Association of Parenteral and Enteral Nutrition. Some were designed specifically for the elderly, such as the MNA from the Nestle Institute or the SNAQ65+. Finally, some were designed for specific conditions; the SGA was developed in the 1980s for patients with liver disease or cancer. However, only one has been found to be both reliable and valid for identifying undernutrition in a variety of patients and settings: the MST from Abbott (Skipper et al., 2012) (Fig. 11.8).

For malnourished adults with chronic starvation: Order meals and snacks according to appetite and preferences; encourage a small snack approximately every 2 to 3 hours. Some individuals may need feeding assistance.

For recent acute illness or injury with inflammation: Offer balanced, nutritious meals in small amounts. Use oral supplements between meals if intake is poor at mealtime and for patients who are frail or have infections, impaired wound healing, or pressure ulcers.

For sarcopenia: Oral diet is best, but enteral or parenteral routes may also be needed. Extra dietary protein or amino acids may be useful; whey protein powder is a good source. Some individuals may need feeding assistance.

Drug Interactions With Food and Nutrients

One of the key aspects of nutrition assessment and patient care includes ongoing review of potential or actual food-drug and drug-nutrient interactions. All drugs have physiologic effects, some of which are unintended side effects and constitute the risks of medication use. The amount and rate of drug absorption can be affected by the composition and timing of food intake. Conversely, food intake, absorption, and metabolism can be altered by medication. Drug-nutrient interactions may reduce drug efficacy, interfere with disease control, and foster nutritional deficiencies. Key interventions may involve a change in foods or nutrient administration, patient education or counseling, and coordination of care with the dietitian.

TJC strongly recommends evaluation of drug and diet combinations. Documentation of these interactions, which may be done by the RD or nurse, is essential in complying with TJC standards. In addition to medications, the use of alcohol and street drugs affects nutrition status and nutrient requirements.

Risk Factors for Drug-Nutrient Interactions

Determination of risk for drug-nutrient reactions depends on characteristics of the individual, including age, physiologic status, multiple-drug intake, hepatic and renal function, and typical dietary intake.

Age. Older adults are more at risk for drug-nutrient reactions because of the greater variety of medications used and the reduced physiologic functioning, which affects drug absorption and efficacy. Older patients often experience several different disorders simultaneously, each with complications and medications that may interact. Young children also can be affected by drug-nutrient interactions. Use in children of vitamins/minerals, dietary supplements, and over-the-counter (OTC) medications intended for adults can result in drug-nutrient reactions because the substances will be metabolized differently.

Physiologic status. Impaired ability to absorb, metabolize, or excrete nutrients and medications because of disorders of the GI tract and reduction in hepatic and renal functioning increases the risk of drug-nutrient reactions. Postoperative trauma or injury may also trigger atypical physiologic responses to drug-nutrient interactions. Age alters physiologic status as the body matures. Drug doses can vary according to a person's weight and metabolic function as an aspect of age-related physiologic status. Use of medications during pregnancy requires caution because of the multiple effects on the fetus and on the nutritional status of the mother.

Polypharmacy (multiple-drug intake). Certain types of illnesses or disease groups tend to require combinations of therapeutic drugs plus other medications, including OTC drugs, for relief of symptoms. The resulting drug-nutrient reactions may be related to the disease itself or be a reaction to medications. For example, intestinal bleeding often causes iron-deficiency anemia among patients with arthritis. This intestinal bleeding is a common side effect of long-term use of nonsteroidal antiinflammatory drugs (NSAIDs), either prescribed or OTC, taken to reduce the symptoms of arthritis.

Influence of typical dietary intake. The basis of a person's nutritional status depends on foods regularly consumed; the nutritional content of these foods affects body functions. A well-nourished individual is better able to withstand a medical regimen that may affect nutrient functioning. In contrast, individuals who are malnourished or marginally deficient in nutrient intake are more at risk for complications of drug-nutrient reactions as the body's stores of nutrients are diminished. For example, individuals who excessively consume alcohol tend to be marginally deficient in several nutrients either because of inadequate food intake (alcohol is an appetite suppressant) or because of drug (alcohol)–nutrient interactions.

Prescription and Over-the-Counter Medications

Television, radio, and print media present numerous advertisements about prescription drugs. Patients now approach primary health care providers requesting prescriptions for drugs that treat conditions for which they have not yet been diagnosed. Although the public has become more educated about prescription drugs, OTC medications seem harmless because prescriptions are not required, but harmless they are not. Interactions may occur between OTC drugs and other medications, foods, nutrients, and herbs and other supplements.

Malnutrition Screening Tool (MST)

STEP 1: Screen with the MST

❶ Have you recently lost weight without trying?

No	0
Unsure	2

If yes, how much weight have you lost?

2-13 lb	1
14-23 lb	2
24-33 lb	3
34 lb or more	4
Unsure	2

Weight loss score:

❷ Have you been eating poorly because of a decreased appetite?

No	0
Yes	1

Appetite score:

Add weight loss and appetite scores

MST SCORE:

STEP 2: Score to determine risk

MST = 0 OR 1
NOT AT RISK
Eating well with little or no weight loss

If length of stay exceeds 7 days, then rescreen, repeating weekly as needed.

MST = 2 OR MORE
AT RISK
Eating poorly and/or recent weight loss

Rapidly implement nutrition interventions. Perform nutrition consult within 24-72 hrs, depending on risk.

STEP 3: Intervene with nutritional support for your patients at risk of malnutrition.

Notes:

Ferguson, M et al. *Nutrition* 1999 15:458-464

©2013 Abbott Laboratories
88205/May 2013 LITHO IN USA
www.abbottnutrition.com/rdtoolkit

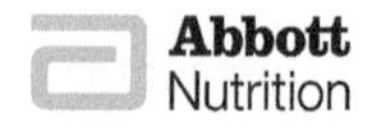

Fig. 11.8 The Malnutrition Screening Tool. (Reprinted from Ferguson M, Capra S, Bauer J, Banks M: Development of a valid and reliable malnutrition screening tool for adult acute hospital patients, *Nutrition* 15:458–464, 1999.)

Effects of Drugs on Food and Nutrients

Most drug absorption occurs through the GI mucosa, predominantly in the small intestine. Before a drug can be absorbed, it must first be metabolized and dissolved in the gastric juices of the stomach. The speed with which the drug leaves the stomach depends on the gastric emptying time, which affects the rate of drug absorption. This rate may either increase or decrease according to the amount of food in the GI tract. In the fasting state, the medication leaves the empty stomach quickly and is absorbed from the small intestine. For some drugs that is too quick, because time is needed for their disintegration into absorbable particles. For those drugs, it is better to take the medication in the fed state, in which the stomach, containing food, empties more slowly, especially after the consumption of large meals, heated food, and meals with fat, all of which slow emptying time.

Drugs can alter food intake, nutrient absorption, metabolism, and excretion. These drugs include prescription medications, OTC drugs, and even alcohol. Drugs used to lower serum cholesterol levels bind with fat-soluble vitamins and bile salts. As a result, both the bile salts and vitamins are excreted. Some drugs can decrease the number of digestive enzymes available and thereby decrease nutrient absorption. The tables in this chapter provide information on selected drug-nutrient interactions.

Mineral status can be affected by drugs. Depletion may occur from the simultaneous use of several medications that have the side effect of mineral depletion. Potassium-depleting diuretics along with laxatives may cause significant loss. Older adults often use these products; their dietary intake may be marginal in mineral content as well. Potassium overload may occur in instances in which renal function is compromised and potassium-sparing diuretics (e.g., spironolactone) and potassium supplements are used. Patient education is vital regarding the use of potassium supplements. Clear information is essential. Patients should be taught about the kind of diuretic they are taking and its potential side effects to reduce inappropriate supplementation.

Medications can alter food intake by acting as appetite suppressants or stimulants (Box 11.4), altering taste sensations (Box 11.5), or producing nausea and vomiting, which further decrease appetite. The *Teaching Tool* box Minimizing Drug Side Effects provides a number of specific suggestions.

BOX 11.4 Selected Drugs That Affect Appetite

Appetite Stimulants

Antidepressants
Amitriptyline (Elavil, Endep)
Clomipramine HCl (Anafranil)
Monoamine oxidase inhibitor (MAOIs)
Tranylcypromine sulfate (Parnate)

Antihistamines
Astemizole (Hismanal)
Cyproheptadine HCl (Periactin)

Bronchodilator
Albuterol sulfate (Proventil, Ventolin)

Steroids
Anabolic steroids
Oxandrolone (Anavar)
Corticosteroids
Hydrocortisone (Cortef)
Glucocorticoids
Dexamethasone (Decadron)
Methylprednisolone (Medrol)

Tranquilizers
Lithium carbonate (Lithane)
Benzodiazepines
Chlordiazepoxide HCl (Librium)
Diazepam (Valium)
Prazepam (Centrax)
Phenothiazines
Chlorpromazine HCl (Thorazine)
Promethazine HCl (Phenergan)

Appetite Suppressants

Amphetamines
Benzphetamine HCl (Didrex)
Fenfluramine HCl (Pondimin)
Phenylpropanolamine (Dexatrim, Dimetapp, Triaminic)

Antidysrhythmics
Digitalis
Digitoxin (Crystodigin, Digitoxin)
Digoxin (Digoxin, Lanoxin)

Antibiotics
Amphotericin B (Fungizone)
Gentamicin (Garamycin)
Metronidazole (Flagyl)
Zidovudine (AZT)

Antidepressant
Fluoxetine HCl (Prozac)

Antihistamine
Azatadine maleate (Optimine)

Antihypertensives
Amiloride and hydrochlorothiazide (Moduretic)
Captopril (Capoten)
Chlorthalidone (Hygroton)

Muscle Relaxant
Dantrolene sodium (Dantrium)

Stimulant/Antiattention Deficit Disorder Agent
Methylphenidate HCl (Ritalin)

Data from Pronsky ZM: *Food-medication interactions*, ed 189, Birchrunville, PA, 2018, Food-Medication Interactions.

BOX 11.5 Selected Drugs That Alter Taste

Antidysrhythmics
Amiodarone (Cordarone)
Antiarthritic/Chelating agent
Penicillamine (Cuprimine, Depen)

Antibiotics
Ampicillin
Clarithromycin (Biaxin)

Anticonvulsant
Phenytoin (Dilantin)

Antidepressants
Clomipramine HCl (Anafranil)
Fluoxetine HCl (Prozac)

Antifungal
Griseofulvin (Fulvicin, Grifulvin V, Grisacrin)

Antigout Agent
Allopurinol (Zyloprim)

Antihypertensives
Captopril (Capoten)
Labetalol HCl (Normodyne, Trandate)

Antimanics
Lithium carbonate (Eskalith, Lithane, Lithobid)
Lithium citrate (Cibalith-S)

Antiparkinsonian
Levodopa (Dopar, Larodopa)

Antiviral/Anti–Human Immunodeficiency Virus Agent
Didanosine (Videx)

Muscle Relaxant
Dantrolene sodium (Dantrium)

Muscle Relaxant/Antispasmodic
Baclofen (Lioresal)

Stimulant/Amphetamine
Dextroamphetamine sulfate (Dexedrine)

Data from Pronsky ZM: *Food-medication interactions*, ed 18, Birchrunville, PA, 2015, Food-Medication Interactions.

TEACHING TOOL

Minimizing Side Effects

Many drugs have side effects—symptoms that are not caused by the illness for which the drugs have been prescribed but are physiologic responses of the body to the drugs themselves. The side effects may be mild or quite bothersome. Some may be serious enough to warrant a change in medication. Before using these strategies as education tools, consult the client's primary health care provider to ascertain whether additional medical intervention is required.

Side Effect: Diminished Appetite
- Consider serving several small meals or snacks throughout the day.
- Establish a setting and atmosphere for mealtimes that enhances appetite. Assist the client in exploring approaches to encourage an optimum eating environment.
- Discuss client's favorite foods. Brainstorm about how recipes can be adapted to comply with dietary therapeutic plans.

Side Effect: Modified Taste Sensations
- Visit a dentist regularly to maintain or improve oral hygiene.
- Mask the taste of medications, if needed, with fruit sauces such as applesauce, crushed pineapple, or milk products. First determine whether combinations are acceptable and not contraindicated.

Side Effect: Increased Appetite
- Alert client to the appetite stimulant effect of certain medications.
- Evaluate client's typical dietary intake. Suggest high-fiber foods to provide a quick sense of feeling full.
- Advise limiting availability of high-kcal foods and drinks to minimize excess kcal intake.
- Increase activity.

Side Effect: Gastrointestinal Tract Irritation and Discomfort
- Advise client to sit up or stand after taking medications that have the potential to cause heartburn or indigestion.
- Reduce intake of fat, greasy, and/or highly acidic foods, including citrus juices and tomato products.
- Limit food intake in the evening to prevent reflux.
- Control consumption of spicy foods, peppermint, colas, chocolate, alcohol, pepper, decaffeinated coffee, and caffeine if they produce gastric discomfort.

Side Effect: Nausea
- Control liquid intake by serving after meals, or drink only small quantities with meals.
- Sustain adequate fluid volume; cold, carbonated, or clear liquids are easier to tolerate.

Side Effect: Dry or Sore Mouth
- Consume softer, moist foods such as applesauce, puddings, pureed foods, and mashed potatoes.
- Include iced and cold foods throughout the day; consider ice pops, frozen yogurt, ice cream, sorbets, and cooled melons.
- Encourage oral hygiene before and after eating.
- Avoid mouthwashes, which can further dry the oral mucosa.

Data from Pronsky ZM: *Food-medication interactions*, ed 18, Birchrunville, PA, 2015, Food-Medication Interactions.

Drugs may cause additional nutrition problems by affecting GI tract motility (which can change nutrient absorption) or GI tract pH. Drugs also may cause injury of GI mucosa, development of drug-nutrient compounds, decreased bile acid function, and depressed nutrient transport mechanisms. The metabolic and excretion rates of the drug itself may also interfere with nutrient metabolism and excretion. Oral contraceptives may cause marginal deficiencies of B vitamins and vitamin C by increasing the body's use of these vitamins. Table 11.6 presents information on how various drug classes affect food intake, nutrient absorption, metabolism, and excretion.

TABLE 11.6 Medications That Affect Food and/or Nutrients

Drug or Class	Examples	Action	Nutrients Affected	How to Avoid
Alcohol, particularly excessive use	Beer, wine, spirits	Increases turnover of some vitamins; substitution of alcohol for food	Vitamin B_{12}, folate, and magnesium	Limit alcohol consumption to two drinks per day for men or one drink per day for women
Analgesics, nonsteroidal antiinflammatory drugs	Salicylates (aspirin), ibuprofen (Motrin, Advil), naproxen (Anaprox, Aleve, Naprosyn), acetaminophen (Tylenol)	Increase loss of vitamin C and compete with folate and vitamin K	Vitamin C, folate, vitamin K	Increase intake of foods high in vitamin C, folate, and vitamin K; take with 8 oz of water
Antacids	Aluminum antacids, histamine H_2 blockers	Inactivates thiamin; decreased absorption of some nutrients	Thiamin (vitamin B_1)	Foods containing thiamin (B_1) should be consumed at a different time: Take antacid after meals; take iron, magnesium, or folate supplements separately 2 hours before or after; take antacid separately 3 hours before or after citrus fruit or juices or calcium citrate
Antiulcer agents (histamine blockers)	Ranitidine (Zantac), cimetidine (Tagamet), famotidine (Pepcid)	Decreases vitamin absorption	Vitamin B_{12}	Consult physician or registered dietitian regarding vitamin B_{12} supplementation
Antibiotics	Tetracycline, ciprofloxacin (Cipro)	Chelation of minerals; ingestion with caffeine may increase excitability and nervousness	Calcium, magnesium, iron, and zinc; caffeine	Take tetracycline at least 1 hour before or 2 hours after a meal; do not take with caffeine-containing products
Antineoplastic drugs	Methotrexate	Cause mucosal damage, which may lead to decreased nutrient absorption	Folate and vitamin B_{12}; also see Antibiotics	Consult physician or registered dietitian regarding supplementation
Anticholinergics	Amitriptyline (Elavil), chlorpromazine (Thorazine)	Thicken saliva, which loses its ability to prevent tooth decay	Fluids	Increase intake of fluids
Anticonvulsants	Phenobarbital, phenytoin (Dilantin)	Increase metabolism of folate (possibly leading to megaloblastic anemia), vitamin D (especially in children), and vitamin K	Folate, vitamin D, and vitamin K	Increase folate, vitamins D and K intake
Antidepressants	Lithium carbonate (Lithane, Lithobid, Lithonate, Lithotabs, Eskalith)	May cause metallic taste, nausea, vomiting, dry mouth, anorexia, weight gain, and increased thirst	Fluids	Drink 2–3 L of water per day and take with food; have a consistent sodium intake
Antihyperlipidemics	Cholestyramine (Questran), colestipol (Colestid)	Bind bile salts and nutrients	Fat-soluble vitamins (A, D, E, K), folate, vitamin B_{12}, and iron	Include rich sources of these vitamins and minerals in diet
Antituberculosis	Isoniazid (INH)	Inhibits conversion of vitamin B_6 to active form	Vitamin B_6	Vitamin B_6 supplementation is necessary to prevent deficiency and peripheral neuropathy

Continued

TABLE 11.6 Medications That Affect Food and/or Nutrients—cont'd

Drug or Class	Examples	Action	Nutrients Affected	How to Avoid
Corticosteroids	Prednisone, Solu-Medrol, hydrocortisone	Increase excretion	Protein, potassium, calcium, magnesium, zinc, vitamin C, and vitamin B_6	Increase intake of foods high in protein, potassium, calcium, magnesium, zinc, vitamin C, and vitamin B_6
Loop diuretics	Furosemide (Lasix)	Increase mineral excretion in urine	Potassium, calcium, magnesium, zinc, sodium, and chloride	Include fresh fruits and vegetables in diet
Thiazide diuretics	Hydrochlorothiazide (HCTZ)	Increase excretion of most electrolytes but enhance reabsorption of calcium	Potassium, calcium, magnesium, zinc, sodium, chloride, and calcium	Increase intake of foods high in potassium, calcium, magnesium, zinc, sodium, chloride, and calcium
Potassium-sparing diuretics	Triamterene (Dyrenium)	Hyperkalemia	Potassium	Avoid potassium-based salt substitutes
Laxatives	Fibercon, Mitrolan	Decrease nutrient absorption	Vitamins and minerals	Consult physician or registered dietitian regarding supplementation
Sedatives	Barbiturates	Increases metabolism of vitamins	Folate, vitamin D, vitamin B_{12}, thiamine, and vitamin C	Increase intake of foods high in folate, vitamin D, vitamin B_{12}, thiamine, and vitamin C
Mineral oil	Agoral Plain	Decreases absorption	Fat-soluble vitamins (A, D, E, K), beta carotene, calcium, phosphorus, and potassium	Take 2 hours before or after food and fat-soluble vitamins
Oral contraceptives	Estrogen/progestin	May cause selective malabsorption or increased metabolism and turnover	Vitamin B_6 and folate	Increase foods high in B_6 and folate

From Drug-nutrient interactions. In Schlenker ED, Gilbert J, editors: *Williams' essentials of nutrition & diet therapy*, ed 12, St. Louis, 2018, Elsevier.

Effects of Food and Nutrients on Drugs

Foods and nutrients may also affect drug action, producing uncomfortable side effects. Most noteworthy are the adverse side effects associated with monoamine oxidase inhibitors (MAOIs). MAOIs, such as phenelzine (Nardil) and tranylcypromine (Parnate), which may be prescribed to treat depression. These drugs inhibit the enzyme monoamine oxidase, the function of which is to inactivate tyramine found in some foods. Without monoamine oxidase, the level of tyramine increases the release of norepinephrine. Elevations of norepinephrine may cause headache, pallor, heart palpitations, and life-threatening severe hypertension. Patients who take MAOIs should avoid foods and drugs that contain tyramine, such as Chianti wine, aged cheese, and several fermented foods. Locate the list in your facility's diet manual and discuss any concerns with the dietitian.

Medications must be absorbed to have a therapeutic effect. Food intake and composition of the food may affect drug absorption. Table 11.7 lists some common drug classes in which absorption is affected by food. A specific food example is grapefruit juice. Grapefruit juice, which patients sometimes use to take medications, can affect the bioavailability of certain drugs (Box 11.6). Table 11.8 lists foods and nutrients that affect medications.

Timing of Medication Administration

The timing of drug administration and meals also has clinical significance. If its absorption is increased by the presence of food, the medication should be taken with a meal or a snack. If the drug's absorption is depressed by the presence of food in the stomach, optimum absorption occurs if the medication is taken at least 1 hour before or 2 hours after eating or tube feeding.

The established drug administration schedules in health care facilities often conflict with the optimal bioavailability of a prescribed drug. As a general guideline, drugs should be given at least 1 hour before or 2 hours after a meal unless the medication causes GI distress when taken on an empty stomach. Such timing should enhance drug absorption and decrease hindrance of nutrient absorption. Tube feedings present other issues of drug-nutrient interactions (Box 11.7).

Effects of Herbs on Food, Nutrients, and Drugs

Herbs are not innocuous; they can have significant effects on the bioavailability of foods, nutrients, and drugs. Of concern are the effects of commonly used herbs on a body undergoing surgery. Ginkgo, feverfew, garlic, ginger, ginseng, dong quai, and danshen affect blood clotting. Other herbs, such as valerian, kava kava (which may also cause liver damage), and St. John's wort, can prolong the effects of narcotic and anesthetic drugs.

Nurses should ask detailed questions about a patient's supplement intake, such as the following:

- Do you use any dietary supplements? (Direct patient to include in the answer vitamins, minerals, botanicals, amino acids, concentrates, and extracts.)
  - If so, what dosage do you take? What other directions do you follow, such as taking with meals or at bedtime?

TABLE 11.7 Drugs That May Cause Nutrition Problems

Nutrition Problem	Drugs	Use
Depression that results in weight fluctuation	Carbidopa/levodopa	Antiparkinsonian
	Beta-blockers	Antihypertensive
	Clonidine	Antihypertensive
	Benzodiazepines	Antianxiety
	Barbiturates	Antianxiety
	Anticonvulsants	Antiepileptic
	Histamine H_2 blockers	Peptic ulcer disease
	Calcium channel blockers	Antihypertensive
	Thiazide diuretics	Antihypertensive
	Digoxin	Antidysrhythmic
Delayed gastric emptying time	Anesthetic agents	Anesthesia
	Opiates	Narcotic
	Tricyclic antidepressant	Antidepressant
	Clonidine	Antihypertensive
	Calcium channel blockers	Antihypertensive
	Nitrates	Antianginal
	Meperidine	Analgesic
	Theophylline	Bronchodilator
	Caffeine	Stimulant
Increased gastric emptying time	Metoclopramide	Antiemetic
	Cisapride	Cholinergic enhancer
	Bethanechol	Cholinergic
	Erythromycin	Antibacterial
Folate deficiency	Phenytoin	Seizures
	Methotrexate	Antimetabolite
	Trimethoprim	Antibacterial
Drowsiness and, possibly, missed meals	Antihistamines	Allergies
	Beta-blockers	Antihypertensive
	Skeletal muscle relaxants	Relieve stiffness, pain, discomfort
	Antiemetics	Nausea and vomiting
	Benzodiazepines	Antianxiety
	Antipsychotics	Psychotic disorders
	Antidepressants	Depression
Nausea and vomiting	Selective serotonin reuptake inhibitors (SSRIs)	Antidepressant
	Antibiotics	Antibacterial
	Antineoplastic agents	Chemotherapy
	Digitalis	Antidysrhythmic
	General anesthetics	Anesthesia
	Theophylline	Bronchodilator
	Opioid derivatives	Narcotic

Data from Losben N: Dietitians and consultant pharmacists: A team approach to improved quality care (in *The Consultant Pharmacist*), Alexandria, VA, 1997, American Society of Consultant Pharmacists. MedlinePlus: *Drugs & supplements*, Bethesda, MD (updated January 2006), U.S. National Library of Medicine and National Institutes of Health. Accessed 20 August, 2020, from http://medlineplus.gov.

BOX 11.6 Grapefruit "Juices Up" Certain Medications

Almost all oral drugs (including alcohol) go through the liver via hepatic portal circulation, which removes some of the active substance from the blood before entering the general circulation. This means that a fraction of the original dose of the drug will not be "available" because bioavailability of the drug has been lowered. One mechanism responsible for this effect is an enzyme system found in the intestinal wall and liver called the cytochrome P450 3A4 system. Most medications are lipid soluble and readily absorbed. To eliminate toxins (i.e., drugs) from the body, however, the cytochrome P450 system either breaks them down in the gut or changes them into more water-soluble versions in the liver, allowing them to be eliminated via urine.

Grapefruit juice blocks the CYP3A4 enzyme in the wall of the small intestine, thus increasing bioavailability of the drugs. The serum drug level is then higher, which may have unpleasant consequences or even cause toxicity. It is believed that more than one component present in grapefruit juice may contribute to this effect. A single glass (8 oz) of grapefruit juice has the potential to increase bioavailability and enhance beneficial or adverse effects for up to 72 hours after consumption. The following table indicates drugs that are influenced by grapefruit juice:

Continued

BOX 11.6 Grapefruit "Juices Up" Certain Medications—cont'd

INTERACTIONS BETWEEN GRAPEFRUIT JUICE AND MEDICATIONS

Category	Generic Name	Brand Name	Effect(s) of Grapefruit Juice
Antihypertensive (calcium channel blockers)	Felodipine	Plendil	Flushing, headache, tachycardia, decreased blood pressure
	Nifedipine	Procardia, Adalat	
	Nimodipine	Nimotop	
	Nisoldipine	Sular	
	Nicardipine	Cardene	
	Isradipine	DynaCirc	
	Verapamil	Calan, Isoptin	Same as above plus bradycardia and atrioventricular (AV) block
Immunosuppressant	Cyclosporine	Neoral, Sandimmune, SangCya	Kidney toxicity, increased susceptibility to infections
	Tacrolimus	Prograf	
Statin (HMG-CoA reductase inhibitors)	Atorvastatin	Lipitor	Headache, gastrointestinal complaints, muscle pain, increased risk of myopathy
	Lovastatin	Mevacor	
	Simvastatin	Zocor	Nervousness, overstimulation
Antianxiety, insomnia, or depression	Buspirone	BuSpar	Increased sedation
	Diazepam	Valium	
	Alprazolam	Xanax	
	Midazolam	Versed	
	Triazolam	Halcion	
	Zaleplon	Sonata	
	Carbamazepine	Tegretol	
	Clomipramine	Anafranil	
	Trazodone	Desyrel	
Protease inhibitors	Saquinavir	Fortovase, Invirase	Doubles bioavailability, resulting in increased efficacy or toxicity depending on dose and patient variability
Sexual dysfunction	Sildenafil	Viagra	Delayed absorption (takes longer to become effective)

MEDICATIONS CONSIDERED SAFE FOR USE WITH GRAPEFRUIT

Cetirizine	Zyrtec, Reactine
Fexofenadine	Allegra
Fluvastatin	Lescol
Loratadine	Claritin
Pravastatin	Pravachol

From Drug-nutrient interactions. In Schlenker ED, Gilbert J, editors: *Williams' essentials of nutrition & diet therapy*, ed 12, St. Louis, 2018, Elsevier.

TABLE 11.8 Foods and Nutrients That Affect Medications

Drug Class	Examples	Use	Food(s)/ Nutrient(s)	Action(s) or Effect(s)	How to Avoid
Alcohol, particularly excessive use	Beer, wine, spirits	Lowers inhibitions; central nervous system (CNS) depressant	Food	Slowing of absorption	Consume alcohol with food or meals
Analgesics and nonsteroidal antiinflammatory drugs	Salicylates (aspirin), ibuprofen (Motrin, Advil), naproxen (Anaprox, Aleve, Naprosyn), acetaminophen (Tylenol)	Pain and fever	Alcohol	Increase in hepatotoxicity, liver damage, or stomach bleeding	Limit alcohol intake to two drinks per day for men, one drink per day for women
Antiulcer agents (histamine blockers)	Cimetidine (Tagamet)	Ulcers	Alcohol	Increased blood alcohol levels	Limit alcohol intake to two drinks per day for men, one drink per day for women
			Caffeine-containing foods and beverages	Reduced caffeine clearance	Limit caffeine intake
Antibiotics	Ciprofloxacin (Cipro)	Infection	Dairy products	Decrease absorption	Avoid dairy products

Continued

TABLE 11.8 Foods and Nutrients That Affect Medications—cont'd

Drug Class	Examples	Use	Food(s)/ Nutrient(s)	Action(s) or Effect(s)	How to Avoid
Anticoagulants	Warfarin (Coumadin)	Blood clots	Vitamins K and E (supplements)	May reduce efficacy	Limit foods high in vitamin K: broccoli, spinach, kale, turnip greens, cauliflower, Brussels sprouts; avoid high dose of vitamin E (400 IU or more)
			Alcohol and garlic	May increase anticoagulation	Avoid alcohol and garlic
Antineoplastic drugs	Methotrexate	Cancer	Alcohol	Increased hepatotoxicity with chronic alcohol use	Avoid alcohol
Antiemetics	Amitriptyline HCl (Elavil), chlorpromazine HCl (Thorazine)	Antidepressant; antipsychotic/ antiemetic	Alcohol	Increased sedation	Avoid alcohol
Anticonvulsants	Phenobarbital	Seizures, epilepsy	Alcohol	Increased sedation	Avoid alcohol
Antidepressants: monoamine oxidase inhibitors (MAOIs)	Phenelzine (Nardil), tranylcypromine (Parnate)	Depression, anxiety	Foods or alcoholic beverages containing tyramine	Rapid, potentially fatal increase in blood pressure	Avoid beer; red wine; Camembert and aged blue cheeses; aged Cheddar, bleu, Brie, mozzarella, and Parmesan cheeses; yogurt; sour cream; beef or chicken liver; cured meats such as sausage and salami; game meats; caviar; dried fish; yeast extracts; sauerkraut; kimchee; fish or shrimp sauce; soy sauce; miso soup; broad (fava) beans
Antihistamines	Fexofenadine (Allegra), loratadine (Claritin), cetirizine (Zyrtec), astemizole (Hismanal)	Allergies	Alcohol	Increases drowsiness and slows mental and motor performance	Use caution when operating machinery or driving
Antihypertensives	Angiotensin-converting enzyme inhibitors, angiotensin II receptor antagonists, beta blockers, verapamil HCl	Hypertension	Natural licorice *(Glycyrrhiza glabra)* and tyramine-rich foods	Reduced effectiveness	Avoid natural licorice and tyramine-containing foods (see previous list for Antidepressants)
Antihyperlipidemics such as statins	Atorvastatin (Lipitor), lovastatin (Mevacor), pravastatin (Pravachol), simvastatin (Zocor)	High serum cholesterol	Food/meals	Altered absorption	Lovastatin should be taken with evening meal to enhance absorption
			Alcohol	Increased risk of liver damage	Avoid large amounts of alcohol
Antiparkinsonian	Levodopa (Dopar, Larodopa)	Parkinson's disease	High-protein foods (eggs, meat, protein supplements); vitamin B_6	Decreased absorption	Spread protein intake equally in three to six meals per day to minimize reaction; avoid B_6 supplements and multivitamin supplements
Antituberculosis agent	Isoniazid (INH)	Tuberculosis	Food	Reduced absorption	Take on empty stomach
			Alcohol	Increased hepatotoxicity and reduced INH levels	Avoid alcohol
Bronchodilators	Theophylline (Slo-bid, Theo-Dur)	Asthma, chronic bronchitis, and emphysema	Caffeine	Increased stimulation of CNS	Limit caffeine-containing foods/ beverages (chocolate, colas, teas, coffee)
			Alcohol	Can increase nausea, vomiting, headache, and irritability	Avoid alcohol
Corticosteroids	Prednisolone (Pediapred, Prelone), methylprednisolone (Solu-Medrol), hydrocortisone	Inflammation and itching	Food	Stomach irritation	Take with food or milk to decrease stomach upset
Hypoglycemic agents	Chlorpropamide (Diabinese), metformin (Glucophage)	Diabetes	Alcohol	Severe nausea and vomiting	Avoid alcohol

From Drug-nutrient interactions. In Schlenker ED, Gilbert J, editors: *Williams' essentials of nutrition & diet therapy*, ed 12, St. Louis, 2018, Elsevier.

BOX 11.7 Tube Feedings and Drug-Nutrient Interactions

Drug-nutrient interactions can compromise pharmacologic and nutritional objectives of safety, efficacy, and quality of care. Moreover, these interactions can affect cost effectiveness of health care. Before administering an oral drug through a gastric or nasogastric feeding tube, ask yourself the following questions:

1. Is the feeding tube placed correctly?
2. Can the medication be crushed and delivered through a feeding tube?
3. Will there be an interaction between the medication and the feeding solution?
   - If so, will the interaction degrade the nutritional components of the feeding solution?
   - Or alter the medication's availability?
   - Or clog the tube?
4. Will the medication change the osmolality or pH in the feeding system?
   - Or cause nausea, vomiting, cramping, or diarrhea?

Pharmacists have valuable expertise in optimizing prescriptions. The number of potential drug–feeding formula interactions is nearly endless, and new medications and feeding formulas are marketed almost daily. Consultation with pharmacy services is recommended to detect possible incompatibilities and recommendations for appropriate alternative forms of medications if necessary. Questions regarding specific feeding formulas and adverse drug reactions can be directed to the dietitian. The following chart offers solutions to potential problems that may occur.

Potential Problem	Solution
Should I administer the tablet or liquid form of the medication?	Whenever possible, use the liquid form of a drug because it bypasses the dissolution process. But be aware that many liquid medications are formulated for pediatric patients; therefore, large volumes must be dispensed to meet the required dose for adults. This often leads to diarrhea as a result of excessive amounts of sorbitol in the adjusted dose.
Okay, I checked and the only form of the medication available is a tablet. What should I do?	If a tablet is the only preparation available, consultation with the pharmacist is mandatory. Some tablets can be crushed if they are simple, compressed tablets designed to dissolve immediately in the gastrointestinal (GI) tract. Keep in mind that crushing the tablet allows it to enter the bloodstream faster. The difference may or may not be clinically significant. Always confirm the type of coating on the tablet with the pharmacy.
I've checked with the pharmacy and was told the tablet could be crushed. How do I do that?	Ideally, medication(s) should be crushed in the pharmacy. But if you must do it yourself, the best technique is to position a unit-dose tablet in a mortar without removing it from the package. Then crush the tablet by tapping it through the package with a pestle (to avoid tearing the package, don't grind). If the medication isn't packaged as a unit-dose, place it between two paper medicine cups and pulverize the tablet with the mortar and pestle. Mix the crushed tablet thoroughly with 15–30 mL water (5–10 mL for children), and administer through the feeding tube. Tubing must be flushed with a minimum of 30 mL of room temperature sterile water before and after administration of each medication.
It seems like it would be easier to add the medication to the feeding formula.	Never add medications directly to the feeding formula. This can alter the medication's therapeutic effect and disrupt the integrity of the feeding formula, causing it to resemble curdled milk.
The pharmacy has the prescribed medications in liquid form. Is there anything special I need to do?	Check whether dilution of the medication formulation before administration is required. Hypertonic, irritating, or viscous medications should be diluted in at least 30 mL of water immediately before infusion to avoid gastric irritation and diarrhea. In some cases, 90 mL of water may be necessary for dilution. Adjust water amounts appropriately for pediatric patients and patients on fluid restrictions. Document the amount of water used on the patient's intake and output records.
If sugar-coated tablets can be crushed, are there tablets that cannot be crushed?	Some types of tablets must not be crushed. These include Buccal or sublingual tablets (e.g., nitroglycerin or isosorbide) are intended to be absorbed by veins under the tongue or in the cheek, thus bypassing the liver (avoiding first-pass effect) and protecting the medication from contact with other drugs, foods, and GI secretions that could affect the medication's potency or bioavailability. Enteric-coated tablets (e.g., bisacodyl [Dulcolax] and ferrous sulfate [Feosol]) are formulated to inhibit release of the active drug until after the tablet has passed from the stomach into the small intestine. Moreover, the tablet's coating protects the stomach from irritation from the medication. Crushing the tablet would put an end to the protective coating. Uncoated gastric irritants (including aspirin) remain effective after crushing, but they are more apt to trigger undesirable GI reactions such as cramping and bleeding. Ask for an alternative form or different medication. Sustained-release or effervescent tablets (e.g., Slow-L, Procan SR, Theolair-SR, Inderal LA) were designed to dissolve and release medication gradually (they contain two or three doses of the medication). As a result, if such a tablet were crushed, the patient would receive an overdose. In addition, the planned beneficial effects would not be maintained throughout the dosing interval.
The prescribed medication is in the form of a capsule. Can't I just place it in the tube and flush it down with some water?	Capsules should not be crushed, but you can open some and mix the contents with water: Hard gelatin capsules (e.g., ampicillin and doxycycline) contain a medication in a powdered form. The capsule can be opened (it's designed to separate in the middle), and the powder mixed thoroughly with water. Spansules release the active medication slowly, over time, through sustained-release capsules (e.g., Slo-bid and Feosol), coated beads or pellets inside the capsules. They are designed to dissolve in the GI tract at different rates, lengthening the medication's duration of action. Obviously, crushing capsules or their contents would damage the timed-release coatings. A better alternative would be a liquid form or a simple compressed tablet that can be crushed (ascertain that dosage frequency is increased appropriately). Soft gel capsules (e.g., chloral hydrate, some vitamin preparations) can be dispensed through a feeding tube by poking a pinhole in one end and squeezing out the liquid contents. The liquid contents can also be drawn up in a syringe. Neither method should be used if delivering an exact dose is important. Some of the drug will always remain inside the capsule. Dissolve the capsule in 15–30 mL of warm water (5–10 mL for pediatric patients), then administer. The drug-water mixture will also work if you plan ahead—dissolving the capsule can take as long as 1 hour.

Developed from Roveron G et al. Clinical Practice Guidelines for the Nursing Management of Percutaneous Endoscopic Gastrostomy and Jejunostomy (PEG/PEJ) in Adult Patients: An Executive Summary. *J Wound Ostomy Continence Nurs* 7(45):326–344, 2018.

- What is the purpose of taking the dietary supplement? (Avoid questions like "What is that supposed to do?" because such implied skepticism can embarrass the patient and discourage honest reporting of supplement use.)
- Have you experienced any side effects?
- Do you take an herbal product, herbal supplement, or other "natural remedy"?
  - If so, do you take any prescription or nonprescription medications for the same purpose as the herbal product?
- Have you used this herbal product before?
- Are you allergic to any plant products?
- Are you pregnant or breastfeeding?
- Are you seeing an herbalist, naturopathic practitioner, nutritionist, or natural healer?
- Is your physician or primary health care provider aware that you take these supplements (in addition to any prescribed medications)?

It is useful to keep an open mind and remain current in this quickly changing area. Table 11.9 lists herbs and the potential drug interactions that are of concern.

TABLE 11.9 Commonly Used Herbal Products and Nutraceuticals That May Be Used to Treat Selected Conditions[a]

Condition/Herb	Use or Action	Associated Adverse Effects; Comments
Asthma		
Tylophora indica, T. asthmatica	Inhibits histamine release	Sore mouth, loss of taste for salt, morning nausea and vomiting
Adhatoda vasica	Bronchodilator	Vomiting and diarrhea; lack of conclusive efficacy data
Picrorhiza kurroa	Bronchodilator	Vomiting, cutaneous rash, anorexia, diarrhea, itching, giddiness, headache, abdominal pain, increased dyspnea
Khellin	Bronchodilator	Avoid taking with prescription bronchodilators
Onion extract *(Allium cepa)*	May inhibit leukotriene and thromboxane	Delirium, tachycardia, nausea, high incidence of gastrointestinal (GI) side effects
Ginkgo *(Ginkgo biloba)*	Smooth muscle relaxant	Clinical efficacy unproven
Anxiety and Depression		
Chamomile *(Chamaemelum nobile, Matricaria chamomilla, M. recutita)*	GI spasm or irritation, sedative	Therapeutic amounts may vary depending on effect chamomile has on an individual; side effects infrequent
Valerian *(Valeriana officinalis)*	Insomnia, mild to moderate anxiety, stress and tension, premenstrual tension, hyperactivity, depression, insomnia, migraine headaches	Side effects not reported, but if used in too large a dose initially, it may cause excitability
Passion flower *(Passiflora incarnate)*	Relaxation and sleep	Not recommended for children <2 years; use of decreased initial dose recommended for those >65 years
Kava *(Piper methysticum)*	Sedative, anticonvulsive, antispasmodic, central muscular relaxant	Prolonged use causes a temporary yellow coloring of skin, hair, and nails; may cause liver damage; not recommended for use with other central nervous system depressants, including alcohol
Hops *(Humulus lupulus)*	Insomnia, digestive aid, treatment of intestinal ailments	
Ginseng *(Panax quinquefolius, P. ginseng, Eleutherococcus senticosus)*	Increase energy, improve stamina, enhance memory	Typically, mild and dose related; most commonly observed are nervousness, sleeplessness, nausea, and occasionally headache
St. John's wort *(Hypericum perforatum)*	Depression	Fatigue, pruritus, weight gain, emotional vulnerability; photosensitivity; decreased effectiveness of oral contraceptive therapy possible
Black cohosh *(Cimicifuga racemosa)*	Sedative, relaxant	Not for use in pregnancy
California poppy *(Eschscholzia californica)*	Hypnotic, tranquilizer	
Damask rose *(Rosa damascene)*	Antidepressant	Use only good-quality damask rose
Jamaican dogwood *(Piscidia erythrina)*	Insomnia, migraine	
Linden *(Tifia europaea)*	Reduces nervous tension	
Gotu kola *(Centella asiatica)*	Relaxant	Gotu kola may cause rash; avoid during pregnancy and breastfeeding
Pasque flower *(Anemone pulsatilla)*	Sedative action	Use only dried plant
Lavender (*Lavandula* species)	Sedative	Avoid high doses in pregnancy
Wild lettuce *(Lactuca virosa)*		Excess amounts can lead to insomnia
Wood betony *(Stachys officinalis)*		Large doses can cause vomiting; avoid high doses in pregnancy
Cancer Prevention and Treatment		
Shark cartilage	Antiangiogenic effect	Doubtful oral bioavailability of biologically active components
Aloe vera	May stimulate macrophage function (antitumor activity)	May have deleterious effects in patients with acquired immunodeficiency syndrome (AIDS)

Continued

TABLE 11.9 **Commonly Used Herbal Products and Nutraceuticals That May Be Used to Treat Selected Conditions[a]—cont'd**

Condition/Herb	Use or Action	Associated Adverse Effects; Comments
Echinacea *(Echinacea angustifolia, E. pallida)*	Immunostimulatory activity	Unknown whether effective orally
Mistletoe *(Phoradendron* species and *Viscum* species)	Potent inducer of cytokines stimulating release of tumor necrosis factor-α and interleukin-1	
Antioxidant vitamins A and E	May reduce risk of lung cancer by reducing formation of free radicals	Vitamin A can be toxic
Garlic and onion (*Allium sativum* and *A. cepa*)	May decrease nitrosamine formation	
Green tea	Antioxidant properties, inhibits nucleoside transport	Contradictory epidemiologic studies regarding efficacy in cancer
Chaparral *(Larrea tridentate, L. divaricata, L. mexicana)*	Antioxidant properties	Hepatoxic; unproven and dangerous
Ginseng *(Panax quinquefolius, P. ginseng, Eleutherococcus senticosus)*	Antiestrogen properties	More data needed
Laetrile	May have tumor static activity	Unproven
Goldenseal *(Hydrastis canadensis)*	May prevent carcinogenesis	Use may be limited by toxicity
Pineapple	May cause tumor regression	More study needed
Sweet and red clover *(Trifolium pretense)*	Stimulates macrophage activity	
Cloud fungus	Immunostimulatory activity	
Colds and Flu		
Anise *(Pimpinella anisum)*	Expectorant action	May cause contact dermatitis; avoid use during pregnancy and breastfeeding
Boneset *(Eupatorium perfoliatum)*	Antipyretic; influenza	Individuals with hypersensitivity to the Asteraceae family (e.g., chamomile, feverfew) should avoid use
Coltsfoot *(Tussilago farfara)*	Antitussive	Possible hepatotoxicity; has abortifacient effects, should not be taken during pregnancy and breastfeeding
Echinacea *(Echinacea angustifolia, E. pallida)*	Prophylaxis and treatment of cold and flu symptoms	Continuous use (>6–8 weeks) may lead to immunosuppression; contraindicated in autoimmune diseases Purple coneflower *(E. purpurea)* is a different species with similar properties
Horehound *(Marrubium vulgare)*	Controversial use as expectorant, antitussive, cough suppressant, digestive aid, appetite stimulant	Large doses have produced cardiac irregularities
Slippery elm *(Ulmus rubra)*	Demulcent and emollient to treat sore throats	Pollen can be an allergen; may cause contact dermatitis
Zinc lozenges	Reduce duration and severity of cold symptoms	Possible nausea, unpleasant taste
Diabetes		
Karela *(Momordica charantia)*	Hypoglycemic	May sufficiently lower blood glucose to merit decrease in insulin or oral medications to avoid or minimize incidence of hypoglycemia; karela juice will cause greater decrease in blood glucose than when slices of karela are fried
Ginseng *(Panax quinquefolius, P. ginseng, Eleutherococcus senticosus)*	Hypoglycemic	Korean or Chinese ginseng may exert greater hypoglycemic effect than Japanese ginseng
Brewer's yeast	Hypoglycemic	May cause unfavorable variability in blood glucose control if medical staff is unaware of concomitant use with chromium
GS_4 *(Gymnema sylvestre)*	Hypoglycemic	May decrease insulin and glyburide requirements but should not be relied on for blood glucose control
Devil's claw *(Harpagophytum procumbens)*		May cause hyperglycemia
Ephedra or ma huang *(Ephedra sinica)*		
Dyslipidemia and Atherosclerosis		
Nicotine acid (niacin)	Reduces total serum cholesterol, low-density lipoprotein (LDL) cholesterol, and triglycerides; increases high-density lipoprotein (HDL) cholesterol	Should be used only under physician's supervision; may raise blood glucose levels; severe hepatotoxicity may occur, especially with sustained-release nicotinic acid products

Continued

TABLE 11.9 Commonly Used Herbal Products and Nutraceuticals That May Be Used to Treat Selected Conditions[a]—cont'd

Condition/Herb	Use or Action	Associated Adverse Effects; Comments
Soluble fiber products (oat bran, guar gum, psyllium, and other dietary sources)	Can lower total serum cholesterol and LDL cholesterol depending on product and amount consumed	Flatulence, cramping, bloating, nausea, diarrhea, indigestion, heartburn
Fish oils (omega-3 fatty acids)	Inhibit platelet aggregation, lower triglyceride levels when consumed in high doses (20–30 g/day)	Triglyceride-lowering effect may diminish with continued use; variable effects (decreases and increases) on blood cholesterol levels; may increase bleeding risk
Vitamin E	200 International Units or more per day *may* reduce risk of coronary heart disease	
Garlic *(Allium sativum)*	Standardized powdered garlic products may produce modest reduction in total cholesterol	
Nuts	Lower plasma lipoprotein levels	
Beta-sitosterol	May produce modest reductions in total and LDL cholesterol	
Alfalfa seed *(Medicago sativa)*	May produce modest reduction in cholesterol	Potential toxic effects outweigh any advantages that might be obtained
Chromium	May produce modest cholesterol reductions; administration as picolinate salt seems to increase bioavailability	
Gastrointestinal Problems		
Aloes *(Aloe barbadensis, Aloe ferox, Aloe africana, Aloe spicata)*	Orally a powerful cathartic and not generally recommended	A harsh purgative; less toxic laxatives are available Contraindicated in patients with hemorrhoids, kidney disease, intestinal obstruction, abdominal pain, nausea, or vomiting
Bilberry fruit *(Vaccinium myrtillus)*	Treatment of diarrhea	No known side effects or interactions
Cascara *(Rhamnus purshiana)*	Stimulant laxative	Avoid during pregnancy and breastfeeding Fresh bark may cause severe vomiting Electrolyte imbalance with misuse; potentiates toxicities of cardiac glycosides and thiazide diuretics
Ginger *(Zingiber officinale)*	Treatment of motion sickness and nausea	May cause prolonged bleeding times; should be used with caution by patients on anticoagulant therapy
Licorice *(Glycyrrhiza glabra; G. uralensis)*	Treatment of peptic ulcer, expectorant	Considered unsafe Contraindicated in patients taking cardiac glycosides or thiazide diuretics
Peppermint *(Mentha piperita)*	Decreases muscle spasms of the GI tract Treatment of abdominal pain Enteric-coated capsules used to treat irritable bowel syndrome	Should not be used by infants or small children; tea from leaves can cause laryngeal and bronchial spasms Overuse can lead to heartburn and relaxation of laryngoesophageal sphincter
Psyllium *(Plantago arenaria, P. psyllium, P. indica, P. ovata)*	Bulk-forming laxative for constipation, irritable bowel syndrome	Possibly interferes with absorption of other drugs Bezoars (fibrous masses in GI tract) may occur if liquid intake is inadequate
Senna *(Cassia acutifolia, C. angustifolia, Senna alexandrina)*	Cathartic; used to treat constipation	Long-term use can result in electrolyte imbalance and potassium loss May increase toxicity of cardiac glycosides and thiazide diuretics
Hypertension		
Garlic *(Allium sativum)*	Antihypertensive	Routine use not recommended Avoid use of garlic with nonsteroidal antiinflammatory drugs, anticoagulants, drugs that inhibit liver metabolism (e.g., cimetidine), and drugs that may be affected by liver inhibition (e.g., propranolol, diazepam)
Grapefruit juice		May cause significant decrease in blood pressure if taken with nifedipine
Licorice *(Glycyrrhiza glabra; G. uralensis)*		May induce hypertension accompanied by hypokalemia Patients taking oral contraceptives or thiazide diuretics may be predisposed to licorice toxicity if taken concomitantly
Yohimbine *(Pausinystalia yohimbe)*	May be used to treat impotence secondary to antihypertensive medications	May increase blood pressure Should not be co-administered with tricyclic antidepressants or clonidine

[a]This table does not provide information on how to use herbs, nor is it an exhaustive look at every herbal product that may be used. Rather, the intent is to provide information regarding herbal products that patients may use.

Data from Bonakdar RA. The H.E.R.B.A.L. *Guide: Dietary Supplement Resources for the Clinician*, 2012, St Louis, MO, Lippincott Williams & Wilkins; and Tyler VE: *The honest herbal*, ed 3, New York, 1993, Pharmaceutical Products Press.

SUMMARY

- The capacity for recovery from illness or disease depends heavily on nutrition status.
- Nurses often perform basic nutrition screening, nutrition education, and monitoring.
- The nutrition status of patients may be compromised by acute care hospital or nursing home stays; nurses must evaluate whether patients receive the nutrients they are served.
- Psychological and physiologic alterations of illness, the effects of bed rest, the risks of malnutrition, food-drug interactions, and the effects of poor intake on immunity and healing require nutrition screening and monitoring.
- It is important to refer patients at nutrition risk to the nutrition team members who can enhance meals or offer alternative methods of intake.
- The registered dietitian (RD/RDN) is best qualified to provide in-depth knowledge about nutrition care, to consult individually with patients, and to participate in team meetings.
- A comprehensive nutrition assessment is conducted by dietitians to determine appropriate nutrition therapy based on identified needs (nutrition diagnoses) of the patient.
- Data are collected from several sources to assess patients' nutrition needs using the ABCD approach: **A**nthropometrics, **B**iochemical tests, **C**linical observations, and **D**iet evaluation.
- The Nutrition Care Process (NCP) addresses the unique nutrition needs of each patient.
- The NCP is similar to the nursing process and involves four steps to identify and solve nutrition-related problems: Assessment, Nutrition Diagnosis, Nutrition Intervention, and Monitoring-Evaluation.
- The NCP process is repeated as often as needed until the nutrition diagnoses have been resolved.
- Specific food or nutrient alterations may be required, or a patient may need education on how to choose foods wisely.
- Drug-nutrient interactions are common.
- Nutrients and foods may interact with drug function; drugs may affect the use of food and nutrients.
- Timing of meals and medication administration is sometimes in conflict in health care facilities.
- Knowledge of all types of potential interactions among food, nutrients, and drugs helps nurses provide more comprehensive patient care.

THE NURSING APPROACH

Clinical Judgment and Next-Generation NCLEX® Examination-Style Questions

Case Study 1

A Comparison of the Nursing Process, the Nutrition Care Process, and the NBSBN Model of Clinical Judgment

The Nursing Process, the Nutrition Care Process (NCP), and the National Council of State Boards of Nursing (NBSBN) Model of Clinical Judgment are systematic problem-solving methods that use critical thinking skills to develop a framework for the plan of care. The following is a case study used to compare the Nursing Process, NCP, and the NBSBN.

James is a 37-year-old Black male with a history of hypertension. He has been noncompliant with his medications for the past 2 years because of the high cost of medications and their unpleasant side effects. He smokes one pack of cigarettes per day but does not drink alcohol. He presents to the clinic today because he has been feeling tired and has had a headache for the past few days.

	Nursing Process		Nutrition Care Process
Assessment/Recognize Cues	Subjective "I work a lot, so I usually eat fast food or frozen meals for breakfast and dinner." "I've been really tired lately, and I've had this headache that won't go away." "I've gained about 10 pounds within the past 3 months." "I don't like to exercise." Objective Height 5′ 9″, weight 205 pounds BP 178/94 mm Hg, pulse 92	Assessment/ Recognize Cues	Anthropometric Measurements Height 5′ 9″, weight 205 pounds "I've gained about 10 pounds within the past 3 months." Biochemical, Medical Tests, and Procedures BP 178/94 mm Hg, pulse 92 Laboratory tests have not been ordered yet Client History Hypertension Food/Nutrition-Related History "I work a lot, so I usually eat fast food or frozen meals for breakfast and dinner." "I've been really tired lately, and I've had this headache that won't go away." "I don't like to exercise." Based on the patient's 24-hour recall, he consumes approximately 3500 kcal/day Sodium intake of approximately 4000 mg/day Consumes 1–2 servings of fruits and vegetables per day Nutrition-Focused Physical Findings Obese

Continued

THE NURSING APPROACH—cont'd

	Nursing Process		Nutrition Care Process
Diagnosis/Analyze Cues	1. Ineffective self-health maintenance related to lack of knowledge, difficulty modifying personal habits, and insufficient financial resources 2. Imbalanced nutrition: more than body requirements related to excessive intake in relation to physical activity as evidenced by body mass index (BMI) >30	Diagnosis/Analyze Cues	1. Excessive energy intake related to food- and nutrition-related knowledge deficit concerning energy intake, as evidenced by BMI >30, 10-pound weight gain, and reports of high-calorie meals 2. Excessive sodium intake related to food- and nutrition-related knowledge deficit concerning sodium intake, as evidenced by hypertension 3. Physical inactivity related to time constraints, as evidenced by BMI >30 and reports of infrequent physical activity
Planning/Prioritize Hypotheses	Patient Outcomes Short term (at the end of this visit): • James will verbalize his personal risk factors and the potential complications of having hypertension. • He will commit to taking his blood pressure medication. • He will select low-sodium, low-fat options from a menu. Long term (at follow-up visit in 1 month): Weight 201 pounds; BP 140/85 • Reports taking medication as prescribed • Feels more energized and no longer has a headache • Has started to quit smoking Nursing Interventions 1. Measure blood pressure, pulse, and weight. 2. Review medication and teach him when to notify the doctor. 3. Teach him about general dietary measures to reduce sodium and fat intake. 4. Provide education and information on how to quit smoking.	Intervention/ Generate Solutions	Short-Term Goals • Verbalize understanding of Dietary Approaches to Stop Hypertension (DASH) diet • Demonstrate how to read food labels and choose low-sodium foods • Verbalize plan to begin exercise regimen • Will schedule follow-up appointment Long-Term Goals • Adhere to DASH diet • Reduce sodium intake to 1.5 g/day • Begin playing tennis three times per week Nutrition Education • Provide support, written and verbal instruction on DASH diet • Will instruct patient to limit dietary sodium to 1.5 g/day • Will instruct patient to begin walking for at least 20 minutes three times per week Coordination of Care • Organize referral to cardiac rehab program through local American Heart Association
Implementation/Take Action	1. Explain risk factors and possible complications of developing hypertension. 2. Provide information about medication and the importance of taking it as prescribed. 3. Teach guidelines for following a heart-healthy diet, and provide information on how to lose weight. 4. Provide education and information on how to quit smoking.	Monitoring & Evaluation/ Evaluate Outcomes	• Follow up with patient in 1 month to assess dietary and lifestyle changes: BMI, BP, dietary patterns, physical activity
Evaluation/Evaluate Outcomes	Short term (at the end of the visit): • Verbalized his risk factors and the possible complications of developing hypertension • Committed to taking his medication as prescribed • Verbalized intent to quit smoking • Identified heart-healthy foods • Made follow-up appointment for 1 month • Goals met		

Discussion Questions

1. Because it is difficult to obtain a true intake record, which question might be more effective?
   a. Do you use salt?
   b. For a typical meal, how many times do you shake salt onto a food?
2. Will it be necessary to provide support to this patient for the changes he is facing? Discuss.
3. If he asks, "Which is more important, eating better or quitting cigarettes?" What would your response be? Why?

Continued

THE NURSING APPROACH—cont'd

Case Study 2

The nurse is admitting an elderly female patient with gastroenteritis. The patient states, that she "sometimes has side effects from new medications". The nurse knows risk for drug-nutrient interactions depend upon which patient factors?

Use an X to mark risk factors for drug-nutrient interactions. Select all that apply.

	Risk Factors
	1. Physiologic status
	2. Ethnic status
	3. Hepatic function
	4. Skin color
	5. Age
	6. Number of meals per day
	7. Multiple-drug intake
	8. Typical dietary intake
	9. Neurological status
	10. Renal function

CRITICAL THINKING

Clinical Applications: Role Play

Malnutrition is important to prevent or correct. Select two of the screening or assessment tools from the websites listed here. Invite a friend to help you. Conduct the two screening interviews and time yourself; do not rush the process. When you are finished, identify the pros and cons of each tool and its ease of use.

- Nutrition Risk Screening-2002 (NRS-2002): http://www.sciencedirect.com/science/article/pii/S0261561403000980
- Malnutrition Universal Screening Tool (MUST): http://www.bapen.org.uk/pdfs/must/must_full.pdf
- Mini Nutrition Assessment (MNA): http://www.mna-elderly.com
- Short Nutritional Assessment Questionnaire (SNAQ65+): https://www.fight-malnutrition.eu/
- Subjective Global Assessment (SGA): http://subjectiveglobalassessment.com

What will you do differently the next time you conduct a nutrition screening?

List three reasons why it is important to identify and correct malnutrition.

WEBSITES OF INTEREST

Academy of Nutrition and Dietetics—Evidence Analysis Library

www.andevidencelibrary.com

National Center for Health Statistics, Centers for Disease Prevention and Control

www.cdc.gov/nchs

Collects statistical data on every aspect of health status and use of health services by socioeconomic status, region, race or ethnicity, and other population attributes.

NCMND Center of Excellence for Nutritional Genomics, University of California, Davis

http://nutrigenomics.ucdavis.edu/

Useful website that addresses the human genome and interactions with diet.

REFERENCES

Academy of Nutrition and Dietetics. *Evidence Analysis Library: Nutrition Screening for Adults*. From: <https://www.andeal.org/topic.cfm?menu=5382#:~:text=Nutrition%20screening%20is%20the%20process,registered%20dietitian%20nutritionist%20(RDN)> (Accessed 20 August, 2020).

Amoroso, L. (2016). The second international conference on nutrition: Implications for hidden hunger. *World Review of Nutrition and Dietetics*, *115*, 142–152.

Ashwell, M., et al. (2012). Waist-to-height ratio is a better screening tool than waist circumference and BMI for adult cardiometabolic risk factors: Systematic review and meta-analysis. *Obesity Reviews: An Official Journal of the International Association for the Study of Obesity*, *13*, 275–286.

Aune, D., et al. (2016). BMI and all-cause mortality: Systematic review and non-linear dose-response meta-analysis of 230 cohort studies with 3.74 million deaths among 30.3 million participants. *British Medical Journal*, *353*, i2156.

Aziz, E. F., et al. (2011). Malnutrition as assessed by nutritional risk index is associated with worse outcome in patients admitted with acute decompensated heart failure: An ACAP-HF data analysis. *Heart International*, *6*, e2.

Barnes, K. L., & Bendixsen, C. G. (2017). "When This Breaks Down, It's Black Gold": Race and gender in agricultural health and safety. *Journal of Agromedicine*, *22*, 56–65.

Berglund, S. K., et al. (2017). Effects of iron supplementation of low-birth-weight infants on cognition and behavior at 7 years: a randomized controlled trial. *Pediatric Research*, *83*, 111–118.

Burgos, R., et al. (2020). Disease-related malnutrition in hospitalized chronic patients with complex needs. *Clinical Nutrition*, *39*, 1440–1453.

Chien, S. C., et al. (2017). Association of low serum albumin concentration and adverse cardiovascular events in stable coronary heart disease. *International Journal of Cardiology*, *241*, 1–5.

Chumlea, W. C., et al. (1988). Prediction of body weight for the non-ambulatory elderly from anthropometry. *Journal of the American Dietetic Association*, *88*, 564–568.

Cui. Z., et al. (2016). Prediction of body mass index using concurrently self-reported or previously measured height and weight. *PLoS ONE*, *11*(11), e0167288.

Eggersdorfer, M., et al. (2018). Hidden hunger: Solutions for America's aging populations. *Nutrients*, *10*, 1210.

English, K. L., et al. (2016). Leucine partially protects muscle mass and function during bed rest in middle-aged adults. *The American Journal of Clinical Nutrition, 103*, 465–473.

Esper, D. H. (2015). Utilization of nutrition-focused physical assessment in identifying micronutrient deficiencies. *Nutrition in Clinical Practice, 30*, 194–202.

FAO (Food and Agriculture Organization of the United Nations). *Hunger and Food Insecurity*, n.d. From: <http://www.fao.org/hunger/en/> (Accessed 20 August, 2020).

Galvan, E., et al. (2016). Protecting skeletal muscle with protein and amino acid during periods of disuse. *Nutrients, 8*, 404.

Gray, D. (1985). Accuracy of recumbent height measurement. *Journal of Parenteral and Enteral Nutrition, 9*, 712–715.

Heymsfield, S., et al. (2016). Why are there race/ethnic differences in adult body mass index-adiposity relationships? A quantitative critical review. *Obesity Reviews: An Official Journal of the International Association for the Study of Obesity, 17*, 262–275.

Jensen, G. L., et al. (2010). Adult starvation and disease-related malnutrition: A proposal for etiology-based diagnosis in the clinical practice setting from the International Consensus Guideline Committee. *Clinical Nutrition, 29*, 151–153.

Lefton, J., & Malone, A. M. (2015). Anthropometric assessment. In P. Charney & A. M. Malone (Eds.), *Academy of nutrition and dietetics pocket guide to nutrition assessment* (3rd ed.). Chicago: Academy of Nutrition and Dietetics.

McCauley, P. A., & Beavers, K. M. (2014). Contribution of cardiorespiratory fitness to the obesity paradox. *Progress in Cardiovascular Diseases, 56*, 434–440.

Millward, D. J. (2017). Nutrition, infection and stunting: The roles of deficiencies of individual nutrients and foods, and of inflammation, as determinants of reduced linear growth of children. *Nutrition Research Reviews, 30*, 50–72.

Mueller, C., et al. (2011). A.S.P.E.N. clinical guidelines: Nutrition screening, assessment, and intervention in adults. *Journal of Parenteral and Enteral Nutrition, 35*, 16–24.

National Heart, Lung, and Blood Institute. (1998). *Clinical guidelines on the identification, evaluation, and treatment of overweight and obesity in adults: the evidence report*. Bethesda, MD: Author. (Pub. No. 98-4083).

National Heart, Lung, and Blood Institute. *Obesity education initiative*, n.d. From: www.nhlbi.nih.gov/health/public/heart/obesity/lose_wt/risk.htm (Accessed 20 August, 2020).

National Institutes of Health, Office of Dietary Supplements (NIH). *Vitamin D: fact sheet for health professionals*. From: ods.od.nih.gov/factsheets/VitaminD-HealthProfessional. (Accessed 20 August, 2020).

Peralta R. *Hypoalbuminemia*. From: http://emedicine.medscape.com/article/166724-overview. (Accessed 20 August, 2020).

Psota, T., & Chen, K. Y. (2013). Measuring energy expenditure in clinical populations: Rewards and challenges. *European Journal of Clinical Nutrition, 67*, 436–442.

Rasmussen, H. H., et al. (2010). Measuring nutritional risk in hospitals. *Clinical Epidemiology, 2*, 209–216.

Reber, E., et al. (2019). Nutritional risk screening and assessment. *Journal of Clinical Medicine, 8*, 1065.

Schnurr, T. M., et al. (2016). Genetic correlation between body fat percentage and cardiorespiratory fitness suggests common genetic etiology. *PLoS ONE, 11*, e0166738.

Semba, R. D., et al. (2016). Perspective: The potential role of essential amino acids and the mechanistic target of rapamycin complex 1 (mTORC1) pathway in the pathogenesis of child stunting. *Advances in Nutrition, 7*, 853–865.

Simeoni, U., et al. (2018). Perinatal origins of adult disease. *Neonatology, 113*, 39–399.

Skipper, A., et al. (2012). Nutrition screening tools: an analysis of the evidence. *Journal of Parenteral and Enteral Nutrition, 36*, 292–298.

The Joint Commission (TJC). *Standards FAQ Details*. From: https://www.jointcommission.org/standards/standard-faqs/critical-access-hospital/provision-of-care-treatment-and-services-pc/000001652/. (Accessed 20 August, 2020).

U.S. Department of Agriculture (USDA). *Food deserts*, n.d. From: https://www.ers.usda.gov/data/fooddesert/. (Accessed 20 August, 2020).

White, J. V., et al. (2012). Consensus statement of the Academy of Nutrition and Dietetics/American Society for Parenteral and Enteral Nutrition: Characteristics recommended for the identification and documentation of adult malnutrition (undernutrition). *Journal of the Academy of Nutrition and Dietetics, 112*, 730–738.

Whitley, A., et al. (2017). Changes in nutritional and functional status in longer stay patients admitted to a geriatric evaluation and management unit. *The Journal of Nutrition, Health & Aging, 21*, 686.

Wilson, L. R., et al. (2017). Vitamin D deficiency as a public health issue: Using vitamin D2 or vitamin D3 in future fortification strategies. *The Proceedings of the Nutrition Society, 76*, 392–399.

World Health Organization. *What is malnutrition?* From: https://www.who.int/news-room/fact-sheets/detail/malnutrition. (Accessed 20 August, 2020).

Xu. X., et al. (2017). Where is the nurse in nutritional care? *Contemporary Nurse, 53*, 267–270.

12

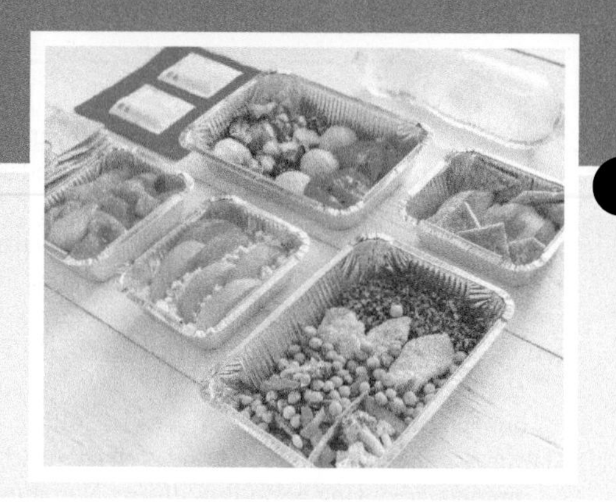

Food-Related Issues

During trying times, food becomes very important, both physiologically and psychologically. It may be one of the few pleasant experiences that patients encounter in a hospital. Having a special problem, such as not being able to eat orally or having a food allergy, can make the hospital stay quite stressful. The sudden onset of food poisoning can be frightening or even life threatening. In addition, the prior use of dietary or herbal supplements may cause unexpected interactions that must be addressed. Through these food-related issues, teamwork between nurses and dietitians can ease the stress and promote recovery.

http://evolve.elsevier.com/GRODNER/FOUNDATIONS

LEARNING OBJECTIVES

- Describe the nutritional therapy rationale for diet orders that have qualitative or quantitative changes.
- Explain appropriate interventions to prevent or resolve incidents that involve food allergies or food poisoning.
- List the risks and benefits of nutritional components of integrative medicine, also called TCAM (traditional, complementary, and alternative medicine).
- Distinguish between alternative medical therapies and integrative medical therapies.
- Summarize potential interactions of herbal dietary supplements with the bioavailability of foods, nutrients, and drugs.
- Compare or contrast the feeding modes of enteral nutrition (EN) and parenteral nutrition (PN).

DIMENSIONS OF HEALTH

Food affects each dimension of health. Careful nursing supervision can ensure adequate nutrient intake to maintain or improve physical health. Effects can be detrimental when dietary supplements interact with medications and inadvertently alter the effects of medications.

The intellectual dimension is tested when nurses and caregivers observe patient intake, determine whether problems are caused by illness or food availability, and choose when to alert the clinical dietitian. Critical thinking skills are also needed to evaluate appropriateness of herbs and therapies that have been used by patients. The effects of nonoral feeding modalities also require awareness by the nurse; side effects are often insidious, but staff reactions must be quick and accurate.

Emotional health is challenged by the stress of dietary modifications that may be long term or permanent. Complementary nutrition approaches are often chosen by the patient who is coping with a chronic disorder (Foley and Steel, 2017). Social health can be altered when patients are served meals in their rooms; they often feel isolated and eat less as a result. The same is true when a patient is given a tube feeding or parenteral nutrition. Instead of being able to eat orally, the patient experiences the loss of a basic human right. Beyond this, food is significant for spiritual health. Many foods have religious significance, such as bread and wine used for Communion or matzo used during the Jewish holiday of Passover. When such foods are restricted because of medical problems, patients may need spiritual or religious advice and support. When sensitive to these issues, nurses can help patients adjust and establish new meanings related to body and spiritual nourishment. The environmental health dimension requires having access to refrigeration to keep foods at their proper cooling temperatures to reduce the risk of food poisoning.

DIETARY GUIDELINES

Most country governments have produced dietary guidelines for their citizens. In the United States the Dietary Guidelines for Americans (DGAs) are updated every 5 years, the most recent (9th edition) was published in 2020. Five key messages are listed here (Office of Disease Prevention and Health Promotion. https://www.dietaryguidelines.gov/):

1. Follow a healthy eating pattern across the life span. All food and beverage choices matter. Choose a healthy eating pattern at an appropriate calorie level to help achieve and maintain a healthy body weight, support nutrient adequacy, and reduce the risk of chronic disease.

2. Focus on variety, nutrient density, and amount. To meet nutrient needs within calorie limits, choose a variety of nutrient-dense foods across and within all food groups in recommended amounts.
3. Limit calories from added sugars and saturated fats, and reduce sodium intake. Consume an eating pattern low in added sugars, saturated fats, and sodium. Cut back on foods and beverages higher in these components to amounts that fit within healthy eating patterns.
4. Shift to healthier food and beverage choices. Choose nutrient-dense foods and beverages across and within all food groups in place of less healthy choices. Consider cultural and personal preferences to make these shifts easier to accomplish and maintain.
5. Support healthy eating patterns for all. Everyone has a role in helping to create and support healthy eating patterns in multiple settings nationwide, from home to school to work to communities.

These messages are the foundation for menu planning. A healthy eating pattern includes a variety of vegetables from all subgroups—dark green, red and orange, legumes (beans and peas), starchy and others; fruits, especially whole fruits; grains, at least half of which are whole grains; fat-free or low-fat dairy, including milk, yogurt, cheese, and fortified soy beverages; a variety of protein foods, including seafood, lean meats and poultry, eggs, legumes (beans and peas), and nuts, seeds, and soy products; and oils.

The healthy eating pattern limits saturated fats and *trans* fats, added sugars, and sodium. The current guidelines do not limit dietary cholesterol. If alcohol is consumed, it should be consumed in moderation—up to one drink per day for women and up to two drinks per day for men—and only by adults of legal drinking age.

One of the most important tools is the nutrition label. A **nutrition facts label** is required on packaged food in most countries. The label helps consumers check calories, serving sizes, specific nutrients (calcium, iron, vitamins A and C), and any health claims. Nurses may find that using a nutrition facts label is helpful, especially when discussing management of conditions such as diabetes or heart disease. Guidance on how to use the label can be found at https://www.fda.gov/food/new-nutrition-facts-label/how-understand-and-use-nutrition-facts-label.

DIETARY MODIFICATIONS

Sometimes dietary modifications are required to allow the body to heal, adjust to physical disability, or prepare for diagnostic tests or surgical procedures. Therapy may require texture changes to liquefied or pureed foods. Nutrients may also be modified, as when a low-sodium diet is used to lower blood pressure or when carbohydrates are controlled for diabetes management. Liquid diets are no longer mandated before surgery, but a patient with a wired jaw will need to sip liquids from a straw. If someone cannot or will not eat for a week or longer, enteral (tube) feeding or parenteral (intravenous) nourishment may be needed. In extreme cases (such as short bowel syndrome), a patient may never again be able to eat orally. This chapter discusses typical hospital diets, enteral formulas, and parenteral nutrition.

DIET ORDERS

Specific diseases or conditions require modifications of the normal (regular, general, house) diet. Each modified diet has a purpose and rationale, and its use is usually determined by the physician or registered dietitian (RD).

Generally, doctors must order diets, including modifications. The Centers for Medicare & Medicaid Services (CMS) announced a rule change in 2014 that would allow "privileged" RDs to independently order patient diets without requiring the supervision or approval of a physician or other practitioner, and to order laboratory tests to monitor the effectiveness of dietary plans and orders. The rule applies only to RDs who are granted privileges by the hospital in which they work (i.e., "privileged registered dietitians"). Implementation of this CMS rule expedites the correction of diet orders that are not effective for the patient because the RD would not have to wait for a change written by the physician.

To appreciate the modified diets described in the following chapters, it is helpful to understand the basis for the diet order called regular, general, or house diet. The regular diet is designed to attain or maintain optimal nutritional status in people who do not require dietary alterations. Individual requirements for specific nutrients vary and are adjusted according to gender, age, height, weight, and activity level. A healthful regular diet is used to reduce risks for chronic diet-related diseases such as cardiovascular diseases and certain cancers.

Depending on individual food choices and intake, a regular diet is designed to be adequate in all recommended dietary allowances (RDAs) of nutrients. In fact, the dietitian or manager who plans nonselect menus must document for regulatory agencies that the house diet meets these minimum requirements for good health. Dietary modifications of the regular diet may then be designed in two ways: quantitative or qualitative. Qualitative changes modify consistency, texture, or nutrients. Quantitative changes involve modifications in number or size of meals served or amounts of specific nutrients; examples might be written as "six small feedings" or "4-gram sodium" diets.

Whatever kind of diet order is prescribed, the patient's acceptance is influenced by nursing personnel. For example, if a caregiver expresses criticism about the food or its service, the patient is likely to do the same. Acceptance of the modified diet is also influenced by patient perception about food and nutrition as a part of the medical treatment. Thus, genuine concern and education from the nursing team can make a difference. By explaining the rationale of why some foods are allowed and others not, the staff may enhance patient adherence to the modified diet. It is important to remember that food provides the energy and nutrients to heal and recover from illness. Food left on the tray does not help the healing process.

Food Service Delivery Systems

Nursing personnel are often involved with meal distribution. Thus, it is important for them to understand how meals are prepared and delivered in different health care facilities. Food service in a health care setting is the responsibility of the director of the food and nutrition services. This person may be either an

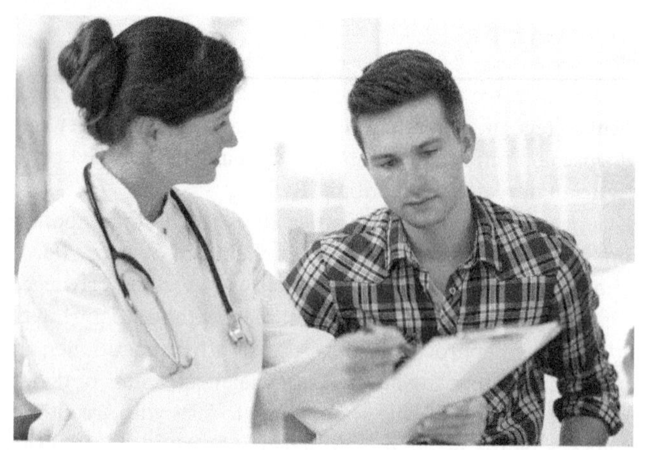

Fig. 12.1 Selective menu planning often requires nursing assistance. (From www.thinkstockphotos.com)

administrative dietitian or a specially trained food service manager. They are responsible for hiring, terminating, and supervising staff; ordering and purchasing food and supplies; delivering food to patients and staff; and overseeing quality improvements. This person is also responsible for patient satisfaction and quality improvements.

Clinical dietitians work with the food service director to assess patients' nutritional status, plan appropriate diets and nutrition intervention, and provide nutrition education. Other personnel from the food and nutrition department include cooks, clerks, dishwashers, aides, and dietetic technicians. Clinical dietitians may be members of the food service department or may work for a separate nutrition department, especially in larger facilities. Their jobs involve direct patient care.

Typically, only RDs (management or clinical) have the appropriate education and training in clinical nutrition with its contextual applications. Other nutrition team members work under the direction of the RD when it comes to the implementation of diet orders, altering fluids or nutrients, and making recommendations. Dietetic technicians, registered (DTRs), work most closely with the RD in direct patient care services.

A selective menu system affords patients the feeling of some control over their lives while hospitalized. Even if the most nutritious meals are planned, malnutrition is a risk when patients do not eat well for several days or more. A standardized house diet is planned, and then options are modified according to special nutritional needs. Some institutions provide selective menus for modified as well as regular diets. The menu for a modified diet lists only foods that are appropriate for that diet order, allowing a choice of foods that the patient will eat. If a selective menu is not available, simple changes or substitutions are allowed (Fig. 12.1).

Many hospitals offer hotel-style room service instead of preplated meal service delivered by carts to nursing units. With this service, patients can order from their menu when hungry, and not just within mealtimes organized by the foodservice department. Greater satisfaction occurs when patients can choose when and what they eat within the constraints of a diet order (McCray et al., 2018). (See the *Teaching Tool* box Assisting Patients with Menu Selections for more suggestions.)

TEACHING TOOL

Assisting Patients With Menu Selections

When we select food items from a restaurant menu while socializing with friends or family, the process is fun. However, choosing foods from the restricted hospital selections, often with little descriptive information, can be a difficult or intimidating chore. Some hospitals use paperless menu planning, with iPads or handheld computers for patients to make their selections. Other hospitals have the patient or family call in their menu choices, especially when room service is available. We understand forms and computers that require us to choose quickly, but our patients may not share that ability and may need our help. Following are potential menu selection problems and possible solutions.

Problem	Solution
Patient is illiterate, too ill to read and write, or has reduced visual abilities.	Read menu items to patient and mark his or her selections.
Patient does not understand the terms used on menu (menu names are not always common knowledge).	Clarify for patient or ask for clarification from dietetic technician, dietitian, or food service personnel.
Patient must select foods from menu a day in advance, often resulting in delivery of too much or too little food.	Remind patients they are selecting food for the next day. If they have not selected enough food, offer them foods kept on the nursing unit for snacks or order additional foods from food service. If they have selected too much food, cover, date, and store appropriate foods for use later in the day; discard if not consumed within 24 hours.
Patient has a poor appetite (particularly when diminished from drug-nutrient interactions or the effects of the illness).	Suggest small frequent meals and snacks every 2 to 3 hours. Choose energy-dense foods like meats, dried fruit, nuts and starches. Have gravy, mayonnaise, or sauces added to menu items. Schedule between-meal supplement drinks, such as Instant Breakfast. Choose whole milk rather than skim milk or water as a beverage.
Patient does not understand why some of their favorite foods are not included on the menu, why smaller amounts are served, or why textures are modified. (Note that when we are ill, familiar foods are comforting.)	Discuss dietary concerns of the patient's illness, explaining why specific foods are not included or only limited amounts allowed. Menus are a great teaching tool for modified diets. Contact the dietitian to provide more education or counseling for the patient.

Nursing personnel, on behalf of their patients, often interact with the foodservice staff at their facility. It is useful to access the following information in your facility:

- Phone number or pager for the clinical dietitian to request assessments or education.
- Time schedule of meal service so requests or changes can be made before meal delivery.

- Location of the diet manual on the nursing unit, required by the Medicare Conditions of Participation for Hospitals and by The Joint Commission (TJC). In some facilities, a diet or nutrition care manual is available on a computer in the nursing stations. This manual is the reference that describes the rationale and indications for using a specific diet; it lists allowed and restricted foods and sample menus. Most diets list key nutrients affected by the modifications. For example, a clear liquid diet is low in protein and should not be used longer than 24 hours.

Modified diets include protein-altered diets for liver or renal disease, low sodium, carbohydrate control for diabetes, food allergies, ketogenic, gluten-free, renal, FODMAPs (fermentable oligosaccharides, disaccharides, monosaccharides, and polyols) for irritable bowel syndrome, and calorie controlled for weight management, bariatric surgery, and other conditions. Each facility has its own set of handouts for patient education.

Meals in Long-Term Care

Most dietary information applies to long-term care facilities, but there are a few additional concerns. Food service supplied to residents in long-term care facilities often relies exclusively on the foodservice department for nutritious foods and meals. Repetition and monotony will influence acceptance of foods and meals as served. Therefore, it is important that these residents be given food they can and will eat because they are at high nutritional risk. (See the *Personal Perspectives* box How We Should Care for One Another.)

PERSONAL PERSPECTIVES

How We Should Care for One Another

Working in long-term care facilities made me aware of how important food is to all people. Every day, three times a day, the residents would make their way to the dining room for meals. Seated next to favorite friends, or sometimes newly admitted strangers, the social event of a meal was the highlight of their day. Whenever possible, serving meals family style would make it more like home. Holidays were extra special, and guests would be invited for the festivities. The biggest celebrations were Thanksgiving, Mother's Day, and Father's Day. The Activities staff would have special musicians and singers come for the events. The meals were always beautifully prepared and served, with an emphasis on memorable choices and exquisite flavors. Knowing that the residents were living in their final "home" made us feel like a family. Our goal of adding comfort to their lives made the work very rewarding.

These experiences also prepared me to care for my own mother for the last 5 years of her life. During that time, she experienced the limitations of Parkinson's disease, hearing loss, cataracts, and a broken hip. Despite these frustrating events, she maintained a bright outlook and her spiritual faith. Having her live with us deepened empathy and compassion in our children, showing them a good example of how an extended family works and how we should care for one another ... in good times and in bad.

Sylvia Escott-Stump
Winterville, NC

Basic Hospital Diets

For the appropriate content of diets served in your facility, check the diet manual. Table 12.1 lists the types of diets available in hospitals and some indications for and contraindications to those diets, as well as providing sample lists of allowed foods for each.

Clear liquid diets. Historically, clear liquid diets were used in preparation for any type of surgery. More recently, it was thought that they were needed before gastrointestinal (GI) surgery or colonoscopy. A clear liquid diet consists of foods that are clear and liquid at room or body temperature, such as popsicles, plain gelatin, ice chips, and apple or grape juices. This diet helps prevent dehydration and keeps colon residue to a minimum. The clear liquid diet is inadequate in protein, fat, fiber, and energy. Evidenced-based guidelines (EBG) recommend a low-residue diet (LRD) before and after colonoscopy to improve tolerability by patients with no adverse effects (Nguyen et al., 2016; Rattray et al., 2017). Use of a clear liquid diet longer than a day can lead to compromised nutritional status and possible nutrient deficiencies. Therefore, your facility should have a policy that orders for clear liquid diets are valid for only 24 hours (much like time-restricted orders for antibiotics).

Full liquid diets. A full liquid diet consists of foods that are liquid at room or body temperature. It is used to provide oral nourishment for patients with wired jaws and those who have difficulty chewing or swallowing solid foods. Unlike the clear liquid diet, the full liquid diet offers more variety, and commercial nutritional supplements and milk can be used to supply adequate amounts of energy and nutrients to make it nutritionally complete. Full liquid diets can be nutritionally complete if they are well planned and include between-meal snacks. Amounts of the diet consumed by patients should be recorded and monitored daily to ensure adequate energy and nutrient consumption.

Lactose-containing (milk-based) foods are allowed on a full liquid diet. Note that patients who are lactose intolerant may experience nausea, vomiting, distention, or diarrhea when given lactose-rich liquids. It is possible to obtain lactose-free milk products for these individuals, especially to provide sufficient calcium and to avoid unnecessary avoidance of dairy products.

Raw eggs and unpasteurized milk should not be used in the preparation of any food served to patients. Patients and their families should be educated about the possible dangers of consuming homemade eggnog and similar items.

Another special concern is for patients who cannot swallow thin liquids. A patient receiving a full liquid diet should be carefully assessed if there are any signs of dysphagia.

Dysphagia diets. With amyotrophic lateral sclerosis (ALS), some forms of stroke, head and neck cancer, and other conditions in which swallowing is impaired, a diet altered in consistency may be needed to prevent aspiration into the lungs. Signs of swallowing difficulty (dysphagia) include drooling, pocketing of food, choking, gagging, and taking longer than 2 to 10 seconds to swallow food.

In 2015, the International Dysphagia Diet Standardization Initiative (IDDSI) classified foods and thickened liquids specifically to ensure safe swallowing in vulnerable patients, regardless of age or facility (IDDSI, 2020). Training is essential; the foodservice staff, nurses, physicians, and aides need to understand the relevance of the diet and any changes that are required to implement the IDDSI.

TABLE 12.1 **Types of Diets**

Diet	Indications	Contraindications	Sample Foods Allowed
Liquid diet	Provide oral fluids; before/after surgery; prepare bowel for diagnostic tests (colonoscopic examination, barium enema, and other procedures); acute gastrointestinal (GI) disturbances	Should not be used more than 24 hours; inadequate GI function; nutrient needs requiring parenteral nutrition	Broths, bouillon, apple juice, grape juice, gelatin made without fruit, 7-Up, ginger ale, coffee and tea without milk/cream
Full liquid	Provide oral fluids; after surgery; transition between clear liquids and solid food; oral or plastic surgery to the face and neck; mandibular fractures; patients who have chewing or swallowing difficulties; esophageal or GI strictures; diarrhea	Dysphagia, wired jaw	Same as clear liquids and add all other juices, milk, ice cream, cooked eggs, eggnog, oral supplements, or milkshakes
Pureed diet	Neurologic changes; inflammation or ulcerations of the oral cavity and/or esophagus; edentulous patients; fractured jaw; head and neck abnormalities; cerebrovascular accident	Situations in which ground or chopped foods are appropriate	Any foods that can be blended and served without particles or strands that might cause choking Sufficient but not excessive fluids should be used for the blending process
Mechanical soft diet	Poorly fitting dentures; edentulous patients; limited chewing or swallowing ability; dysphagia; strictures of intestinal tract; radiation treatment to oral cavity; progression from enteral tube feedings or parenteral nutrition to solid foods	Situations in which regular foods are appropriate	All foods that are easily cut with a fork, chopped or blended Hard, stringy, or tough foods such as celery, broccoli, nuts, popcorn, and meat strands should be omitted because they may cause choking Depending on the reason for the modification, more foods might be eliminated or added back to the diet as the patient progresses
Soft diet	Debilitated patients unable to consume a regular diet; mild GI problems	Situations in which regular foods are appropriate	All foods served on the general diet, with the exception of highly fibrous fruits and vegetables Most cooked or canned foods are acceptable choices Omit chewy, stringy, and tough foods

The Dysphagia Diet has multiple levels. The most restrictive is a Pureed Diet; no coarse textures are allowed, and foods are totally blended without lumps. For the Minced and Moist Diet, foods are to be moist, softened, and easily chewed. Meats are ground and served with a gravy or sauce, or soft salads may be used (tuna or chicken salad, for example). At the next level, foods are Soft and Bite-Sized; no hard, dry, sticky, or crunchy foods are offered. When possible, patients can return to the diet with easy-to-chew foods, or even a regular diet.

Liquids are ordered separately; they may be thinned or thickened according to the evaluation by a speech-language pathologist. Thickeners are usually modified starch or xanthan gum, and orders will state one specific viscosity. In most facilities, bedside thickening by the nursing staff is best to ensure that the liquids are consumed at the proper consistency. Fig. 12.2 shows the IDDSI framework, and each facility documents how orders are implemented.

Mechanically altered diets

When a patient has problems chewing, foods can be chopped, ground, mashed, or pureed. Consistency of food can be varied according to the patient's ability. The nurse, dietitian, and patient should work together to evaluate the need for modifying consistency according to food preferences and diet orders. If needed, the speech-language pathologist should be consulted if swallowing problems also exists.

Some foods, such as mashed potatoes and ice cream, are already a smooth consistency. For other foods, small amounts of liquid (e.g., broth, milk, gravies) can be added to reach the appropriate consistency needed. Any liquid added to pureed foods should complement the food and should not conceal the food's original flavor. Care should be taken to add only enough liquid to achieve desired consistency yet allow the nutritional quality of the food to be retained. Butter, margarine, gravies, sugar, or honey may be added to foods to increase energy density.

To make pureed foods more attractive, **component pureeing** may be used. For example, a cake-decorating tool (icing bag and tips) can be used to make pureed peas look like regular peas. Molds are also used to shape foods. However, scooped or unmolded pureed foods are equally acceptable and identifiable (Lepore et al., 2014).

The exact composition and consistency of a mechanically altered diet will vary according to the patient's needs. These diets can be modified for additional changes, such as lowering sodium, carbohydrate, or fat content.

It is important to remember the patient's quality of life depends on receiving foods that are appealing, tasty, and served with an appropriate consistency. **Edentulous** patients can often chew solid or soft foods. Sometimes, foods just need to be chopped, either coarsely or finely. The general rule of thumb is to serve the least modified consistency that the patient can safely consume. When a patient needs only the meat pureed,

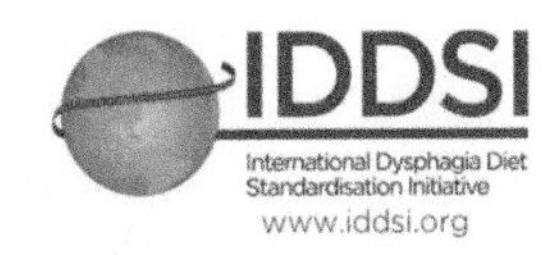

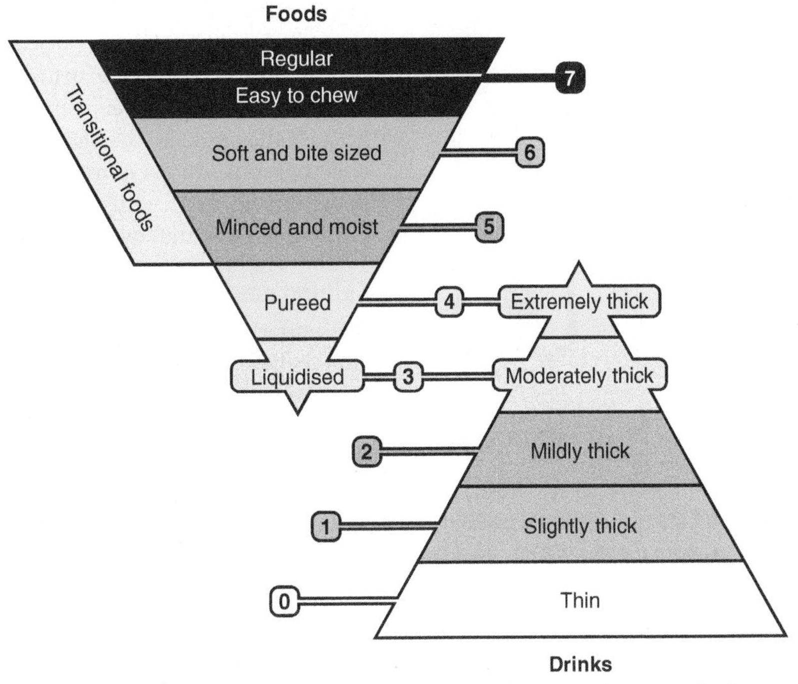

Fig. 12.2 The International Dysphagia Diet Standardization Initiative framework shows the various levels of food and liquid consistencies for safe swallowing.

then puree only the meats. When a patient needs chopped or ground foods, the foods should not be pureed.

Soft diets. Soft diets are sometimes ordered after surgery or as transition from liquid diets to regular diets. Whole foods that are low in fiber and only lightly seasoned are used. Food supplements or between-meals snacks may be used to add extra energy. This diet often has a nebulous meaning and is not appropriate for patients requiring mechanically altered diets.

"Diet as tolerated." Occasionally when patients are admitted, the physician writes an order for "diet as tolerated." It is also common for this diet to be ordered postoperatively. It permits the patient's preferences and situation to be taken into consideration. This diet order provides an excellent opportunity for collaboration by the nurse, dietitian, and patient to plan and provide food that is eaten, tolerated, and nourishing while observing the progression of the patient.

Vegetarian diets. A vegetarian diet is a normal diet but does not include meat, poultry, fish or seafood, or products containing those foods, and it can be healthful and nutritionally adequate if planned well (Melina et al., 2016). Note that Hindus, Seventh Day Adventists, Buddhists, and some other religious groups suggest following a vegetarian lifestyle. For patients who wish to follow this type of plan, the RD should be consulted. Important nutrients that must be planned include protein, vitamins B_{12} and D, iron, zinc, iodine, and calcium.

A vegan diet omits all animal proteins, including dairy products and eggs. In a study of intakes among meat eaters and vegans, meat eaters had the highest intakes of energy, saturated fat, protein, riboflavin, zinc, iodine, and vitamins B_{12} and D; vegans had the highest intakes of polyunsaturated fatty acids, dietary fiber, vitamins C and E, folate, magnesium, iron, and copper (Sobiecki et al, 2016). Thus, the differences in nutrient intake may have implications for heart disease and other chronic conditions.

Other modified diets. Modified diets, such as those limiting carbohydrates or salt, are described in relevant chapters in this text.

OTHER FOOD CONSIDERATIONS

Food Allergy or Intolerance

A true food allergy is caused by the release of histamine and serotonin, which can be reproduced in a double-blind food challenge (Ho et al., 2014). These responses usually occur quickly every time the food is eaten. In a hospital or nursing home setting, an allergic reaction can be quickly addressed if staff members know the typical symptoms and how to respond. The most common symptoms of food allergies are diarrhea, nausea, vomiting, cramping, abdominal distention, and pain. Although nearly 200 different foods have been known to produce an allergy or intolerance, only 8 foods (eggs, milk, wheat, soy, fish, shellfish, peanuts, and tree nuts) are major triggers in adults. Infants may react to cow's milk and soy, but most of them outgrow this sensitivity by age 4 years.

It is important to assess true food allergies (documented by a physician) versus food dislikes or intolerances. Food intolerance is a nonallergic reaction; it may be caused by toxins, drugs, or conditions such as lactose and gluten intolerances. Intolerances are often dose responsive, occurring after a large amount has been consumed. Often patients state, "I am allergic to milk" but will say they can use it on cereal; thus, they do not have a milk allergy. Most patients who

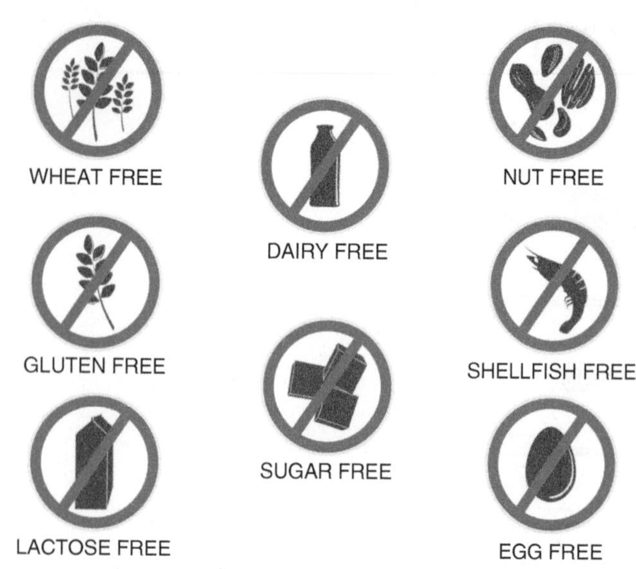
WHEAT FREE
DAIRY FREE
NUT FREE
GLUTEN FREE
SHELLFISH FREE
SUGAR FREE
LACTOSE FREE
EGG FREE

Fig. 12.3 Common diet orders that may include food allergens.

are lactose intolerant can use treated milk (Lactaid), cheeses, and yogurt. Ask the RD to evaluate such patients further because it is important to find ways to include calcium for individuals who are lactose intolerant. See Fig. 12.3 for some of the more common diet orders that include allergens and food sensitivities.

Food Safety and Sanitation

Foodborne illness (food poisoning) can occur in any setting. Personal hygiene and hand washing are the most important factors in prevention. Food temperatures should be maintained at 40° F or lower for refrigerated items, 165° F for most hot foods. Foods should be handled, stored, and held at proper temperatures. Refrigerators on nursing units should be checked regularly, and hot foods should be served to patients as soon as possible after they have been cooked.

Any protein-rich food (milk, eggs, cheese, meat/poultry/fish) should be discarded if left at room temperature longer than 2 hours. Items that are not consumed should be labeled, dated, refrigerated, then used within 24 hours. To prevent cross-contamination, refrigerators on nursing units should not mix drugs, staff foods, and patient foods.

A foodborne outbreak occurs when two or more individuals have the same symptoms over the same time period—such as nausea, vomiting, diarrhea, abdominal cramping, vision problems, fever, chills, dizziness, and headaches. When there is an outbreak, it must be reported (by the food service director or director of nursing) to the local health department authorities. Suspected foods should be tested for microbial contamination.

The top causes of food poisoning are norovirus, *Salmonella, Clostridium perfringens, Campylobacter* spp., and *Staphylococcus aureus.* The U.S. Food and Drug Administration (FDA) Food Safety Modernization Act (FSMA) aims to ensure that the U.S. food supply is safe by shifting the focus of federal regulator from responding to contamination to preventing it, from farm to table (FDA, 2020). The Centers for Disease Control and Prevention (CDC) website offers a useful pictorial of food outbreak investigations along the food chain at www.cdc.gov/outbreaknet/investigations/figure_food_production.html.

At the institutional level, all food service employees are taught about HACCP (hazard analysis and critical control points). In HACCP, biological, chemical, and physical hazards from raw material production, procurement, and handling to manufacturing, distribution, and consumption of the finished product are controlled. HACCP training discusses receiving, cooking, serving, and handling of high-risk foods and how to prevent illness.

Nursing staff members benefit from food safety education because they prepare the patients for meals, handle their trays, open beverages, unwrap food, and sometimes handle the food items during the feeding process. In-service sessions can be given to nursing staff by the RD on request.

Cultural and Religious Implications of Food

It is important to ask a patient about cultural, ethnic, and religious beliefs and preferences related to food. All of us grow up in families and communities in which certain patterns and rituals are considered "the norm." Asking questions and understanding these individual needs and expectations are basic and important parts of the nursing assessment.

Cultural food patterns. Understanding the common food preferences and patterns used by different cultures helps nurses identify better food choices and lower the number of meal refusals. With the diversity of food choices in grocery stores and restaurants, Americans have adopted many foods into their daily lives that would have been considered "foreign food" to past generations.

Many older adults prefer simple choices and "comfort foods" over exotic and unfamiliar options. At the same time, enhancement of meals with simple herbs and spices (dill, onion, garlic, parsley) often helps increase intake for those individuals who have lost their sense of smell or taste. It is important to remember, as well, that medications and treatments such as chemotherapy alter taste buds. The patient who complains that the food "tastes lousy" should be given the opportunity to select something else during mealtimes to avoid the potential for nutritional decline. To read more about foods and various cultures, the following websites are useful.

- Countries and their cultures: www.everyculture.com
- Culinary History Timeline (social history, manners, and menus) www.foodtimeline.org/food1.html
- Health Resources and Services Administration's Cultural Competence website: www.hrsa.gov/culturalcompetence/index.html
- Think Cultural Health: www.thinkculturalhealth.hhs.gov

Religious implications for dietary patterns. Beliefs of several major religions include practices that affect or prescribe specific dietary patterns or prohibit consumption of certain foods. Individuals practicing these religions may or may not adhere to all customs. A brief review of some of these practices is found here.

Western and Near-Eastern Religions

Christianity: Some sects may not eat meat on holy days; others prohibit alcohol and caffeine consumption.

Seventh-Day Adventist: General restrictions of pork and pork-related products, shellfish, alcohol, coffee, and tea are followed. Some followers are ovo-lacto vegetarians or vegans.

Church of Latter-Day Saints/Mormon: Alcohol and caffeine are prohibited or strongly discouraged.

Islam: Pork and pork-related products are not eaten. Meats that are consumed must be slaughtered by a prescribed ritual called halal. Because these procedures are similar to the Judaic kosher slaughtering of animals, Muslims may eat kosher meats. Coffee, tea, and alcohol are not consumed. During the month of Ramadan, Muslims fast during the day from dawn to sunset. Exemptions are made for pregnant women or people with serious medical conditions, including diabetes, but many will still participate against medical advice (Hassanein et al., 2017).

Judaism: No pork or pork-related products or fish without scales and fins are eaten. Dairy foods are not consumed with meat or animal-related foods (excludes fish). Once meat or dairy is eaten, 6 hours must pass for the other to be consumed. Animals are slaughtered according to ritual, in which blood is drained and the carcass is salted and rinsed; meat prepared this way is *kosher*. Preparation of processed foods must adhere to guidelines. Because meat and dairy must not mix, two sets of dishes and utensils are used at home and in kosher restaurants. Foods that are neither meat nor dairy are called *pareve* and labeled by food manufacturers. Additional customs affect food consumption on Saturday (the Sabbath), during which no cooking occurs. Fasting (no water or food) for 24 hours occurs during Yom Kippur (Day of Atonement). During Passover, an 8-day holiday, no leavened bread is consumed—only matzo (made from flour and water) and products made from matzo flour.

Eastern Religions

Hinduism and Buddhism: Animal foods of beef, pork, lamb, and poultry are not eaten. Monks participate in fasting, as may some followers. Followers are often lacto-vegetarians or vegans.

Complementary-Alternative Medicine

TCAM (traditional, complementary, and alternative medicine) has become a part of life for many Americans. To address this increased interest, the National Institutes of Health created the National Center for Complementary and Alternative Medicine (NCCAM). TCAM consists of a cluster of medical and health care approaches, methods, and items not associated with conventional medicine (NCCAM, 2020).

The Eastern traditional cultures base their system on the forces of nature, understood through the fundamental concept of *yin* and *yang*. Illness is viewed as an imbalance of these two forces, which are opposites of each other. Yin is dark, night, feminine, and contracting; yang is light, day, masculine, and expanding. The imbalance of these two forces affects *Qi*, the life force.

Acupuncture, energy work, body work, and herbal medicine have been part of traditional medicine for thousands of years. Eastern medicine treats the person as a whole, whereas conventional western medicine treats organ systems. Mind-body, nutrition, and exercise are applied for daily wellness.

Complementary medicine refers to non-Western healing approaches used at the same time as conventional medicine (allopathy). For instance, the patient who attempts to lower hypertension takes prescription medications (conventional) but also attends yoga classes (complementary) for physical and psychologic benefits.

Naturopathic medicine is based on noninvasive, natural healing to recover from disease and to achieve wellness (NCCAM, 2020). This system incorporates techniques from Eastern and Western traditions. Techniques include acupuncture, exercise, massage, and dietary alterations.

Alternative medicine therapies are used instead of conventional medicine (NCCAM, 2020). An example is the use of herbal supplements or shark cartilage to treat cancer instead of chemotherapy or surgery.

Integrative medicine merges conventional medical therapies with TCAM modalities for which safety and efficacy have been demonstrated (NCCAM, 2020). Integrative medical centers are often available in larger or teaching hospitals. Advanced practice nurses with a Master of Science degree in holistic health can provide levels of integrative care. Insurance companies have gradually increased coverage for such treatments, recognizing the cost benefits of many of these approaches.

A person-centered therapeutic process helps people take charge of their own health and well-being (Prescott & Logan, 2019). An example is given here when a patient recovering from heart bypass surgery can be referred to a center for integrative medicine. There, a board-certified nurse practitioner or physician evaluates the patient and may prescribe therapeutic massage for stress reduction and yoga to assist recovery. All services are provided within the same health care facility.

Complementary-Alternative Medicine: Herbs and Botanicals

Biologically based therapies encompass materials found in nature. These materials include functional foods, botanicals, and herbs. Previously, the efficacy of these therapies tended to be anecdotal, based on the self-reported experiences of individuals. Well-designed studies continue to identify the active ingredients in herbs, botanical products, and functional foods. For example, yogurt and kefir with active bacterial cultures are natural probiotics that enhance intestinal health.

There are benefits and risks with herbs, botanicals, and dietary supplements, including efficacy, safety versus harm, and potential drug-supplement interactions. Box 12.1 discusses the safety of some natural remedies.

BOX 12.1 Natural Does Not Equal Safe!

Herbal remedies and dietary supplements are not regulated by the U.S. Food and Drug Administration (FDA), so the purity, potency, and safety of these products can and do vary. Manufacturers' claims of efficacy and safety are not subject to the rigorous testing that is mandatory for medications. Herbs and dietary supplements may be contaminated with other herbs, pesticides, herbicides, and other products during growth, harvesting, preparation, and storage. Moreover, active chemical components in the herb may not be standardized, leading to dissimilar potencies from lot to lot, or even from capsule to capsule within the same lot. Safety, toxicity, and the likelihood of adverse interactions with other medications or treatments often have not been tested, particularly in children. Patients contemplating use of herbs and dietary supplements should proceed with caution and should seek out products only from reliable manufacturers.

Functional foods contain physiologically active (bioactive) substances. These foods may have been modified to increase nutrient density when being fortified, enriched, or enhanced. Some functional food components are marketed as dietary supplements, such as herb-enriched beverages. An enhanced beverage may contain St. John's wort; consuming a small amount would be ineffective for depression treatment and pointless for any other purpose. Care must be taken when selecting a product for "functional" health purposes because the amounts and sources of ingredients are not well regulated and few controlled clinical trials have been completed.

Dietary supplements are consumed orally as tablets, liquids, capsules, extracts, powders, concentrates, gel caps, liquids, or powders. There are special requirements for supplement labeling for these products. Under the Dietary Supplement Health and Education Act of 1994 (DSHEA), dietary supplements are considered foods, not drugs. DSHEA established the definition of dietary supplements as products that supplement dietary intake and contain one or more of the following (Center for Food Safety and Applied Nutrition [CFSAN], 2017):

- A vitamin or a mineral
- An herb or other botanical
- An amino acid
- A dietary substance for use to supplement the diet by increasing the total dietary intake
- A concentrate, metabolite, constituent, extract, or a combination of the preceding ingredients

Based on this definition, dietary supplements are not drugs or food additives. This distinction affects the way they are regulated and facilitates the approval process. Drugs and food additives require more stringent testing for safety and efficacy. Consequently, dietary supplements can enter the marketplace much more quickly, with fewer data confirming their function and effectiveness. Consumers may spend money needlessly, or they may delay medical treatments if choosing unproven, untested supplements or herbal remedies. Nurses will want to include questions about the use of such products during patient assessments and physicians should be informed accordingly.

Physicians and dietitians strongly recommend that nutrients be consumed through food rather than single supplements. Specific supplement combinations may be recommended as a safety net for infants, children, teens, pregnant women, or the elderly. As a safety net, vitamin/mineral supplements at 100% or less of the Dietary Reference Intake (DRI) are appropriate.

Labeling of dietary supplements must follow the regulated format for nutrition labels (see Chapter 2). This means that the label needs to identify the product as a dietary supplement and must include the name and amount of each item contained in the product. Labels may also include approved statements of health claims such as are allowable on food product labels. For example, a claim may be made that a diet containing soluble fiber from whole oats and psyllium may reduce the risk of coronary heart disease. If claims are made by supplements, the label must include the statement "This statement has not been evaluated by the FDA. This product is not intended to diagnose, treat, cure, or prevent any disease" (NCCAM, 2020).

Genetically Modified Foods

Another area of discussion is the category of genetically modified foods. A **genetically modified organism (GMO)** has had its DNA altered or modified in some way through genetic engineering, mostly with DNA from a bacterium, plant, virus, or animal (Live Science, 2020). The purpose of creating GMO foods is to increase the food supply, make foods more shelf stable, and improve quality. The major drawback is that some individuals could have an allergic reaction to a modified food item.

Overall, consuming foods containing ingredients derived from genetically modified crops is no riskier than consuming the same foods containing ingredients from crop plants modified by conventional plant improvement techniques (Live Science, 2020). Corn, soybeans, summer squash, apples, potatoes, and canola are examples of crops that have been improved by genetic modifications. GM crops have been altered to increase economic value, conserve biodiversity, decrease carbon emissions and support human health (IFIC, 2020).

Application to nursing. Familiarity with alternative therapies and their efficacy is important. Acceptance without judgment provides support for patients in their quest for health. The nurse may be the first person to document the patient's use of products that could interfere with other medical therapies or medications. Drawing attention to these concerns may prevent an unexpected medical incident.

If patients use supplements instead of conventional medications because of high prescription costs, they can be referred to social services or pharmaceutical company programs for financial assistance. Referral to registered dietitians for nutrition therapy involving dietary supplements or for general nutrition counseling is another option. Additional concerns are discussed in the *Cultural Diversity and Nutrition* box Complementary Medicine and Cultural Implications.

CULTURAL DIVERSITY AND NUTRITION

Complementary Medicine and Cultural Implications

Global Strategies

The World Health Organization (WHO) provides guidelines for countries to develop policies to evaluate and regulate traditional, complementary, and alternative medicine (TCAM). The global plan supports strategies to expand the availability and uniformity of traditional medicine. Cultures where traditional medicine may prevail include those in the Middle East, India, China, western Africa, Latin America, Appalachia, and the Caribbean; Native American cultures; and the Maori culture of New Zealand.

Application to Nursing

TCAM may be inappropriately applied when translated from one culture to another. Nurses working with diverse cultural groups should become aware of the TCAM practices of their patients' culture of origin. A prime example is the herb *ma huang* (ephedra), used in China for short periods to reduce respiratory congestion. In the United States, *ma huang* was marketed as a weight-loss product, causing strokes, heart attacks, or death when it was used long term.

In the United States, Hispanic immigrants are quite heterogeneous in their approaches to medical treatment. Language differences, cultural values, religion, historical experiences, and health beliefs are part of the tapestry that underpins complementary medicine. Sensitivity and respect are fundamental for a positive patient-provider relationship.

Nonoral Feeding

Any time the GI tract is used to provide nourishment, the feeding is a form of enteral nutrition (EN). This includes liquid diets, soft and solid food diets, and special nutritionally complete formulas administered orally or via tubes. When a patient is not able to eat orally for more than a few days, a nonoral method must be used. If medical personnel talk about "enteral nutrition," they are referring to tube feedings.

Tube Feeding

Often patients are unable or unwilling to consume adequate nutrients and calories by mouth. When this is the case and the GI tract is functioning, nutrients can be provided via feeding tubes placed into the alimentary tract. (See the *Teaching Tool* box Tube Feeding the Infant or Child.)

TEACHING TOOL

Tube Feeding the Infant or Child

Parents and caregivers need special support when their infants and children are tube fed. Assure them that the children can still be cuddled and can play without interfering with the tube nourishment. Teach the adults how the process works; they can be allies in helping young children accept and understand these procedures. Be sure to explain the procedures to the children as well. Dolls or stuffed animals can be used to explain how tube feeding helps speed the healing process.

Each infant and child has individual nutritional requirements based on growth, allergies, and medical conditions. Check with the nurse or dietitian for appropriate rate, concentration, and volume of feedings. The following are some specific techniques to share with the parent or caregiver to ensure adequate nutrient intake and food safety:

- Wash your hands with soap and water for at least 20 seconds (the time it takes to sing the "Happy Birthday" song twice).
- Flush feeding tube with 1 to 5 mL of water before and after each feeding and before and after giving medications to prevent the feeding tube from clogging.
- Never add new formula to formula already in the feeding container.
- Change the entire feeding setup every 24 hours.
- Place only 8 hours of formula or 4 hours of breast milk in the feeding container at any given time.
- Make sure your infant or child has pleasant sensations during feedings: Hold your child during feedings, and allow them to suck on a pacifier, sit in a high chair, and be a part of family meals.
- Give medications only in liquid form.
- Elevate the head of the bed 30 to 45 degrees if the child cannot be held.

(Data from Cincinnati Children's Hospital Medical Center, *Nasojejunal tube feeding with enteral pump.* Accessed 26 August, 2020, from www.cincinnatichildrens.org/health/info/abdomen/home/nasojejunal-kangaroo.htm.)

When the GI tract is functional, accessible, and safe to use, enteral feedings are preferred over parenteral nutrition (PN) because they are physiologically beneficial in maintaining the integrity and function of the gut. Enteral tube feedings are much less costly than PN for both the patient and the health care institution.

Tube feeding can be part of routine care when a patient experiences inadequate or reduced oral intake over the previous week. Other conditions warranting tube feeding are severe dysphagia, major burns, short bowel syndrome after resection, and intestinal fistulas (abnormal passages between the intestines). Conditions under which tube feedings are helpful, but not routine, include major trauma, radiation therapy, chemotherapeutic regimens, acute or chronic liver failure, and severe renal dysfunction.

Tube feeding is of limited value if intensive chemotherapy leads to GI tract dysfunction or if adequate postoperative oral intake is expected to resume within 5 to 7 days. If EN is not contraindicated (e.g., by hemodynamic instability, bowel obstruction, high-output fistula, or severe ileus), then the RD should recommend that EN be started within 24 to 48 hours after injury or admission to the intensive care unit (Academy of Nutrition and Dietetics, Evidence Analysis Library [EAL], 2020). The benefits of starting EN early include less risk for malnutrition, fewer complications, faster wound healing, and shorter length of hospital stay.

Types of formulas. For years, enteral formulas were prepared with the use of foodstuffs, vitamin/mineral preparations, and a blender. Today an extensive variety of commercially prepared formulas are used. Some formulas are nutritionally complete, some are formulated for specific diseases or conditions, and others (modular) provide specific nutrients to supplement a diet or other formula. Commercial products are preferred over hospital or home-blended solutions because they provide a known nutrient composition, controlled osmolality and consistency, and bacteriologic safety. They are also much easier to prepare and store. Many are nutritionally complete if consumed in the volumes recommended by the manufacturers.

Standard formulas. Standard (polymeric) formulas are composed of intact nutrients that require a functioning GI tract for digestion and absorption of nutrients. There are several categories of polymeric formulas that provide 1 to 2 kcal/mL. Standard formulas can be categorized into blenderized food products, milk-based products, high-kcal lactose-free products, and normocaloric lactose-free products. Normocaloric (1 kcal/mL) lactose-free formulas have low osmolality, which generally makes them well tolerated. Fiber-containing products are low osmolality and are used for patients with abnormal bowel regulation. These formulas contain fiber from natural food sources or soy polysaccharide.

Hypercaloric (1.5–2 kcal/mL) formulas are designed to meet kcal and protein demands in a reduced volume and have moderate to high osmolality. High-nitrogen lactose-free formulas (1–2 kcal/mL) are designed to meet higher protein demands at usual or increased energy needs. They have low to moderate osmolality.

Elemental formulas are also called predigested or hydrolyzed formulas (1–1.3 kcal/mL). They are composed of partially or fully hydrolyzed nutrients that can be used for the patient with a partially functioning GI tract, impaired capacity to digest foods or absorb nutrients, pancreatic insufficiency, or bile salt deficiency. These products are lactose-free and are usually hyperosmolar. They are not palatable and are best suited only for administration by tube. These products are used less often because most patients can tolerate standard formulas.

Modular formulas (3.8–4 kcal/mL) are not nutritionally complete by themselves because they are single macronutrients, such as glucose polymers, protein, or lipids. They are added to foods or other enteral products to change composition when nutritional needs cannot otherwise be met.

Specialty formulas (1–2 kcal/mL) are designed to meet specialized nutrient demands for specific disease states, such as diabetes, renal failure, liver failure, pulmonary disease, and human immunodeficiency virus/acquired immunodeficiency syndrome (HIV/AIDS). For critically ill patients, immune-enhancing formulas may be considered (EAL, 2020). These products contain omega-3 fatty acids, borage oil, antioxidants, and other additives. Some specialty formulas require additional supplementation with vitamins, minerals, or trace elements. Some are unpalatable, and all are more expensive than standard formulas.

Formula selection. The numerous types and brands of enteral feeding products on the market can make product selection a complex process. Whether a patient can digest and absorb nutrients indicates whether an elemental or polymeric formula should be used. Individual nutrient requirements determine the type and amount of tube-feeding formula. The RD will assist the physician with ongoing assessment of nutritional status and formula tolerance.

Feeding routes. Like the choice of an appropriate tube-feeding formula, selection of the correct feeding tube and feeding route involves consideration of various factors. If the tube feeding will be used for short duration, a nonsurgical placement can be made. If the feeding tube will be in place long term or permanently, surgical placement is necessary. Routes for tube feeding include the following (Fig. 12.4):

Nasogastric: Tube is passed through the nose to the stomach.

Nasoduodenal: Tube is passed from the nose to the duodenum (small intestine).

Nasojejunal: Tube is passed through the nose to the jejunum (small intestine).

Esophagostomy: Tube is surgically inserted into the neck and extends to the stomach.

Gastrostomy: Tube is surgically inserted into the stomach.

Jejunostomy: Tube is surgically inserted into the small intestine.

Placing the feeding tube into the stomach, duodenum, or jejunum through the nose is the simplest and most common feeding technique. This technique is preferred for patients who will resume oral feedings in a few days. Feeding through a tube placed in the stomach simulates normal GI function but should be reserved for patients who are alert, with intact gag and cough reflexes. Tube placement into the small intestine has less risk of aspiration, but elemental formulas are often required for easier absorption, and continuous feedings are better tolerated.

Surgical placement of the feeding tube is preferred when long-term use is anticipated or when obstruction makes insertion through the nose impossible. These procedures require surgery with general anesthesia. Placement of a **percutaneous endoscopic gastrostomy (PEG)** tube can be performed with

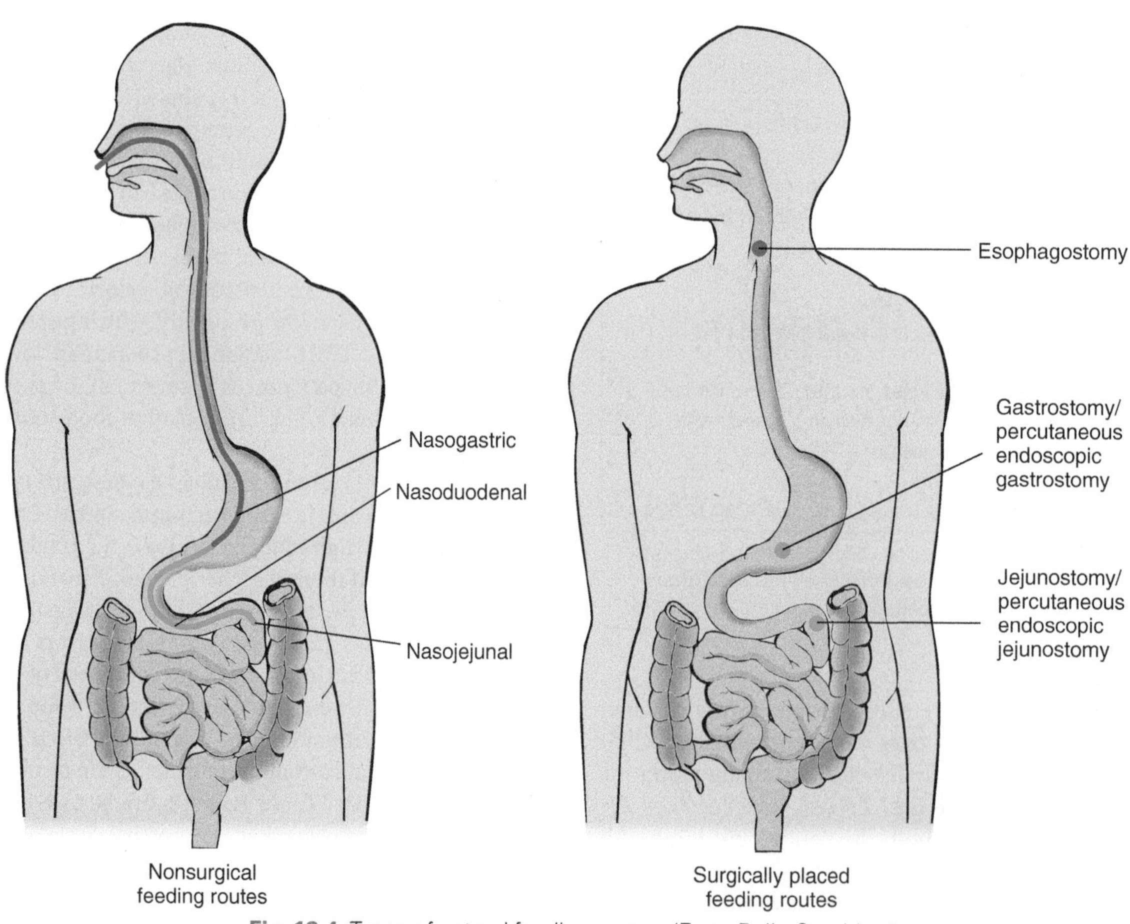

Fig. 12.4 Types of enteral feeding routes. (From Rolin Graphics.)

TABLE 12.2 **Advantages and Disadvantages of Enteral Feeding Routes**

Feeding Route	Characteristics	Advantages	Disadvantages
Nasogastric	Tube extends from nose into stomach	Easy to place/easy to remove No surgery necessary Less expensive Medications can be administered	Greater risk of aspiration (compared with nasointestinal feeding) Gastric emptying must be monitored
Nasoduodenal or nasojejunal	*Nasoduodenal:* Tube extends from nose through pylorus into duodenum; tube must be advanced by peristalsis or videofluoroscopy *Nasojejunal:* Tube extends from nose through pylorus into jejunum and is usually placed by videofluoroscopy or endoscopy	Less aspiration (compared with nasogastric feedings) Helpful in patients with gastroparesis	Requires placement via endoscopy Gastric motility cannot be monitored
Gastrostomy or percutaneous endoscopic gastrostomy (PEG)	*Gastrostomy:* Tube placed through incision in abdominal wall into stomach *PEG:* Tube percutaneously placed in stomach under endoscopic guidance, secured by rubber "bumpers" or inflated balloon catheter	Intermediate/bolus feedings possible Patient comfort Size of tube allows medication administration and/or gastric decompression	Increased risk of aspiration in some individuals Stoma care required Potential for dislodgment of tube
Jejunostomy or percutaneous endoscopic jejunostomy (PEJ)	*Jejunostomy:* Types include needle catheter placement, direct tube placement, and creation of jejunal stoma that is catheterized intermittently *PEJ:* Weighted feeding tube (from PEG insertion) passed into duodenum; peristaltic action advances tube into jejunum	Early postoperative feeding possible Decreased aspiration risk	Smaller tube used, so tube may clog easily Stoma care required Intraperitoneal leakage possible Volvulus possible

minimal sedation and has fewer complications than surgical placement. PEG involves placing a feeding tube into stomach via the esophagus and then drawing it through the abdominal skin using a stab incision. Table 12.2 describes the classifications, advantages, and disadvantages of different feeding routes.

Positioning. Unless contraindicated, patients should be positioned with the head of the bed elevated 30 to 45 degrees for tube feedings; this practice decreases the incidence of aspiration pneumonia and reflux of gastric contents into the esophagus and pharynx (EAL, 2020).

Method of administration. Proper administration safeguards delivery of the desired nutrients, enhances patient tolerance, and provides optimal nutrition support. Factors affecting decisions about appropriate methods of formula infusion include the patient's medical status and GI function and the feeding route. Tube feedings can be administered by three methods: continuous, intermittent, or bolus infusion. Table 12.3 summarizes indications for and advantages and disadvantages of each feeding method.

Continuous infusion is a common method of feeding. It provides controlled delivery of a prescribed volume of formula at a constant rate over a continuous period using an infusion pump. This method requires use of special equipment but is preferred when feeding into the small intestine; its effect mimics typical gastric emptying.

Intermittent infusion involves delivering the total quantity of formulas needed for a 24-hour period in three to six equal feedings. Each feeding is usually delivered by gravity over 30 to 60 minutes. This method represents a more normal feeding pattern, but patients often do not tolerate it if the rate is too rapid. Although equipment needs are minimal, this method is time-consuming because feedings must be closely monitored to ensure proper delivery rate.

Bolus feedings involve infusing volumes of formula (250–500 mL) by gravity or syringe over short periods. This method requires minimal equipment and time but is associated with greater potential for aspiration, regurgitation, and GI side effects. It should not be used for intestinal feedings.

Starting the tube feeding. Before initiation of enteral tube feedings, placement of the feeding tube must be confirmed and documented. Tube placement is often confirmed radiologically after initial insertion. Thereafter, aspiration of gastric contents with a large syringe (60-mL) is used to reconfirm tube placement.

The high osmolality of a hypertonic formula can lead to GI distress, such as intestinal distention and osmotic diarrhea. Diluting tube feedings will lengthen the amount of time necessary before nutritional requirements can be met. Therefore, most formulas are started at full strength but infused at a lower rate than goal. The rate of the feedings can be advanced to meet the desired volume, and then concentration can be gradually increased until kcal and protein needs are met.

Rate and concentration should never be advanced at the same time. If the feeding is not tolerated, rate or concentration can be reduced to the last level of tolerance, then gradually increased again. Other criteria to be considered to ensure optimal tolerance of the formula and safety of the feedings are solution temperature, prevention of bacterial contamination, prevention of aspiration, patency of tubing, administration of medications, and patient monitoring (Table 12.4).

Complications of tube feeding. Most problems in tube feeding can be prevented simply through good handwashing techniques by the nursing staff administering the feeding.

TABLE 12.3 Administration of Enteral Tube Feedings

Method	Indications	Advantages	Disadvantages
Continuous	Patients who have not eaten for a significant period; debilitated patients; patients with impaired gastrointestinal (GI) function; patients with uncontrolled T1D mellitus; intestinal feedings	Feedings can be administered at constant rate over 24-hour period; feedings can be cycled (allows formula to be delivered over shorter period, allowing patients freedom of movement, and to promote oral intake if appropriate); gastric pooling minimized and fewer GI side effects experienced; continuous feeding into jejunum is similar to normal gastric emptying	Requires feeding pump if accuracy of volume delivered is required; continuous drip by gravity is possible, but less accurate
Intermittent	Feedings that are infused at specific intervals throughout the day (total volume of feeding divided and given four to six times per day)	Requires only simple equipment; can be used in home settings; may be more physiologic than continuous infusion; feedings can be administered by gravity over 30–90 minutes	In absence of pumps, feedings must be monitored vigilantly; may become time consuming depending on number of scheduled feedings per day; rate of intermittent infusion (rather than volume) seems to be a major reason for intolerance of tube feedings
Bolus	Appropriate only for feeding into the stomach; involves feeding large volumes of formula intermittently over short periods, usually by syringe	More manageable for the patient; rate of 30 mL/min or volume of 500–700 mL per feeding seems to be cutoff of physical tolerance	Associated with increased risk of aspiration, regurgitation, and GI side effects; not appropriate for postpyloric feedings

(Data from Moore, M.C. *Pocket guide to nutrition assessment and care*, ed 6, St. Louis, 2016, Mosby/Elsevier.)

TABLE 12.4 Criteria for Safe Administration of Enteral Tube Feedings

Criterion	Considerations
Temperature	Administer solutions infused by continuous drip chilled Administer intermittent and bolus feedings at room temperature to decrease incidence of gastrointestinal (GI) side effects
Prevention of bacterial contamination	Use closed feeding containers Prefilled, ready-to-feed closed systems are available for some products (less chance of contamination) Change extension tubing administration set and bag daily Never add new formula to old formula Do not hang feedings for longer than 4–8 hours Keep ice in pouch of bag at all times while formula is running
Prevention of aspiration	Check tube placement before administration Tubes placed into small bowel are associated with decreased risk for aspiration Head of bed (HOB) should be elevated 30–45 degrees Consider adding vegetable food coloring to formula to allow for detection of aspirated tube feeding from pulmonary secretions (Remember: This does not protect against aspiration)
Patency of tubing	Irrigate tubes every 6–8 hours with 40–50 mL of warm water (continuous feeds) For intermittent or bolus feedings, irrigate tubes after each feeding with 40–50 mL of warm water Flush tube with 40–50 mL of water each time feeding is stopped If tubing clogs, flush with 30–50 mL of warm water Systems are available that allow for self-flushing of the feeding tube (e.g., from Ross Laboratories)
Medications	Medications administered through the feeding tube should be in liquid form Flush tubing before and after giving the medication with 20 mL of water to prevent clogging If medication is not available in liquid form, consult the pharmacist before crushing or diluting the medication (some medications are pharmacologically altered by mechanical manipulation) Never crush time-released, liquid-filled capsules or enteric-coated medications Do not give sublingual medications through the tubing Because hyperosmolar liquid medications (KCl) may cause gastric irritation or diarrhea, dilute with water before administration Supplemental electrolyte preparations (KCl, NaCl, $NaPO_4$) increase the osmolality of the formula and may cause feeding tubes to clog Do not mix together multiple medications and deliver simultaneously unless the compatibility of the medications is known If feeding into the duodenum or jejunum instead of the stomach, check the effect of medication absorption Monitor patient response to medications given through the feeding tube, and make the changes needed

Continued

TABLE 12.4 Criteria for Safe Administration of Enteral Tube Feedings—cont'd

Criterion	Considerations
Monitoring	Confirm tube placement before initiating feeding and before each intermittent feeding Record urine glucose level every shift until final feeding rate and concentration are established Record gastric residuals every 4 hours (gastric feedings only) Record bowel movements and consistency Record tolerance to feedings Record daily: Weight Intake and output Record weekly: • Serum electrolytes and blood counts Chemistry profile (including liver function tests, phosphorus, calcium, magnesium, total protein, and albumin) Nitrogen balance, if appropriate Reassess nutrition indexes weekly, adjusting energy and protein as needed

(Data from Moore, M.C. *Pocket guide to nutrition assessment and care*, ed 6, St. Louis, 2016, Mosby/Elsevier.)

GI problems include diarrhea, nausea and vomiting, cramping, distention, and constipation. In past efforts to check for aspirated contents, blue dye was added to enteral formulas. However, the dye contributed to several deaths, so it should no longer be used to check for aspiration (EAL, 2020).

Mechanical complications consist of tube displacement or obstruction, pulmonary aspiration, and mucosal damage. Metabolic difficulties involve hyperosmolar dehydration or overhydration; abnormal (too high or too low) blood concentration levels of sodium, potassium, phosphorus, and magnesium; hyperglycemia; respiratory insufficiency; and rapid weight gain. Table 12.5 summarizes possible complications of tube feeding, probable causes, and corrective actions.

Diarrhea, a common complication of enteral feedings, was once thought to be caused by the feeding solutions; however, other factors may contribute to this problem. Patients receiving tube feedings are often also started on liquid medications that contain sorbitol, which can cause diarrhea. Bacterial dysentery from *Clostridium difficile* is also a common cause of diarrhea. Diarrhea should not be attributed to tube-feeding formulas until other causes have been ruled out.

Home enteral nutrition. The demand for home tube feeding has been growing steadily. Although it provides opportunity and convenience for patients, home enteral nutrition (HEN) imparts responsibility on the patient or home caregiver and involves risks that must be anticipated. In addition to criteria already discussed, requirements that should be considered in the decision to send a patient home on EN include the following:

- Patient's nutritional needs cannot be met orally.
- Appropriate enteral access is in place and functioning, and patient is tolerating tube-feeding regimen.
- Patient and/or significant other are able and willing to perform HEN techniques safely and effectively.
- Underlying disease state is stable, and patient is ready for discharge and can be monitored in the home setting.
- Affordable HEN supplies are available.

Once a patient is considered an appropriate candidate for HEN, the nutrition care plan must be modified to an appropriate home plan that includes tailoring the enteral formula, route and method of administration, and feeding schedule. The amount or type of formula may need to be adjusted to meet the patient's long-term nutritional requirements.

Homemade, blenderized formulas are strongly discouraged because of reasons previously discussed. Feeding schedules may need to be arranged around family members' schedules or other daily routines. They should be planned to augment patient comfort and convenience and to maximize nutritional benefit.

The patient should be stabilized on the home feeding regimen while still hospitalized before patient education is initiated. Education should include oral instructions, written guidelines, staff demonstration, return demonstration by the patient and caregiver, and their assumption of full responsibility for tube feeding before the patients is discharged. Fig. 12.5 is a sample HEN training checklist.

Patients should also be referred to a source for obtaining supplies such as formula and administration equipment before discharge. Some patients may need help in obtaining financial assistance for purchase of supplies. Most often, referral to home health agencies provides the necessary supplies, equipment, and staff for home follow-up visits, as well as assistance with third-party payers.

Parenteral Nutrition

Fortunately, there are alternatives for providing nutrients to patients when they cannot or won't eat and tube feedings are contraindicated. Parenteral nutrition (PN) involves the provision of energy and nutrients intravenously. When nutrients are infused into a large-diameter vein, such as the superior vena cava or subclavian vein (Fig. 12.6), the method is called total parenteral nutrition (TPN) or central parenteral nutrition (CPN). When a smaller, peripheral vein is used (usually in the forearm), it is called peripheral parenteral nutrition (PPN).

TPN may mean the difference between life and death for patients who cannot be adequately nourished via the GI tract. Factors that should be considered before initiating TPN are the nature of the patient's GI dysfunction, severity of malnutrition, degree of hypercatabolism, medical prognosis, and patient wishes.

TABLE 12.5 **Tube-Feeding Complications and Management**

Complication	Cause	Prevention/treatment
Diarrhea	Too rapid increase in amount of feed per day	Observe adaptation phase
	Too rapid infusion rate	Reduce/control infusion rate
	Feed temperature too cold	Increase to room temperature
	Hyperosmolar feedings (>300 mOsm)	Use isotonic feeding solution, initially dilute hyperosmolar feeding solutions
	Lactose intolerance	Use low-lactose or lactose-free diet
	Fat malabsorption	Use low-fat or MCT-containing diet
	Hypoalbuminemia	Use chemically defined diet and/or feed
	Antibiotic therapy or medications	Review medications
	Chemotherapy/radiotherapy	Prescribe antidiarrheal medications
Nausea/vomiting	Too rapid infusion rate	Reduce/control infusion rate
	Bacterial contamination of formula feed/delivery equipment contamination	Handle administration systems hygienically, change delivery equipment every 24 hours, keep opened bottles of formula no more than 24 hours in refrigerator
Cramps/bloating	Too rapid infusion rate	Reduce/control infusion rate
	Lactose intolerance	Use low-lactose or lactose-free diet
	Fat malabsorption	Use low-fat or MCT-containing diet
Regurgitation/aspiration	Gastric retention	Reduce/control infusion rate, use duodenal tubes, incline patient during food administration
Constipation	Inadequate fluid intake	Increase fluid intake, check fluid balance
	Fiber intake too low	Use fiber-containing formulas
	Fecal impaction	Enemas
	Electrolyte and hormonal derangement	Osmotic laxatives (lactulose 15–60 mL),

MCT, Medium-chain triglycerides.
(Data from Blumenstein, I., et al. Gastroenteric tube feeding: Techniques, problems and solutions. *World J Gastroenterol* 20:8505–8524, 2014. From: https://www.ncbi.nlm.nih.gov/pmc/articles/PMC4093701/ (Accessed 26 August, 2020). https://stanfordhealthcare.org/medical-treatments/f/feeding-tube/complications.html, https://www.nursingtimes.net/clinical-archive/nutrition/peg-tubes-dealing-with-complications-31-10-2014/, https://www.myamericannurse.com/enteral-feeding-indications-complications-and-nursing-care/.)

Components of Parenteral Nutrition Solutions

PN solutions contain the same nutrients and components found in any EN source: water, amino acids, dextrose, electrolytes, vitamins, and trace elements. Fat is also included, often by means of piggyback administration or by adding it directly to the PN solution (called a three-in-one solution).

Carbohydrates. The most common carbohydrate used in PN is dextrose monohydrate. Used as an energy source, it yields 3.4 kcal/g because of its hydrated form. Dextrose solutions are available in initial concentrations of 5% through 70%. Higher glucose concentrations are useful when a patient's fluids need to be restricted; lower concentrations are often used to help control hyperglycemia. Concentrations greater than 10% (final concentration) are hypertonic and must be delivered via the larger central vein.

Amino acids. Protein is provided in PN solutions as a mixture of essential and nonessential crystalline amino acids that are available with or without added electrolytes. It is important that the amino acids be used for protein synthesis and not as an energy (kcal) source. Amino acid solutions are available in different concentrations as well as in various amino acid compositions.

Fats. Intravenous (IV) lipid emulsions are used as concentrated energy sources and to prevent development of an essential fatty acid (EFA) deficiency. Commercial lipid emulsions are formulations of safflower oil, soybean oil, or a combination of the two, with glycerol added for isotonicity and egg phospholipid added as an emulsifying agent. Some newer formulas also add olive oil, or fish oil as a source of omega-3 fatty acids. The kcal density of lipid solutions is useful when volume restriction is necessary. A 10% fat emulsion yields 1.1 kcal/mL or 550 kcal per 500-mL bottle, and a 20% solution yields 2 kcal/mL or 1000 kcal per 500-mL bottle. Use of lipids increases calories without increasing osmolality as much.

Traditionally, lipid emulsions have been delivered peripherally with a piggyback system. Baseline serum triglyceride levels should be confirmed before administration of IV lipid emulsions and should be monitored according to institutional policy. If a lipid profile is ordered for a patient receiving lipids, the patient should not have received lipid emulsion for the 12 hours before the blood specimen is drawn.

Total nutrient admixtures. When lipid emulsions are added to dextrose and amino acid mixtures, the resulting solution is called a three-in-one mixture, or a total nutrient admixture (TNA) (Fig. 12.7). Such solutions allow lipid infusion over 24 hours, decreasing carbon dioxide production and reducing hepatic accumulation of fat.

Electrolytes. Electrolytes and minerals can be provided by the general amino acid solution or as a combined electrolyte concentrate, or they can be added separately as individual salts. Commercial electrolyte solutions are available. Magnesium,

PURPOSE AND INSTRUCTIONS: This checklist will assist in identifying instructional responsibilities and aid in training patients in the skills needed for performing home enteral nutrition (HEN).

The nurse and dietitian will jointly instruct the patient on tube feeding administration and care.

Date and initial section when instruction/demonstration is completed.

RNs: Document training in Nursing Notes.

RDs: Document training in Progress Notes.

STAGE I: INITIATION OF HEN PROGRAM

_____ Patient assessment (Dietitian-Nurse)
Medical-social-nutritional history
_____ Plan of care outlined (Dietitian-Nurse)
_____ Identification of dismissal date _____ (Nurse)
_____ Home enteral coordinator notified (Dietitian)

STAGE II: IMPLEMENTATION OF HEN TRAINING (Dietitian)

INTRODUCTION TO HEN PROGRAM (Dietitian)

_____ Discuss purpose
_____ Introduce manual *Instructions for Tube Feeding at Home*

EQUIPMENT (Dietitian-Nurse)

Discuss purpose, assembly, use, care, and cleaning of equipment.

	Discuss	Demonstrate	Patient Demonstrate
Feeding tube	_____	_____	_____
Feeding bag	_____	_____	_____
Gavage syringe	_____	_____	_____
Enteral pump (if needed)	_____	_____	_____

FORMULA—FLUIDS (Dietitian)

_____ Show formula.
_____ Discuss purpose, type, amount, formula concentrations, fluid needs.
_____ Discuss preparation.
_____ Discuss administration schedule.
_____ Discuss weight expectations.

Fig. 12.5 Home enteral training checklist. (From Nelson, J.K., Weckworth, J.A. Home enteral nutrition. In Skipper, A., editor: *Dietitian's handbook of enteral and parenteral nutrition*, Rockville, MD, 1989, Aspen.)

phosphate, and potassium requirements must be monitored carefully to prevent overfeeding and underfeeding of malnourished individuals.

Trace elements. Trace element formulations contain zinc, copper, manganese, chromium, and selenium. Already combined commercial solutions may be used, or an institutional pharmacy may develop its own IV injectable formula.

Vitamins. Adult and pediatric multivitamin formulations for IV use are commercially available. In clear vitamin deficiency, multiples of daily doses can be given in accordance with clinical status.

Bioactive substances. Evidence suggests that additives such as prebiotics or probiotics, antioxidants, and glutamine may benefit certain patients. An individual assessment must be done.

Peripheral Parenteral Nutrition

PPN solutions composed of more than 10% (final concentration) dextrose and/or more than 5% (final concentration) amino acids are hypertonic and can be administered only into central veins. These solutions administered via peripheral veins must be isotonic to prevent damage to the veins. Isotonic PN solutions usually contain 5% to 10% dextrose (final concentration) and 3% to 5% amino acids, plus electrolytes, vitamins, minerals, and fat as needed. PPN is most often used when only short-term nutrition support is needed.

Monitoring Guidelines and Complications

Monitoring needs and protocols vary among institutions and patient populations. Frequency of monitoring ranges from every 6 hours to a one-time baseline reading, from biweekly

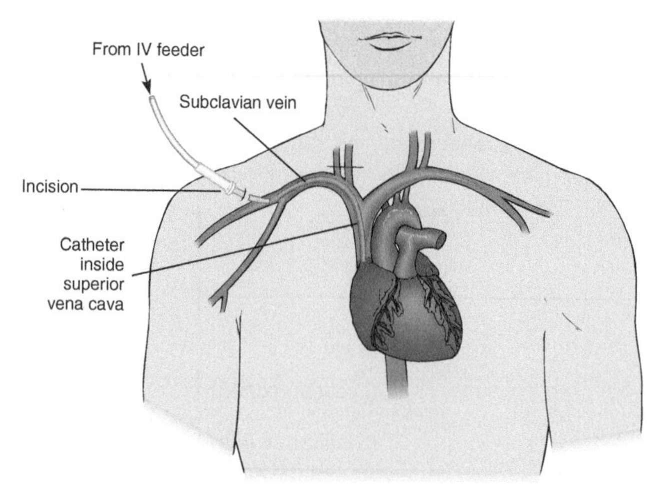

Fig. 12.6 Placement of catheter for central parenteral nutrition, via the subclavian vein to the superior vena cava. *IV*, Intravenous. (From Rolin Graphics.)

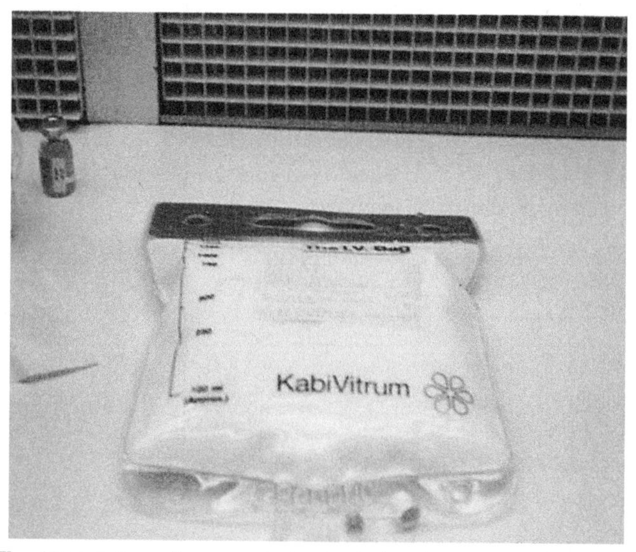

Fig. 12.7 A three-in-one solution includes dextrose, amino acids, and lipids. (From Morgan, S.L., Weinsier, R.L. *Fundamentals of clinical nutrition*, ed 2, St. Louis, 1998, Mosby.)

to "as needed." Specific parameters and recommendations are listed in Box 12.2.

As with enteral tube feedings, complications can occur with PN. Most can be averted by following the monitoring recommendations. Others can be circumvented by adhering to stringent technique. Technical complications are related to catheter placement; pneumothorax can be prevented by careful insertion of the central line using proper technique. Septic complications, like technical complications, are not unique to parenteral nutrition. Infections can be local or systemic, and they usually occur because of poor technique in aseptic catheter care.

Metabolic complications are common because metabolic requirements (electrolytes and energy) differ from patient to patient. Hyperglycemia is common and can be treated by administering insulin or by adding it to the solution, reducing the dextrose load, or ensuring that the total calorie load is not excessive. Box 12.3 summarizes possible complications.

BOX 12.2 Nurses' Guide for Monitoring Patients on Total Parenteral Nutrition

Factor	Rationale
Monitor vital signs, observing for signs of infection such as elevated temperature.	Bacteria may grow in high-glucose and high-protein solutions.
Use strict aseptic technique with IV tubing, dressing changes, and TPN solution, and refrigerate solution until 30 minutes before using.	Infusion site is at high risk for development of infection.
Monitor blood glucose levels. Observe for signs of hyperglycemia or hypoglycemia and administer insulin as directed.	Blood glucose levels may be affected if TPN is turned off, if the rate is reduced, or if excess levels of insulin are added to the solution.
Monitor for signs of fluid overload.	TPN is a hypertonic solution and can create intravascular shifting of extracellular fluid.
Monitor renal status. Document intake and output ratio, daily weights.	Report unexpected changes. Laboratory studies such as serum creatinine and BUN are used to assess renal function.
Maintain accurate infusion rate with infusion pump, make rate changes gradually, and never discontinue TPN abruptly.	Abrupt discontinuation may cause hypoglycemia, and a sudden change in flow rate can cause fluctuations in blood glucose levels.

BUN, Blood urea nitrogen; *IV*, intravenous; *TPN*, total parental nutrition.
(Data from: Banusanm J.B. *Nursing care for patients receiving total parenteral nutrition (TPN)*. From: https://www.rn101.net/single-post/2018/03/03/Nursing-Care-For-Patients-Receiving-Total-Parenteral-Nutrition-TPN. (Accessed 26 August, 2020).)

Home Parenteral Nutrition

Home parenteral nutrition (HPN) enables selected patients who depend on PN to return to a reasonably normal lifestyle. A specialized catheter is used to reduce possibility of infection. The catheter is placed through a tunnel under the skin and exits the chest at a place where the patient or caretaker can care for it conveniently. As with HEN, HPN requires that both patient and caregiver are willing and able to perform daily procedures involved in administering the PN, which include monitoring laboratory values, temperature, weights, glucose measurements, and fluids. Home health care agencies may be used to provide equipment, supplies, and services.

Patients may be scheduled to receive HPN at night during sleep (cyclic CPN) to allow freedom to leave home or even work during the day. Sometimes, if the GI tract is functional, HPN is administered only on selected nights per week to supplement oral intake. Although expensive, HPN costs less than hospitalization, allows the patient to leave the hospital sooner, and in many cases allows the patient to resume a productive lifestyle.

Transitional Feedings

A period of adjustment, or weaning, is necessary before discontinuation of nutritional support or for conversion from

BOX 12.3 Complications of Parenteral Nutrition

Mechanical/Technical Complications

Subclavian artery puncture, carotid artery puncture, or catheter obstruction

Improper initial placement of a central venous catheter can lead to pneumothorax, vascular injury with hemothorax, brachial plexus injury or cardiac arrhythmia.

Venous thrombosis can occur after central venous access is established. Signs include distended neck veins and swelling of the face and ipsilateral arm. The risk of venous thrombosis is greater with dehydration, certain malignancies, prolonged bed rest, venous stasis, sepsis, hypercoagulation, morbid obesity, history of smoking or ongoing estrogen therapy.

Septic Complications

Catheter-related sepsis or septic thrombosis

Metabolic complications

Early complications	Late complications
Volume overload	Essential fatty acid deficiency
Hyperglycemia	Trace mineral deficiency
Refeeding syndrome	Vitamin deficiency
Hypokalemia	Metabolic bone disease
Hypophosphatemia	Hepatic steatosis
Hypomagnesemia	Hepatic cholestasis
Hyperchloremic acidosis	

(Data from *Complications of TPN*. From: http://www.rxkinetics.com/tpntutorial/3_3.html. (Accessed 26 August, 2020).)

one form of nutritional support to another. Transition to an adequate oral intake to maintain nutritional status differs from patient to patient. Although the GI tract responds quickly to enteral feeding, patients who have been receiving TPN usually have decreased appetites and it may take 1 to 2 weeks after complete cessation of TPN for them to feel hungry. This early satiety necessitates gradual weaning from PN as oral or tube feeding progresses to ensure continued adequate intake. Moreover, stopping TPN too quickly can result in hypoglycemia.

Parenteral Nutrition to Oral or Tube Feeding

Long periods of PN without enteral feedings result in atrophy of the GI tract. If not contraindicated, minimal enteral intake (sips of diluted fruit juice) helps maintain normal GI tract physiology and gut mucosal immunity. Before weaning from TPN, judicious assessment of GI function is recommended to prevent problems with delayed gastric emptying, nausea, vomiting, or diarrhea. As TPN is tapered and oral or tube-feeding intake increases, it is important to document actual enteral intake, including fluids, to facilitate nutrient sufficiency. If oral feedings or isotonic formulas are not well tolerated, an elemental formula may be needed.

Tube Feeding to Oral Feeding

In addition to documentation of intake per tube and orally, it will be important to assess the patient's swallowing ability before offering oral feedings. A full liquid diet is usually offered first, followed by pureed or soft foods. Tube feedings should be stopped at least 1 hour before and after mealtime to promote appetite. As oral intake increases, tube-feeding volume should be decreased. When oral intake consistently exceeds two-thirds of energy requirements, the tube feedings can be discontinued.

SUMMARY

- All patient nutrition is provided through food service delivery systems of acute care hospitals and long-term care facilities.
- Foodservice staff includes a director of the food and nutrition services department, clinical dietitians, as well as cooks, clerks, dishwashers, aides, and dietetic technicians, registered.
- To provide nutritional therapy, regular or modified diets are developed to meet specific needs of patients as determined by the physician or registered dietitian.
- Qualitative diet changes include modifications in consistency, texture, or nutrients.
- Quantitative diet changes include modifications in size and number of meals served or amounts of specific nutrients.
- Incidents related to food allergy or food poisoning require appropriate interventions to address those incidents while promoting rapid recovery and a continuation of the healing process.
- Traditional complementary and alternative medicine (TCAM) is a significant component of health care in the United States.
- TCAM consists of a cluster of medical and health care approaches, methods, and items not associated with conventional medicine.
- Complementary medicine refers to nonWestern healing approaches used at the same time as conventional medicine.
- Alternative medicine practices replace conventional medical treatment.
- Integrative medicine merges conventional medical therapies with TCAM modalities for which safety and efficacy have been demonstrated by scientific data.
- Use of herbs as dietary supplements or as natural medications can interact with bioavailability of foods, nutrients, and drugs.
- Dietary supplements are substances consumed orally as an addition to dietary intake.
- The Dietary Supplement Health and Education Act of 1994 regulates supplement identity, potency, contents, and labeling under the supervision of the U.S. Food and Drug Administration.
- Supplement use has grown substantially; some may interact with other medications and treatments.

- Oral and tube feedings are the preferred methods of nutritional intake because the gastrointestinal (GI) tract maintains its integrity.
- Feeding patients via the GI tract is safer and easier to administer, aids in maintaining GI tract integrity, and is much less expensive than parenteral nutrition (PN).
- Commercial tube-feeding products supply intact nutrients and are readily available.
- When tube feedings are administered in the appropriate volume, 100% of the daily requirements for vitamins and minerals can be provided, as well as adequate amounts of energy and protein.
- When patients are unable to obtain nutrition by oral or tube feeding, parenteral nutrition can literally be lifesaving.
- Peripheral or central infusions of amino acids, dextrose, fat emulsions, vitamins, and minerals can provide the ordinary or extraordinary nutrient needs of patients.
- When managed through a team approach and routine monitoring, PN can provide a safe vehicle for meeting patients' nutritional goals.
- By working together, nurses and dietetic professionals can efficiently meet the nutritional and medical needs of patients.

THE NURSING APPROACH

Clinical Judgment and Next-Generation NCLEX® Examination-Style Questions

Case Study 1

Empathy and Dietary Teaching: Experiencing Modified Diets

An effective way for nursing students to learn about medical nutrition is to research modified dietary pattern guidelines and resources for specific disorders and conditions and then experience these diets personally. Following a modified diet even for 1 day gives students empathy with patients who need to change their regular eating habits and adhere to special dietary intakes. This dietary experience also supplies nursing students with strategies to reinforce teaching by dietitians.

Purposes of the Experience

- Experience a modified diet (for health promotion or nutrition therapy) for 1 day (24 hours).
- Identify components or principles of the diet and the specific foods allowed or restricted.
- Gain empathy for patients who are beginning nutrition therapy for disorders or conditions and need to adhere to modified dietary patterns.
- Reflect on teaching ideas for use with patients.

Choose One Diet and Follow It for a 24-Hour Period or Longer

- High fiber and adequate liquid (for diverticulosis)
- Gluten-free (for celiac disease)
- Carbohydrate counting (for diabetes)
- Dietary Approaches to Stop Hypertension (DASH) diet (for hypertension)

Answer These Questions

1. List three health problems that may make this diet modification necessary or desirable.
2. What general guidelines were followed?
   a. What types of food were consumed?
      i. Food groups and temperature of foods; textures, such as solid, pureed, or liquid.
      ii. Examples of foods.
   b. What amounts of food were consumed? Number of calories or specific measurements.
   c. At what time of day were foods consumed? Create a food diary. Include times and types of meals (e.g., breakfast, 7 AM).
   d. What foods/beverages were avoided or restricted?
      i. What foods/beverages were avoided or restricted? List specific foods/beverages.
      ii. Rationale.
3. What resources besides this textbook were used to learn about the diet? Were any Internet sites especially useful?
4. What was your experience?
   a. How did you feel physically and/or emotionally?
   b. What did you learn by paying attention to food labels?
   c. What surprised you the most about this diet?
   d. What foods were challenging to include or eliminate?
   e. What were other personal barriers that made following this diet difficult?
5. Are there special dietary products that may help people with this diet?
   a. Are special products needed? Why?
   b. What products (helpful or not) are available?
   c. Which of these products would you buy if on this diet for a month?
6. What are the pros and cons of this diet?
   a. Benefits
   b. Disadvantages and/or risks
7. What aspect of this experience gave you empathy for a patient who is following this diet?
   a. What dietary guidelines would be especially difficult if you followed this diet for 1 month? Why (e.g., cost, not wanting to be different from peers)?
   b. Was it necessary to learn a large amount of new information? Explain the steps taken to gain this information.
   c. Would it be difficult to follow this diet indefinitely? Discuss.
8. How would you teach a patient about this diet?
   a. What would you do to promote understanding of this diet (which foods and why)?
   b. What patient education materials would assist a patient to make wise food choices?
   c. What would be a reasonable goal that a patient could successfully achieve by the end of the first week?
   d. What would you recommend as the first step a patient should take when beginning this dietary pattern?

Continued

THE NURSING APPROACH—cont'd

Case Study 2
Safe Administration of Enteral Tube Feedings
Place an X in the boxes of correct guidelines for the safe administration of enteral tube feedings.

1. Confirm tube placement before initiating feeding and before each intermittent feeding
2. Record urine glucose level daily until final feeding rate and concentration are established
3. Record gastric residuals every 6 hours (gastric feedings only)
4. Record bowel movements and consistency
5. Record tolerance to feedings after every feeding
6. Record daily:
   Intake and output
7. Record daily:
   Serum electrolytes and blood counts
8. Reassess nutrition indexes every 2–3 days, adjusting energy and protein as needed
9. Record weekly:
   Weight
10. Record weekly:
    Chemistry profile (including liver function tests, phosphorus, calcium, magnesium, total protein, and albumin)
    Nitrogen balance, if appropriate

Data fom Moore MC: *Pocket guide to nutrition assessment and care*, ed 6, St. Louis, 2016, Mosby/Elsevier.)

CRITICAL THINKING

Clinical Applications

Faye, a 20-year-old student from Germany, seeks medical attention at the urging of her roommates, who report that her mood has become increasingly depressed during the past two semesters. She has become withdrawn and moody—a significant change from her affect since first coming to the United States to attend college. She is otherwise healthy. Faye reports a 5-pound weight loss during the past 3 months. She takes oral contraceptives for regulation of menses. Her mother has been treated for depression with *Hypericum perforatum* (St. John's wort) by the family physician for the past 10 years. Faye reports smoking a pack of cigarettes per day. Plans are to treat her with 50 mg sertraline (Zoloft) per day and to provide counseling therapy. During the diet history, the dietitian asks Faye whether she uses any over-the-counter vitamins, minerals, or herbal supplements. She tells the dietitian that her mother suggested she try St. John's wort, because in Germany it is prescribed to treat depression. Faye did as her mother suggested because it is available without prescription in the United States.

1. Faye's depression will be treated with sertraline, a selective serotonin reuptake inhibitor (SSRI). How do SSRIs work?
2. What is St. John's wort?
3. How is St. John's wort used in the United States? How is it regulated?
4. How does St. John's wort work as an antidepressant?
5. Does St. John's wort have any side effects?
6. How is St. John's wort used in Europe?
7. Why do you think people are interested in alternative medicine and herbal treatments?
8. What is your immediate concern regarding Faye's use of St. John's wort?

CRITICAL THINKING

Clinical Applications

Advances in medical technology have provided mechanisms to feed or nourish patients who once could not otherwise be fed or nourished. However, like most medical advances, the advances also engender dilemmas and difficult decisions about patient care. Nutrition care dilemmas occur when this technology will keep the patient alive even though the patient has no hope of ever living a normal life. What happens if a person loses decision-making capacity? Who should decide? What should be decided? Who should the surrogate be? What should that person do?

In a perfect world, the person should be someone designated by the patient while the patient still has decision-making capacity (durable power of attorney for health care). In the world we live in, when a patient does not have the capacity to make decisions or has not made an advanced directive, some family member without legal authority has to make decisions about life and death matters, often in a time of crisis. And what happens if family members of the patient do not agree on what should be done? Often, the dilemma requires legal action for resolution.

Such was the situation in the case of 41-year-old Terri Schiavo. Schiavo collapsed at home and experienced several minutes of oxygen deprivation to the brain in 1990, leaving her in a persistent vegetative state (PVS). In 1993 her husband decided to withdraw artificial nutrition, hydration, and life support on the grounds that she would not want to be kept alive this way. Her mother and father, the Schindlers, disagreed, and a controversy began in 1993 that lasted more than 12 years, going back and forth to court. What made the Schiavo case different from its predecessors (those of Karen Ann Quinlan of New Jersey and Nancy Cruzan of Missouri) was the involvement of Jeb Bush, then governor of Florida; the Florida state legislature; U.S. Congress; and 19 judges in six courts, including the Florida Supreme Court and federal courts. The courts continually sided with Terri's husband, whereas Bush and the Florida legislature sided with the Schindlers. Her feeding tube was removed on March 18, 2005, and Terri Schiavo died 13 days later. What are your thoughts about the following circumstances?

- An 85-year-old man, who suffers from many physical problems but is not terminally ill, refuses to be tube fed.
- A 57-year-old woman is hospitalized as a result of a severe psychiatric disorder that prohibits her from speaking or eating. She is bedridden in a fetal position and has a gastrostomy tube. She repeatedly dislodges the feeding tube and is combative when it is replaced.
- A 75-year-old woman's husband has requested termination of her nasogastric feedings. She is brain dead and has no living will.

WEBSITES OF INTEREST

Academy of Nutrition and Dietetics
https://www.eatrightpro.org/
Tips for managing diets, educating patients, working with dietitians.

American Botanical Council
www.herbalgram.org
Information and research findings to encourage appropriate use of phytomedicines and medicinal plants.

American Society of Parenteral and Enteral Nutrition (ASPEN)
www.nutritioncare.org
Dedicated to making sure patients receive the most appropriate nutritional therapy. Interactive features on the site allow users to post questions, register for conferences, and view links to other related organizations.

Dietary Guidelines for Americans
https://health.gov/our-work/food-nutrition/about-dietary-guidelines
U.S. Department of Health and Human Services and U.S. Department of Agriculture provide multiple resources for teaching the guidelines.

Food and Drug Administration—Nutrition Facts Label
https://www.fda.gov/food/ingredientspackaginglabeling/labelingnutrition/ucm274593.htm
This website provides information about the Nutrition Facts label, especially as the science of nutrition evolves and as packaging rules change.

Food Safety
https://www.foodsafety.gov
Tips for keeping food safe while preparing or serving food. The site also provides charts for the four simple steps of food safety—clean, separate, cook, and chill.

National Center for Complementary and Alternative Medicine (NCCAM)
www.nccam.nih.gov
Promotes scientific research on complementary and alternative medicine (CAM) and distributes information to the public and health professionals on the efficacy of CAM modalities.

REFERENCES

Academy of Nutrition and Dietetics, Evidence Analysis Library: *Critical illness nutrition practice recommendations.* From: www.adaevidencelibrary.com. (Accessed 26 August, 2020).

Center for Food Safety and Applied Nutrition, Office of Nutritional Products, Labeling, and Dietary Supplements, Food and Drug Administration: *Dietary supplement labeling,* College Park, MD, Author. From: www.fda.gov/Food/DietarySupplements/default.htm. (Accessed 26 August, 2020).

Foley, H., & Steel, A. (2017). The nexus between patient-centered care and complementary medicine: Allies in the era of chronic disease? *Journal of Alternative and Complementary Medicine, 23* (3), 158–163.

Food and Drug Administration (FDA): *Food Safety Modernization Act.* From: https://www.fda.gov/food/guidance-regulation-food-and-dietary-supplements/food-safety-modernization-act-fsma. (Accessed 25 August, 2020).

Hassanein, M., et al. (2017). Diabetes and Ramadan: practical guidelines. *Diabetes Research and Clinical Practice, 126,* 303–316.

Ho, M. H., et al. (2014). Clinical spectrum of food allergies: a comprehensive review. *Clinical Reviews in Allergy & Immunology, 46,* 225–240.

IDDSI. International Dysphagia Diet Standardization Initiative: A global initiative to improve the lives of over 590 million people worldwide living with dysphagia. From: https://iddsi.org/. (Accessed 25 August, 2020).

IFIC. International Food Information Council: *A Useful Guide to Understanding GMOs.* From: https://foodinsight.org/a-useful-guide-to-understanding-gmos/. (Accessed 26 August, 2020).

Lepore, J. R., et al. (2014). Acceptability and identification of scooped versus molded puréed foods. *Canadian Journal Of Dietetic Practice, 75,* 145–147.

Live Science: *GMOs: Facts About Genetically Modified Food,* 2019. From https://www.livescience.com/40895-gmo-facts.html. (Accessed 26 August, 2020).

McCray, S., et al. (2018). Room service improves nutritional intake and increases patient satisfaction while decreasing food waste and cost. *Journal of the Academy of Nutrition and Dietetics, 118,* 284–293.

Melina, V., et al. (2016). Position of the academy of nutrition and dietetics: Vegetarian diets. *Journal of the Academy of Nutrition and Dietetics, 116,* 1970–1980.

National Center for Complementary and Alternative Medicine (NCCAM): *What's in a name?* (Publication No. D347). From: http://nccam.nih.gov/health/whatiscam. (Accessed 25 August, 2020).

Nguyen, D. L., et al. (2016). Low-residue versus clear liquid diet before colonoscopy: A meta-analysis of randomized, controlled trials. *Gastrointestinal Endoscopy, 83,* 499–507.

Prescott, S. L., & Logan, A. C. (2019). Planetary Health: From the wellspring of holistic medicine to personal and public health imperative. *Explore (NY), 15,* 98–106.

Rattray, M., et al. (2017). A systematic review of feeding practices among postoperative patients: Is practice in-line with evidenced-based guidelines? *Journal of Human Nutrition and Dietetics, 31,* 151–167.

Sobiecki, J. G., et al. (2016). High compliance with dietary recommendations in a cohort of meat eaters, fish eaters, vegetarians, and vegans: results from the European Prospective Investigation into Cancer and Nutrition-Oxford study. *Nut Res, 36*(5), 464–477.

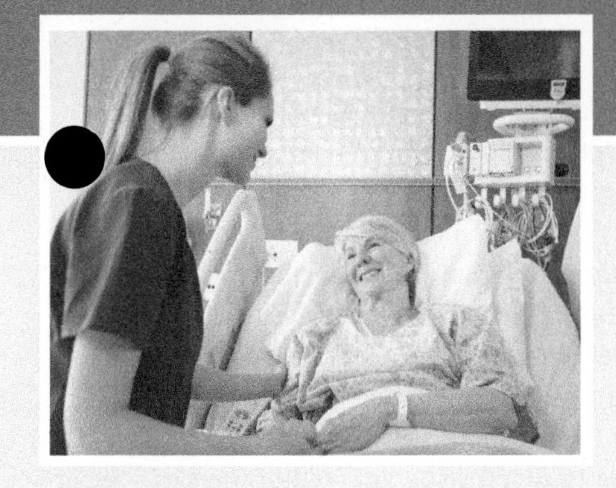

13

Nutrition for Disorders of the Gastrointestinal Tract

The ability to chew, swallow, digest, and absorb nutrients, while passing fiber and other substances on for elimination, may be compromised by disorders of the gastrointestinal (GI) tract. Almost everyone experiences intermittent GI complaints from time to time. Indigestion, gas, bloating, nausea, abdominal pain or cramping, diarrhea, and esophageal reflux are some of the symptoms occasionally experienced by healthy people.

http://evolve.elsevier.com/GRODNER/FOUNDATIONS

LEARNING OBJECTIVES

- List the organs affected by disorders of the gastrointestinal (GI) tract.
- Describe disorders that affect the flow of sustenance through the GI tract.
- Discuss the microbiome and identify pros and cons of using prebiotic or probiotic foods.
- Identify how and why certain disorders cause site-specific tissue inflammation.
- Compare and contrast disorders caused by the inability to produce digestive enzymes and those caused by the inability to metabolize substances.
- Explain how inflammatory bowel disorders have autoimmune properties.
- Discuss individualized nutrition therapy for GI disorders.

DIMENSIONS OF GI HEALTH

Consider the six dimensions of health. Physical health is most affected when a gastrointestinal (GI) disorder is chronic and intensive. Eventually, weight loss and nutrient deficiencies pose health risks in addition to the primary disorder. Intellectual health is tested as the patient tries to find food combinations and textures that are aesthetically pleasing. Some disorders require constant vigilance to restrict inadvertent consumption of problematic foods (e.g., gluten in celiac disease). Emotional health is taxed when patients struggle with acceptance of their dietary or physical limitations. Poorly managed symptoms diminish psychological well-being and overall quality of life. Social health strategies are needed to help patients handle the personal ramifications of colostomies, dumping syndrome, and other disorders. Spiritual health can be enhanced through yoga and meditation, which are tied to mind and body wellness. For those with GI disorders that may cause unexpected need for access to a bathroom, the environmental health dimension of facilities at home, at work, during a commute, or when traveling may alter one's sense of wellness.

COMMON DIGESTIVE DISORDERS

Many GI disorders have significant nutritional implications where diet is the cornerstone of therapy. Evaluation of a patient's GI symptoms requires a team effort to separate symptoms associated with dietary practices from those associated with disease or dysfunction. The registered dietitian can identify unusual dietary practices, nutritional inadequacies, or food intolerances through an in-depth diet history assessment.

The simple act of eating an apple may no longer be easy for individuals with disorders of the GI tract. The ability to chew, swallow, digest, and absorb nutrients, while passing along fiber and other substances for elimination, may be compromised (Fig. 13.1). GI disorders affect the availability of nutrients to all other organs and body systems, thereby influencing overall health.

THE MICROBIOME, PREBIOTICS, AND PROBIOTICS

The human GI tract has a complex ecosystem (the microbiome) colonized by more than 10 trillion microorganisms (Mills et al., 2019). The first 1000 days of life is an important time when the neonate acquires either a healthy microbiome, or one that is lacking in diversity. Caesarean birth versus vaginal delivery, formula feeding versus breast milk, early introduction of complementary foods or cow's milk – any of these factors can negatively alter the infant's microbiome.

All throughout life, healthy interactions between gut microbes and their host are needed to maintain homeostasis. These

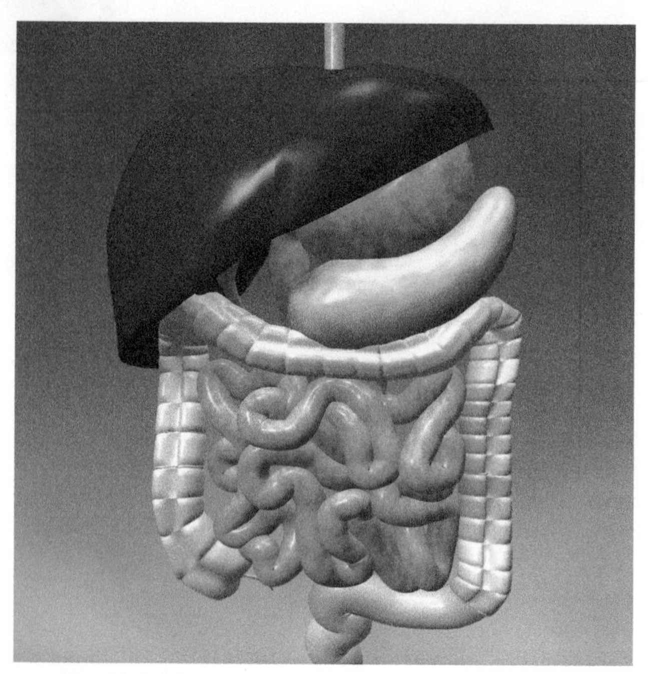

Fig. 13.1 Major organs of the gastrointestinal tract.

microbes may contribute to low-grade inflammation through gut barrier dysfunctions that affect the crosstalk between the brain, muscles, liver, brain, and even adipose tissue (Geurts et al., 2014) Changes in microbiome structure lead to dysbiosis. With advancing chronological age, the gut microbiota decreases in richness; dysbiosis can trigger an innate immune response and chronic low-grade inflammation, leading to many age-related degenerative pathologies and unhealthy aging (Kim & Jazwinski, 2018).

Prebiotics are a special form of dietary fiber that acts as a fertilizer for the healthy gut bacteria. Examples include raw asparagus or onions and garlic, jicama, Jerusalem artichokes (sunchokes), honey, slightly unripe bananas, and raw dandelion greens. Probiotics are live bacteria found in yogurt, kefir, aged cheeses, kimchi, miso soup, sauerkraut, tempeh, and sweet acidophilus milk. The use of prebiotic and probiotic therapy shows great promise for many of the disorders described in this chapter.

ANTIINFLAMMATORY DIETS

Because of the health benefits of a diet that reduces inflammation, all members of the health team can promote its features. Two diets have the most evidence for their protective qualities: the traditional Mediterranean diet and the DASH (Dietary Approaches to Stop Hypertension) diet. Both encourage the use of antioxidant foods rich in carotenes, vitamins C and E, and selenium. People are calling these superfoods: avocado, blueberries, cherries, green tea, coffee, dark chocolate and cocoa powder, whole grains, strawberries, raspberries, cloves, ginger, turmeric, mint, cinnamon, beans and legumes, pecans and other nuts, seeds, artichokes, mango, cranberries, chili peppers, watermelon, and so on.

Foods rich in zinc, copper, iron, and manganese protect against free radical damage from pollution, radiation, burned food, or excessive sunlight. Omega-3 fatty acids (specifically docosahexaenoic acid [DHA] and eicosatetraenoic acid [EPA]) are antiinflammatory and are found in salmon, tuna, mackerel, sardines.

Extra-virgin olive oil (EVOO) is a special food with multiple plant chemicals (phytochemicals) that reduce inflammation. EVOO is a fundamental food in the world's healthiest diet—the Mediterranean diet! The Mediterranean diet encourages EVOO, fruits, vegetables, whole grains, legumes, herbs, and spices. It recommends lean proteins from fish and poultry and red wine in moderate amounts. Note that red wine and red grape skins are rich sources of resveratrol, a phytochemical that may lower blood pressure, decrease low-density lipoprotein cholesterol, protect the brain, even increase insulin sensitivity.

The DASH diet is a dietary pattern promoted by the National Heart, Lung, and Blood Institute to prevent and control hypertension. Like the Mediterranean plan, it promotes an abundance of fruits and vegetables, whole grains, and fiber-rich foods. Low-fat dairy products are included, and the plan normalizes the ratio of sodium to potassium, magnesium, and calcium. This diet is useful for weight management, cardiac patients, and general healthy eating.

ESOPHAGEAL DISORDERS

Dysphagia

Swallowing is often an involuntary activity that is not contemplated, just like breathing or the beating of a heart. Swallowing takes place in three stages: oral preparation and transit, pharyngeal transit, and esophageal transit (Fig. 13.2). A disorder affecting any of these stages may require specific nutrition interventions. For patients with chewing or swallowing difficulties, diets must meet individual nutritional needs while preventing aspiration. Box 13.1 lists some conditions that may cause dysphagia.

Proper diagnosis and treatment of oral-pharyngeal dysphagia involve a multidisciplinary health care team effort; it starts with systematic screening of at-risk patients (McGinnis et al., 2019). There is a 10-item swallowing screening tool, the Eating Assessment Tool (EAT-10) from the Nestlé Nutrition Institute, available at https://www.nestlehealthscience.com/health-management/gastro-intestinal/dysphagia/eat-10. Above all, remember that the onset of dysphagia can be frightening for both patients and family members. See the *Personal Perspectives* box The Pain of Parkinson's Disease.

Food and Nutrition Therapies

Systematic screening for dysphagia and resulting malnutrition among at-risk older adults is important. Nurses often witness the following warning signs that suggest swallowing problems (Mayo Clinic, 2020):

Pain while swallowing (odynophagia)
Inability to swallow
Sensation of food getting stuck in the throat or chest
Drooling
Hoarseness
Bringing food back up (regurgitation)

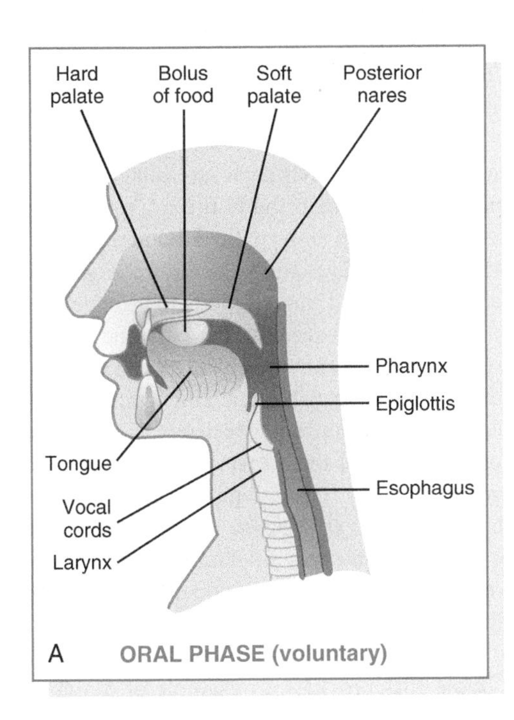

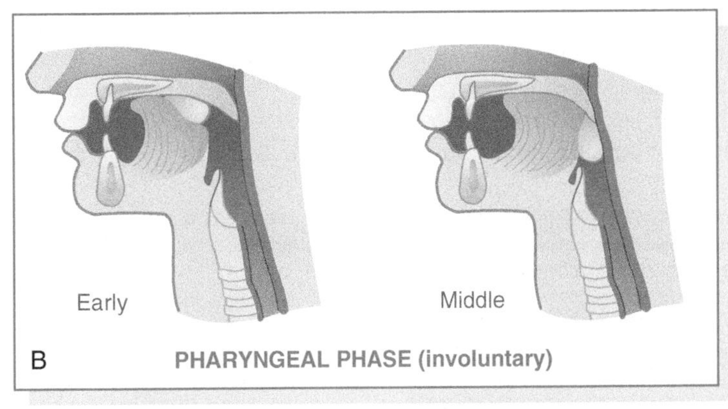

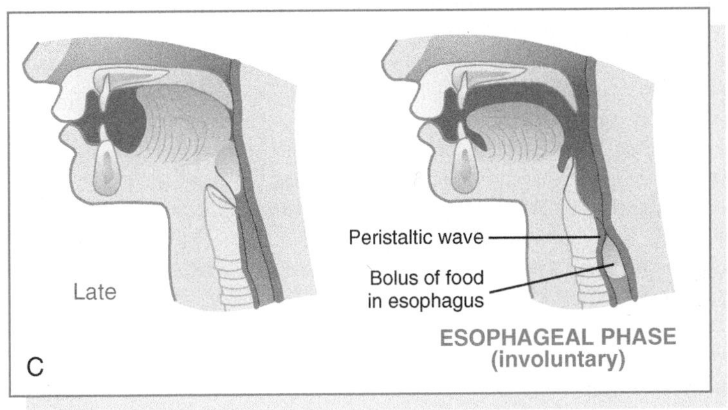

Fig. 13.2 Swallowing occurs in three phases: (A) Voluntary or oral phase. The tongue presses food against the hard palate, forcing it toward the pharynx. (B) Involuntary, pharyngeal phase. Early: wave of peristalsis forces a bolus between the tonsillar pillars. Middle: soft palate draws upward to close posterior nares and respirations cease momentarily. Late: vocal cords approximate and the larynx pulls upward, covering the airway and stretching the esophagus open. (C) Involuntary, esophageal phase. Relaxation of the upper esophageal (hypopharyngeal) sphincter allows the peristaltic wave to move the bolus down the esophagus. (From Mahan LK, Raymond KL: *Krause's food & nutrition therapy*, ed 14, Philadelphia, 2016, Elsevier.)

BOX 13.1 Conditions That May Cause Dysphagia

Achalasia
Acute cervical spinal cord injury
Alzheimer's disease and dementia
Amyloidosis
Amyotrophic lateral sclerosis (ALS, Lou Gehrig's disease)
Anoxia
Botulism
Cerebrovascular accident (CVA)/stroke
Chagas disease
Diabetes, type 1 (long term)
Esophageal cancer
Esophageal varices
Gastroesophageal reflux (GERD)
Gastroparesis
Goiter
Guillain-Barré syndrome
Head and/or neck cancer, including brainstem tumors
Head injury
Human immunodeficiency virus (HIV) infection
Huntington's disease
Inflammatory masses
Intrinsic and extrinsic structural lesions
Lung inflammation, including chronic obstructive pulmonary disease (COPD), with excessive secretions
Multiple sclerosis (MS)
Multiple system atrophy (MSA)
Muscular dystrophies (MDs)
Myasthenia gravis
Parkinson's disease
Poliomyelitis
Postintubation trauma
Presbyphagia (swallowing difficulty of old age)
Scleroderma
Stricture or inflammation of pharynx or esophagus
Tumor or obstruction of throat

(Data from Academy of Nutrition and Dietetics: *Nutrition care manual*, Chicago, Author. From https://www.nutritioncaremanual.org/auth.cfm. (Accessed 26 August, 2020).)

Frequent heartburn
Food or stomach acid backing up into the throat
Unplanned weight loss
Coughing or gagging when swallowing
Avoidance of certain foods because of trouble swallowing

PERSONAL PERSPECTIVES

The Pain of Parkinson's Disease

When Don Kaemmer met his soon-to-be second wife, Yetta, he was a physically active 70-year-old widower. A few years after they wed, he was diagnosed with a quickly advancing condition of Parkinson's disease that significantly affected his ability to speak and swallow. Here are some of Mrs. Kaemmer's reflections on her husband's dysphagia.

The doctor approached me and said, "I know what your husband had for dinner tonight." I just stared at him and thought, how does he know? Hours after dinner that night, an ambulance brought Don to the hospital because of a kidney infection. While examining my husband, the doctor found partially chewed chicken in Don's mouth and throat. I thought Don swallowed his dinner but apparently not. An example of Parkinson's effect on daily activity became clear.

As the effects of the disorder progressed, my husband had trouble chewing and swallowing food and medications. I don't know if he was just too tired, too depressed, or didn't have an appetite to eat. He often looked as if he was wearing a mask with no emotion and said little. I often felt like a cheerleader trying to boost his spirits to get him to eat. How could he stay well if he didn't eat? I made soft foods like chicken soup with pieces of cut-up chicken and vegetables, split pea soup, puddings, and ice cream. During one hospital stay he had a supplement drink that he was willing to drink at home. It was expensive, so we would get a supply of it from the Veterans Administration because Don was entitled to benefits, having served in WWII. But toward the end, only small spoonfuls of ice cream or sherbet felt good. It took too much energy to drink. Instead of feeding with food, I nourished him by being there.

Yetta Kaemmer
Tamarac, FL

A videofluoroscopy swallow study (VFSS) determines the level of bolus consistency the patient can tolerate. Solid foods and liquids are evaluated separately. Dietary modifications are based on texture, cohesiveness, density, viscosity, consistency, temperature, and taste. Different physiologic problems will dictate the necessity for different consistencies of food.

No two patients with dysphagia are alike. Therefore, diet must be individualized according to the swallowing ability and personal food preferences of the patient. Food must be served in a form that fits the specific anatomic and functional needs of the patient. Patients may need pureed foods to provide stimulation that provokes the reflex to swallow. For patients whose pharyngeal swallow is reduced (but not delayed or absent), liquids tend to be the most difficult consistency. Thickening agents can be used to acquire the appropriate consistency. For patients who have lost coordination of the upper esophageal sphincter (cricopharyngeal dysfunction), thin liquids are more appropriate.

Patients may require changes in food consistency during a hospital or nursing home stay. Thickening agents provide varying levels of consistency to accommodate individual needs. A nutritionally adequate diet for dysphagia considers these characteristics, along with careful planning to ensure nutritional adequacy. Table 13.1 provides an example of dysphagia diets; each institution should have a clear description available for all team members to learn.

Application to nursing. Enlisting the aid of a speech-language pathologist (SLP) is usually necessary to teach the patient various techniques to compensate for swallowing problems. The supraglottic swallow technique is appropriate for patients with reduced laryngeal function. This method involves teaching the patient to take a breath before swallowing, consciously hold the breath during the swallow, exhale forcefully or cough gently after the swallow, and swallow again to clear the mouth. The Mendelsohn maneuver is helpful for individuals with

TABLE 13.1 Sample Dysphagia Diet

Level	Rationale	Description
Pureed	Suitable for people with severely reduced oral preparatory-stage abilities, impaired lip and tongue control, delayed swallow reflex triggering, oral hypersensitivity, reduced pharyngeal peristalsis, and/or cricopharyngeal dysfunction.	Thick homogeneous textures are emphasized. Pureed foods should be "spoon-thick" or "pudding-like" consistency. No coarse textures, nuts, raw fruits, or raw vegetables are allowed. Liquid or crushed medications (refer to physician or pharmacist for pharmoefficacy of medications) are required and may be mixed with pureed fruits. Liquids and water are thickened with commercial thickening agent as needed to recommended consistency.
Mechanically altered	Intended for patients who can tolerate a minimum amount of easily chewed foods. May be suitable for people with moderately impaired oral preparatory-stage abilities, edentulous oral cavity, decreased pharyngeal peristalsis, and/or cricopharyngeal muscle dysfunction.	No coarse textures, nuts, raw fruits (except ripe or mashed bananas), or vegetables, except as noted. Pureed or slurried bread, if necessary. Liquid or crushed medications may still be required (refer to physician or pharmacist for pharmoefficacy of medications). Liquids and water thickened as needed with commercial thickening agent to recommended consistency.
Advanced	Designed for patients who chew soft textures. Based on a soft diet; may be appropriate for individuals with mild oral preparatory-stage deficits.	Textures are soft with no tough skins, no nuts or dry, crispy, raw, or stringy foods. Meats should be moist and tender or casseroles with small chunks of meat allowed. Fluid consistency ordered separately: may be thin, nectar-thick, honey-like, or spoon-thick. Moist potatoes, rice, and dressing allowed. All soups except those with tough meat or vegetables. Soft, peeled fruit without seeds. Moist breads and cereals allowed. All fats except those with chunky additives.

(Data from Academy of Nutrition and Dietetics: *Nutrition care manual.* From https://www.nutritioncaremanual.org/auth.cfm. (Accessed 26 August, 2020).)

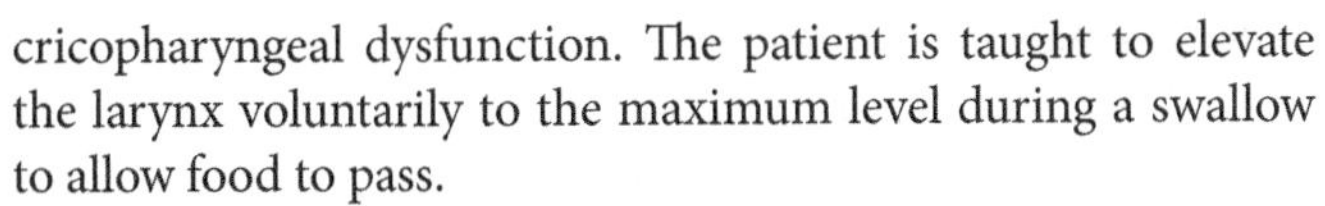

cricopharyngeal dysfunction. The patient is taught to elevate the larynx voluntarily to the maximum level during a swallow to allow food to pass.

In the care of patients with dysphagia at mealtime, several aspects are of concern: bolus consistency, feeding rate, specific swallowing techniques, and patient positioning. One of the safest eating positions for patients who have dysphagia is upright. If patients cannot sit up by themselves, the head of the bed should be raised to provide support. Add pillows and wedges to support arms, head, neck, or trunk when necessary. The upright position allows gravity to assist with the passage of food along the esophagus and helps prevent choking and aspiration.

Aspiration of foreign materials (food, liquids) can lead to pneumonia and other upper respiratory infections. A patient who has aspirated may have a bluish tinge in the skin, wheeze, cough with foul sputum, rapid pulse, excessive sweating, or chest pain. Generally, antibiotics are first-line treatment for aspiration pneumonia.

Dehydration is another concern. Patients with dysphagia are usually not permitted to drink liquids on their own. Thus, attention must be paid to their total fluid intake throughout the day. Intake and output (I&O) records are very important for this population. As needed, the SLP or the registered dietitian can request changes to the diet.

Residents in long-term care facilities often experience serious difficulties with swallowing solid oral dosage forms (SODFs). Crushing the product can lead to medication errors and changes in efficacy (van Welie et al., 2016). The best way to administer medications to a patient with dysphagia should be discussed with the pharmacist.

When dry mouth is a problem, nursing personnel can use several techniques: Encourage the patient to think or talk about food before mealtime; this helps stimulate the flow of saliva for chewing and swallowing. Tart or sour foods can also stimulate saliva production. Have the patient practice oral swallowing exercises. Many exercises can be found at this resource: http://www.swallowingdisorderfoundation.com/oral-swallowing-exercises (National Foundation of Swallowing Disorders, 2020).

During meals, supervision is necessary to prevent or minimize swallowing problems. Patients should be reevaluated regularly to determine whether any changes need to be made in the consistency of fluids or food. Sometimes patients eat too quickly and then choke when trying to swallow. Staff can observe and supervise patients while they eat to remind them to complete the swallowing sequence before taking the next bite of food.

Evaluating and documenting the patient's food intake are prudent to ensure adequate nutritional intake and status. Make sure meals are as relaxing as possible; let patients eat at their own pace. Patience on the part of the feeding team is rewarded when patients eat with minimal difficulty while maintaining their nutritional status. Consider a tube feeding if intake is continuously less than 50% at meals. See the *Teaching Tool* box Recommendations for Feeding Patients with Dysphasia.

Heartburn and Gastroesophageal Reflux Disorder

Heartburn is a burning sensation felt in the esophagus when acid refluxes after food has already been passed to the stomach; it may pass back up through the cardiac sphincter into the esophagus. Some people consider it normal and never report the symptoms to their physicians.

Unlike the stomach, the esophagus is not lined with acid-resistant mucus, so the acidic mixture of food burns the walls of the esophagus and causes pain. Heartburn is also called gastroesophageal reflux. Depending on the frequency and severity of heartburn—including symptoms such as severe burning sensation under the sternum; asthma; chronic cough; and other ear, nose, and throat ailments—either gastroesophageal reflux disorder (GERD) or laryngopharyngeal reflux (LPR) (in which reflux affects the larynx or pharynx) may be diagnosed. The reflux usually takes place within 1 to 4 hours after a meal.

TEACHING TOOL

Recommendations for Feeding Patients With Dysphagia

1. Position patient upright, bent slightly forward, with the chin tucked and head tilted forward.
2. Eliminate distractions so the patient can focus all attention on the meal.
3. The feeding assistant should sit at or below patient's eye level while feeding.
4. Avoid asking patient to talk while eating.
5. Instruct the patient not to use liquids to clear the mouth of foods. Liquids should be used only after the patient has cleared food from the mouth.
6. Encourage frequent dry swallows or coughing to help clear food from the mouth between bites.
7. Encourage small bites (½ to 1 teaspoon solid food or about 10–15 mL liquid), especially if patient's ability to manage food is impaired.
8. Allow adequate time (e.g., 20–30 minutes) to feed the patient.
9. Use spoons rather than cups; patients have less difficulty taking food and liquid this way.
10. A straw may be used by some patients to drink liquids and thinned foods.
11. While patient eats, check for voice quality. A wet or gurgled voice indicates food may be resting on the vocal cords.

(Academy of Nutrition and Dietetics: *Nutrition care manual.* From https://www.nutritioncaremanual.org/auth.cfm (Accessed 26 August, 2020).)

Food and Nutrition Therapies

It is important for patients with GERD to avoid large or high-fat meals. Slow emptying of the stomach from eating high-fat food increases sphincter relaxation, leading to potential reflux. Foods such as chocolate, alcohol, peppermint, spearmint, liqueurs, and caffeine and high-acid foods (tomatoes, vinegar-based foods, citrus fruits, and juices) may irritate the esophagus and cause heartburn. Patients should also avoid overeating, which slows gastric emptying.

Application to nursing. Suggest prevention and treatment strategies to reduce pressure in the stomach so that the cardiac sphincter is not opened by excessive pressure from stomach contents. Straining to defecate affects the contents of the stomach by creating additional pressure; prevention and management of constipation are important. See the *Teaching Tool* box Recommendations for Managing Symptoms of Gastroesophageal Reflux Disorder.

TEACHING TOOL

Recommendations for Managing Symptoms of Gastroesophageal Reflux Disorder

- Avoid lying down shortly after eating: Resting or sleeping with a full stomach may push contents against the cardiac sphincter. Wait several hours after a meal before lying flat or keep head and shoulders elevated when reclining.
- Avoid tight clothing: Wearing restrictive clothing around the waist and midriff affects the functioning of the stomach and may increase stomach pressure.
- Avoid eating "on the run": Eating meals while under stress or trying to do other activities at the same time may cause food to not be chewed enough. Big clumps of foods in the stomach force the stomach muscles to react strongly, which may cause reflux.
- Avoid some medications: Taking certain medications regularly may initiate heartburn. If heartburn often occurs when taking birth control pills, antihistamines, tranquilizers (e.g., diazepam [Valium]), or any drug taken often, check with the primary care provider.

ESOPHAGITIS AND HIATAL HERNIA

Normally the lower esophageal sphincter (LES) prevents stomach contents from entering the esophagus. Factors that may decrease sphincter pressure include smoking, chocolate, alcohol, caffeine, and some medications (Fig. 13.3).

Unlike gastric mucosa, the esophageal mucosa can be damaged when exposed to gastric contents. If not treated, chronic reflux can result in esophagitis (inflammation of the lower esophagus). Reflux is aggravated by increased intra-abdominal pressure from excessive coughing, straining, bending, vomiting, obesity, pregnancy, trauma, ascites, reclining after eating, lifting heavy objects, and strenuous exercise.

Hiatal hernia is a condition in which part of the stomach bulges upward through the diaphragm. Patients may experience respiratory symptoms, such as pneumonitis, chronic bronchitis, and asthma.

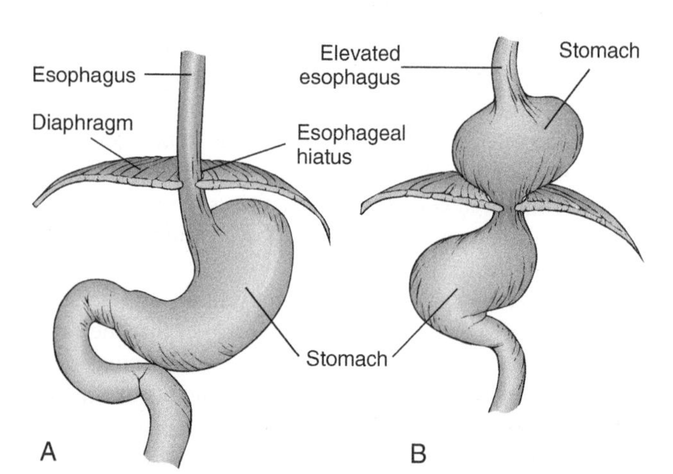

Fig. 13.3 Normal stomach (A) compared with hiatal hernia (B). (From Rolin Graphics.)

Food and Nutrition Therapies

Patients may be able to minimize symptoms of esophagitis or hiatal hernia by manipulating the way they eat and by avoiding certain foods, especially those high in fat. See the previous section on heartburn for more guidance.

Application to nursing. Esophagitis is treated medically by reducing intra-abdominal pressure and gastric acid production. Medical management can be divided into six stages (Box 13.2 and Fig. 13.4).

Table 13.2 summarizes medications that may be used. Attention to metabolism of these medications and their interaction with other prescribed and over-the-counter medications should be considered, particularly among members of different populations. (See the *Cultural Diversity and Nutrition* box Biologic Variations of Medication Metabolism.) If medical management does not work, surgical intervention may be necessary. See the *Teaching Tool* box Recommendations for Living With a Hiatal Hernia.

BOX 13.2 Management of Gastroesophageal Reflux Disease

Lifestyle Modifications
- Head of bed elevated 6 inches
- Decreased fat intake
- Smoking cessation
- Weight reduction for obese patients
- Avoidance of recumbent positions for 3 hours postprandially
- Small, frequent meals
- Avoidance of alcohol, chocolate, caffeine
- Avoidance of tight, waist-constricting clothing

Pharmacologic Therapy
- Antacid or antacid product
- Over-the-counter histamine H_2 receptor blocker
- With documented erosive esophagitis, a proton pump inhibitor may be used as first-line therapy
- Stool softeners

Surgery
- May be appropriate in patient with severe symptoms, erosive esophagitis, or disease complications
- Laparoscopic fundoplication procedure

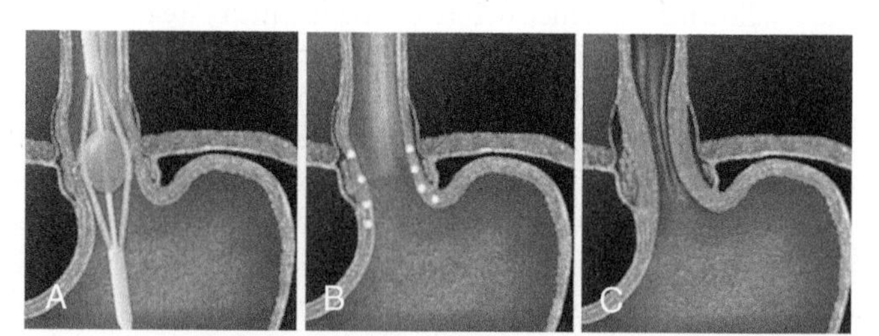

Fig. 13.4 Stretta procedure used to treat gastroesophageal reflux disease (GERD). (A) Catheter positioned. (B) Multiple sites treated with radiofrequency energy. (C) Remodeling occurs with collagen formation. (Courtesy Curon Medical, Inc., Freemont, CA.)

TABLE 13.2 Medications Used to Treat Gastroesophageal Reflux Disease

Medication and Purpose	Potential Adverse Effects and Comments
Antacids: Neutralize gastric acid	
Aluminum salts (AlternaGEL, Alu-Cap, Amphojel, Basaljel)	Constipation, hypophosphatemia, accumulation in patients with renal impairment
Calcium salts, Tums, Tums E-X, Titralac (Amitone)	Constipation, milk-alkali syndrome with high doses, rebound hyperacidity (depending on dosage)
Magnesium salts (Phillips' Milk of Magnesia, Mygel, Almacone)	Diarrhea
Sodium bicarbonate (Citrocarbonate)	Milk-alkali syndrome with high doses
Magnesium-aluminum combinations (Maalox, Maalox Plus, Mylanta, Mylanta Double Strength, Di-Gel, Gelusil)	Take iron or folic acid supplement separately by 2 hours; take separately from citrus fruit/juice or calcium citrate by 3 hours; minor changes in bowel function Magnesium-containing products may accumulate in patients with renal impairment Magnesium-containing products may cause diarrhea
Histamine H_2 Receptor Blockers: Inhibit histamine stimulation of gastric parietal cells, suppressing gastric acid secretion Nizatidine (Axid AR) Famotidine (Pepcid AC) Cimetidine (Tagamet HB) Ranitidine (Zantac)	Take at least 2 hours after iron supplement; take magnesium supplement or magnesium-aluminum antacids separately by at least 2 hours; limit caffeine/xanthine; avoid alcohol Liquid cimetidine precipitates tube feeding
Prokinetic Agents – Increase gastric emptying and lower esophageal sphincter pressure Metoclopramide (Reglan) Bethanechol (Urecholine)	Most effective when used in combination with acid-suppression therapy; drowsiness, psychiatric symptoms, and extrapyramidal reactions may occur with long-term use
Proton Pump Inhibitors – Strongly inhibits gastric acid secretion by inhibiting H^+-K^+ adenosine triphosphatase pump of parietal cells Lansoprazole (Prevacid) Omeprazole (Prilosec) Pantoprazole (Protonix) Rabeprazole (Aciphex) Esomeprazole (Nexium)	Uncommon; include diarrhea, nausea, dizziness, and headaches Optimal: take 30–60 minutes before a meal; swallow whole, do not crush; omeprazole only—capsule may be opened and granules sprinkled on 1 tbsp applesauce; avoid alcohol

(Data from Pronsky ZM, Elbe D: *Food-medication interactions*, ed 18, Birchrunville, PA, 2015, Food-Medication Interactions.)

CULTURAL DIVERSITY AND NUTRITION

Biologic Variations of Medication Metabolism

Ethnic differences in medication metabolism exist because of unique genetics and pharmacokinetics. The result can be different therapeutic consequences and unexpected side effects. Individuals are slow metabolizers when the drug-metabolizing liver enzymes are slowed or impaired by deoxyribonucleic acid (DNA) mutations (allele differences). Others may be considered extensive metabolizers if they have normally functioning enzymes, and even others may be identified as ultra-rapid metabolizers (Borba et al., 2016). Because significant disparities remain in health, health quality, and access to health care within the United States, more research on these biologic variations is needed.

TEACHING TOOL

Recommendations for Living With a Hiatal Hernia

- Avoid large meals. If additional calories are needed for weight gain or maintenance, include midmorning and midafternoon snacks.
- Avoid eating meals and snacks for at least 2 hours before lying down.
- Avoid vigorous activity soon after eating.
- Avoid or limit foods and beverages that relax the lower esophageal sphincter (allowing stomach contents to back up), such as alcohol, carminatives (oil of peppermint or spearmint, garlic, onion), chocolate, and high-fat foods (fried foods, high-fat meats, cream sauces, gravies, margarine and butter, cream, oil, salad dressings).
- Avoid or limit foods and beverages that can irritate damaged esophageal mucosa. These will vary individually and may include carbonated beverages, citrus fruit and juices, coffee (regular and decaffeinated), herbs, pepper, spices, tomato products, and very hot or very cold foods.
- Increase intake of protein foods with low-fat content (lean meats, skim or 1% milk, cheeses, and yogurt made from skim milk) and carbohydrate foods with low-fat content (breads, cereals, crackers, fruit, noodles, potatoes, rice, and vegetables prepared without added fat).
- Achieve and maintain a desirable body weight.

STOMACH DISORDERS

Vomiting

Vomiting is reverse peristalsis. Instead of food moving down the GI tract, the peristalsis muscles move the contents of the stomach back through the esophagus and forcefully out the mouth. It is an involuntary muscular action that cannot be easily controlled. Often it is painful; the contents of the stomach already consist of acidic gastric juices that can burn the unprotected esophagus.

Vomiting is one way the body protects itself. When an intruding virus or toxin has entered the GI tract, vomiting removes the offending substance. Nausea and vomiting may occur in GI diseases as well as other conditions. An altered sense of equilibrium during air or sea travel can result in motion sickness with nausea and vomiting. Pregnant women are affected with hormonal shifts and vomiting, especially during the first trimester. In addition, some patients with cancer suffer from episodes of vomiting because of chemotherapy, radiation treatments, or use of medicines such as opioids. A primary health care provider should be consulted to determine the cause of chronic or persistent vomiting and to recommend a treatment method.

Individuals who force vomiting to control their weight may suffer from eating disorders such as anorexia nervosa and bulimia. Repetitive self-induced vomiting can injure the esophagus and wear away tooth enamel. Anyone practicing this self-destructive behavior should consult a primary care provider and a mental health professional as soon as possible.

Food and Nutrition Therapies

Dehydration is a concern when vomiting is continual. Vomiting causes a loss of fluid and electrolytes (magnesium, potassium, sodium), stressing body functions. Infants are at high risk for dehydration because their bodies contain a high percentage of fluids.

When patients are experiencing nausea or vomiting, small cold meals may be better tolerated than large hot meals. For example, crackers and cheese, gelatin, fruit, or lemonade might be tolerated. Avoid mixing hot and cold foods, which may aggravate the problem. Hot, fried, spicy, and strong-smelling foods should also be avoided. Some patients find relief with broth-based soups, warm tea with mint, and ginger ale or other carbonated beverages.

Application to nursing. Nursing personnel will care for many patients who are experiencing nausea and vomiting. Offering small meals at frequent intervals is a good place to start. Breathing exercises and repositioning may be helpful in some patients. Eliminate strong odors when possible. Good oral health is important, and patients may be prescribed antiemetics (e.g., Zofran, Compazine, or Phenergan) 30 to 60 minutes before meals are served. See the *Teaching Tool* box Recommendations for Managing Nausea and Vomiting.

TEACHING TOOL

Recommendations for Managing Nausea and Vomiting

- Chew foods slowly and thoroughly.
- Use ice chips.
- Sip on cool, clear, carbonated (allow to become "flat") beverages such as 7-Up and ginger ale.
- Avoid the caffeine of colas unless tolerated.
- Limit or omit acidic fruit juices such as orange, tomato, and grapefruit.
- Rest before and after meals. However, keep the head elevated to avoid reflux.

Peptic Ulcer Disease

Peptic ulcer disease (PUD) is the term used to describe a break or ulceration in the protective mucosal lining of the lower esophagus, stomach, or duodenum. Such ulcerations expose the submucosal areas to gastric secretions and autodigestion. Peptic ulcers can be acute or chronic and superficial (erosions) or deep. Deep ulcers may penetrate the mucosa and damage blood vessels, causing hemorrhage or perforation of the GI wall.

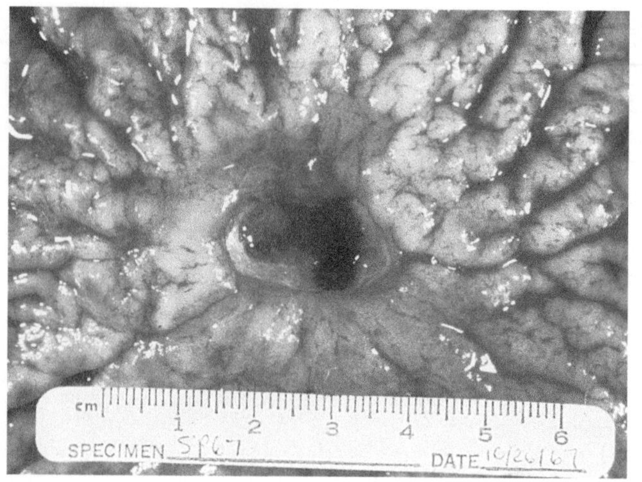

Fig. 13.5 Chronic peptic ulcer. (From Damjanov I, Linder J, editors: *Anderson's pathology*, ed 10, vol 2, St. Louis, 1996, Mosby.)

Infection with *Helicobacter pylori* and use of nonsteroidal antiinflammatory drugs (NSAIDs) are major causes of duodenal ulcers (Fig. 13.5). *H. pylori* weakens the protective mucosal layer of the stomach and duodenum, allowing gastric acid to damage epithelial tissues, which leads to ulcerogenesis. Treatment goals focus largely on eradicating *H. pylori*, reducing stomach acidity, relieving symptoms, healing the ulcer, preventing reoccurrence, and avoiding complications. Goals are accomplished through triple therapy, a combination of two antibiotics and acid-reducing medications (see Table 13.2) taken for at least 10 to 14 days. The acid-reducing medications help relieve pain and help the antibiotics work more effectively.

NSAIDs are likely to promote mucosal inflammation and ulcer formation through cellular damage, reducing gastric blood flow, reducing mucus and HCO_3 (bicarbonate) secretion and decreasing the ability of cells to repair and replicate, leading to breakdown of mucosal defense mechanisms. Low-dose aspirin (75–325 mg daily) is widely used for cardiovascular protection and patients with a high risk for ulcers may also need proton pump inhibitors (Hsu & Tsai, 2015).

Food and Nutrition Therapies

There is no evidence that a "bland diet" (or any specific diet) improves symptoms of ulcers or promotes their healing. Any dietary modifications must be individualized to include avoidance of foods that a patient can associate with symptoms. Some individuals avoid red and black pepper, chili pepper, coffee (caffeinated and decaffeinated), other caffeinated beverages, and alcohol.

Application to nursing. Foods and spices that are irritants, cause superficial mucosal damage, or worsen existing disease should be omitted. Patients need encouragement to take prescribed medications. Triple therapy often requires more than one round of treatment to eradicate *H. pylori* completely. See the *Teaching Tool* box Recommendations for Managing Ulcer Symptoms.

TEACHING TOOL

Recommendations for Managing Ulcer Symptoms

- Regardless of the cause of an ulcer, smoking aggravates peptic ulcer disease. A smoking cessation program should be considered.
- Eating a high-quality diet is also important.

Dumping Syndrome

One of the functions of the stomach is to control the rate of gastric emptying of nutrients into the small intestine. Emptying occurs according to signals from the stomach and duodenum. This process ensures efficient digestion, absorption, and metabolism. With partial or total stomach removal (gastrectomy) or with a bypass for obesity (Fig. 13.6), dumping syndrome may develop. Impairment of the normal stomach reservoir causes a large volume of particles to be dumped rapidly into the small intestine. These hyperosmolar contents draw water into the lumen and stimulate bowel motility.

Early-phase dumping syndrome occurs 10 to 20 minutes postprandially (after a meal) with epigastric fullness, abdominal cramps, nausea, or diarrhea. Vasomotor symptoms may also occur: tachycardia, postural hypotension, profuse sweating, weakness, flushing, and syncope. Patients may experience intestinal symptoms but not vasomotor symptoms, or vice versa. A late phase may occur 1 to 3 hours postprandially. Less common than the early phase, its symptoms include perspiration, hunger, nausea, anxiety, tremors, and weakness.

Food and Nutrition Therapies

Food and meals can be manipulated or restricted to help alleviate the symptoms of patients with dumping syndrome. Liquids should be consumed between rather than with meals to slow the movement of food from the stomach into the duodenum. Simple carbohydrates are limited because they may worsen the syndrome. Protein, fat, and complex carbohydrates are better tolerated.

Patients will lose weight from early dumping syndrome after gastric bypass (Roux-en-Y) surgery, and this is considered a protection against overconsumption (Laurenius & Engstrom, 2016). Other patients who experience dumping syndrome should be evaluated regularly by a registered dietitian; deficiencies of iron, vitamin B_{12}, protein, and vitamin D can occur over time (Academy of Nutrition and Dietetics, 2020).

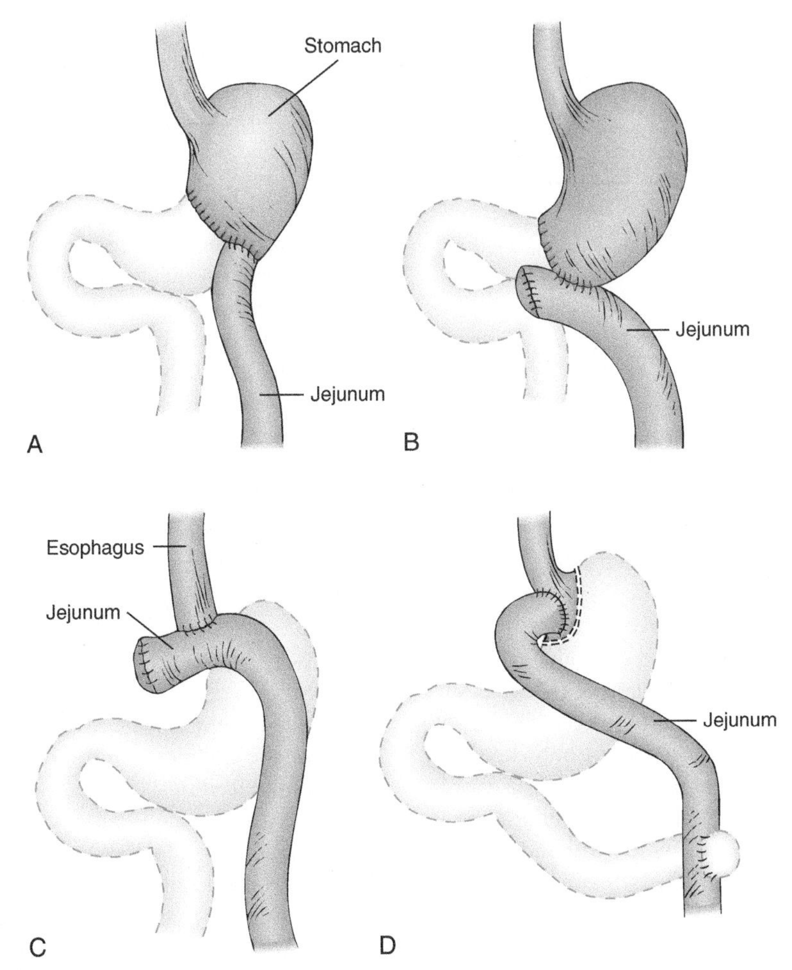

Fig. 13.6 Typical gastric surgery resections. (A) Partial gastrectomy, Billroth I (gastroduodenostomy). (B) Partial gastrectomy, Billroth II (gastrojejunostomy). (C) Total gastrectomy. (D) Roux-en-Y bypass procedure. (A–C from Rolin Graphics.)

Application to nursing. Coping with dumping syndrome may seem overwhelming to newly diagnosed clients. Help them understand what is happening; discuss foods to avoid. Make sure patients consume adequate fluids between meals to prevent dehydration; I&O records will be important. See the *Teaching Tool* box Recommendations for Managing Dumping Syndrome.

TEACHING TOOL

Recommendations for Managing Dumping Syndrome

- Avoid drinking liquids with meals. Drink liquids 30 minutes before or 30 minutes after meals and limit servings to ½ to 1 cup.
- Carbonated beverages may cause excess gas formation and therefore are not recommended.
- Eat small, frequent meals to decrease intestinal distention caused by rapid emptying of large meals.
- Eat foods slowly, chew them well, and relax while eating.
- Avoid any foods that are not tolerated.
- Keep simple sugars (monosaccharides and disaccharides) to a minimum. Initially avoid sugar, honey, syrup, and other foods high in sugar; they may need long-term limitation.
- Food and liquids should be consumed at moderate temperatures (not too hot or too cold).
- Milk and milk products containing lactose may not be tolerated. Establish tolerance by gradually introducing them into the diet over time.
- Lie down for 15 to 30 minutes after meals to help decrease symptoms of dumping. If bothered by reflux, recline (at an angle) rather than lying flat.
- Pectin, a dietary fiber, may be helpful in delaying gastric emptying. Pectin can be purchased in powder form in grocery stores and supermarkets. One teaspoon of pectin powder three times daily may be beneficial.

(From Academy of Nutrition and Dietetics: *Nutrition care manual.* From https://www.nutritioncaremanual.org/auth.cfm. (Accessed 26 August, 2020).)

INTESTINAL DISORDERS

Intestinal Gas (Flatus)

Everyone produces and releases gas from the lower intestinal tract, mostly without our awareness because it is odorless. Gas in the GI tract is caused by swallowing air, or by the fermentation of indigestible carbohydrates by bacteria in the large intestine. Everyone swallows a small amount of air when eating and drinking; however, the amount increases when people eat or drink too fast, smoke, chew gum, or drink carbonated beverages.

Some individuals cannot tolerate gas-producing foods. Indigestible carbohydrates are found in legumes or lentils, such as soybeans and black beans, and cruciferous vegetables, such as broccoli and cabbage. Another indigestible carbohydrate may be the lactose in milk. When the patient is missing the enzyme lactase, lactose begins to ferment, causing gas buildup, bloating, and diarrhea. Fructose, found in some fruits and used as a sweetener in soft drinks and other products, may also contribute to intestinal gas. For many people, alcohol may be a problem.

Food and Nutrition Therapies

Intestinal gas can be decreased through some simple changes of food-related behaviors. Increase fluid intake and consume sufficient amounts of fiber to prevent constipation. To increase fiber intake, gradually add more fibrous foods to allow the system to adjust and tolerate the increase. Patients should omit alcoholic beverages and products containing fructose as needed.

If there are effects after drinking milk, drink small quantities over several weeks, working up to an 8-ounce glass. Note at what level gas develops. If a problem persists, consider other dairy products such as yogurt, cheese, or lactose-reduced milk. Lactase enzyme is available in forms such as pills, tablets or drops.

Application to nursing. Encourage the patient to identify foods that are problematic. The cause of flatulence will be unique for each person. Over-the-counter products can be suggested, including Gas-X, simethicone, and Mylanta. Nurses can teach patients how to manage the intricacies of digestive enzyme replacement therapies and ensure their effectiveness (Felicilda-Reynaldo & Kenneally, 2016). See the *Teaching Tool* box Recommendations for Reducing Intestinal Gas.

TEACHING TOOL

Recommendations for Reducing Intestinal Gas

- Eat slower, and chew foods more thoroughly.
- Avoid gum, carbonated beverages, and drinking out of a straw.
- Add new fiber-rich foods one at a time; evaluate for any discomfort before adding more new items.
- Drink plenty of liquids each day.
- Evaluate the effects of lactose from drinking milk. Use enzyme replacements if needed.

Diarrhea

Diarrhea is the passing of loose, watery bowel movements that result when the contents of the GI tract move through too quickly to allow water to be reabsorbed in the colon. An occasional bout is not a problem. However, if diarrhea persists, fluid and electrolytes may be lost, leading to dehydration.

Acute diarrhea is typically of short duration and is usually the result of enteritis, effects of medications, changes in dietary habits or intake, or emotional stress. Diarrhea that lasts longer than 4 weeks is considered chronic and should be evaluated by a physician (Centers for Disease Control and Prevention, 2020). If it is the result of malabsorption or inflammatory bowel disease, dietary changes may be required.

Food and Nutrition Therapies

Nutrition therapy is based on the cause of diarrhea. In severe cases, the patient may be restricted to taking nothing by mouth to allow the GI tract to rest; however, it is usually unnecessary to withhold feedings.

Infants, young children, and older adults with diarrhea are at high risk for dehydration. Thus, carbohydrate and electrolytes may be administered as enteral or intravenous (IV) fluids. Enteral therapy may consist of oral rehydration solutions for 1 or 2 days before progressing to a low-fat, low-fiber, or low-lactose diet. Small, frequent meals are often better tolerated than three larger meals. The patient may return to the normal diet as soon as tolerated.

Application to nursing. Adequate hydration is essential in high-risk populations with diarrhea. Infants cannot easily communicate their thirst, and a greater proportion of their bodies consists of fluid; the excessive loss of fluid has serious consequences, such as electrolyte imbalance and a distorted ability to maintain body temperature and functions. In older adults, the ability to detect thirst may be diminished. Disorientation, sometimes mistaken as senility, may be a sign of dehydration.

Because it is a symptom of illness, diarrhea that lasts more than a few days should be discussed with the primary care provider. In a patient receiving a tube feeding, check contributors such as antibiotic and medication use before assuming the diarrhea was caused by the feeding. See the *Teaching Tool* box Recommendations for Managing Diarrhea.

Constipation

Individuals vary in their natural urge to defecate. Not everyone needs to pass a bowel movement daily. Normal functioning ranges from three times a day to every 3 days. Constipation means having fewer than three stools per week; in addition, afflicted people strain to pass hard, dry stools (National Institute of Diabetes and Digestive and Kidney Diseases, 2020).

TEACHING TOOL

Recommendations for Managing Diarrhea

- Eat small meals frequently throughout the day.
- Chew with a closed mouth to avoid swallowing too much air.
- Drink liquids 30 minutes before or after meals.
- Limit use of apple juice, which may aggravate diarrhea (especially in children).
- Include foods that are low in fiber (bananas, rice, applesauce, dry toast, crackers) during the acute phase.
- Progress to foods that are high in potassium when tolerated. Include oranges, grapefruit, bananas, apples, potatoes, dairy products, apricot nectar, baked squash, and sweet potatoes.
- Electrolyte solutions (Gatorade, Pedialyte, etc.) may be prescribed with medical advisement to replenish lost sodium and potassium.
- If diarrhea is severe, the doctor may prescribe medication such as loperamide (Imodium).
- Get plenty of rest—lie down for 30 to 60 minutes after meals.
- Avoid foods during periods of severe diarrhea that are:
  - Very hot—which might increase natural movement of the intestines
  - High in caffeine—such as coffee, colas, chocolate
  - High in fiber—whole-grain breads or cereals, raw fruits and vegetables, nuts, dried fruit, popcorn, salads, and bran
  - Gas-forming—cabbage, onions, dried beans or lentils, carbonated beverages, broccoli, cauliflower, chewing gum.
- Milk contains lactose, a natural sugar that may not be digested properly. For some, this is a temporary situation.
- Polyols are carbohydrates not well tolerated by individuals who have irritable bowel syndrome with primarily diarrhea. Natural sources are found in apples, apricots, nectarines, pears, plums, prunes, and mushrooms. Other sources include additives such as sorbitol, mannitol, xylitol, maltitol, and isomalt.
- Excess fructose is found naturally in honey, apples, mango, pear, and watermelon. Products made with high-fructose corn syrup should be eliminated when not well tolerated.

Food and Nutrition Therapies

Water helps lubricate the intestines, making bowel movements easier to pass. To prevent dehydration and constipation, fluid intake should be approximately 8 to 10 glasses a day. Most of us need to consciously remember to drink water and other liquids to fulfill this need. In fact, as we grow older, we tend to lose our thirst sensation and may need reminding to drink more liquids.

The patient should use fiber-rich products such psyllium (Metamucil), whole-grain breads and cereals, fruits, and vegetables. After fermentation, short-chain fatty acids and gas are produced that support intestinal health (Alexander et al., 2019).

Application to nursing. Chronic constipation is a distressing condition. Most patients in the hospital are at risk for constipation from decreased activity and the medications they are taking (especially opioids). Increasing physical activity and fluid are key factors.

Bulking agents, stool softeners, laxatives, and probiotics may be prescribed to prevent or alleviate constipation. Gastroenterologists may recommend over-the-counter products by brand name, or a pharmacist can offer other suggestions. Mineral oil should not be used because it depletes fat-soluble vitamins (A, D, E, and K) when used over time.

Behavioral and psychological approaches or biofeedback techniques may be useful (Bharucha et al., 2016). If these strategies do not relieve constipation, the physician should be consulted to rule out more serious disorders. (See the *Personal Perspectives* box Constipation as a Warning?)

PERSONAL PERSPECTIVES

Constipation as a Warning?

A spouse or significant other is an observer of the health and illness of one's partner. As such, a spouse may note physical changes and remember medical history more clearly than the partner experiencing the symptoms. This is the perspective of a spouse about an early symptom of a neurologic disorder in her husband.

I remember the look of panic on his face. The simple act of "having a bowel movement" just wasn't happening for my husband. It had been several days. This was never a problem before, so the discomfort and panic increased. In 5 days, we were to fly to the Netherlands to visit our son, whom we hadn't seen in almost a year.

After trying the usual over-the-counter laxatives with no reaction, he called his internist, who said to go to the emergency room. Emergency room! Now I have to admit I thought my husband was overreacting. Because he was so uncomfortable, I agreed we should go to the nearby hospital. After many hours of enemas, an overnight stay, and an emergency colonoscopy, my husband was released with follow-up instructions from a gastroenterologist. Diagnosis: unknown cause (an isolated incident). Nonetheless, he continues to need to use a prescriptive laxative.

We did visit our son in the Netherlands without any medical mishaps. However, about 2 years later, my husband was diagnosed with multiple system atrophy, a rare degenerative neurologic movement disorder. The original constipation problem was an early symptom of this serious disorder, which affects the sympathetic nervous system.

The moral of this story? A cluster of seemingly unrelated symptoms may be related and are important to communicate to health care providers. Keeping a record of symptoms, treatments, medications, and dates can be quite valuable.

Michele Grodner
Montclair, NJ

Copious amounts of fiber, particularly wheat bran, may result in the formation of bezoars in some people. Bezoars are physical obstacles created by tangles of fibrous material in the GI tract that may cause dangerous GI obstructions. They tend to occur more commonly in individuals who have diabetes and who suffer from gastroparesis. See the *Teaching Tool* box Recommendation for Managing Constipation.

TEACHING TOOL

Recommendations for Managing Constipation

- Listen to the body's signals and follow a schedule that allows time for a bowel movement to occur. Ignoring the natural urge to defecate causes feces to remain in the colon longer. This allows more water to be withdrawn, resulting in harder, drier feces.
- Exercise regularly. Lack of exercise can lead to a loss of tone in the muscles of the lower gastrointestinal tract.
- Relax. Stress tightens muscles throughout the body and may inhibit proper bowel functioning.
- Consume regular meals. The body works best with an intake of nutrients and fiber throughout the day. Skipping meals should be avoided.

Celiac Disease and Gluten Sensitivity

Celiac disease is a chronic autoimmune disorder in which the mucosa of the small intestine, especially the duodenum and proximal jejunum, is damaged by dietary gluten. The gliadin fraction in wheat, secalin in rye, and hordein in barley are the specific prolamins (storage proteins), collectively known as gluten, that trigger the toxic reaction in genetically predisposed individuals (Escott-Stump, 2015). The resulting malabsorption of nutrients causes symptoms that can vary greatly depending on the duration and severity of the disease, the person's age, and the presence of extraintestinal conditions.

Although the classic symptoms are diarrhea, abdominal distention, fat malabsorption, and weight loss, many patients do not present with GI symptoms or are asymptomatic. Others may experience anemia, osteoporosis, infertility, or even lymphoma if their disease is untreated. In mild stages, steatorrhea (fat malabsorption) is common. In severe cases the digestion and absorption of proteins, fats, carbohydrates (especially lactose), calcium, vitamin D, vitamin K, iron, folate, and vitamin B_{12}, as well as other nutrients, become impaired. Studies suggest that folate, magnesium, and zinc intakes may be deficient (DiNardo et al., 2019). Severe nutritional deficiencies lead to osteopenia or osteoporosis, inadequate blood coagulation, easy bruising of skin as a result of lack of vitamin K, iron-deficiency anemia, and macrocytic anemia as a result of vitamin B_{12} and folate malabsorption (Escott-Stump, 2015). Thus, it is wise to use a multivitamin-mineral supplement while following the gluten-free diet.

Food and Nutrition Therapies

Once gluten is removed from the diet, symptoms gradually improve over the following weeks and months. Intestinal mucosa subsequently returns to a near normal condition. There is only one catch: Maintaining an asymptomatic state depends on lifelong avoidance of gluten. A diet that restricts these four grains can become monotonous. Table 13.3 summarizes sources of gluten.

Application to nursing. The restrictive diet required by celiac disease can be frustrating because of its limitations. Abstaining from wheat, oats, rye, and barley is difficult. Patients may need new coping skills. The diet will change many routines at home, school, and work for the patient and family as well. See the *Teaching Tool* box Recommendations for Managing Celiac Disease.

TEACHING TOOL

Recommendations for Managing Celiac Disease

- Gluten-containing grains and products made from these grains are staples in the American diet. They are used as emulsifiers, thickeners, and other additives in commercially processed foods.
- Patients, with the help of registered dietitians and celiac disease support groups, must become ardent label readers to avoid unintentional ingestion of gluten.
- Availability of alternatives to wheat-based breads, crackers, and pasta is limited when one is eating away from home. Patients may need to pack lunches or snacks for a variety of events.

Lactose Intolerance

The most common disaccharidase disorder is a deficiency of lactase, the intestinal brush-border enzyme that hydrolyzes lactose into glucose and galactose (see Chapter 4). This lactase deficiency leads to lactose intolerance, which is prevalent worldwide, mostly in non-European countries.

Lactose intolerance is investigated with a hydrogen breath test or with genotyping in patients who have abdominal symptoms (Misselwitz et al., 2019). Undigested lactose remaining in the intestine will, through osmotic effect, draw water into the digestive tract, resulting in abdominal cramping, flatulence, and diarrhea. The severity of these symptoms often depends on the amount of lactose ingested and the degree of intolerance an individual has. Lactase deficiency is sometimes secondary to acute or chronic diseases, such as celiac disease and Crohn's disease, or to small bowel or gastric surgery.

Food and Nutrition Therapies

Tolerance for lactose varies from population to population and from person to person. For individuals who have lactose intolerance or in whom it is suspected, health care professionals need to establish tolerance by gradually adding small amounts of lactose-containing foods to a lactose-free diet (Box 13.3). Most people can tolerate 6 to 9 g of lactose at a given time, which is the amount in 4 to 6 ounces of milk. These small amounts of lactose can generally be consumed on several occasions throughout the day. Individuals usually tolerate lactose if it is consumed along with other foods, rather than alone as a beverage or a snack. Yogurt may be better tolerated than milk, depending on brand and processing method. Cocoa and chocolate milk may also be better tolerated. *Lactobacillus acidophilus* milk is generally not tolerated, because it still contains lactose.

Application to nursing. Limiting lactose-containing foods poses a risk for calcium, riboflavin, and vitamin D deficiencies,

TABLE 13.3 Sources of Gluten

Foods to include	Rice Corn Amaranth Quinoa Teff (or Tef) Millet Finger millet (ragi) Sorghum Indian rice grass (Montina) Arrowroot Buckwheat Flax Job's tears Sago Potato Soy Legumes Mesquite Tapioca Wild rice Cassava (Manloc) Yucca Nuts Seeds
Grains to avoid	Wheat, all varieties, including: • Einkorn • Emmer • Spelt • Kamut • Wheat bran • Wheat germ • Cracked wheat • Hydrolyzed wheat protein Barley Rye Cross-bread varieties such as triticale (cross between wheat and rye)
Processed foods that may contain wheat, barley, or rye	Bouillon cubes Brown rice syrup Candy Cold cuts Communion wafers[a] French fries Gravy Hot dogs Imitation fish Licorice Matzoh Rice mixes Salami Sauces Sausage Seasoned snack foods (e.g., tortilla chips, potato chips) Seitan Self-basting turkey Soups Soy sauce Vegetables in sauce

[a]Communion wafers are generally made from wheat, although gluten-free wafers are manufactured by Ener-G Foods (www.ener-g.com). Low-gluten Communion wafers that conform to (Catholic) Canon law have been developed by the Benedictine Sisters of Perpetual Adoration (www.benedictinesisters.org).

© Academy of Nutrition and Dietetics, Celiac Disease Nutrition Therapy, taken from the Nutrition Care Manual, Accessed [26 August 2020] Used with permission.

depending on the degree of restriction. These nutrients can be provided at the recommended dietary allowance (RDA) level with lactase-treated milk and milk products or with supplementation. Calcium is especially important for children and women of childbearing age. Supplementation is necessary for individuals with low serum levels of vitamin D. See the *Teaching Tool* box Recommendations for Lactose Intolerance.

Irritable Bowel Syndrome

Irritable bowel syndrome (IBS) is a GI disorder involving disturbed gut microbiota with abdominal discomfort, changes in bowel habits, and pain (Hadjivasilis et al., 2019). Patients with IBS can be divided into those who have alternating bowel habits (IBS-A), constipation-predominant IBS (IBS-C), or diarrhea-predominant IBS (IBS-D). Some patients with IBS may have a nonceliac wheat or gluten sensitivity, lactose intolerance, or food allergies.

TEACHING TOOL

Recommendations for Lactose Intolerance

- Lactase enzyme is available as Lactaid or Dairy Ease and may be added to milk 24 hours in advance of ingestion. The tablet form is available and can be ingested just before eating a lactose-containing meal. Depending on the degree of intolerance, patients may use one half to three tablets (Academy of Nutrition and Dietetics, 2020).
- Cheese and yogurt are dairy foods that are likely well tolerated; they can be used daily for calcium and riboflavin if milk is not included in the diet.

BOX 13.3 Lactose Content of Foods

Lactose content will vary, depending on portion size and product preparation. Most individuals can experiment with different lactose-containing foods to determine their level of tolerance. Although dairy products all contain lactose, processing reduces the lactose in some products.

High-Lactose Foods
Buttermilk
Cheesecake, cream pies
Cold cuts and hot dogs (some may contain varying amounts of lactose)
Cottage cheese (nonfat, low-fat, regular)
Cream
Cream cheese
Cream or milk soups
Creamy sauces (white sauce, Alfredo sauce, vegetables au gratin)
Evaporated milk
Half and half
Ice cream (regular and low-fat), ice milk, frozen yogurt
Milk (nonfat, skim, low-fat, whole)
Milk-related products
Powdered milk
Pudding, custard
Ricotta cheese
Salad dressings with milk
Sour cream
Yogurt

Low-Lactose Dairy Foods
Aged cheese (cheddar, Swiss)
Butter/margarine
Commercial bread and cake products (bread, muffins, pancakes, waffles, biscuits)
Drug preparations (tablets) (may contain lactose as filler, but usually tolerated)
Lactose-reduced milk (nonfat, skim, low-fat, whole)
Processed cheese (depending on milk solids added)
Processed foods containing dry milk solids or whey
Ready-to-eat cereals containing milk/lactose
Sherbet
Yogurt (may be tolerated)

Over the past decade, pathophysiology and treatment have changed for patients with IBS. The latest research suggests fecal microbiota transplantation (FMT). In FMT, stool from a healthy donor is liquified and transferred to the colon of the afflicted patient to introduce helpful bacteria. Research needs to identify the exact microbial strains needed by an individual patient to be effective.

Food and Nutrition Therapies

Depending on the individual's symptoms and food diary, lactose, gluten, or sugars may be eliminated from the diet. The low-FODMAP (fermentable oligosaccharides, disaccharides, monosaccharides, and polyols) diet is one strategy. This diet limits sugar intake, which increases osmolarity. Foods containing fructose, sucrose, polyols (sorbitol and mannitol), and related carbohydrates are restricted. In addition, note that a diet with higher protein and healthy fats (such as olive oil) should be suggested.

Application to nursing. Treatment may include both pharmacologic and nonpharmacologic interventions, mostly based on symptom management (Weaver et al., 2017). Dietary changes may be needed. Patients with IBS require medical attention when they have a fever, persistent diarrhea, anemia, rectal bleeding, palpable abdominal masses, unintended weight loss or symptoms at night. See the *Teaching Tool* box Irritable Bowel Syndrome.

TEACHING TOOL
Irritable Bowel Syndrome

- Use a food diary to note symptoms, specific foods, or dietary practices that cause problems.
- Prebiotic or probiotic therapy may be beneficial.
- Patients should be taught when to contact their physician with pain, fever and other symptoms or changes in quality of life.
- Dietitian-led education is necessary for use of the FODMAPs diet plan. This chart is a highly simplified version:

	Type	Foods Found in:
Fermentable Oligosaccharides	Fructans & galacto-oligosaccharides	Wheat, rye, barley, onions, garlic, leeks, legumes, lentils
Disaccharides	Lactose	Milk, yogurt, custard, ice cream
Monosaccharides	Fructose (in excess of glucose)	Honey, mango, watermelon, pears, high-fructose corn syrup
And Polyols	Alcohol sugars: Sorbitol, Mannitol, Maltitol, Xylitol	Apples, pears, apricots, plums, cauliflower, chewing gum

(Data from IBS Diets at https://www.ibsdiets.org/fodmap-diet/fodmap-diet-chart/. (Accessed 27 August, 2020).)

Inflammatory Bowel Disease

Inflammatory bowel disease refers to two chronic inflammatory conditions of the intestines—ulcerative colitis (UC) and Crohn's disease (regional enteritis). UC is an inflammatory process confined to the mucosa of the large intestine. Crohn's disease is an inflammatory disorder that involves all layers of the intestinal wall and may affect the small intestine, large intestine, or both. It is associated with stricture formation, fistulous tracts, and abscesses.

Inflammatory bowel disorders are considered autoimmune conditions caused by a genetic predisposition followed by an environmental trigger. Both cause diarrhea, which may be profuse and bloody. Abdominal pain, intestinal bleeding, protein loss, and fever often result in nutritional depletion. Thus, decreased oral intake, malabsorption, increased nutrient loss, increased nutrient requirements, and drug-nutrient interactions must be addressed. Attention must be given to intestinal function, including any previous intestinal resections, site and extent of disease process (Fig. 13.7), and anticipated medical and surgical treatment.

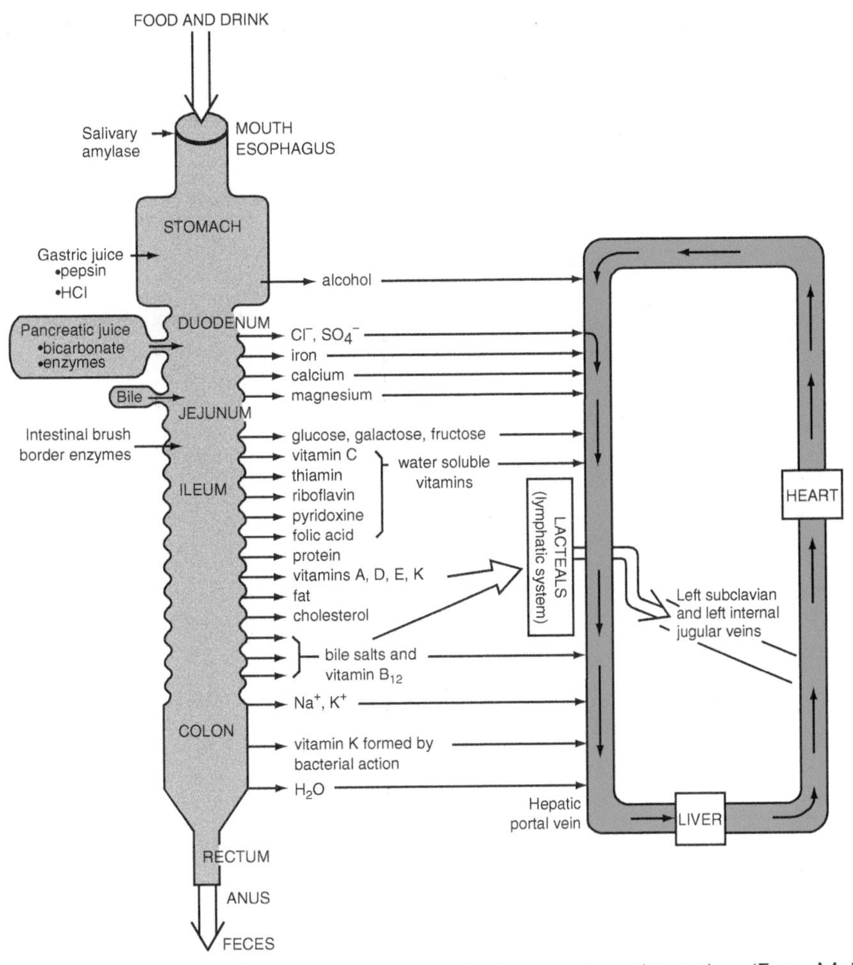

Fig. 13.7 Site and extent of disease process and effect on nutrient absorption. (From Mahan LK, Raymond JL: *Krause's food & nutrition therapy*, ed 14, Philadelphia, 2016, Elsevier.)

Food and Nutrition Therapies

The goals of nutrition therapy are to replace lost nutrients, correct deficits, and achieve energy, nitrogen, fluid, and electrolyte balance. During acute stages of IBD, nutrition therapy is individualized based on food tolerance and affected portions of the GI tract. Diet and weight histories are essential to evaluate potential nutrient deficiencies. The nutrients that most commonly may be poorly absorbed are minerals (iron, calcium, zinc, magnesium, selenium) and vitamins (folate, thiamine, riboflavin, pyridoxine, vitamins A, B_{12}, D, and E). A high-calorie, high-protein diet divided into small, frequent meals is often recommended (Academy of Nutrition and Dietetics, 2020).

Application to nursing. Proper management requires nutritional maintenance and repletion, along with therapies to facilitate healing of the inflamed bowel. Precise body weight measurements are necessary to detect the onset of malnutrition risk. Specific pharmacotherapy, surgery, and nutritional support are used. Although surgery is curative in ulcerative colitis, Crohn's disease tends to recur after surgical resection of affected sections. Box 13.4 and Table 13.4 summarize diets used for these disorders.

Ileostomies and Colostomies

Occasionally, when disease or obstruction cannot be resolved, all or a segment of the colon, including the rectum, is removed. An ileostomy consists of the removal of the entire colon and rectum. A surgical opening of the ileum onto the surface of the abdomen is created, through which fecal matter is emptied. A colostomy consists of the surgical creation of an artificial anus on the abdominal wall by incising the colon and bringing it out to the surface. It may be single barreled (one opening) or double barreled (distal and proximal loops open onto the abdomen).

Food and Nutrition Therapies

Appropriate nutrition therapy depends on the type of ostomy performed. Goals are related to the liquidity of the effluent. In the case of an ileostomy, the effluent is more liquid because the ileocecal valve, which controls rate of movement from the small intestine to the large, is absent. Water, sodium, and other minerals that would otherwise be absorbed are lost, making fluid and electrolyte replacement an important goal. With a colostomy, the effluent liquid is proportional to the length of the remaining bowel (Fig. 13.8).

BOX 13.4 Increasing Fiber Intake[a]

Excellent Sources of Fiber (10–16 g/cup)
All-Bran cereal
Bran Buds cereal
Grape Nuts cereal
Fiber One cereal
Baked beans
Black beans
Chickpeas (garbanzo)
Kidney beans, cooked
Split peas or lentils
Artichokes

Good Sources of Fiber (4–9 g per cup)
Apple with skin
Blueberries
Broccoli, cooked
Pear, with skin
Prunes
Raspberries
Green beans, frozen
Lima beans, cooked (1 cup)
Sweet potato with skin
Turnip greens, boiled (1 cup)
Barley, pearl, cooked (1cup)
Peas, cooked
Black-eyed peas
Bran muffin
Bran Chex cereal
Corn Bran cereal
Graham crackers
Raisin Bran cereal
Oatmeal, cooked
Whole-wheat bread
Shredded wheat cereal
Sunflower seeds (1/4 cup)
Spaghetti, whole wheat

Fair Sources of Fiber (1–3 g/serving)
Banana
Pineapple, canned
Cheerios
Corn, whole kernel canned
Cauliflower
Carrots
Figs. (2 medium dried)
Nuts—almonds, pistachios, pecans (1 oz)
Tomato, raw
Tomato paste (1/4 cup)
Brown rice (1 cup)
Potato with skin
Popcorn, air popped (3 cups)
Raisins (1 oz)
Strawberries, raw (1 cup)
Rye bread

Poor Sources
Celery
Cucumber
Lettuce (iceberg)
Mushrooms
Onions
Grapefruit
Fruit juices
Vegetable juices
Crisped rice cereal
Corn flakes cereal
Refined white flour products (white breads, rolls, bagels, most pastas, pizza crust, crackers)

Note: Increasing fiber without increasing fluid can lead to more constipation, abdominal pain, bloating, and gas. Fiber intake should be increased gradually, over a period of weeks, while fluids are simultaneously increased.

[a]Recommendations for Adequate Intake (AI) are for 25–38 g/day. This goal can be met by eating a well-balanced diet containing a variety of foods: 2–4 servings of fruit, 3–5 servings of vegetables, 6–11 servings of whole-grain breads or cereals, plenty of fluids.
(Data from Academy of Nutrition and Dietetics: *Nutrition care manual*, Chicago, Author. From https://www.nutritioncaremanual.org/auth.cfm (Accessed 26 August, 2020); U.S. Department of Agriculture: *National nutrient database for standard reference, 2012.* From http://ndb.nal.usda.gov. (Accessed 27 August, 2020).)

Application to nursing. The more liquid the stool, the greater the loss of fluid and electrolytes. Any restrictions placed on the patient should be based solely on individual tolerance. See the *Teaching Tool* box Inflammatory Bowel Disease and the *Teaching Tool* box Recommendations for Colostomy and Ileostomy.

Short Bowel Syndrome

When large portions of the small intestine must be resected because of illness or injury, short bowel syndrome (SBS) may occur. The severity of SBS depends on the length and anatomy of the bowel resected and the health of the remaining tissue (Matarese, 2013). An inadequate absorptive surface results in malabsorption of vitamin B_{12} and other vitamins and less than optimal nutritional status. Patients with SBS are at risk for deficiencies in vitamins, minerals, and essential fatty acids; serum levels of these nutrients should be periodically monitored and supplements provided as needed (Matarese, 2013).

TEACHING TOOL

Inflammatory Bowel Disease

- During acute episodes, bowel rest and a low-fiber diet (see Table 13.4) are often suggested to minimize symptoms.
- During periods of remission, avoid unwarranted restrictions. A high-fiber diet (see Box 13.4) can stimulate peristalsis and improve muscular tone of the walls of the gastrointestinal tract, especially the colon.
- Prebiotic or probiotic therapy may be beneficial. The nurse should work with the medical and nutrition teams to evaluate product options.

TABLE 13.4 Guidelines for Ostomy Patients

Food Group	Recommended Foods	Foods Not Recommended
Dairy	Buttermilk Evaporated, skim, and low-fat milk Soy milk Yogurt with live active cultures Powdered milk Cheese	Yogurts with nuts or dried fruits Whole milk Half-and-half Cream Sour cream Regular (whole milk) ice cream
Grains Choose grains with <2 g dietary fiber/serving	White flour Bread, bagels, rolls, crackers, pasta made from white or refined flour Cold or hot cereals made from white or refined flour	Whole-wheat or whole grain breads, rolls, crackers, or pasta Brown or wild rice Barley, oats, and other whole grains Cereals made from whole grains or bran Breads or cereals made with seeds or nuts Popcorn
Fruits and vegetables	Fruit juice without pulp, except prune juice Ripe bananas Canned soft fruits Most well-cooked vegetables without seeds or skins Potatoes without skin Lettuce Strained vegetable juice	All raw fruits and vegetables (except banana, melons, lettuce) Dried fruits, including prunes and raisins Fruit juice with pulp Canned fruit in heavy syrup Any fruits sweetened with sorbitol Prune juice Fried vegetables Beets Cruciferous vegetables (broccoli, Brussels sprouts, cabbage, cauliflower) Greens (collard, mustard, turnip) Corn Potato skins
Proteins	Tender, well-cooked meat, poultry, fish, eggs, or soy foods made without added fat Smooth nut butters	Fried meat, poultry, or fish Luncheon meats, such as bologna or salami Sausage or bacon Hot dogs Fatty meats Nuts Chunky nut butters
Beverages 8–10 cups of fluid are recommended each day; more may be needed to replace fluids lost to diarrhea	Decaffeinated coffee Caffeine-free teas Soft drinks without caffeine Rehydration beverages	Caffeinated beverages (coffee, tea, colas, energy drinks) Limit beverages containing high fructose corn syrup to 12 oz/day Avoid beverages sweetened with sorbitol Alcoholic beverages
Fats		Limit to <8 tsp/day
Other foods		Sugar alcohol such as xylitol and sorbitol Honey

(Modified from Academy of Nutrition and Dietetics: Fiber-restricted nutrition therapy. In *Nutrition care manual*, Chicago, Author. From https://www.nutritioncaremanual.org/auth.cfm. (Accessed 26 August, 2020).)

TEACHING TOOL

Recommendations for a Colostomy or Ileostomy

Meals can still be an enjoyable experience for patients with colostomies and ileostomies. Individual experimentation works best to determine the most appropriate dietary restrictions. The following are some strategies to share:

- **Eat meals regularly**. Eat three or more times a day; an ostomy works best this way and produces less gas.
- **Chew food well to avoid a blockage**. If you have an ileostomy, be especially careful when chewing foods that may be hard to digest or foods that have a high fiber content.
- **Try new foods one at a time**. Learn which foods may give you annoying side effects such as excess gas, constipation, a looser stool, or odor. If a new food seems to give you problems, eliminate it for a few weeks, but try it again later. You may find something else was causing your problem.
- **Avoid gaining excess weight**. Extra weight is not good for your ostomy, and it can cause health problems in general.
- **Drink a lot of fluid daily**. Ileostomy patients and colostomy patients who have lost a large part of their large intestine will especially notice more fluid loss.
- **No two people will react the same to foods**. You will learn through experience which foods, if any, you should avoid.

(Data from University of Pittsburgh Medical Center: *Living with an Ostomy*, Pittsburgh, 2020, Author. From https://www.upmc.com/health-library/article?hwid=ug2186 (Accessed 27 August, 2020).)

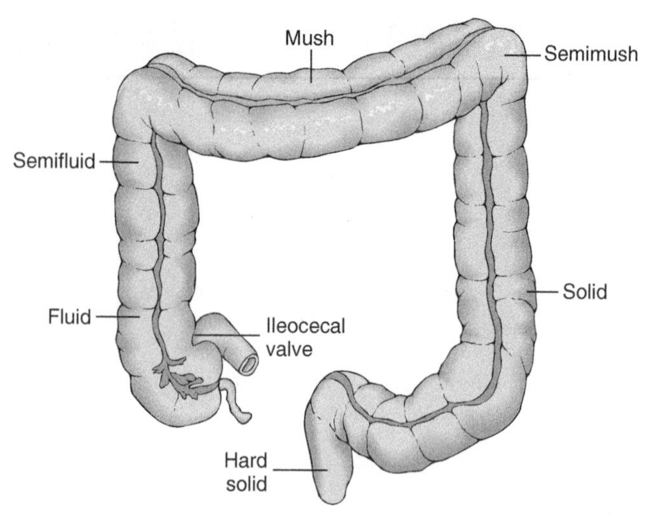

Fig. 13.8 Colostomy site and its effect on output. Excess motility causes less absorption and diarrhea or loose feces. Poor motility causes more absorption, resulting in hard feces and constipation. (From Rolin Graphics. Modified from Guyton AC: *Textbook of medical physiology*, ed 11, Philadelphia, 2005, Saunders.)

Food and Nutrition Therapies

Nutritional management of the patient with SBS with intestinal failure (IF) should consider the individual's digestive and absorptive capabilities. Patients require parenteral nutrition (PN) or IV fluids in the immediate postresection period. Use of GLP-2 analogues can reduce PN requirements in formerly PN-dependent patients (Carroll et al., 2016).

Diet and enteral nutrition (EN) should be reintroduced as soon as possible (Matarese, 2013). Complex carbohydrates from whole grains, fruits, and vegetables should be used, but simple sugars should not. **Medium-chain triglyceride (MCT) oils** are specialized modular formulas that do not require pancreatic lipase or bile for digestion and absorption. They are absorbed directly into the portal vein (like amino acids and monosaccharides) rather than the lymphatic system like other lipids. Many SBS patients will be given MCT oil in their enteral formula.

Application to nursing. Patients with SBS are at high risk of dehydration. Offer oral rehydration solutions to sip throughout the day. If patients are on PN, they should be monitored closely for any signs of complications. See the *Teaching Tool* box Recommendations for Managing Short-Bowel Syndrome.

Diverticular Diseases

When the musculature of the bowel walls weakens, **diverticula** (pouchlike herniations protruding from the muscular layer of the colon) often develop, resulting in the condition **diverticulosis**. It develops as the result of long-term eating habits low in fiber and increased intracolonic pressure such as that created with straining to have a bowel movement. Usually, this condition remains undetected until the diverticula become infected and inflamed from trapped fecal material and colon bacteria; the condition is then known as **diverticulitis**.

> **TEACHING TOOL**
>
> ***Recommendations for Managing Short-Bowel Syndrome***
>
> During the 2 years after resection, the remnant bowel undergoes an adaptation process that increases its absorptive capacity (Matarese, 2013). Frequent monitoring of nutritional status, especially fluid and electrolyte balance, is crucial. If a patient continues to fail on an oral diet, long-term parenteral nutrition at home may be indicated. Prebiotic or probiotic therapy may prove to be beneficial, but more research is needed.

Food and Nutrition Therapies

When diverticula are inflamed, patients are given nothing by mouth, and then progress to liquids. After the inflammation abates, a high-fiber diet is recommended to reduce straining during defecation. High-fiber diets increase fiber-rich foods in the general diet by including fruits, vegetables, legumes, whole-grain breads, and cereals. Current recommendations for fiber are noted as Adequate Intakes (AI) of 25 to 38 g/day.

Application to nursing. During periods of inflammation, the medical goal is to rest the bowel, allowing the infection to resolve. If constipation is a problem, stool softeners may be needed to avoid straining. Remember to encourage adequate fluid intake. See the *Teaching Tool* box Recommendations for Managing Diverticular Disorders.

> **TEACHING TOOL**
>
> ***Recommendations for Managing Diverticular Disorders***
>
> - Eating high-fiber foods is the only treatment for diverticulosis; see Box 13.4. Americans should consume at least five servings or cups of fruits and vegetables and six servings or ounces of whole-grain breads, cereals, or legumes per day.
> - Add more fiber gradually to allow the intestinal tract to adapt. This approach minimizes side effects such as abdominal distress, bloating, flatulence, cramps, and diarrhea, which are usually temporary.
> - There is no evidence-based research indicating that nuts and seeds or popcorn worsen diverticular symptoms.
> - Care should also be taken to consume adequate amounts of fluid—at least 8 to 12 cups per day (Academy of Nutrition and Dietetics, 2020).
>
> (From Academy of Nutrition and Dietetics: Nutrition care manual. From https://www.nutritioncaremanual.org/auth.cfm (Accessed 26 August, 2020).)

SUMMARY

- Disorders of the gastrointestinal (GI) tract include those that affect the esophagus, stomach, small intestine, and large intestine.
- Some disorders affect the muscular action of these sections of the GI tract, thereby affecting flow of sustenance through the GI tract; they include dysphagia and hiatal hernia.
- Peptic ulcer and diverticulitis can lead to site-specific tissue inflammation and pain.
- Several disorders may be caused by inability of the body to produce necessary digestive enzymes (e.g., lactase in lactose intolerance) or inability to metabolize nutrient substances (e.g., gliadin, resulting in severe reactions caused by celiac disease).
- Most disorders are also influenced by lifestyle behaviors that affect stress levels and alter dietary patterns.
- Prebiotics and probiotics show promise for the management of lower GI disorders, but the exact strains are not yet identified.
- Inflammatory bowel disorders are considered autoimmune conditions that have a genetic predisposition and an environmental trigger.
- All GI disorders require some level of nutrition therapy, individualized to meet the needs of each patient.

THE NURSING APPROACH

Clinical Judgment and Next-Generation NCLEX® Examination-Style Questions

Case Study 1

Dysphagia and Feeding Self-Care Deficit

Pierre, age 80 years, had a left-sided stroke 1 month ago and is in a rehabilitation center. He has been getting physical therapy for hemiparesis (one-sided weakness) in his right arm and leg. Initially after the stroke, he was evaluated by a speech therapist and received nourishment through a small-bore nasoduodenal feeding tube because of aphasia (language problems) and dysphagia (swallowing difficulties). Pierre has since been advanced to a soft diet (per doctor's orders), and he continues to work with a speech therapist in relation to expressive aphasia (knows what he wants to say but has trouble saying or writing what he means).

Assessment/Recognize Cues

Subjective (From Patient Statements)

The nurse is unable to understand Pierre's attempts to speak.

Objective (From Physical Examination)

- Coughs and chokes frequently when trying to eat or drink
- Clear lung sounds
- Pockets food in his cheeks
- Fed by nursing staff, does not assist with feeding, eats very slowly
- Can follow directions but has difficulty expressing himself

Diagnoses (Nursing)/Analyze Cues

Potential for aspiration related to impaired swallowing

1. Decreased functional ability related to weakness of right hand and arm

Planning/Prioritize Hypotheses

Patient Outcomes

Short term (within 2 weeks):

- Pierre will be able to eat with minimal or no choking.
- Lung sounds will remain clear.
- He will not pocket food in his cheeks.
- He will be able to assist with his own feeding.

Long term (by discharge):

- He will not develop aspiration pneumonia.
- Pierre will be able to feed himself using adaptive equipment and assistance in setting up his food.

Nursing Interventions/Generate Solutions

1. Implement aspiration precautions.
2. Reinforce rehabilitation efforts by the health care team.

Implementation/Take Action

1. Met with the health care team to design and implement an individualized rehabilitation care plan.
   The doctor prescribed the diet and therapies:
   - The dietitian planned nourishment consistent with physical limitations and nutrient needs.
   - The physical therapist strengthened the patient's weak arm to help with self-feeding.
   - The speech therapist taught the patient how to chew and swallow safely and to communicate needs.
   - The occupational therapist provided adaptive equipment for self-feeding and taught the patient how to become more independent.
   - The nurse helped facilitate schedules for the various therapies, helped feed the patient when team members from the other disciplines were not there, and reinforced teaching.

   Team efforts enhance rehabilitation measures. Nurses are with the patient 24 hours per day and thus are in a position to coordinate necessary therapies and help implement the plan of care.
2. Tested Pierre's gag reflex and listened to lung sounds every morning before feeding him.
   Presence of the gag reflex reduces risk for aspiration. Assessment should be ongoing for any signs of aspiration pneumonia.
3. Positioned him in an upright position (high Fowler's) during meals and for 30 minutes after the meal.
   Gravity assists the passage of food and reduces the risk of choking and aspiration.
4. Reduced distractions such as television during mealtimes.
   Creating a focus for eating helps the patient concentrate on new swallowing and feeding techniques.
5. Assessed Pierre's food preferences by having him point to pictures of foods he likes that are part of the soft diet prescribed by the physician and at the recommendation of the dietitian.
   When the patient is able to make decisions about what to eat, he may feel some control of his situation. Foods that are easiest to chew and swallow include finely chopped meat and smooth textures. Nuts, tough skins, and dry, crispy, raw, or stringy foods are not allowed.
6. Added a commercial thickening agent to juices and water.
   Thin liquids provoke choking; thicker liquids are easier to swallow.
7. Used custard, gelatin, and liquid nutritional supplements between meals two or three times a day.

Continued

THE NURSING APPROACH—cont'd

Intake at mealtime is limited by patient tolerance and time. Between-meal snacks provide extra calories and fluids.

8. Instructed Pierre to follow specific steps when swallowing:
   A. Take a breath before swallowing
   B. Hold breath during swallowing
   C. Exhale forcefully after swallowing
   D. Swallow again
   This maneuver decreases the potential for aspiration by closing off the trachea.
9. Had suction equipment available during feedings.
   The nurse may need to remove fluids from the patient's mouth and throat by suction to prevent aspiration.
10. Provided mouth care before and after meals.
   A fresh mouth encourages appetite. Removal of pocketed food (food remaining in the weak side of the mouth) reduces danger of choking.
11. Encouraged Pierre to feed himself, using special plates and utensils. *Adaptive equipment may facilitate success of the patient's attempts to feed himself.*

Evaluation/Evaluate Outcomes

Short term (at the end of 2 weeks):

- Pierre was beginning to feed himself.
- He was no longer pocketing food in his cheeks.
- He was still choking occasionally on his food and liquids, but his lungs remained clear.

Goals partially met.

Discussion Questions

As Pierre started feeding himself, he sometimes left food on the same side of the plate as his weak arm. He also failed to see the nurse when she would come to assist feeding him if the nurse stood at his weak side. The nurse added the patient problem of unilateral neglect.

1. What causes this problem?
2. How could the nurse teach Pierre to compensate for this condition?

Note that periodic swallowing reevaluation is recommended. Swallowing dysfunction is different for every patient, and appropriate dietary modifications are determined by speech pathologists and registered dietitians.

Swallowing Exercise: Put Yourself in a Dysphagic Patient's Shoes

Most people take normal activities of daily living for granted. When something as simple as swallowing is impaired, eating and drinking become more difficult. To experience difficulty swallowing, tilt your head all the way backward so that you are looking up at the ceiling. Now try to swallow. Next, put your chin down toward your chest so that you are looking down. Again, try to swallow. Next, tilt your head all the way to the right side, and then swallow. Finally, look straight ahead with your head at a normal 90-degree angle and swallow. Can you tell the difference? Which was the easiest? As you can tell, it is much harder to swallow when your head is not aligned properly.

This is a simple exercise to demonstrate how difficult it can be for a patient with dysphagia to swallow. It also emphasizes the importance of ensuring that patients are sitting upright with their heads at a normal angle while eating and drinking. Not only does this positioning make swallowing easier, it also may allow for more independence and ease in self-feeding.

Case Study 2

The nurse is discharging a patient who was admitted with gastroesophageal reflux disease (GERD). What are some lifestyle modifications the nurse teaches the patient?

Teaching Tool for Gastroesophageal Reflux Disease (GERD)

For each lifestyle modification, use an **X** to indicate whether the lifestyle modification would be **Effective** (helped to meet expected outcomes), **Ineffective** (did not help to meet expected outcomes), or **Unrelated** (not related to the expected outcomes).

Lifestyle Modifications	Effective	Ineffective	Unrelated
1. Avoid lying down shortly after eating.			
2. Elevate head of bed by 2 inches			
3. Avoid tight clothing			
4. Limit smoking to no more than a pack a day			
5. Avoid eating ice cream or other frozen foods			
6. Eat three normal meals a day			
7. Drink three 8-oz glasses of milk a day			

(Data from *Nursing diagnoses—definitions and classification 2012–2014*. Copyright © 2012, 1994–2012 by NANDA International. Used by arrangement with Blackwell Publishing Limited, a company of John Wiley & Sons, Inc.)

CRITICAL THINKING

Clinical Applications

Theresa, aged 35 years, is admitted with microcytic anemia. Her medical history indicates that she underwent a total gastrectomy 2 years ago to treat bleeding ulcers. On admission she weighs 120 pounds, and she is 5 feet 9 inches tall. She has lost 30 pounds since the surgery. She has been taking ferrous sulfate and monthly injections of vitamin B_{12}. On admission, her laboratory findings are as follows: hemoglobin 8 g/dL, hematocrit 26%, and serum albumin 2.7 g/dL. Her typical dietary intake is as follows:

Breakfast

1 egg scrambled in 1 teaspoon margarine
½ cup cream of wheat with 1 teaspoon margarine
1 slice white toast with 1 teaspoon margarine
1 cup black coffee

10 AM

6 saltine crackers
12-ounce can diet cola

Lunch

2 baked chicken wings
1 cup cooked carrots
1 medium boiled red potato
1 medium banana
12 ounces diet lemon-lime soda

3 PM

½ bagel with 1 tablespoon cream cheese
8 ounces chocolate milk

Continued

CRITICAL THINKING—cont'd

Dinner
1 broiled chicken breast
½ cup steamed broccoli
1 cup hot tea with artificial sweetener

9 PM
6 saltine crackers
1 tablespoon peanut butter
1 cup black coffee

1. What are common nutrition problems found in patients who have gastrectomies?
2. Which of these problems has Theresa experienced?
3. What factors explain the iron-deficiency anemia that develops after a gastrectomy? What is used to treat this anemia?
4. How do Theresa's laboratory values compare with normal values? What do they indicate?
5. Why is Theresa receiving monthly injections of vitamin B12? Would you advise her to eat more foods high in B12? Explain your rationale.
6. Review Theresa's usual dietary intake; what food groups and/or nutrients are lacking in her diet?
7. What suggestions would you offer Theresa concerning her dietary habits?
8. Should Theresa continue to consume six smaller meals and snacks? Why or why not?

WEBSITES OF INTEREST

Crohn's Disease/Ulcerative Colitis/Inflammatory Bowel Disease
https://www.crohnsandcolitis.com/crohns
Provides information on several digestive diseases; includes resources and links.

International Foundation for Functional Gastrointestinal Disorders (IFFGD)
www.iffgd.org
Provides updates and information to manage dysphagia, irritable bowel syndrome, and other GI disorders.

Medline Plus—DASH Diet
https://medlineplus.gov/dashdiet.html
Provides tips for the DASH diet plan and offers multiple resources.

National Digestive Diseases Information Clearinghouse (NDDIC)
https://www.niddk.nih.gov/health-information/community-health-outreach/information-clearinghouses
Sponsored by the National Institute of Digestive Diseases, this database contains health promotion and education materials not indexed elsewhere.

National Institute of Diabetes and Digestive and Kidney Diseases (NIDDK)
www.niddk.nih.gov
Contains information, resources, and related links on digestive diseases, diabetes, kidney and urologic diseases, and nutrition.

Oldways
https://oldwayspt.org/traditional-diets/mediterranean-diet
This website shares the original Mediterranean diet pyramid and other resources. Oldways is a nonprofit food and nutrition education organization that promotes healthy eating through traditional patterns.

REFERENCES

Academy of Nutrition and Dietetics. (2020). *Nutrition care manual.* Chicago: Author. From: https://www.nutritioncaremanual.org/auth.cfm. (Accessed 26 August, 2020).

Alexander, C., et al. (2019). Perspective: Physiologic importance of short-chain fatty acids from nondigestible carbohydrate fermentation. *Advances in Nutrition, 10*, 576–589.

Bharucha, A. E., et al. (2016). Common functional gastroenterological disorders associated with abdominal pain. *Mayo Clinic Proceedings. Mayo Clinic, 91*, 1118–1132.

Carroll, R. E., et al. (2016). Management and complications of short bowel syndrome: an updated review. *Current Gastroenterology Reports, 18*, 40.

Centers for Disease Control and Prevention (CDC): Chronic Diarrhea. From https://www.cdc.gov/healthywater/hygiene/disease/chronic_diarrhea.html. (Accessed 26 August, 2020).

DiNardo, G., et al. (2019). Nutritional deficiencies in children with celiac disease resulting from a gluten-free diet: A systematic review. *Nutrients, 11*, 1588.

Escott-Stump, S. (2015). *Nutrition and diagnosis-related care* (ed. 8). Baltimore: Lippincott Williams & Wilkins.

Felicilda-Reynaldo, R. F., & Kenneally, M. (2016). Digestive enzyme replacement therapy: pancreatic enzymes and lactase. *Medsurg Nursing, 25*, 182–185.

Geurts, S., et al. (2014). Gut microbiota controls adipose tissue expansion, gut barrier and glucose metabolism: novel insights into molecular targets and interventions using prebiotics. *Benef Microbes, 5*(1), 3–17.

Hadjivasilis. A., et al. (2019). New insights into irritable bowel syndrome: from pathophysiology to treatment. *Annals of Gastroenterology, 32*, 554–564.

Hsu, P. I., & Tsai, J. (2015). Epidemiology of upper gastrointestinal damage associated with low-dose aspirin. *Current Pharmaceutical Design, 21*, 5049–5055.

Kim, S., & Jazwinski, S. M. (2018). The gut microbiota and healthy aging: A mini-review. *Gerontology, 64*, 513–520.

Laurenius, A., & Engstrom, M. (2016). Early dumping syndrome is not a complication but a desirable feature of Roux-en-Y gastric bypass surgery *Clinical Obesity 6*, 332–340.

Matarese, L. E. (2013). Nutrition and fluid optimization for patients with short bowel syndrome. *Journal of Parenteral and Enteral Nutrition, 37*, 161–170.

Mayo Clinic: *Dysphagia*. From: https://www.mayoclinic.org/diseases-conditions/dysphagia/symptoms-causes/syc-20372028. (Accessed 26 August, 2020).

McGinnis, C. M., et al. (2019). Dysphagia: interprofessional management, impact, and patient-centered care. *Nutrition in Clinical Practice, 34*, 90–95.

Mills, S., et al. (2019). Precision nutrition and the microbiome, Part I: Current state of the science. *Nutrients, 11*, 923.

Misselwitz. B., et al. (2019). Update on lactose malabsorption and intolerance: pathogenesis, diagnosis and clinical management. *Gut, 68*, 2080–2091.

National Foundation of Swallowing Disorders: *Oral swallowing exercises*. From: www.swallowingdisorderfoundation.com/oral-swallowing-exercises/. (Accessed 26 August, 2020).

NIDDK. National Institute of Diabetes and Digestive and Kidney Diseases: *Constipation*. From: https://www.niddk.nih.gov/health-information/digestive-diseases/constipation/treatment. (Accessed 26 August, 2020).

van Welie, S., et al. (2016). Effect of warning symbols in combination with education on the frequency of erroneously crushing medication in nursing homes: an uncontrolled before and after study. *BMJ Open*, *6*, e012286.

Weaver, K. R., et al. (2017). Irritable bowel syndrome. *The American Journal of Nursing*, *117*, 48–55.

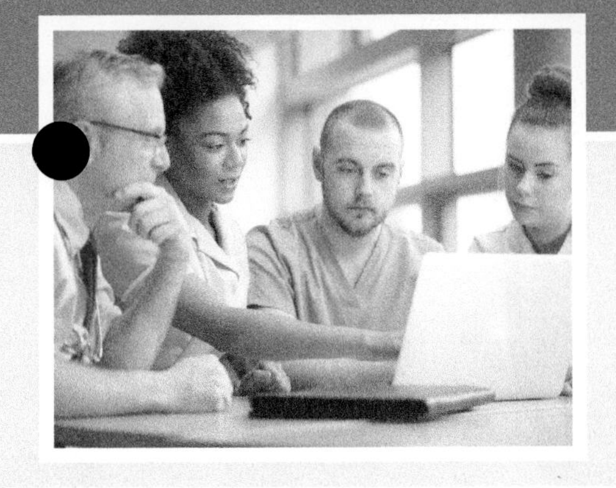

14

Nutrition for Disorders of the Liver, Gallbladder, and Pancreas

Although the liver, gallbladder, and pancreas are not part of the digestive tract proper, little digestion, absorption, or metabolism would take place without them. You can live without a lung, but you cannot survive without a liver or a pancreas.

http://evolve.elsevier.com/GRODNER/FOUNDATIONS

LEARNING OBJECTIVES

- Identify the importance of the liver, the gallbladder, and the pancreas for proper digestion.
- Describe disorders of the liver and the nutritional therapy to treat each disorder.
- Outline the specific nutrition therapy needs of each stage of liver transplantation.
- Discuss the nutrition approaches to reduce the symptoms of gallbladder disorders.
- Explain how pancreatitis alters digestion and absorption of dietary fats and protein.
- Review the potential need for enteral or parenteral nutrition support during treatment of pancreatitis.

NUTRITION IN LIVER HEALTH

Wellness requires well-functioning body organs. Physical health is crucially dependent on the liver, pancreas, and gallbladder; one malfunction can devastate nutritional status. Reasoning, an aspect of intellectual health, is required to make lifestyle decisions related to alcohol when a person is at risk for cirrhosis. A chronic life-threatening illness, such as pancreatitis, challenges emotional health. Restrictive dietary guidelines inhibit the ability to easily socialize with others, thereby diminishing social health. Spiritual health and religious beliefs will provide comfort when one is coping with serious physical disorders. The environmental health dimension encompasses striving for work and living surroundings that are free of toxic substances that could contaminate food, water, and air. Consumption of toxic substances can affect the health of the liver, which acts as a filter of toxins for the body.

LIVER DISORDERS

The liver, the largest organ in the body, lies beneath the diaphragm in the right upper quadrant of the abdomen and is responsible for most biochemical functions that take place in the body. The liver manages bile production and its role in metabolism of carbohydrates, protein, lipids, and vitamins. Because this organ is such a workhorse, impaired liver function can result in major imbalances in metabolism and nutritional status. Progressive decline in nutritional status further impairs liver function. Fig. 14.1 summarizes only a few of the liver's many roles in metabolism and nutritional status.

Hepatitis

Hepatitis is inflammation of the liver. Acute hepatitis can occur as the result of infectious mononucleosis, cirrhosis, toxic chemicals, or viral infection. Five types of hepatitis have been characterized. Their symptoms, signs, and presentation are similar, but their immunologic and epidemiologic characteristics are different (Table 14.1).

Hepatitis A virus (HAV) is typically transmitted through the fecal-oral route (contaminated food or water) but occasionally can be spread by transfusion of infected blood. It is often the result of poor hand washing or stool precautions and is widespread in overcrowded areas with poor sanitation (Box 14.1). Vaccination is recommended for persons at risk for HAV. Onset of HAV is rapid—4 to 6 weeks—and time to onset of symptoms may be dose related. Occurrence of disease manifestations and severity of symptoms directly correlate with the patient's age. Treatment of acute HAV is generally supportive as bed rest; no antiviral therapy is available. Hospitalization and intravenous (IV) fluids may be necessary for dehydration caused by nausea and vomiting. A balanced diet that excludes alcohol is recommended.

Hepatitis B virus (HBV) is an exceptionally resistant virus capable of surviving extreme temperatures and humidity. HBV is transmitted via blood, semen, vaginal mucus, saliva, and tears. IV drug users, patients with hemophilia, those undergoing renal

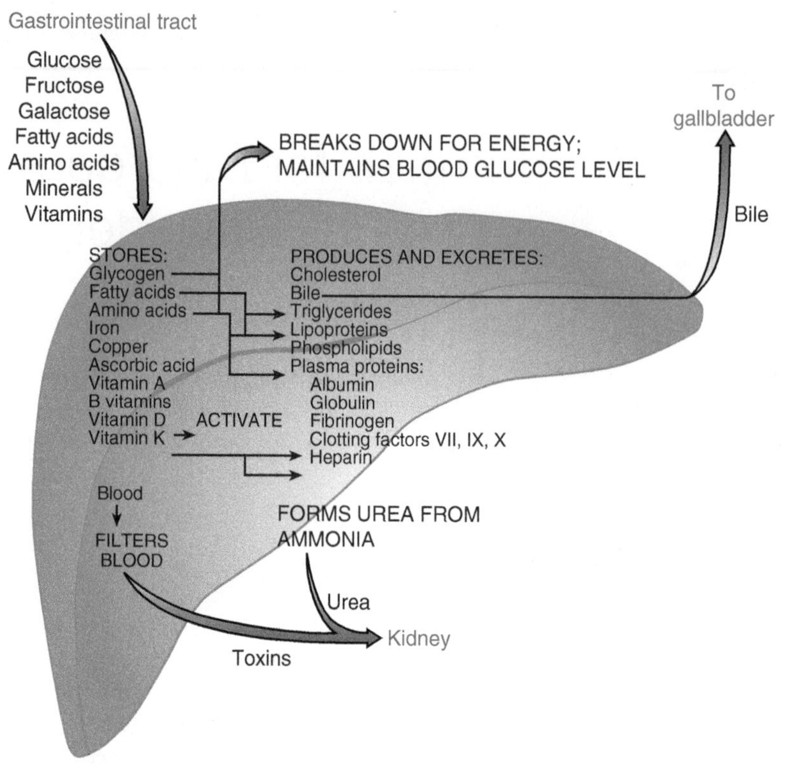

Fig. 14.1 Role of the liver in metabolism and nutrition. Any damage to the liver may affect nutritional status. (From Rolin Graphics.)

TABLE 14.1 Comparison of Hepatitis Viruses

Symptoms	Hepatitis A (HAV)	Hepatitis B (HBV)	Hepatitis C (HCV)	Hepatitis D (HDV)	Hepatitis E (HEV)
Jaundice	X	X	X	X	X
Low-grade fever	X	X	X	X	
Malaise	X	X	X	X	
Anorexia	X	X	X	X	
Dark urine	X	X	X	X	
Diarrhea	X	X	X	X	
Pale stools	X	X	X	X	
Hepatitis B surface antigen (HbsAg) in serum		X	X	X	
Can be asymptomatic			X	X	
Flulike aches and pains					X
Transmission					
Fecal-oral	X				X
Foodborne	X				X
Sexual	X	X		X	
Parenteral		X		X	
Perinatal		Rare			
Contaminated food or water	X				X
Blood or serum			X		
Sharing contaminated needles, tattooing/piercing equipment			X		
Co-infected with HBV				X	

BOX 14.1 Risk Factors for Hepatitis A Virus

- Travelers to areas where hepatitis A virus (HAV) is common
- Homosexual and male
- Sexual contact with infected people
- Use of injectable and noninjectable drugs
- Household contact with infected people
- Health care and public safety workers
- People, especially children, living in regions of the United States that have consistently increased rates of HAV

(Data from Centers for Disease Control and Prevention: *Hepatitis A*, Atlanta, Author. Accessed 31 August, 2020, from https://www.cdc.gov/hepatitis/hav/index.htm.)

BOX 14.2 Risk Factors for Hepatitis B Virus

- People with multiple sex partners or partners diagnosed with a sexually transmitted disease
- Homosexual men
- Sexual contact with infected people
- Use of injectable drugs
- Household contact with chronically infected people
- Infants born to infected mothers
- Infants and children of immigrants from areas with high rates of hepatitis B virus infection
- Health care and public safety workers
- Patients receiving hemodialysis treatments

(Data from Centers for Disease Control and Prevention: *Hepatitis B*, Atlanta, Author. Accessed 31 August, 2020, from https://www.cdc.gov/hepatitis/hbv/index.htm.)

dialysis, and those who have undergone organ transplantation are at increased risk for HBV (Box 14.2). As a result, routine HBV vaccination is recommended for risk groups of all ages and for children up to age 18. The average incubation time of HBV is approximately 12 weeks. As with HAV, most patients are asymptomatic. Those who acquire chronic HBV infection (determined by biopsy) can be healthy, asymptomatic carriers but remain infectious to others through parenteral or sexual transmission.

Chronic HBV is a major risk factor predisposing to hepatocellular carcinoma (HCC) (Sayiner et al., 2019). Chronic HBV is treated with interferon-α and lamivudine to reduce symptoms and prevent or delay progression of chronic hepatitis to cirrhosis or HCC. Hepatitis B immunoglobulin (HBIG) provides passive immunization. The hepatitis B vaccine is targeted to adolescents and adults in high-risk groups. Patients who need repeated transfusions, health care workers, patients and employees in hemodialysis centers, and nurses working in emergency departments or operating rooms should be vaccinated against HBV. Travelers to areas of the world where HBV is prevalent should be vaccinated; see the *Cultural Diversity and Nutrition* box Hepatitis B Virus Prevalence Among Underserved Areas.

CULTURAL DIVERSITY AND NUTRITION

Hepatitis B Virus Prevalence in Underserved Areas

Hepatitis B virus (HBV) occurs worldwide, especially where there are limited or primitive medical services. In Africa and Asia, widespread infection may occur in infancy and childhood. The overall carrier rates may be as high as 10% to 15%. HBV infection is prevalent in sub-Saharan Africa where many barriers prevent containment of the epidemic. An estimated 325 million people worldwide live with hepatitis B and/or C; for most, testing and treatment are not available (World Health Organization, 2020). In the United States, HBV infection is a significant racial health disparity; Asian Americans and Pacific Islanders make up more than 50% of those with HBV infection (Tang et al, 2018). Generally, in developed countries, HBV is more common in high-risk groups. Contaminated and inadequately sterilized syringes and needles have led to outbreaks of hepatitis B among patients in clinics, physicians' offices, tattoo parlors, and acupuncturists' offices. Occult HBV infection may occur in blood donors, especially immigrants.

Application to Nursing

Nurses working with clients who are at high risk for HBV can advocate for hepatitis B vaccinations for these individuals. Such clients include foreign-born individuals, individuals with alternative sexual orientation, people with histories of current or past drug abuse, and those exposed to or already diagnosed with human immunodeficiency virus.

(Data from Tang AS, et al: Disparities in Hepatitis B Virus Infection and Immunity Among New York City Asian American Patients, 1997 to 2017. *Am J Public Health* 108:S327–S335, 2018; World Health Organization: *Hepatitis.* Accessed 30 August, 2020, from https://www.who.int/health-topics/hepatits.)

Hepatitis C virus (HCV) infection is increasing worldwide and is the major form of hepatitis in the United States. It can be transmitted through contaminated saliva and semen, but HCV is predominantly associated with blood exposure (e.g., transfusion, IV drug use, acupuncture, tattooing, and sharing razors). Onset is usually slow (i.e., ~8 weeks). HCV can develop into some form of chronic liver disease and is a risk factor for liver cancer.

Most cases of acute HCV are asymptomatic and infrequently detected. Chronic infection develops in 70% to 80% of infected people. Progression from HCV to cirrhosis may take 10 to 40 years. A more rapid disease progression is observed in older persons, those infected with human immunodeficiency virus (HIV) or HBV, and alcoholics. Chronic HCV is treated with a combination therapy of interferon-α and ribavirin. No special diet is recommended.

Hepatitis D virus (HDV) can occur only if an individual with HBV is subsequently exposed to HDV (co-infection or superinfection). The incubation period is 21 to 45 days but may be shorter in cases of superinfection. Clinical course varies, ranging from acute, self-limiting infection to acute fulminant liver failure. HDV is most prevalent in the Mediterranean basin, Middle East, Amazon basin, and Asia. Of persons infected with HDV, 90% are likely to be asymptomatic. Parenteral transmission is understood to be the most common means of infection, making IV drug use a risk factor. Patients co-infected with HBV and HDV are less responsive to interferon therapy than patients infected with HBV alone. Diet does not need to be restricted.

Hepatitis E virus (HEV) is an enterically transmitted (oral-fecal route), self-limiting infection. The prevalence of HEV is generally attributed to travel in tropical climates, inadequate sanitation, and poor personal hygiene. The incubation period ranges from 15 to 60 days, and symptoms include myalgia, anorexia, nausea/vomiting, weight loss (typically 5–10 pounds), dehydration, jaundice, dark urine, and light-colored stools. Therapy should be predominantly preventive.

Travelers to endemic areas should avoid drinking water or other beverages that may be contaminated. Uncooked fruits and vegetables should not be eaten. No vaccines are available for HEV. Once infection occurs, therapy is limited to support.

Food and Nutrition Therapies

During periods of nausea and vomiting in patients with hepatitis, hydration via IV fluids may be necessary. Oral feedings should be initiated as soon as possible, with frequent feedings high in energy and high-quality protein to minimize loss of muscle mass. Adequate protein, 1.0 to 1.2 g/kg body weight, is recommended for most persons. Dietary fats should not be limited unless they are not well tolerated (e.g., steatorrhea).

Fluid intake should be adequate to accommodate the high protein intake unless otherwise contraindicated. Supplementation with a multivitamin that includes vitamin B complex (especially thiamin and vitamin B_{12} because of decreased absorption and hepatic uptake), vitamin K (to normalize bleeding tendency), vitamin C, and zinc for poor appetite is recommended. Abstinence from alcohol is imperative.

Application to nursing. Patients should receive adequate hydration and electrolyte repletion. Hospitalization may be necessary for those unable to maintain an adequate oral intake. Bed rest and proper nutrition are the major constituents of therapy for all types of hepatitis. Treatment goals are as follows:

- Decrease viral replication or eradicate the infection
- Delay fibrosis and progression to cirrhosis
- Decrease incidence of liver cancer
- Ameliorate fatigue and joint pain
- Prevent hepatic decompensation and the need for liver transplantation. See the *Teaching Tool* box Suggestions for Coping with Hepatitis.

Fatty Liver and Nonalcoholic Fatty Liver Disease

Fatty liver (hepatic steatosis) is an early form of liver disease that can be caused by alcoholism, obesity, complications of drug therapy (e.g., corticosteroids, tetracyclines), excessive parenteral nutrition, pregnancy, diabetes mellitus, inadequate intake of protein (in malnutrition), infection, or malignancy.

Nonalcoholic fatty liver disease (NAFLD) includes a spectrum of disorders from nonalcoholic fatty liver (NAFL) to nonalcoholic steatohepatitis (NASH), fibrosis, and eventually cirrhosis (Kabbany et al., 2017). NAFLD has become the most common form of liver disease in the United States and is the most frequent reason for liver transplantation (Sheka et al., 2020).

Food and Nutrition Therapies

A thorough diet history is essential, and a nutrition plan should be developed according to the etiology of the condition. If the problem is related to diabetes, glucose management requires carbohydrate counting. If the fatty liver occurs after initiation of parenteral nutrition, the amount and rate of administration should be altered.

Because there is no effective drug therapy for NAFLD, lifestyle interventions remain the first line of treatment. Some studies suggest exclusion of high-sugar foods and beverages (Schwimmer et al., 2019). Weight loss may be needed, but meals should not be skipped to lose weight rapidly.

Because this condition is common among the morbidly obese (body mass index [BMI] >40), bariatric surgery may be required. The effects of bariatric surgery, nutrition, pharmacotherapy, and immunosuppressive agents must be considered for patients who have NAFLD.

Application to nursing. A calorie-controlled diet limiting fats, simple sugars, fructose, and alcohol may be ordered. Adequate tracking of glucose and lipid levels will be needed. Whatever the cause, proper nutrition in the form of a well-balanced diet is important in reversing fatty infiltration. See the *Teaching Tool* box Suggestions for Coping With Fatty Liver or Nonalcoholic Steatohepatitis.

TEACHING TOOL

Suggestions for Coping With Hepatitis

- A nutritious diet that excludes alcohol is important.
- For many individuals, loss of appetite, weight loss, and fatigue are common problems. Recommend rest periods before and after meals.
- Offer guidance and tips for increasing protein and calories without adding more total food volume. Sauces, gravies, desserts, milkshakes, and similar enhancements will help.

TEACHING TOOL

Suggestions for Coping With Fatty Liver or Nonalcoholic Steatohepatitis

- A balanced diet is important. Eliminate alcohol and limit total intake of fat and fructose.
- The assistance of a registered dietitian will be needed to guide this nutrition care plan successfully.
- Probiotics or prebiotics may be beneficial, but the most effective strains have yet to be identified.

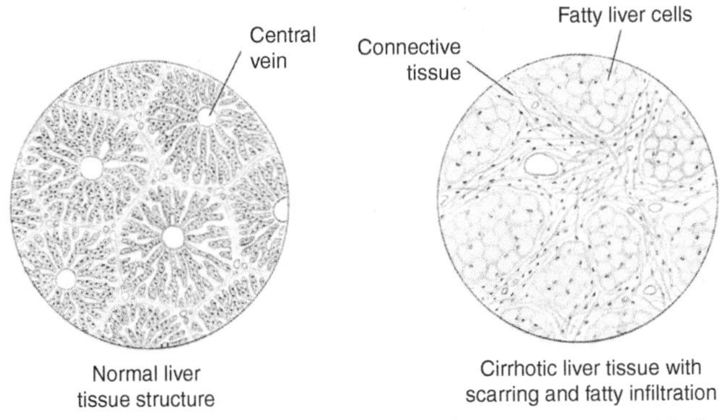

Fig. 14.2 Comparison of normal liver tissue structure with liver tissue changes from cirrhosis. (Medical and Scientific Illustration. From Nix S: *Williams' Basic nutrition and diet therapy*, ed 15, St. Louis, 2017, Elsevier Science.)

Cirrhosis

In cirrhosis, liver cells are replaced by fibrous connective tissue and fat infiltration (Fig. 14.2). This damage can occur for a variety of reasons, including the following:

- Hepatitis (postnecrotic cirrhosis)
- Biliary cirrhosis disorders
- Chronic autoimmune disease
- Metabolic disorders (Wilson's disease or hemochromatosis)
- Chronic hepatotoxic drug use
- Alcoholic cirrhosis (see the *Health Debate* box Alcohol: Prescribe? Proscribe?)

HEALTH DEBATE

Alcohol: Prescribe? Proscribe?

Alcohol is probably the most commonly-used hepatotoxic drug. Next to caffeine, it is the most socially acceptable drug in the United States. Alcohol is legal, but its sales are regulated by state-controlled establishments. One drink equals 12 ounces beer, 5 ounces wine, or 1½ ounces hard liquor.

Alcohol use is linked with birth defects, domestic violence, and traffic accidents. Heavy alcohol intake (3+ drinks daily) causes damage to the liver, brain, and heart and increases the risk of cancer. Chronic, heavy drinking is associated with cancers of the mouth, throat, larynx, and liver. Moderate drinking has been linked with breast, prostate, and rectal cancers.

Could any possible good come from such a drug? Studies suggest a lower coronary artery disease mortality risk among moderate drinkers (one or two drinks daily) than among nondrinkers. Resveratrol, flavonoids, and other antioxidants in red wine can potentially reduce heart disease risk, but they can also be found in other foods like grapes or red grape juice or blueberries (American Heart Association [AHA], 2020). Note that heavy drinking may lead to hypertension, obesity or stroke.

Remember, alcohol is a drug and the dangers of excess outweigh any benefits. The American Heart Association does not recommend drinking wine or any other form of alcohol to gain potential health benefits (AHA, 2020). The message is this: do not begin if you do not currently drink, have hypertension, are pregnant or trying to conceive, are taking medications, are driving, or are unable to control your drinking.

(Data from American Heart Association, https://www.heart.org/en/healthy-living/healthy-eating/eat-smart/nutrition-basics/alcohol-and-heart-health (Accessed 31 August, 2020).)

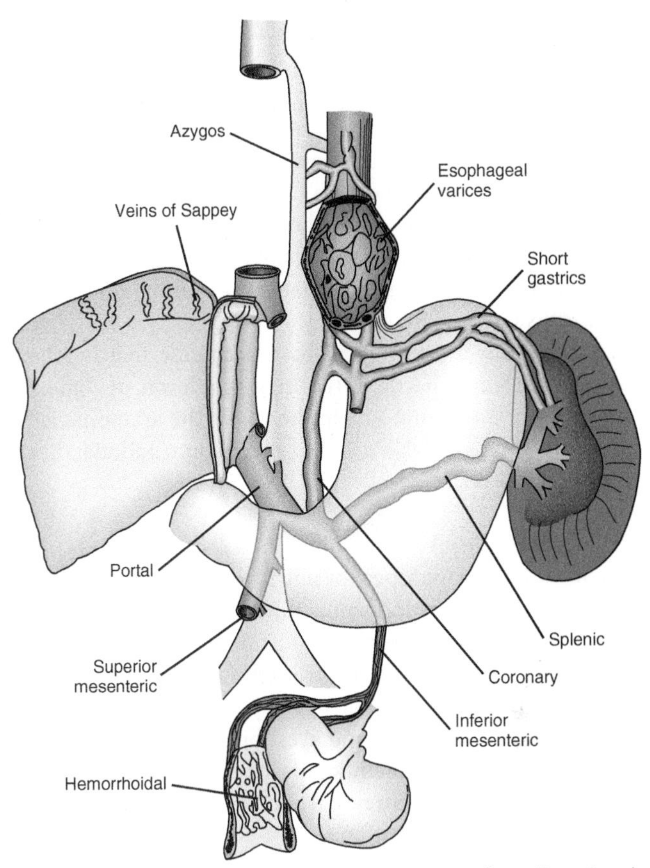

Fig. 14.3 Varices related to portal hypertension. Portal vein, its major tributaries, and the most important shunts (collateral veins) between the portal and caval systems. (Redrawn from Linder J, Damjanov I, editors: *Anderson's pathology*, ed 10, St. Louis, 1996, Elsevier.)

Liver cell scarring can cause congestion of hepatic circulation (backing up of blood in the portal vein), which results in further decline of liver function and portal hypertension. Blood vessels tend to enlarge and bulge into the lumen of the esophagus, where they may rupture. Esophageal varices can occur; they are the result of collateral circulation that develops around the esophagus when normal blood flow through the liver is blocked (Fig. 14.3). The bleeding tends to recur and can eventually be fatal.

Another complication, ascites, is the accumulation of fluid in the peritoneal cavity. Fluid is trapped in the characteristic swollen or distended abdomen seen in patients with cirrhosis. As liver disease continues to progress, blood is shunted from portal circulation to systemic circulation. This causes blood to bypass the liver, perhaps even leading to hepatic coma.

Hepatic encephalopathy is a "cerebral intoxication" caused by intestinal contents that have not been metabolized by the liver. In this condition, ammonia cannot be eliminated from the body. Patients experience changes in consciousness and behavior, loss of concentration and memory, confusion, apathy, personality changes, and other psychiatric symptoms. Neurologic changes include spasticity, muscle spasms, asterixis or flapping (involuntary jerky movements, especially of the hands), and rigidity of the limbs with flexion withdrawal of the lower limbs.

Neomycin is used to reduce the numbers of bacteria in the gastrointestinal (GI) tract, thus decreasing the amount of urea that can be converted to ammonia. Neomycin treatment allows more protein to be included in the diet for tissue regeneration, although protein intake might be mildly restricted. One disadvantage of neomycin is that it contributes to malabsorption of most nutrients and can cause nausea, vomiting, diarrhea, and nephrotoxicity.

Lactulose is a nonabsorbable disaccharide that is metabolized by intestinal bacteria, resulting in a lower-pH stool. The lowered pH traps ammonia in the colon; the ammonia is then excreted. This agent also has a laxative action, and diarrhea is a common side effect.

Food and Nutrition Therapies

The most important aspect of nutrition therapy for cirrhosis is that each patient has individual nutritional needs that must be addressed. Protein-energy malnutrition is common in patients with end-stage liver disease with cirrhosis. A minimum of 0.8 g protein per kg body weight per day is essential. To promote positive nitrogen balance and avert breakdown of endogenous protein stores, 1.2 g protein/kg dry or appropriate body weight is recommended. Protein restriction should be avoided because it could worsen malnutrition.

If a patient appears to be protein-sensitive with increased encephalopathy, branched-chain amino acid–based formulas with restricted aromatic amino acids can ensure a sustained level of protein intake. Plant proteins from legumes or vegetables also produce less ammonia.

Patients with esophageal varices should eat soft, low-fiber foods. For ascites, a dietary sodium restriction (2000 mg) is used, usually with a fluid restriction. When diuretics are used, attention should be given to whether the drug depletes or spares potassium. If a potassium-depleting diuretic is used, potassium levels must be monitored carefully.

Application to nursing. Fluids are given in accordance with input and output (I&O), shifts in daily weights, and electrolyte values. Fluid restrictions are often necessary, starting with 1500 mL per day. Limits may decrease to 1000 to 1200 mL per day, depending on the patient's response. The nurse may provide suggestions on how to cope with thirst to improve patient compliance with these kinds of fluid restrictions. See the *Teaching Tool* box Suggestions for Coping With Fluid Restriction.

TEACHING TOOL

Suggestions for Coping With Fluid Restriction

1. Salty and spicy foods make you thirsty; limit the amount of sodium and spicy foods in your diet.
2. Be aware of hidden fluids in foods: gelatin, watermelon, soup, gravy, and frozen treats like popsicles and ice cream.
3. Stay cool, especially in warmer weather. Try drinking cold liquids instead of hot beverages.
4. Try snacking on approved vegetables and fruits that are ice cold.
5. Sip your beverages; use small cups or glasses for your beverages.
6. Drink to quench thirst only. Avoid drinking from habit or to be sociable.
7. Sliced lemon wedges can stimulate saliva and moisten a dry mouth.
8. Keep your mouth clean by brushing teeth frequently and rinsing mouth with water (do not swallow rinse water).
9. Battle dry mouth. Chew gum, suck sour hard candies, or use mints to stimulate saliva flow.
10. Freeze the allotted amount of fluid as ice. Sucking on ice is satisfying because it stays in the mouth longer. Add lemon to the ice cubes.
11. Limit fluids at mealtime; when appropriate, take medications with mealtime liquids or soft foods like applesauce.
12. Take medications with applesauce instead of liquid.
13. Take a small amount of fluid at one time.
14. If allowable, use high-fat foods such as gravies and margarine to moisten foods and make them easier to swallow.
15. If you have diabetes, maintain good blood glucose levels. High blood glucose levels will increase your thirst.

(Data from Davita: *Fluid control for kidney disease patients on dialysis.* From https://www.davita.com/diet-nutrition/articles/basics/fluid-control-for-kidney-disease-patients-on-dialysis. Accessed 31 August, 2020; National Kidney Foundation. *Thirst Tips for Dialysis Patients.* From https://www.kidney.org/newsletter/thirst-tips-dialysis-patients. Accessed 31 August, 2020.)

Liver Transplantation

Liver transplantation is regarded as an appropriate treatment for end-stage liver disease. Nutritional goals for the patient awaiting a liver transplant depend on the individual's weight history and status. Most patients in this condition show some indications of compromised nutritional status and therefore require special attention to nutritional needs.

It is difficult to assess nutritional status in patients with liver disorders because many parameters (e.g., body weight, nitrogen balance determination, total lymphocyte count, serum protein levels) are affected by edema, ascites, and hepatic necrosis. Therefore, it may be more appropriate to use subjective parameters, such as appetite, satiety level, taste changes, diet history, and GI symptoms. Weight change, however, is more often a reflection of fluid shifts rather than true weight loss. Physical examination findings such as temporal wasting of muscle and wasting of the upper extremities can be helpful to estimate the degree of malnutrition.

Food and Nutrition Therapies

Each phase of the transplantation procedure dictates specific nutritional requirements (Table 14.2). The primary objective in pretransplantation nutrition therapy is to provide enough calories and protein to decrease protein catabolism and correct any nutritional deficiencies. The 4 to 8 weeks after surgery—the immediate posttransplantation period—require individualization of nutrition therapy according to the patient's needs. Ascites, edema, and excess fluid make using the patient's actual weight unreliable for determining energy and protein needs. Ideal (desirable) weight is a better reference point.

Adequate calories and protein are necessary for the stresses that result from surgery and high doses of glucocorticoids. Early enteral nutrition is recommended where possible. However, parenteral nutrition may be necessary if nutritional needs cannot be met from oral diet or tube feeding. When oral intake is

TABLE 14.2 Nutrition Care Guidelines After Liver Transplantation

Nutrients/Fluids	Short Term	Long Term
Energy	1.2–1.5 × BEE (use higher range if patient is severely underweight)	1.2–1.3 × BEE or as adequate to maintain weight
Protein	1.5–2 g/kg/day	0.8–1 g/kg
Carbohydrate		20–30 g dietary fiber/day
Fat		25%–35% kcal <10% kcal from saturated fats
Vitamins	History of alcoholism could suggest deficiencies in vitamins A, B_6, and B_{12}, niacin, thiamine, and folate	Recommended dietary allowance (RDA) amounts
	History of cholestatic liver disease could suggest preexisting deficiencies of fat-soluble vitamins and B_{12}	Consider supplementation/restriction based on pretransplantation condition and diagnosis or posttransplantation complications
Minerals	Provide RDA in consideration of medical history	RDA
Electrolytes		Sodium <4 g/day Monitor potassium, phosphorus, magnesium Supplement/restrict as needed
Fluids	30–35 mL/kg, adjusting for increased losses or decreased needs	30–35 mL/kg; requirements higher in hot climates or with fever
Common Long-Term Complications	**Nutrition Care**	
Excessive weight gain	Reduce kcal intake; aerobic exercise three to five times a week; reduce corticosteroid dose as able	
Hyperlipidemia	Recommendations as above; change corticosteroid to tacrolimus; lipid-lowering medication used with caution	
Diabetes mellitus	Diet and insulin or oral hypoglycemic agent to maintain glycemic control (fasting glucose <125 mg/dL, hemoglobin A_{1C} <7%); blood glucose self-monitoring; aerobic exercise three to five times a week; reduction of corticosteroid doses as possible	
Osteoporosis	1000–1500 mg calcium/day; vitamin D supplements; weight-bearing exercise; discontinuation of smoking; moderate sodium and protein intake; hormone replacement therapy when appropriate	

BEE, Basal energy expenditure.
(Data from Hasse JM: Adult liver transplantation. In Hasse JM, Blue LS, editors: *Comprehensive guide to transplant nutrition*, Chicago, 2002, American Dietetic Association.)

initiated, early satiety and altered tastes may prevent adequate intake. In such cases, between-meal feedings or supplements should be used to meet calorie and protein goals. Fluid losses from drains, nasogastric tubes, stool output, and urine should be considered in the determination of postoperative fluid needs.

Application to nursing. Over the long term after liver transplantation, a healthy, well-balanced diet is the nutrition goal. Because of common posttransplantation complications (e.g., excessive weight gain, hypertension, hyperlipidemia, diabetes), adjustments in intake of calories, fat, and concentrated carbohydrates may be necessary. See the *Teaching Tool* box Suggestions for Coping With Transplantation.

TEACHING TOOL

Suggestions for Coping With Transplantation

- Patients will experience anxiety and depression after their transplantation.
- Support groups, social support, or therapy may be needed to improve quality of life.
- Patients will need follow-up nutrition counseling if they have diabetes or are obese.

GALLBLADDER DISORDERS

The gallbladder and the hepatic, cystic, and common bile ducts compose the biliary system (Fig. 14.4). Bile is transported from the liver to the gallbladder via the common hepatic duct system, where

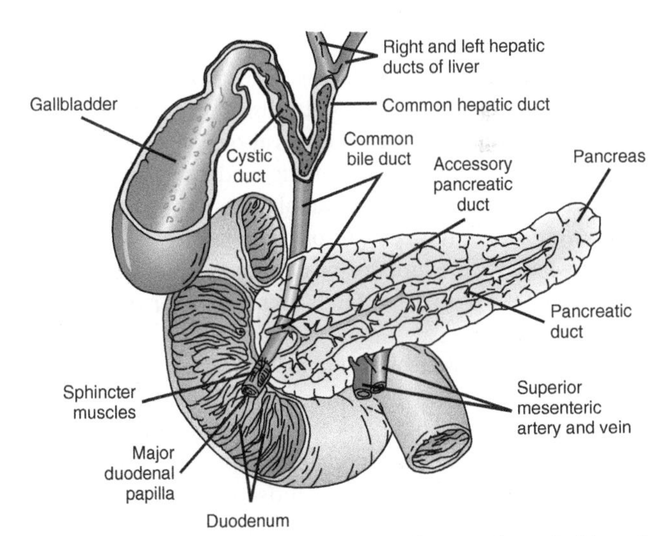

Fig. 14.4 Gallbladder and bile ducts. Obstruction of either the hepatic or the common bile duct by stone or spasm prevents bile from being ejected into the duodenum. (From Rolin Graphics.)

it is concentrated and stored until being released into the duodenum. Bile expedites absorption of fats, fat-soluble vitamins, and certain minerals and activates the release of pancreatic enzymes.

One of the main constituents of bile is cholesterol, which is also a major constituent of gallstones (cholelithiasis). Cholelithiasis affects 15% of the population in the United States, especially women and individuals who are obese or have metabolic syndrome

BOX 14.3 Risk Factors in Gallbladder Disease

- Age ≥60 years
- Diabetes
- Diet that is high fat, high cholesterol, and/or low fiber
- Enzyme defects (mucin) and *LITH* gene
- American Indian or Mexican American ethnicity
- Family history of gallstones
- Female gender
- Hormonal imbalance (estrogen, progestin, insulin)
- Losing weight very quickly
- Medications (estrogen or oral contraceptives; clofibrate, cholestyramine, cholesterol-lowering)
- Obesity
- Pregnancy

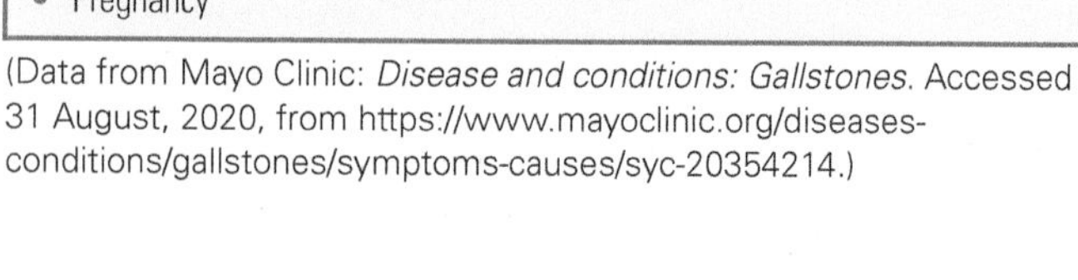

(Data from Mayo Clinic: *Disease and conditions: Gallstones.* Accessed 31 August, 2020, from https://www.mayoclinic.org/diseases-conditions/gallstones/symptoms-causes/syc-20354214.)

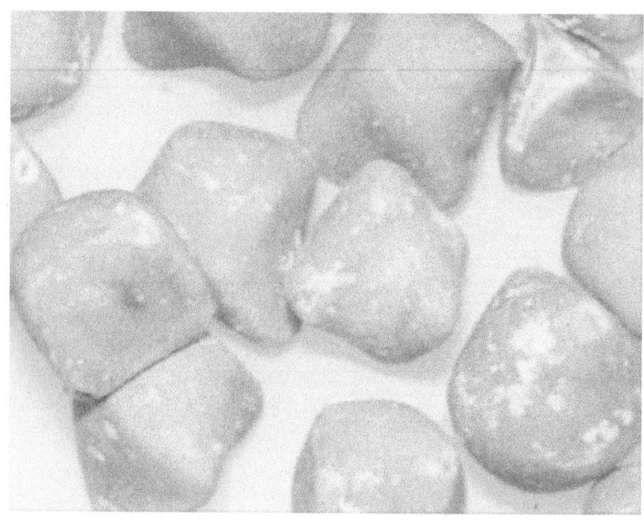

Fig. 14.5 Gallstones. (From Lowe J, Anderson P, Anderson S: *Stevens and Lowes' Human histology*, ed 5, London, 2020, Elsevier.)

(Littlefield & Lenahan, 2019). Gallstones are also found in women who are multiparous, are undergoing estrogen therapy, or use oral contraceptives; individuals with sedentary lifestyles; the aged; and those who have diabetes mellitus (Box 14.3).

Most gallstones are "silent" (asymptomatic). When cholelithiasis is asymptomatic, no specific therapy is necessary. Individuals who experience symptoms may have an inflamed gallbladder (acute cholecystitis). Symptoms usually manifest after consumption of a high-fat meal, with a mild, aching pain in the mid-epigastrium that may increase in intensity. Because the gallbladder lies directly beneath the right lobe of the liver, pain may radiate to the right upper quadrant and right subscapular region. Nausea, vomiting, tachycardia, and diaphoresis also may be present.

Gallstones form because of genetic tendencies, supersaturation of cholesterol in bile, and gallbladder hypomotility (after rapid weight loss). The amount of cholesterol in bile is determined in part by the amount of dietary fat consumed. Thus, long-term intake of high-fat foods increases the risk for cholelithiasis (Fig. 14.5).

People who lose a great deal of weight rapidly through very low-calorie diets (VLCDs) and some commercial weight-loss programs are at a high risk for development of gallstones. Following a diet too low in fat or going for long periods without eating (e.g., skipping breakfast) will decrease gallbladder contractions. If the gallbladder does not contract often enough to empty out the bile, gallstones form. People considering losing a significant amount of weight should see a physician to evaluate their medical history, individual circumstances, and the proposed method of weight loss.

Cholecystitis occurs when gallstones block the cystic duct or as the result of stasis, bacterial infection, or ischemia of the gallbladder. This inflammation is associated with pain, tenderness, and fever. Fat intolerance may manifest as regurgitation, flatulence, belching, epigastric heaviness, indigestion, heartburn, chronic upper abdominal pain, and nausea. Jaundice and steatorrhea may also be present. Recommended therapy for symptomatic cholelithiasis and cholecystitis is surgical removal of the gallbladder (cholecystectomy). Most patients can undergo laparoscopic surgery for this procedure.

Food and Nutrition Therapies

The main objective of nutritional care is to decrease the patient's discomfort. Most patients become acutely aware of foods that cause discomfort and thus avoid them. Individual food intolerances vary widely, but many patients omit foods that cause flatulence and bloating. During an acute attack, the hospitalized patient may receive IV fluids with nothing orally.

Avoiding fat is often advised, but no strong evidence supports this recommendation. It is better to recommend increased intake of fatty fish such as salmon, herring, mackerel, and tuna. Intake of omega-3 polyunsaturated fatty acids (PUFAs) influences bile composition, decreasing biliary cholesterol saturation (Pasternak et al., 2017).

Application to nursing. After cholecystectomy, bile enters the small intestine continually rather than in response to food in the GI tract. Immediately after an open laparotomy cholecystectomy, patients may be given liquids until they can tolerate a regular diet. See the *Teaching Tool* box Suggestions for Coping With Gallbaldder Disorders.

TEACHING TOOL
Suggestions for Coping With Gallbladder Disorders

- Without symptoms, a wait-and-see approach is recommended.
- For mild symptoms, follow a low-fat diet and lose weight slowly; the advice of a registered dietitian may be beneficial.
- For acute symptoms with pain and fever, most patients are hospitalized for antibiotic therapy and pain management.
- If surgery is needed, laparoscopy is quite simple. See the *Personal Perspectives box* Cholecystectomy Before Laparoscopy.

PERSONAL PERSPECTIVES

Cholecystectomy Before Laparoscopy

I was just 25 years old, having taken the Graduate Record Examination (GRE) on a snowy Saturday in Pennsylvania. I lived on the top of a steep hill, so driving to and from the examination on slippery roads had made me even more anxious than the test itself. Finally, relief was in sight ... but not for long! That night, after going to bed, I was awakened with severe colicky pain and nausea. Maybe it was an ulcer, or even a heart attack from the recent stress! Fortunately, I was working as a clinical dietitian at the local hospital and saw my own doctor at work the following Monday. He immediately scheduled an x-ray examination for me. Surprisingly, they found gallstones. The radiologist made a joke (he thought) by saying, "Ah, too many French fries!" But I knew better. My diet was healthy, except for skipping some meals and attempting to maintain a low body weight. I had been taking hormones to manage my irregular periods for several years, and most of the adult women in my family had already had gallbladder surgery.

I had surgery the following summer, certain that it would be an easy recovery. I even asked the doctor whether I could leave the hospital the night before my surgery to go for my usual 2-mile run. Overconfidence about the surgery reigned. But after the procedure, the pain was debilitating. The incision was about 10 inches long, and I had to wear an abdominal support brace to be comfortable at home and back at work. The healing process took longer than I had expected, and I can honestly say there was abdominal pain in the scar area for a year after the surgery. Wearing any type of two-piece bathing suit became a thing of the past. Thus, when laparoscopy became available, I encouraged that procedure for patients who must undergo cholecystectomy.

Sylvia Escott-Stump
Winterville, NC

PANCREATIC DISORDERS

Pancreatitis

The pancreas secretes hormones such as insulin and glucagon for glucose homeostasis. In addition to hormonal functions, the pancreas secretes enzymes necessary for protein, carbohydrate, and fat digestion. The pancreas also secretes sodium bicarbonate to neutralize acidic gastric contents as they enter the duodenum, providing the optimal pH for the activation of these enzymes.

Pancreatitis is an inflammatory process characterized by decreased production of digestive enzymes and bicarbonate, causing malabsorption of fats and proteins. This acute inflammation causes the local blood vessels to become exceptionally permeable, leaking fluid and plasma proteins into spaces between the cells. Edema and damage result.

Pancreatic enzymes are ordinarily secreted into the intestinal lumen, where they are activated. However, if the pancreas is damaged, the enzymes are retained and activated within the pancreas, resulting in a form of autodigestion with severe pain. When the enzymes amylase and lipase cannot be secreted into the intestine, they accumulate in the bloodstream. Thus, a highly elevated serum amylase value is an indication of pancreatitis.

Acute pancreatitis is commonly caused by excessive alcohol consumption or gallbladder disease. Chronic pancreatitis is often associated with chronic alcohol consumption, smoking or genetics and is characterized by chronic pain with exocrine and endocrine insufficiency. Diabetes mellitus can occur as the result of chronic pancreatitis if beta cells are damaged, thus decreasing insulin production. Autoimmune pancreatitis (AIP) is an immunoglobulin systemic disease that may respond to therapy with corticosteroids (Madhani & Farrell, 2016).

Food and Nutrition Therapies

The primary goal in acute pancreatitis is to provide nutrition while minimizing pancreatic secretions. Clinical evidence indicates that parenteral nutrition administered within 24 hours of admission worsens the outcome by increasing inflammation and impairing the immune response. Bowel rest leads to atrophy of intestinal mucosa and bacterial translocation. In contrast, early introduction of enteral nutrition promotes fewer infections, shorter hospital stays, and overall decreased medical costs.

Feeding into the lower small bowel, in the jejunum distal to the ligament of Treitz, bypasses the areas associated with pancreatic stimulation. Low-fat, enteral formulas are recommended. Patients receiving enteral feedings should be closely monitored for increases in pancreatic enzyme levels, abdominal pain, and discomfort. Enteral feedings should be terminated if any of these symptoms occurs.

Chronic pancreatitis patients can experience long-term sequelae, such as diabetes (38%–40%) and exocrine insufficiency (30%–48%), for which dietary changes may be needed (Singh et al., 2019). In general, parenteral nutrition is avoided. The use of pancreatic enzymes and antioxidants (a combination of multivitamins, selenium, and methionine) may control symptoms in up to 50% of patients (Singh et al., 2019). Surgery is a last resort.

Application to nursing. The first 24 hours after admission for acute pancreatitis require rapid response. Evidence-based guidelines are used to manage severe pain, nausea, and vomiting. Goal-directed therapy, nutrition support and management of complications are best practice; surgery is no longer an initial treatment (Hines et al., 2019).

Early enteral feeding within 24 to 48 hours is important, using standard formulas through gastric or jejunal tube placement (Ramanathan & Aadam, 2019). Elemental formulas and parenteral nutrition are not advised. See the *Teaching Tool* box Suggestions for Coping With Pancreatitis.

TEACHING TOOL

Suggestions for Coping With Pancreatitis

- A medium-chain triglyceride (MCT) product such as MCT oil may be used to increase calories if needed.
- Consuming small meals in six feedings daily may facilitate adequate nutritional intake.
- In some cases, replacement pancreatic enzymes are taken orally with meals to control maldigestion and malabsorption.
- Complete abstinence from alcohol is essential.
- Eat a high-protein, nutrient-dense diet that includes fruits, vegetables, whole grains, low-fat dairy, and other lean protein sources. A multivitamin supplement is also beneficial.

SUMMARY

- The liver, gallbladder, and pancreas are important organs for proper digestion.
- Disorders of the liver include hepatitis, an inflammation of the liver, and cirrhosis, a chronic degenerative disease that causes fibrous connective tissue and fat infiltration of the liver.
- Nutrition therapy consists of bed rest and proper nutrition for hepatitis and individual nutrition plans for cirrhosis that ease liver function.
- Meeting nutrition therapy needs while still providing for adequate energy and Recommended Dietary Allowance nutrient levels is challenging.
- Liver transplantations occur as treatment for end-stage liver disease, with specific nutrition therapies at each stage.
- Gallbladder disorders are characterized by the formation of gallstones within the gallbladder. Cholecystitis involves acute inflammation as well.
- Patients with gallbladder disease may require low-fat diets or calorie-controlled diets, but not all individuals gain relief from them.
- Pancreatitis affects production of digestive secretions, resulting in malabsorption of dietary fats and protein.

Note that in serious cases, pancreatitis requires enteral or parenteral nutrition support. If tube feeding is used, tube placement into the jejunum is tolerated.

THE NURSING APPROACH

Clinical Judgment and Next-Generation NCLEX® Examination-Style Questions

Case Study 1

Cirrhosis of the Liver

Eric, aged 50 years, was diagnosed with cirrhosis subsequent to chronic hepatitis. As the liver damage progressed, he had frequent hospitalizations. At this admission, he is being treated with diuretics because of ascites (fluid in the peritoneal cavity) and peripheral edema. He is receiving lactulose to reduce levels of ammonia because of hepatic encephalopathy. The doctor has prescribed a 2000-kcal, 40-g protein, 1-g sodium diet with fluids restricted to 1200 mL per day.

Assessment/Recognize Cues

Subjective (From Patient Statements)

- "I don't have any appetite. You wouldn't either if you were feeling sick to your stomach and throwing up."
- "I'm thirsty."
- "Just leave me alone. Where am I anyway?"
- "Is it nighttime? I can't remember what I was doing."
- Usual weight 205 pounds when he doesn't have ascites.

Objective (From Physical Examination)

- Present weight 210 pounds
- Dark amber urine, jaundice of skin, and sclera
- Abdominal distention, ascites
- Peripheral edema in ankles and lower legs
- Muscle wasting of upper extremities and thighs
- Enlargement of the liver seen on radiograph
- Laboratory test results: Normal blood urea nitrogen, normal hematocrit, low albumin, and elevated liver enzymes
- Disoriented to date, time, and place

Diagnoses (Nursing)/Analyze Cues

1. Imbalanced nutrition: less than body requirements related to anorexia and nausea and vomiting, as evidenced by muscle wasting and loss of true body weight
2. Excess fluid volume related to intrahepatic pressure and decreased colloidal osmotic pressure, as evidenced by ascites and peripheral edema
3. Acute confusion related to toxicities in the brain, as evidenced by agitation; disorientation to date, time, and place; and short-term memory loss

Planning/Prioritize Hypotheses

Patient Outcomes

Short term (at the end of 1 week):

- Eating meals well
- Decrease of jaundice, nausea, and vomiting
- Loss of 1500 mL of body fluids, as evidenced by weight 207 pounds (loss of 3 pounds), output greater than intake on records, and decreases in abdominal girth and ankle edema
- Slight decrease of liver enzymes, and electrolytes within normal ranges
- No further muscle wasting of extremities
- Oriented to date, time, and place and calmer

Nursing Interventions/Generate Solutions

1. Provide 2000-kcal diet with protein, sodium, and water restrictions as ordered.
2. Facilitate loss of excess fluid.
3. Orient Eric frequently.

Implementation/Take Action

1. Asked the dietitian to assess Eric's nutritional status and food preferences to optimally implement the diet of 2000 kcal, 40 g protein, and 1 g sodium, with 1200-mL fluid restriction.
   With patient assessment, the dietitian can individualize complex diets.
2. Helped deliver small frequent meals with high kcal, high carbohydrates, moderate fats, and restricted proteins (following the plan of the dietitian).
   Patients with nausea and distended abdomens usually tolerate small, frequent meals better than large meals. High kcal is needed for healing and prevention of catabolism of body proteins. Fat contains high kcal and fat-soluble vitamins but may not be metabolized well, causing steatorrhea (fat in the stools). Protein is needed for healing, but excess could increase ammonia production and make encephalopathy worse.
3. Removed noxious odors and unpleasant objects from the room before meals and gave antiemetic medication as ordered.
   Unpleasant smells and sights can trigger nausea, thus leading to anorexia. Antiemetics are given to prevent vomiting.
4. Restricted sodium to 1 g and planned with Eric how to restrict fluids to 1200 mL/day (300 mL with meals and 300 mL total between meals). Posted

Continued

THE NURSING APPROACH—cont'd

the plan on the bulletin board by Eric's bed and taught him, his family, and nursing staff the reasons for the fluid restriction.

Sodium is limited to decrease fluid retention. Fluid restriction is necessary to decrease portal hypertension, ascites, and peripheral edema. Involving the patient in planning encourages commitment and a sense of control. Dietary restrictions are easier to follow when purposes are understood. Written communication of the plan helps coordinate efforts.

5. Gave Eric ice, hard candy, and lemon wedges to reduce thirst.
   Thirst is minimized by spacing out fluid intake and providing treats that can dissolve slowly in the mouth.
6. Allowed no alcohol intake.
   Alcohol would further damage the liver and add to the patient's confusion.
7. Oriented Eric frequently to date, time, and place and gave him simple instructions and reminders. Wrote the date and name of the nurse on the white board by the patient's bed and clock.
   Confused patients become less agitated when told where they are, even if they forget quickly what the nurse just told them.
8. Asked dietary staff for herbs and spices that could be put on Eric's low-sodium food for flavoring.
   Low-sodium foods are bland without additional flavoring.
9. Provided supplemental vitamins and liquids (such as Ensure and Ensure Plus).
   Nutrient-dense supplements increase nourishment and kcal. Drinking liquid nourishment requires less energy than chewing foods.
10. Gave diuretic medicines as ordered.
    Diuretics cause increased urine output, thus reducing body fluids, ascites, and peripheral edema.
11. Gave lactulose as ordered.
    Ammonia is produced when intestinal bacteria metabolize protein. Ammonia going to the brain (because the liver cannot detoxify it) contributes to hepatic encephalopathy. Lactulose is a synthetic nonabsorbable disaccharide that is given to reduce ammonia in the intestines. Lactulose is metabolized in the intestines, releasing organic acids and lowering the pH; this enables trapping of ammonia in the stool, where it can be excreted. Lactulose also causes diarrhea, limiting time for intestinal bacteria to produce ammonia.
12. Carefully measured and recorded intake and output each shift; measured and recorded patient weights and abdominal girth daily.
    Ongoing assessment of fluid balance helps evaluate effectiveness of treatment.
13. Monitored laboratory reports for changes.
    Diarrhea from lactulose may lead to loss of fluids and electrolytes. Some diuretics cause loss of potassium.

Evaluation/Evaluate Outcomes

At the end of 1 week:

- Eating meals well
- No change in muscle wasting of extremities
- Jaundice, nausea, and vomiting decreased
- Liver enzymes slightly decreased and electrolytes within normal ranges
- Quickly forgot about his water restriction even with frequent reminders
- Exceeded water intake (about 1400 mL rather than 1200 mL per day)
- Body fluids decreased by 1000 mL, as evidenced by weight of 208 pounds (loss of 2 pounds), output greater than intake on records, and decreased abdominal girth and ankle edema
- Oriented to place but not date and time

Goals partially met.

Discussion Questions

During a follow-up appointment with the physician, the nurse asked Eric how he was doing with his diet. His response was "Not very well. I really don't know what foods I am supposed to eat."

1. What other questions should the nurse ask? What patient problem will the nurse probably identify?
2. Should the nurse suggest to the doctor that he refer Eric to a dietitian? Why?

Case Study 2

The nurse is discharging an adult patient who was admitted with a diagnosis of pancreatitis. To help the patient minimize the risk of redeveloping pancreatitis, the nurse provides health teaching.

Use an **X** for the health teaching below that is **Indicated** (appropriate or necessary), **Contraindicated** (could be harmful), or **Nonessential** (makes no difference or not necessary) before the patient's discharge at this time.

	Health Teaching	Indicated	Contraindicated	Nonessential
1.	Eat a low-protein diet.			
2.	Remember the primary goal in pancreatitis is to provide nutrition while minimizing pancreatic secretions.			
3.	Cut down alcohol intake to one glass of wine a day.			
4.	Get 8–10 hours of sleep a night.			
5.	Take a multivitamin supplement daily.			
6.	Consume small meals in four feedings daily to facilitate adequate nutritional intake.			
7.	Exercise daily as tolerated.			
8.	Take replacement pancreatic enzymes orally between meals to control maldigestion and malabsorption.			

CRITICAL THINKING

Clinical Applications

Chronic alcohol abuse is usually the cause of chronic liver disease (cirrhosis and hepatic encephalopathy) and chronic pancreatitis. One way to evaluate the risk of alcohol-related liver disease is to assess the pattern, quantity, and duration of alcohol intake; usual dietary intake; and socioeconomic factors affecting eating habits. Data can be collected from the patient or a reliable friend or family member and evaluated to determine amount (grams) and the kcal value of alcohol consumed. When consumed in large quantities, alcohol can provide the majority of the day's kcal intake. Professionals working with individuals who consume excessive amounts of alcohol advise that self-reported intakes may constitute about half of what is actually consumed. Therefore, double-checking any information obtained from a patient about alcohol intake with a reliable family member or friend is recommended.

Alcohol provides 7 kcal/g.[a] The average percent alcohol content (based on weight per volume) of various forms of alcoholic beverages is as follows:

Beer = 4% to 6%

Wine = 9% to 12%

Distilled alcohol (whiskey, rum, gin, or brandy) = 35% to 50%

The concentration of alcohol in distilled beverages (hard liquor) is usually referred to as proof. One proof equals 0.5% alcohol, which means that 80-proof tequila contains 40% alcohol. Hard liquor is routinely measured in a jigger or shot, which holds 1½ ounces or 45 mL.

1. How many grams of alcohol and kcal would two shots of 80-proof tequila provide?
2. What is the best way to obtain information from an individual about their alcohol consumption?
3. You obtain the following information from the alcohol intake questionnaire and diet history: Alcohol is consumed 7 days/week at home, work, and bars. A typical day's intake consists of a bloody Mary (1 cup tomato juice, two shots 80-proof vodka) first thing in the morning, followed by 5 cups of black coffee (some at home, some at work). Three more shots of 80-proof vodka are consumed at work. Lunch is usually a fast-food double cheeseburger, small fries, and a cup of black coffee. After work, four 12-ounce bottles of beer 4% alcohol) and pretzels (about 30) are consumed at the local bar with friends. Dinner at home consists of a lunchmeat sandwich (usually two slices white bread, 2 ounces bologna, 1 teaspoon mustard), 10 potato chips, and two more 12-ounce beers. Total intake for the day is approximately 3200 kcal.
   a. How many grams of alcohol are consumed? __________ grams alcohol
   b. How many kcal are provided by the alcohol? __________ kcal from alcohol
   c. What percent of the kcal are provided by alcohol? __________ % energy from alcohol

Alcohol Intake Assessment Tool

1. How many days a week do you drink alcoholic beverages?
   Circle number of days: 0 1 2 3 4 5 6 7
2. Where do you drink? Circle all that apply:
   a. At home
   b. At a friend's
   c. At a bar
   d. At work
   e. In the car
   f. Other (specify)
3. Which alcoholic beverages do you consume? Circle all that apply:
   a. Beer
   b. Wine
   c. Sherry or port
   d. Gin
   e. Whiskey
   f. Vodka
   g. Rum
   h. Other (specify)
4. How do you determine how much you drink? Circle all that apply:
   a. Count the number of beer cans
   b. Count the number of wine glasses
   c. Count the number of shots poured
   d. Count the number of bottles of wine
   e. Count the number of bottles of liquor used a day or week
   f. I don't know exactly how much I drink
   g. Other method of deciding alcohol intake (specify)
5. On any drinking day, how many drinks do you have?
   Circle letter(s) indicating drinks consumed and number within each category consumed to indicate number of drinks per day:

a. Beer	1	2	3	4	5	>5
b. White, red, or rosé wine	1	2	3	4	5	>5
c. Sherry or port	1	2	3	4	5	>5
d. Gin	1	2	3	4	5	>5
e. Whiskey	1	2	3	4	5	>5
f. Vodka	1	2	3	4	5	>5
g. Rum	1	2	3	4	5	>5
h. Other (specify)	1	2	3	4	5	>5

6. For how long have you been drinking this quantity?
7. Do you drink this amount on a regular basis?

[a]Any beverages used as mixers should be included in the estimated kcal intake.

WEBSITES OF INTEREST

Alcoholics Anonymous

http://www.aa.org

Dedicated to the self-help approach for overcoming alcoholism, including links for teenagers, newcomers, health professionals, and the AA Grapevine.

American Liver Foundation

www.liverfoundation.org

Devoted to research, education, and support groups related to hepatitis and all liver diseases.

Centers for Disease Control and Prevention (CDC)

http://www.cdc.gov/hepatitis

Useful for obtaining tips and statistics for the five types of hepatitis.

National Institute on Alcohol Abuse and Alcoholism

https://www.niaaa.nih.gov

Provides leadership for the national effort to reduce alcohol-related problems through research, collaborative endeavors of agencies and organizations, and educational resources.

REFERENCES

Hines, O. J., et al. (2019). Management of severe acute pancreatitis. *BMJ (Clinical Research ed.)*, *2*, 367.

Kabbany, M. N., et al. (2017). Prevalence of nonalcoholic steatohepatitis-associated cirrhosis in the United States: an analysis of national health and nutrition examination survey data. *The American Journal of Gastroenterology*, *112*, 581–587.

Littlefield, A., & Lenahan, C. (2019). Cholelithiasis: Presentation and management. *Journal of Midwifery*, *64*, 289–297.

Madhani, K., & Farrell, J. J. (2016). Autoimmune pancreatitis: an update on diagnosis and management. *Gastroenterology Clinics of North America*, *45*(1), 29–43.

Pasternak, A., et al. (2017). Biliary polyunsaturated fatty acids and telocytes in gallstone disease. *Cell Transplantation*, *26*, 125–133.

Ramanathan, M., & Aadam, A. A. (2019). Nutrition management in acute pancreatitis. *Nutrition in Clinical Practice: Official Publication of the American Society for Parenteral and Enteral Nutrition*, *34*, S7–S12.

Sayiner, M., et al. (2019). Disease burden of hepatocellular carcinoma: a global perspective. *Digestive Diseases and Sciences*, *64*, 910–917.

Schwimmer, J. B., et al. (2019). Effect of a low free sugar diet vs usual diet on nonalcoholic fatty liver disease in adolescent boys: a randomized clinical trial. *JAMA: the Journal of the American Medical Association*, *321*, 256–265.

Sheka, A. C., et al (2020). Nonalcoholic steatohepatitis: a review, 323:1175–1183.

Singh, V. K., et al. (2019). Diagnosis and management of chronic pancreatitis: a review. *JAMA: the Journal of the American Medical Association*, *322*, 2422–2434.

15

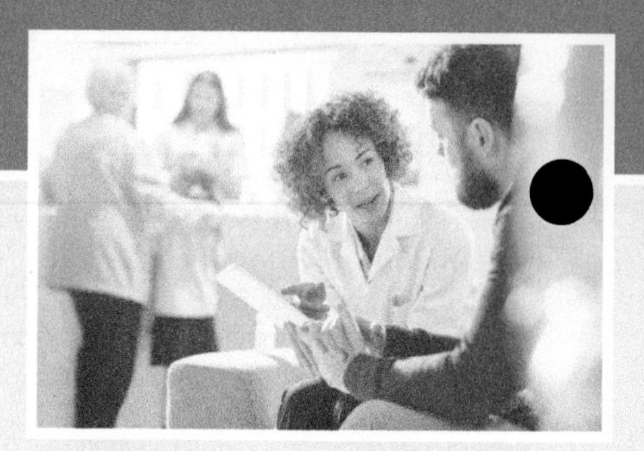

Nutrition for Diabetes Mellitus

Diabetes is a chronic disease that affects how your body turns food into energy. More than 122 million Americans are living with diabetes (34.2 million) or prediabetes (88 million).

Centers for Disease Control and Prevention, 2020

http://evolve.elsevier.com/GRODNER/FOUNDATIONS

LEARNING OBJECTIVES

- Define diabetes mellitus (DM) and its forms.
- Identify the role of vitamin D in the onset of diabetes.
- Compare and contrast T1D mellitus (T1DM) with T2D mellitus (T2DM).
- Explain the main goal of diabetes treatment and how it can be achieved.
- Discuss the composition and process of the diabetes management team.
- Describe current nutrition therapy guidelines.
- Identify groups for whom special care and individualized goals are needed.

WELLNESS AND DIABETES

Serious physical health complications may be avoided if hyperglycemia is controlled through dietary and lifestyle modifications. The ability of the individual to understand the condition; to be compliant on a regular basis regarding insulin injections, if required; and to follow dietary and exercise recommendations depends on intellectual health. Not only must the individual deal with a chronic lifelong condition, but changes in dietary habits may necessitate the loss of favorite foods, which affects emotional health. Support, especially from family members and friends, is a crucial part of social health. Finally, people who eat certain foods according to their religious or spiritual beliefs may need special adaptations for spiritual health while living with diabetes. The environmental health dimension can support diabetes management based on the availability and means to access diabetes management health care.

DEFINITION

Diabetes mellitus represents a group of conditions characterized by either a relative or complete lack of insulin secretion by the beta cells of the pancreas or by defects of cell insulin receptors (Fig. 15.1). This deficit results in disturbances of carbohydrate, protein, and lipid metabolism. Although many cases of diabetes are undiagnosed, the medical community is aware that the condition is prevalent and growing in all age groups.

Diabetes is usually diagnosed by elevated fasting blood glucose values (>126 mg/dL if found on at least two occasions), hemoglobin A_1c 6.5% or more, a random blood glucose level more than 200 mg/dL, or a blood glucose of more than 200 mg/dL 2 hours after eating. The main goal of treatment is achievement of insulin/glucose homeostasis.

In addition to everyday maintenance necessary to control blood glucose levels, diabetes is associated with disability and premature death because of the effect on structural and functional alterations in many body systems, especially large and small blood vessels. Ranked as one of the most expensive health problems in America, diabetes mellitus is often a "silent killer."

PREDIABETES AND INSULIN RESISTANCE

Doctors use the term prediabetes to indicate that blood glucose levels are higher than normal but not high enough for a diagnosis of diabetes. One in three American adults has prediabetes (Fig. 15.2).

In insulin resistance, muscle, fat, and liver cells do not respond properly to insulin and cannot easily absorb glucose from the bloodstream. The body then needs higher levels of insulin to help glucose enter cells. Excess body fat increases the risk for insulin resistance and prediabetes; obese men and women, respectively, have a sevenfold and twelvefold higher risk for developing T2D (Lau & Teoh, 2017).

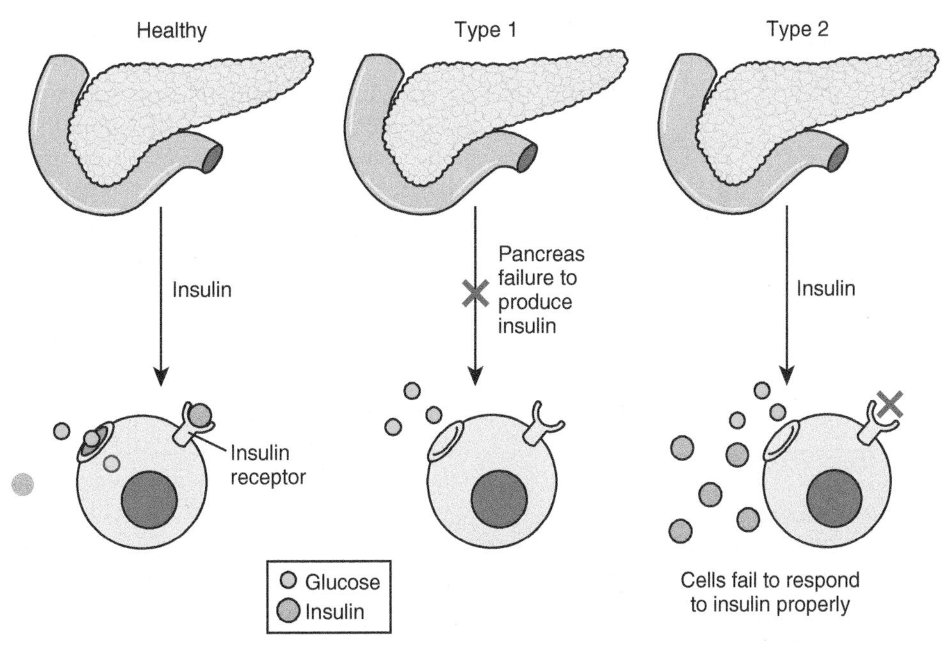

Fig. 15.1 Types of diabetes. News Medical: *Diabetes Mellitus Subtypes.* (Adapted from https://www.news-medical.net/health/Diabetes-Mellitus-Subtypes.aspx Accessed 2 September, 2020.)

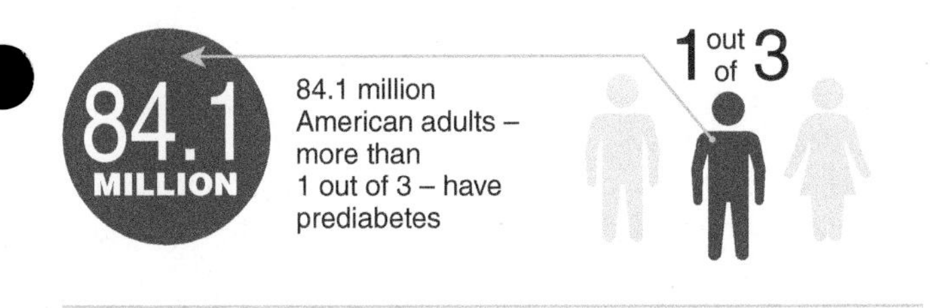

Fig. 15.2 Prediabetes. (Modified from: Centers for Disease Control and Prevention. *Prediabetes: Could It Be You?* https://www.cdc.gov/diabetes/library/socialmedia/infographics/prediabetes.html Accessed 2 September, 2020.)

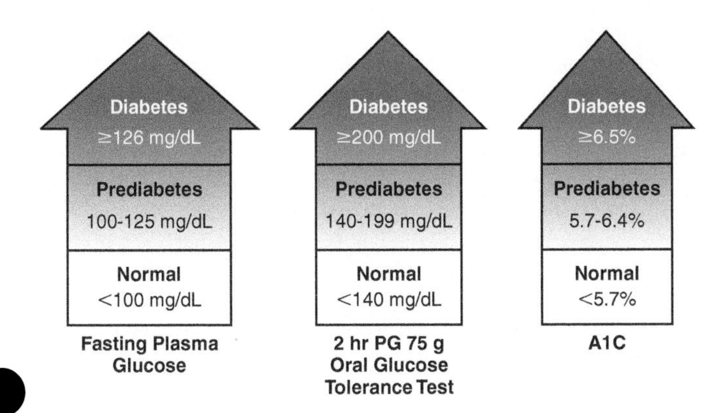

Fig. 15.3 Criteria for diagnosing diabetes and prediabetes. (Modified from American Diabetes Association. From https://www.diabetes.org/a1c/d. Accessed 1 September, 2020.)

A person with certain risk factors is more likely to develop prediabetes and T2D: being older than age 45 years, overweight or obese, leading a sedentary lifestyle, or having a family history of diabetes or certain ethnic background (Black American, Hispanic/Latino, Native American, Asian American, or Pacific Islander) (Liu et al., 2020). Women who have a history of diabetes while pregnant (gestational diabetes) or having given birth to a baby weighing 9 pounds or more are also at risk. Many people are unaware of the presence of prediabetes or diabetes; Fig. 15.3 provides a graphic for assessment.

Fortunately, there are ways to prevent or delay progression to T2D through lifestyle interventions. The National Diabetes Prevention Program, organized by the Centers for Disease Control and Prevention, connects individuals with prediabetes and trained coaches who discuss food choices, physical activity, and coping skills. Pharmacotherapy and bariatric surgery may be necessary for some individuals who cannot achieve weight loss.

Vitamin D and Diabetes

Vitamin D deficiency is linked to the onset of diabetes through its role in maintaining the normal release of insulin by beta cells of the pancreas (Berridge, 2017). Vitamin D plays a significant role in maintaining the epigenome, reducing inflammation that leads to insulin resistance, and protecting the beta cells against destruction; see Figure 15.4 for an image of this relationship.

Vitamin D synthesis takes place in the skin with solar ultraviolet B (UVB) radiation exposure. Because serum levels of vitamin D are low in many breastfeeding mothers, especially dark-skinned women and those who are covered,

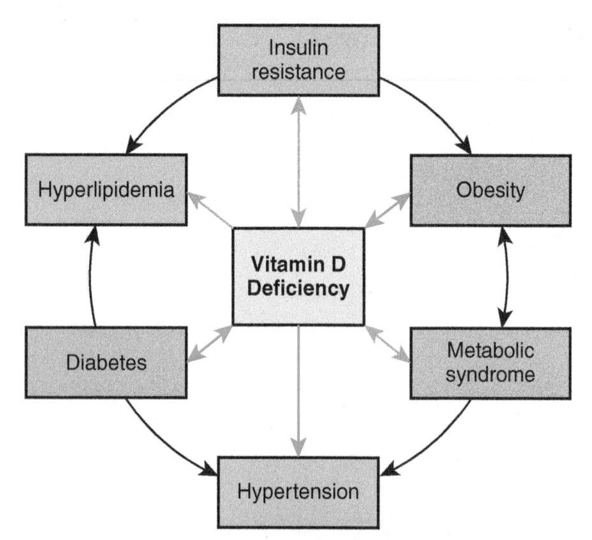

Fig. 15.4 Endocrine effects of vitamin D deficiency. (Modified from Wimalawansa SJ: Associations of vitamin D with insulin resistance, obesity, T2D, and metabolic syndrome, *J Steroid Biochem and Molecular Biol* 175:177–189, 2018.)

it is prudent to use a supplement. It may also be beneficial for individuals who have diabetes and COVID-19 infection (Singh et al., 2020).

Children with T1D mellitus (T1DM) have a generalized 25OHD deficiency; supplementation improves glycemic control and glycosylated hemoglobin (A_1c) levels and should be additional therapy (Savastio et al, 2016).

Vitamin D supplementation may be needed by individuals who cannot obtain enough from safe exposure to sun or from consuming vitamin C-fortified foods (Wimalawansa, 2018). Large randomized, blinded, prospective studies are required to fully evaluate the roles of UVB and vitamin D in preventing diabetes (Altieri et al, 2017).

Complications

Everyone with diabetes is vulnerable to long-term complications (Table 15.1) and premature death. Many of these complications may be preempted with control of hyperglycemia. Macrovascular effects of diabetes increase the risk of coronary artery disease, peripheral vascular disease, and stroke. Unfortunately, cardiovascular disease is often established by the time diabetes is diagnosed. In fact, two out of three people with diabetes die from cardiovascular diseases.

Microvascular effects include nephropathy (changes in the kidney), retinopathy (eye disorder from blood vessel changes), and neuropathy (changes in the nervous system). With nephropathy, chronic kidney disease (CKD) and renal failure requiring dialysis develop in approximately half of all individuals with T1DM. Retinopathy from diabetes is the leading cause of blindness in North America. Neuropathy affects peripheral circulation, causing decreased sensations in extremities that may result in injury without the patient's knowledge. Healing is impaired because of the effects of diabetes on the circulatory system; gangrene may develop, and amputation may be necessary.

Autonomic effects may include orthostatic hypotension, persistent tachycardia, gastroparesis, neurogenic bladder (urinary bladder dysfunction from neurologic damage), impotence, and impairment of visceral pain sensation that can obscure symptoms of angina pectoris or myocardial infarction. Development of these long-term complications is believed to be correlated to the level and frequency of hyperglycemia experiences throughout the life span of a person with diabetes.

CLASSIFICATION

Glucose intolerance is classified primarily as T1DM and T2DM. Other types are latent autoimmune diabetes of adults (LADA), gestational diabetes mellitus (GDM), and impaired glucose tolerance (IGT). These classifications are based on cause, treatment needs, and symptoms. More than 90% of people with diabetes have T2DM.

T1D MELLITUS

T1DM is an autoimmune disease resulting in beta-cell destruction. Autoantibodies to beta-cell proteins form after autoimmune destruction of the beta cells. The rate of beta-cell destruction is variable, being rapid in infants and children and slow in adults. Although most individuals diagnosed with T1DM are usually 20 years of age or younger, a growing number of cases are documented in older individuals. Therefore, note that the terms insulin-dependent or juvenile diabetes are not used to describe T1DM.

Onset of T1DM is usually sudden. Cells use glucose for energy, and without endogenous insulin, they literally begin to starve. The body responds by sending signals to eat because cells are hungry, but because glucose cannot enter cells, it builds up in the bloodstream. It is common for the person to experience weight loss while consuming large quantities of food

PERSONAL PERSPECTIVE

T1D Mellitus: The Bionic Pancreas

Imagine trying to maintain blood glucose levels when the pancreas is producing little if any insulin and the means to self-inject insulin is not yet available or still is being refined as treatment. Over 90 years ago, T1D mellitus (T1DM) was a death sentence. Half of people who developed it died within two years; more than 90% were dead within five years. Thanks to the introduction of insulin therapy in 1922, and numerous advances since then, many people with T1D now live into their 50s and beyond. A bionic pancreas developed at Boston University and Massachusetts General Hospital shows even greater promise for managing this complex disease. Researchers Edward Damiano, an associate professor of biomedical engineering at Boston University, along with Steven Russell, an assistant professor of medicine at Massachusetts General Hospital, have a passion to make this happen. For Damiano, the work is personal: He has a 21-year-old son who has had T1D since he was a baby.

(From Lewine H: "Bionic pancreas" could help people with T1D control blood sugar. Harvard Health Publications, 2014. Accessed 1 September, 2020 from http://www.health.harvard.edu/blog/bionic-pancreas-help-people-type-1-diabetes-control-blood-sugar-201406177215.)

TABLE 15.1 Clinical Complications of Diabetes Mellitus

Complication	Manifestation	Comments
Dental disease	Periodontitis	Those with diabetes mellitus (DM) are often at twice the risk of those without diabetes. Almost 30% of people with diabetes have severe periodontal disease with loss of attachment of gums to the teeth measuring ≥5 mm.
Pregnancy	Congenital malformations	Poorly controlled diabetes before conception and during the first trimester of pregnancy can cause major birth defects in 5%–10% of pregnancies and spontaneous abortions in 15%–20% of pregnancies. Poorly controlled diabetes during second and third trimesters of pregnancy can result in excessively large newborns.
Microvascular[a]	Retinopathy	Diabetes retinopathy is the leading cause of blindness in adults. Glaucoma is 40% more common in adults with diabetes; cataracts are 60% more common.
	Nephropathy	Kidney disease will develop in more than 30% of people with T1D mellitus (T1DM), compared with perhaps 10% of those with T2DM. Risk of end-stage renal disease in people with T1DM is high.
Macrovascular[b]	Coronary artery disease	Patients with DM are two to four times more likely to have heart disease; heart disease deaths are also two to four times higher than in adults without DM.
	Peripheral vascular disease	
	Cerebrovascular disease	Patients with DM are two to four times more likely to suffer stroke than people without DM
Neuropathy	Peripheral	Approximately 60%–70% of people with diabetes have mild to severe forms of nerve damage with tingling, pain, weakness in hands or feet. Neuropathy is a major contributing factor in foot and leg amputations among people with the disease. Risk of leg amputation is 15–40 times greater for a person with DM.
	Autonomic (postural hypotension, persistent tachycardia, neurogenic bladder, incontinence, gastroparesis, impotence)	Diarrhea or constipation is a common complaint. Gastroparesis slows the speed of food through the gastrointestinal tract; bloating or vomiting can result. It is difficult to regulate food and insulin. A neurogenic bladder contributes to frequent urinary tract infections. Erectile dysfunction occurs in approximately 13% of men who have T1DM and 8% of men with T2DM.
Skin conditions	Atherosclerosis	As blood vessels narrow, the skin changes. It becomes hairless, thin, cool, and shiny. Toes become cold. Toenails thicken and discolor.
	Fungal infections *(Candida albicans)*	Common fungal infections are "jock itch," "athlete's foot," ringworm, and vaginal infections, all of which can cause itching.
	Bullosis diabeticorum (diabetic blisters)	Rare condition that can occur on backs of hands, fingers, toes, feet, and sometimes legs or forearms. They look like burn blisters, are painless, and have no redness. Often occur in people with neuropathy; the only treatment is to bring blood glucose levels under control.
	Diabetic dermopathy	Light brown scaly skin patches often mistaken for age spots; occurs most often on the fronts of both legs. Patches do not hurt, open up, or itch.
	Necrobiosis lipoidica diabeticorum (NLD)	Rare condition. Similar to diabetic dermopathy; however, spots are fewer but larger and deeper. Often start as dull, red raised area. Sometimes itchy and painful; spots may crack open.
	Eruptive xanthomatosis	Firm, yellow, pealike enlargements in the skin. Occurs most often on backs of hands, feet, arms, legs, and buttocks. Usually occurs in young men with T1DM who have high serum levels of cholesterol and lipids. Usually disappear when glucose levels are controlled.
	Digital sclerosis	Tight, thick, waxy skin on backs of hands. Finger joints become stiff. Occurs in about 30% of those with T1DM. The only treatment is to control blood glucose levels.
	Disseminated granuloma annulare	Sharply defined ring- or arc-shaped raised areas on skin that can be red, red-brown, or skin colored. Occurs most often on distal parts of the body.
	Acanthosis nigricans	Tan or brown raised areas on sides of the neck, axilla, and groin. May sometimes occur on hands, elbows, and knees. Usually manifests in the obese.

[a]Compounds effects of macrovascular problems.
[b]Exacerbated by concurrent hypertension, dyslipidemia, smoking, and aging.

(Data from American Diabetes Association: *Complications*, n.d., Arlington, VA, Author. From http://www.diabetes.org/living-with-diabetes/complications/?loc=symptoms. Accessed 1 September, 2020.)

(polyphagia). Because glucose cannot enter cells and it builds up in the bloodstream, blood becomes hypertonic, and the body tries to get rid of the excess glucose by increasing urine output (polyuria). In reaction to increased excretion of urine, the body increases thirst (polydipsia) to replace lost fluids. Blood glucose is preferred over A_1c to diagnose acute onset of T1D with symptoms of hyperglycemia.

When a person chooses food and activity wisely, they can live healthfully with T1DM. See the *Personal Perspective* box T1D Mellitus: The Bionic Pancreas.

Treatment

Insulin

Everyone with T1DM requires exogenous insulin to maintain normal blood glucose levels and to survive. Some individuals with T2DM may require insulin to optimize blood glucose control. Regardless of the type of diabetes, the goal of insulin therapy, in conjunction with nutrition therapy and physical activity, is to mimic physiologic insulin delivery. Fig. 15.3 lists the typical metabolic goals for diabetes management.

Optimal insulin management can be realized only by evaluating blood glucose monitoring records, adjusting food and exercise activities, and proposing insulin adjustments.

Bioengineered human insulin is the only insulin available for use in the United States. Types of insulin are classified into three groups according to duration of their action: rapid or short acting, intermediate acting, and long acting; see Table 15.2.

Patterns of insulin administration vary with type of diabetes and desired glycemic control. A single dose of insulin is rarely capable of providing optimal glycemic control in T1DM. The three basic types of insulin administration regimens are described here.

Conventional or standard insulin therapy is composed of a constant dose of intermediate-acting insulin combined with short- or rapid-acting insulin or a mixed dose of insulin. Insulins may be mixed by the patient or purchased premixed (e.g., 30 units of 70/30 insulin). Administration of insulin and food intake must be synchronized to avoid hypoglycemia. Insulin regimen must be truly integrated with the patient's lifestyle.

Flexible or intensive insulin therapy is composed of multiple daily injections (MDIs) of short- or rapid-acting insulin before meals, as well as intermediate-acting insulin once or twice daily. This approach allows insulin to be adjusted to correspond with food intake, imitating endogenous insulin secretion in a person without diabetes. Insulin doses can also be adjusted to treat hyperglycemia, inconsistent carbohydrate intake, or modification in usual physical activity. Individuals who use intensive therapy should know the basic insulin doses for both insulins they use. This knowledge allows them to fine-tune short- and rapid-acting insulin doses when they deviate from usual meal plans and/or exercise programs. Intensive therapy is not appropriate for everyone.

TABLE 15.2 Metabolic Goals in Diabetes Management

	Goal
Glycemic control	<7.0%
Hemoglobin A_1c	
Preprandial capillary plasma glucose (mg/dL)	90–130
Peak postprandial capillary plasma glucose (mg/dL)	<180
Cardiovascular	
Blood pressure (mm Hg)	<139/80
Triglycerides (mg/dL)	<150
Low-density lipoprotein cholesterol (mg/dL)	<100
High-density lipoprotein cholesterol (mg/dL)	
Males	>40
Females	>50

(Data from Evert AB, et al: Nutrition therapy recommendations for the management of adults with diabetes, *Diabetes Care* 36:3821–3842, 2013. Accessed 22 July, 2017, from http://care.diabetesjournals.org/content/diacare/36/11/3821.full.pdf.)

Continuous subcutaneous insulin infusion is a form of intensive therapy. Rapid- or short-acting insulin is pumped continuously in micro-amounts through a subcutaneous catheter and is monitored 24 hours a day. Boluses of rapid- or short-acting insulins are given before meals.

Exercise

Exercise, like insulin, lowers blood glucose levels, helps to maintain normal lipid levels, and increases circulation. For most individuals, consistent and individualized exercise helps reduce the therapeutic dose of insulin. People with T1DM who do not have complications and are in good blood glucose control can perform all levels of exercise, including leisure activities, recreational sports, and competitive sports. To do so safely, the patient must possess the ability to collect self-monitored blood glucose data during exercise and then adjust the regimen (insulin and diet).

General guidelines for regulating the glycemic response to exercise are, as follows:

1. Metabolic control before exercise: Avoid exercise if fasting glucose levels are 250 mg/dL or more and ketosis is present or if glucose levels are greater than 300 mg/dL, regardless of whether ketosis is present. Ingest added carbohydrate if glucose levels are less than 100 mg/dL. Patients with T1DM should not perform exercise at the time insulin is at its peak. Ideally, they should exercise when blood glucose levels are between 100 and 200 mg/dL or about 30 to 60 minutes after meals. They should also avoid exercising when blood glucose is greater than 250 mg/dL or when ketones are present in the urine.
2. Blood glucose monitoring before and after exercise: Identify when changes in insulin or food intake are necessary. Learn the blood glucose response to different exercise conditions.

3. Food intake: Consume added carbohydrate as needed to avoid hypoglycemia. Carbohydrate-based foods should be readily available during and after exercise (Box 15.1). Glucose control can be compromised if proper adjustments are not made in food intake or insulin administration.

T2D MELLITUS

The primary metabolic problem in T2DM is insulin resistance (failure of cells to respond to insulin produced by the body) or defects in insulin secretion. Risk factors for T2DM include overweight or obesity, large waist circumference, inactivity, family history of diabetes, older age, high-risk ethnicity, gestational diabetes, polycystic ovarian syndrome, and genetics (Mayo Clinic, 2020). Upper body obesity, defined as a waist-to-hip ratio greater than 0.8 for women and 0.95 to 1 for men, is a risk factor for diabetes, heart disease, and hypertension.

The genetic tendency for diabetes leads to beta-cell exhaustion and hyperglycemia in many obese individuals. Fortunately, Mediterranean diet food components (extra-virgin olive oil, nuts, vegetables, and other polyphenols) are important environmental factors that can modulate gene expression that affects important metabolic pathways (Mirabelli et al., 2020).

People with T2DM have gradual onset of polyuria and polydipsia, are easily fatigued, and have frequent infections (especially of the urinary tract). Some of the first symptoms that cause individuals to seek medical attention are complications associated with diabetes, such as a stroke or heart attack. It is not uncommon for a person to have T2DM several years before diagnosis. All adults with risk factors should be evaluated for signs of prediabetes or diabetes.

Unfortunately, diabetes is one of the conditions that affects certain populations more than others (see the *Cultural Diversity and Nutrition* box Prevalence of T2D Mellitus).

Treatment: Oral Glucose-Lowering Medications

Oral glucose-lowering medications are used to treat T2DM when diet and physical activity alone cannot control hyperglycemia. Medications used to manage T2DM use different pharmacologic approaches (Table 15.3). Although the variety of new drugs for the treatment of diabetes has greatly expanded during the past several years, metformin continues to be first-line therapy.

BOX 15.1 Foods Containing 15 Grams of Carbohydrate Per Serving

Grains, Breads, Cereals, Starches
1 slice bread
¾ cup dry cereal
½ cup cooked cereal
⅓ cup cooked rice or pasta

Milk and Yogurt
1 cup milk
⅓ cup (6 ounces) unsweetened or sugar-free yogurt

Fruits
1 small fresh fruit
½ cup canned fruit (canned in juice)
1 cup melon or berries
¼ cup dried fruit
½ cup unsweetened fruit juice

Vegetables
½ cup cooked potatoes, peas, or corn
3 cups raw vegetables
1½ cups cooked vegetables
Small portions (½ cup) of nonstarchy vegetables are free

Sweets and Snack Foods
½ cup or ¾ ounce snack food (pretzels, chips)
4 to 6 snack crackers
1-ounce sweet snack (2 small cookies)
½ cup regular ice cream
1 tablespoon sugar

(Modified from American Diabetes Association: *Get to Know Carbs*)

MANAGEMENT OF DIABETES

Blood Glucose Monitoring

Controlled blood glucose levels are the cornerstone of diabetes management. Improved control is correlated with sustained reduced rates of retinopathy, nephropathy, and neuropathy. Follow-up studies of the Diabetes Control and Complications Trial–the Epidemiology of Diabetes Intervention and Complications Study (DCCT-EDIC) and the United Kingdom Prospective Diabetes Study (UKPDS) emphasize the role of glycemic control. Hyperglycemia leads to long-lasting epigenetic modifications (called metabolic memory), with changes in chromatin structure and altered gene expression (Reddy et al., 2015).

Glycemic control can be monitored by measurement of **glycosylated hemoglobin, or hemoglobin A1c**, along with self-monitoring of blood glucose (SMBG). A_1c is formed through an irreversible process. As red blood cells (RBCs) circulate in the bloodstream, hemoglobin combines with glucose, forming glycosylated hemoglobin. The amount of glycosylated hemoglobin formed depends on the amount of glucose in the bloodstream circulation during the 120-day life span of the red blood cells. The more glucose a cell was exposed to, the higher the value. This value is not affected by short-term factors such as food intake, exercise, or stress, so the blood sample can be drawn at any time. A_1c samples are easier to obtain than the fasting blood glucose samples. Table 15.4 shows the correlation between mean plasma glucose levels and A_1c levels.

Self-monitoring and charting are useful in evaluating glycemic control, physical activity, and effectiveness of the meal

CULTURAL DIVERSITY AND NUTRITION

Prevalence of T2D Mellitus

T2D mellitus (T2DM) poses a major health threat worldwide. Diabetes prevalence is high in North America, Oceania, Asia, Latin America, the Caribbean, North Africa, and the Middle East. Among ethnic groups significantly at risk for T2DM in the United States are Black Americans, Hispanics/Latinos, Native Americans, Asian and Pacific Islanders. By the year 2050, it is estimated that 50% of the population will be from these groups (Caballero, 2018). Factors influencing prevention and diabetes management include limited access to health care, cultural attitudes about medicine, as well as behaviors related to diet, immunizations, and self-care. The COVID-19 pandemic has demonstrated the vulnerability of individuals who have diabetes, as deaths have been highest among nonCaucasians for a variety of reasons.

Application to Nursing

Lifestyle changes, weight loss, increased exercise, and bariatric surgery decrease the risk of T2DM. For minority and cultural groups, language barriers, health care access, level of acculturation, practices of diabetes self-care, and genetic variations may contribute to higher risk of long-term diabetes complications. Patient care and education, provider education, and community outreach should encompass physical, mental, spiritual, and emotional needs. Nurses will want to tailor counseling for their patients in culturally appropriate ways.

The American Association of Diabetes Educators (AADE, 2020) suggests **"Five Tips for Improving Self-Care"** to ensure successful cultural encounters are, as follows:

1. **Encourage activity rather than exercise**. Instead of urging patients to partake in traditional exercise, suggest they choose from a variety of activities they find enjoyable. For example, a Black teenager who has diabetes and is overweight may be reluctant to go to a Pilates class, lift weights, or ride her bike, but she may enjoy dancing with her friends.
2. **Emphasize health, not weight loss**. In some cultures, weight loss can have negative implications. Mexican Americans, for example, consider a full figure representative of good health and weight loss a sign of disease. Instead of telling your patients to lose weight, suggest they list their goals, such as playing with their grandchildren or avoiding diabetes complications seen in relatives or friends. Explain how eating healthfully and moving more will lower their blood glucose levels, which in turn will help them achieve their goals.
3. **Include familiar foods**. Patients with diabetes are more likely to follow a healthful diet if it includes familiar foods they like. Adapt favorite foods to make them healthier, such as baking instead of frying chicken or using dry beans, which are lower in sodium than canned beans.
4. **Recruit the family**. Many cultures are family-focused, and the support of family members can help patients with diabetes better manage their condition. Encourage family members to be supportive, not judgmental or scolding, by providing positive feedback such as, "You look great, Mom!" and agreeing to avoid sodas and unhealthful foods.
5. **Partner up**. Work with people from the local community and church groups who can provide tips and help understand the culture.

(Data from AADE. American Association of Diabetes Educators. From https://www.diabeteseducator.org/docs/default-source/legacy-docs/_resources/pdf/general/Five_Tips_for_Improving_Self-Care_v3.pdf. Accessed 1 September 2020.)

TABLE 15.3 Oral Hypoglycemic Agents

Agent	Action
Sulfonylureas (glipizide, glyburide, gliclazide, glimepiride)	Insulin secretagogues. Sulfonylureas increase beta-cell insuloin secretion, decrease hepatic glucose output, and increase insulin receptor sensitivity at peripheral target tissues
Meglitinides (repaglinide and nateglinide)	Insulin secretagogues.
Biguanides (metformin)	Insulin sensitizers. Biguanides decrease hepatic glucose production, decrease gastrointestinal glucose absorption, and increase target cell insulin sensitivity
Thiazolidinediones (pioglitazone, rosiglitazone)	Insulin sensitizers. Thiazolidinediones increase insulin receptor sensitivity and influence the production of gene products involved in lipid and glucose metabolism; their mechanism of action depends on the presence of insulin for activity
α-Glucosidase inhibitors (acarbose, miglitol, voglibose)	Nutrient load reducers (absorption inhibitors). Alpha-glucosidase inhibitors inhibit the upper gastrointestinal enzymes that convert dietary starch and other complex carbohydrates into simple sugars, which can be absorbed
DPP-4 inhibitors (sitagliptin, saxagliptin, vildagliptin, linagliptin, alogliptin)	Insulin secretagogues (indirectly via incretin pathway).
Cycloset (pramlintide, bromocriptine)	Insulin sensitizers (indirectly via counter-regulatory hormone pathways).
SGLT2 inhibitors (dapagliflozin and canagliflozin)	Excretion enhancers.

(Data from MedScape: Oral Hypoglycemia Agents. From https://emedicine.medscape.com/article/2172160-overview. Accessed 1 September, 2020.)

plan in meeting the goals of medical nutrition therapy (MNT). SMBG can be performed in the individual's home with blood glucose meters, which can be purchased at pharmacies. A droplet of blood is obtained through a finger stick on a regular basis to monitor glucose levels before and after meals and at bedtime.

SMBG is recommended three or more times daily for nearly all individuals with T1DM and for pregnant women taking insulin. Individuals with T2DM who take insulin usually need to perform SMBG more often than those not taking it. Records should be kept of SMBG levels for review by

TABLE 15.4 Relationship of Plasma Glucose and Hemoglobin A_{1c} Levels

A_{1c} %	3-Month Average Blood Sugar
4.0	65
4.5	83
5.0	100
5.5	118
6.0	135
6.5	153
7.0	170
7.5	187
8.0	204
8.5	222
9.0	240
9.5	258
10.0	275
10.5	293
11.0	310
11.5	328
12.0	345

(Data from American Diabetes Association. https://professional.diabetes.org/diapro/glucose_calc. Accessed 1 September, 2020.)

the health care team to determine food, insulin, and exercise needs. This approach allows for individualized treatment, especially with meal plans. Blood glucose levels are often regulated as follows:

- Before meals: 70 to 130 mg/dL
- Two hours after meals: less than 180 mg/dL (expect a 30- to 50-point rise from premeal glucose)
- Bedtime: 90 to 150 mg/dL

Hypoglycemia

Hypoglycemia (low blood sugar, <70 mg/dL) usually results from taking too much insulin, skipping meals, or engaging in too much exercise without a concomitant increase in food intake.

Hypoglycemia can occur during exercise that lasts longer than 1 hour or up to 24 hours after unusually strenuous or prolonged exercise. Onset is sudden, and the complication can be fatal if left untreated. Hypoglycemia can occur when plasma insulin (or oral hypoglycemic agents) levels peak or during the night while the patient sleeps (fasting). Box 15.2 lists the symptoms of hypoglycemia.

Consuming 15 to 20 g of a fast-acting carbohydrate is the initial treatment for hypoglycemia. Fast-acting carbohydrates, such as candy, fruit juice, regular soft drinks, or glucose tablets or gel, are easily converted to sugar in the body. Blood glucose levels should be monitored closely. If blood sugar levels 15 minutes after treatment are still low, treat with another 15 to 20 g of fast-acting carbohydrate and recheck the blood sugar level in 15 minutes. Repeat these steps until the blood sugar is greater than 70 mg/dL. Once the blood sugar levels are back to normal, a balanced snack or small meal is needed to replenish glycogen stores that were depleted. Follow-up with a physician is suggested.

BOX 15.2 Symptoms of Hypoglycemia

- Cool, clammy, pale skin
- Confusion
- Erratic behavior
- Hunger
- Trembling, shaking

Diabetic Ketoacidosis

Diabetic ketoacidosis (DKA) occurs when the body cannot produce enough insulin and breaks down fat for fuel, producing high levels of blood acids (ketones). Severe DKA is defined by a pH less than 7.15, a form of metabolic acidosis; hyperglycemia causes osmotic diuresis, dehydration, and lactic acidosis. Lowered pH stimulates the respiratory center and produces deep, rapid respirations known as Kussmaul's respirations. Large amounts of ketone bodies in the body produce a fruity, acetone odor to the breath (a person suffering from DKA could be mistaken for someone who is inebriated). If this condition is not recognized and treated promptly, the acidosis and dehydration may lead to loss of consciousness and possibly coma and death. Box 15.3 lists symptoms and clinical signs of DKA.

DKA may be the initial presentation of T1DM, after missed insulin injections, or from insulin pump failure. DKA is best handled in an intensive care unit for correction of fluid loss with intravenous fluids, hyperglycemia with insulin, electrolyte disturbances (potassium loss) or acid-base balance with appropriate solutions, and treatment of any infections. Once the crisis has been stabilized, drinking low-calorie fluids is recommended to maintain hydration.

Hyperglycemic Hyperosmolar Nonketotic Syndrome

Hyperglycemic hyperosmolar nonketotic syndrome (HHNS), like DKA, is a life-threatening emergency caused by a relative or actual insulin deficiency resulting in severe hyperglycemia. Most often HHNS is triggered by trauma or infection that increases the body's demand for insulin. Although enough insulin may be present in the plasma to prevent formation of ketones and acidosis, there may not be enough to prevent hyperglycemia. If hyperglycemia is left untreated, serum becomes hyperosmolar. Osmotic diuresis causes significant loss of electrolytes via urine. The mortality rate for HHNS is 10% to 25%. Symptoms and clinical signs of HHNS are listed in Box 15.4.

Food and Nutrition Therapies

There is no ideal "diabetic" or "American Diabetes Association (ADA)" diet. In the past, physicians ordered a calorie level. The ADA no longer endorses any meal plan or specific percentages of carbohydrate, protein, and fat based on exchange lists. Diet orders such as "no concentrated sweets," "no sugar added," "low sugar," and "liberal diabetic" are not suitable because they do not reflect current diabetes nutrition recommendations. Old, rigid meal plans propagate the false notion that merely restricting sucrose-sweetened foods will improve blood glucose control.

BOX 15.3 Symptoms and Clinical Signs of Diabetic Ketoacidosis

- Dehydration and metabolic acidosis
- Dry, flushed skin and mucous membranes
- Fruity (acetone) breath
- Generalized weakness
- Nausea
- Polydipsia
- Polyphagia
- Polyuria
- Vomiting
- Weakness, fatigue
- Weight loss

BOX 15.4 Symptoms and Clinical Signs of Hyperglycemic Hyperosmolar Nonketotic Syndrome

- Polyuria
- Polyphagia
- Weight loss
- Nausea
- Dry, flushed skin and mucous membranes
- Dehydration secondary to osmotic diuresis
- Polydipsia
- Possible seizures and tremors
- Generalized weakness
- Vomiting
- Fatigue

Table 15.5 shows an interesting timeline about the history of diet for diabetes management.

Nutrition therapy is an essential element of glycemic control and diabetes self-management education (DSME). Individualized nutrition therapy is required to achieve treatment goals. The basis for nutrition therapy and DSME involves a comprehensive nutrition assessment, a self-care treatment plan, and the client's health status, learning ability, readiness to change, and current lifestyle. The key is to tailor the meal planning approach to individual needs. Individuals using intensive insulin therapy have flexibility in when and what they eat, whereas people using conventional insulin therapy must be consistent with timing of meals and amounts of food consumed.

Recommendations for total fat, saturated fat, cholesterol, fiber, vitamins, and mineral intakes are the same for individuals with diabetes as those for the general population. Carbohydrate control is based on the individual's eating habits, blood glucose, and lipid goals. Carbohydrate counting is a very effective method for most individuals to maintain glycemic control (Fig. 15.5).

Although blood glucose control is not impaired by sucrose in the meal plan, sucrose-containing foods should only be eaten as an occasional substitute for other carbohydrate foods. Protein intake can range from 15% to 20% of daily kcal from animal and vegetable protein sources.

If diabetes is well controlled, blood glucose levels are not affected by moderate alcohol use. Alcohol ought to be regarded as additional energy, and no food should be omitted. Alcohol should be consumed with food to reduce the risk of hypoglycemia.

The latest recommendations are shown in Table 15.6. Goals of nutrition therapy that apply to all individuals with diabetes are as follows:

1. Attain and maintain optimal metabolic outcomes, including the following:
   a. Glucose level in normal range, or as close to normal range as is safely possible to prevent or reduce risk of complications
   b. Lipid or lipoprotein profile that reduces risk for macrovascular disease
   c. Blood pressure levels that reduce risk for vascular disease or stroke (Box 15.5)
2. Modify nutrient intake and lifestyle as appropriate for prevention and treatment of obesity, dyslipidemia, cardiovascular disease, hypertension, and nephropathy.
3. Enhance health using healthy food choices and physical activity.
4. Address individual nutritional needs, cultural preferences, and personal lifestyles while respecting the individual's wishes and willingness to change.

A registered dietitian who is knowledgeable and skilled in nutrition therapy for diabetes is the medical team member responsible for providing MNT, especially if the patient's health care team is coding and billing for services. It is essential that other health care team members be knowledgeable about the implications of dietary choices in diabetes and supportive of the patient with diabetes who needs to make these important lifestyle changes.

Nutrition therapy is an integral component of diabetes management and DSME. It involves conducting a nutrition assessment to evaluate a patient's food intake, metabolic status, lifestyle, and willingness to make changes; goal setting; nutrition education; individualized counseling; and monitoring and evaluation. To enhance compliance, the MNT plan must be individualized. Patients with diabetes require assessment by a registered dietitian to determine an appropriate nutrition prescription and plan for DSME. Nutrition therapy should consider a person's usual eating habits and other lifestyle factors.

Maintaining consistency within an eating pattern, rather than following an arbitrary eating style, will result in lower glycosylated hemoglobin levels. Other issues include use of nutritive and nonnutritive sweeteners. Although fructose creates a smaller rise in plasma glucose than sucrose and other carbohydrates, large amounts of fructose provide no advantage as a sweetener. Other nutritive sweeteners, such as corn sweeteners, fruit juice or juice concentrate, honey, molasses, dextrose, and maltose, affect glycemic response and caloric content much like sucrose does. Sugar alcohols

TABLE 15.5 Historical Perspective of Nutrition Recommendations for Diabetes Mellitus

Year	Carbohydrate	Fat	Protein
Pre-1921	Starvation diets		
1921	20% of total energy	70% of total energy	10% of total energy
1950	40% of total energy	40% of total energy	20% of total energy
1971	45% of total energy	35% of total energy	20% of total energy
1986	≤60% of total energy	<30% of total energy	12%–20% of total energy
1994	Based on nutrition assessment and treatment goal	<10% of energy from saturated fats	10%–20% of total energy
2002	Patients should receive individualized nutrition therapy as needed to achieve treatment goals, preferably provided by a registered dietitian familiar with components of diabetes nutrition therapy (NT).		
	Whole grains, fruits, vegetables, and low-fat milk should be included in a healthy diet. Total amount of carbohydrate in meals or snacks is more important than source or type of carbohydrate. Sucrose and sucrose-containing foods should be eaten in the context of a healthy diet (they do not need to be restricted but should be occasionally consumed instead of other carbohydrate sources or covered with insulin or other glucose-lowering medication). Individuals receiving intensive insulin therapy should adjust their premeal insulin dosages on basis of carbohydrate content of meals. Individuals receiving fixed daily insulin dosages should be consistent in day-to-day carbohydrate intake.	<10% of energy from saturated fat ~10% of energy from polyunsaturated fat Omit *trans* fat <300 mg dietary cholesterol/day Fat intake should be individualized and designed to fit ethnic and cultural backgrounds	Ingested protein is just as potent a stimulant of insulin secretion as carbohydrate Protein requirements may be >0.8 g/kg/day for individuals with less-than-optional glycemic control Usual protein intake (15%–20% of total energy) need not be modified if renal function is normal
2010	About 79 million Americans with prediabetes are at risk for development of diabetes in the next 10 years if they don't make appropriate lifestyle changes.		
2017	Very low-carbohydrate, low-saturated-fat/high-unsaturated-fat diet produces greater improvement in A_1c, lipid levels and blood glucose control and reductions in diabetes medication (Tay et al, 2015).		

(Modified from Gaquin M: *Historical perspectives of dietary recommendations for diabetes.* Wiley Publishers. 2015. Online library https://onlinelibrary.wiley.com/doi/10.1002/9781119121725.ch3 Accessed 1 September, 2020; Tay J et al: Comparison of low- and high-carbohydrate diets for T2D management: a randomized trial, *Am J Clin Nutr* 102:780–790, 2015.)

TABLE 15.6 Nutrition Recommendations for Diabetes During Pregnancy

Nutrient	Recommendations
Medical nutrition therapy	Recommended for all women with gestational or overt diabetes to help achieve and maintain glycemic control and provide nutrient requirements.
Individualized plan	Provide adequate calorie intake to promote fetal/neonatal and maternal health, achieve glycemic goals, and promote appropriate gestational weight gain. There is no definitive research that identifies a specific optimal calorie intake for women with gestational diabetes mellitus (GDM).
Insulin management	Insulin is the preferred agent for management of both T1D and T2D in pregnancy because it does not cross the placenta. Manage insulin with food intake carefully.
Carbohydrate and protein	Limit carbohydrate to 35%–40% of total calories. Distribute in three small- to moderate-sized meals and two to four snacks (including an evening snack). The Dietary Reference Intakes (DRI) suggest a minimum of 175 g of carbohydrate, a minimum of 71 g of protein, and 28 g of fiber.
Nutritional supplements (minerals, vitamins)	Same recommendations as for women without diabetes with the exception of folic acid (5 mg daily starting 3 months before) withdrawing contraceptive measures or attempting conception. Reduce dose of folic acid to 0.4-1.0 mg/d at 12 weeks' gestation; continue this dose until completion of breastfeeding.
Postpartum	Because GDM may represent preexisting undiagnosed type 2 or even T1D, women with GDM should be tested for persistent diabetes or prediabetes at 4–12 weeks postpartum with a 75-g oral glucose tolerance test using nonpregnancy criteria.
Breastfeeding	Because lactation provides benefits to both mother and baby, all women should be encouraged to breastfeed.

(Modified from American Diabetes Association. Management of diabetes in pregnancy: *Standards of Medical Care in Diabetes—2019*. Diabetes Care 42(S1): S165–S172, 2019.)

Diabetes Care and Education
a diecetic practice group of the
eat right. Academy of Nutrition and Dietetics

Ready, Set, Start Counting!

Carbohydrate Counting — a Tool to Help Manage Your Blood Glucose

When you have diabetes, keeping your blood glucose in a healthy range will help you feel your best today and in the future. Carbohydrate counting — or "carb counting" — is a flexible meal-planning tool (not a diet) that helps you understand how your food choices affect your blood glucose level.

Carbohydrate and blood glucose

Any carbohydrate food you eat (e.g., milk, fruit, bread and pasta) is digested into glucose, which causes your blood glucose level to increase. That said, it's still important to eat carbohydrates throughout the day because they provide energy and essential nutrients for your body. To better manage your blood glucose, energy levels and weight, pay attention to how much carbohydrate you eat.

Maintaining the right balance between carbohydrate and insulin (whether you make it or take it) regulates your blood glucose level. Determining when and how much you eat — and whether or not you have snacks — should be based on your lifestyle, medications and meal-planning goals. A registered dietitian (RD) may consider the following factors in helping you determine the healthiest plan for you:

- **Consistency:** If you use diabetes medications or insulin, it is important to eat the same amount of food and carbohydrate at the same time each day. Doing this can keep your blood glucose from getting too high or too low.
- **Maximums:** Setting a meal-time maximum for carbohydrates along with focusing on a healthy lifestyle, and/or taking diabetes medications, is another way you can help keep your blood sugar from getting too high.
- **Matching:** If your insulin plan includes varying your dose based on what you are eating, it is important to know how much carbohydrate you are eating.

Foods that contain carbohydrate:

- Grains (e.g., breads, crackers, rice, hot and cold cereals, tortillas and noodles)
- Starchy vegetables (e.g., potatoes, peas, corn, winter squash, lentils and beans)
- Fruit and juices
- Milk and yogurt
- Sweets and desserts

Non-starchy vegetables (e.g., carrots, broccoli and tomatoes) contain only a small amount of carbohydrates and will not affect blood glucose when eaten in small portions.

Fig. 15.5 Carbohydrate counting.

(sorbitol, mannitol, and xylitol) result in lower glycemic responses than other carbohydrates, but ingesting large amounts of them may have a laxative effect.

Nonnutritive sweeteners approved for use by the U.S. Food and Drug Administration (FDA), such as saccharin, aspartame, and acesulfame K, are considered safe for consumption by individuals with diabetes. Each product has undergone rigorous testing and scrutiny before approval. All have been found to be safe when consumed by the public, including people with diabetes and pregnant women.

BOX 15.5 Strategies for Metabolic Control in T2D Mellitus

- Nutritionally adequate meal plan with a reduction of total fat, especially saturated fats
- Meals spaced throughout the day, consistently from day to day
- Mild to moderate weight loss (5–10 kg [10–20 lb]) even if desirable body weight is not achieved (moderate decrease in energy intake, increase in kcal expenditure)
- Regular exercise
- Monitoring of blood glucose levels, glycosylated hemoglobin, lipids, and blood pressure
- Oral hypoglycemic or insulin if preceding does not work

Nutrition and diet are considered by both patients and health professionals to be the most difficult problems in diabetes management. The plate method and glycemic index are two methods for planning. Glycemic index (GI) planning is rather complicated, and each person responds uniquely to a "low-GI" or "high-GI" food. Thus, an individual person with diabetes may want to keep track of how different foods affect their blood glucose levels.

The plate method (Fig. 15.6) asks you to draw an imaginary line on your plate and then try to fill it with half nonstarchy vegetables; the remaining two sections can be protein foods and starches. Add a glass of low-fat milk and a small portion of fruit to balance the meal nutritionally.

Although no longer mandatory, food exchange lists provide a good estimation of nutrient and calorie content for planning meals. Such lists show foods with their serving sizes, which are usually measured after cooking, and the number of calories they provide from the macronutrients

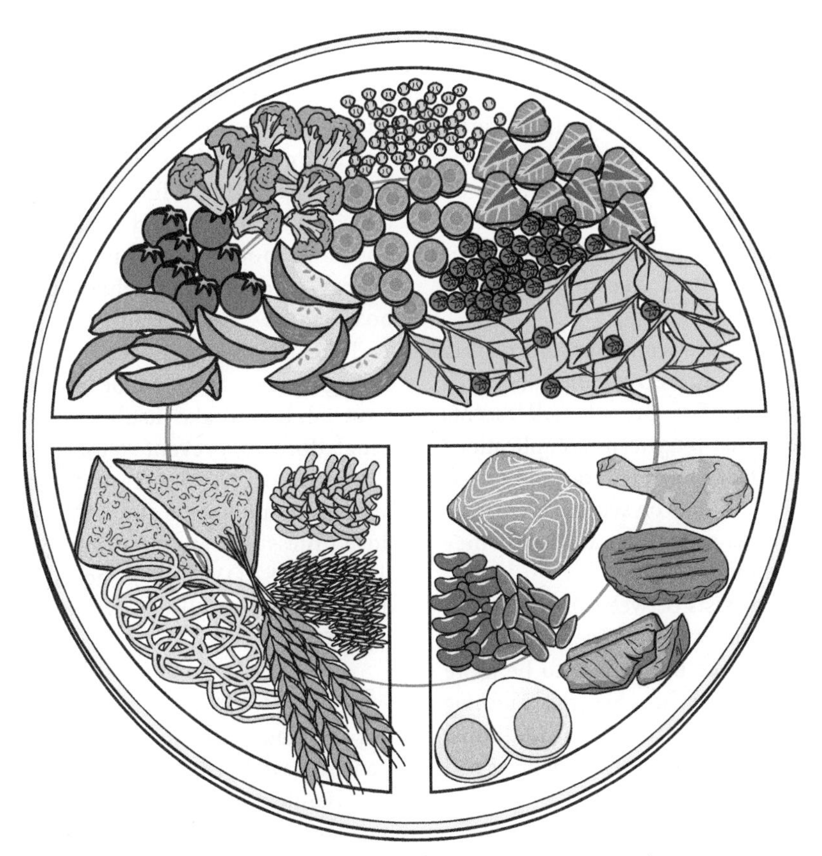

Fig. 15.6 The Plate Method for diabetes meal management. Start with a 9-inch dinner plate:
- Fill half with nonstarchy vegetables, such as salad, green beans, broccoli, cauliflower, cabbage, and carrots.
- Fill one quarter with a lean protein, such as chicken, turkey, beans, tofu, or eggs.
- Fill a quarter with a grain or starchy food, such as potatoes, rice, or pasta (or skip the starch altogether and double up on nonstarchy veggies).

(From Centers for Disease Control & Prevention. "Plate method," from https://www.cdc.gov/diabetes/managing/eat-well/meal-plan-method.html Accessed 1 September, 2020.)

(carbohydrate, protein, and fat). It is useful to measure the size of each serving to learn to "eyeball" correct serving sizes.

The following chart shows the amount of nutrients in one serving from each exchange group or list:

Groups/Lists	Carbohydrate (g)	Protein (g)	Fat (g)	Calories
Carbohydrate Group				
Starch	15	3	0–1	80
Fruit	15	—	—	60
Milk				
Fat-free, low-fat	12	8	0–3	90
Reduced-fat	12	8	5	120
Whole	12	8	8	150
Other carbohydrates	15	Varies	Varies	Varies
Nonstarchy vegetables	5	2	—	25
Meat and Meat Substitutes Group				
Very lean	—	7	0–1	35
Lean	—	7	3	55
Medium-fat	—	7	5	75
High-fat	—	7	8	100
Fat Group	—	—	5	45

(Modified from Diabetes Ed Net. The Diabetic Exchange List. From https://diabetesed.net/page/_files/THE-DIABETIC-EXCHANGE-LIST.pdf Accessed 1 September, 2020.)

Role of the Nurse

The role of the nurse in advising patients with diabetes varies according to the setting and the age of the client. However, the general approach is to help assess the patient's knowledge of, understanding of, and adherence to the prescribed diet. When possible, observing meals and food choices as well as monitoring glucose levels can give important clues to the level of compliance.

When adherence is faulty, the nurse can offer information and support. Knowledge deficits can be remedied, but lack of motivation is harder to handle. For example, adolescents with diabetes may not believe that long-term complications are related to diet and may be more motivated to eat like their peers, or older adults with diabetes may be set in lifelong eating habits and may not want to change them as long as they take medication for hyperglycemia.

When a trusting relationship exists between the nurse and patient, discussions about motivations or concerns can take place. The nurse may then influence the patient to be more concerned about their long-term welfare. See the *Teaching Tool* box Helping Clients Follow Instructions. Additional forms of support may be provided by community agencies and associations (Box 15.6).

SPECIAL CONSIDERATIONS

Illness

During periods of illness, blood glucose values may become elevated, and diabetes control may worsen. These changes are caused by an increase in hepatic production of glucose that has been stimulated by infection, illness, injury, or stress (specifically by the release of epinephrine, norepinephrine, glucagon, and cortisol). Under such conditions, this hyperglycemia increases insulin requirements. Although illness increases the need for insulin, decreased appetite and food intake are common. Liquids and soft foods are often better tolerated, provide some energy, and prevent dehydration. See the *Teaching Tool* box Sick Day Guidelines.

Take the usual medications to control blood glucose. Dosages may need to be adjusted when food intake is reduced. If you take insulin, you must continue to take your usual dose to prevent ketoacidosis. The need for insulin continues or may increase during illness. If you take oral hypoglycemic agents (tablets), continue to take your usual dose unless you are vomiting. Be aware that some medications ("O SADMANS") should be withheld during dehydrating illnesses; discuss with a pharmacist as needed. (See Fig. 15.8.)

Gastroparesis

Approximately 20% to 30% of individuals with diabetes experience delayed gastric emptying (gastroparesis). This condition can manifest as heartburn, nausea, abdominal pain, vomiting, early satiety, and weight loss. Gastroparesis occurs from vagal autonomic neuropathy and occurs more often in T1DM. Gastric electric stimulation (GES) is used to treat patients with refractory gastroparesis symptoms with fairly good results (Heckert et al., 2016).

Dietary treatment involves careful monitoring of intake. Carbohydrates should be replaced with foods of soft or liquid consistency. Six small meals may be better tolerated than three large meals. A low-fat diet may be useful to prevent

TEACHING TOOL

Helping Clients Follow Instructions

Diabetes is on the rise. English is a second language for many patients, and education may be limited for others (e.g., reading at a fourth- or fifth-grade level). Nearly 50% of Americans have low literacy skills, which affect their ability to understand their disease and treatment instructions. Because diabetes requires long-term behavioral changes and monitoring, adherence is important. The following care plan provides guidance for the team. Patients who are empowered with knowledge about their disease and treatment can take an active role in their diabetes care (Sun et al., 2019). Health professionals can improve understanding and compliance by (1) using patient education materials that are simple and concise, (2) using culturally appropriate graphics showing step-by-step instructions, and (3) involving family members.

To be effective, diabetes nutrition therapy must be individualized with consideration of personal preferences (traditions, culture, religion, health beliefs, and economics) and the ability to make lifestyle changes for healthy eating patterns and portions. The whole health care team establishes the care plan, but the patient is the key decision-maker; Fig. 15.7 shows how one hospital system provides diabetes management as a team.

Interdisciplinary Diabetes Care for Nonpregnant Adults

Bedside Nurse
Assesses patient for education needs

Goal: Patient verbalizes understanding of diabetes survival skills

1. Medication
2. Monitoring
3. Hypoglycemia
4. Who to call

Medical and Surgical Provider
Provides effective glycemic control

Goal: Patient has orders for safe and effective diabetes care management

1. Order sets
2. Daily monitoring
3. Discharge Rx and instructions
4. Follow-up appt with diabetes provider

RN/SW Case Manager
Assesses patient for discharge needs

Goal: Patient is connected to resources for post-acute care

1. Assure patient has diabetes supplies
2. Provide patient with outpatient diabetes education resources and contact # (from CM Resource page)

Pharmacist
Resolves medication safety issues

Goal: Patient with complex medication issues is safe

1. U-500 insulin
2. Insulin pumps
3. Alternate meds
4. Learning barriers

Nutritionist
Assesses patient for nutritional needs

Goal: Patient verbalizes understanding of nutrition principles for diabetes

1. All newly diagnosed patients
2. Referrals from medical providers
3. Referrals from nurses

Diabetes Education Community Resources

Goal: Self-management education resources available for patient

- Home health and telehealth
- Vidant wellness centers
- Health coaches
- Public health departments
- Community care plan
- Independent entities

Toolbox

- Basics of diabetes card
- Dashboard-videos
- DM patient education box
- Nutrition care manual
- Mosby patient education
- Patient education

Toolbox

- Diabetes education resources in Eastern NC (on CM resource page)
- Adult diabetes discharge
- Supplies process
- Practical inpatient management of adults with diabetes and hyperglycemia

Fig. 15.7 Interdisciplinary diabetes care. (Modified from Hardee SG et al: Interdisciplinary diabetes care: a new model for inpatient diabetes education, *Diabetes Spectrum* 28: 276–282, 2015. Accessed 1 September, 2020.) *CM*, Case manager; *DM*, diabetes mellitus.

delay in gastric emptying. With metoclopramide (Reglan) to increase gastric contractions and relax the pyloric sphincter, the patient may experience dry mouth and nausea. If the patient complains of dry mouth, fluids can be increased and hot foods may be moistened with broth. Insulin should be matched with meals to regulate delayed absorption and glucose changes.

If constipation or diarrhea occurs, fiber intake is altered according to patient needs. Formation of an indigestible solid mass (a bezoar) can occur after eating oranges, coconuts, green beans, apples, figs, potato skins, Brussels sprouts, or sauerkraut. If problems are severe, a temporary jejunostomy tube feeding may be indicated.

Eating Disorders

Eating disorders in T1DM are somewhat common. Once insulin therapy is initiated, weight gain occurs. Disordered eating from body image problems has been named "diabulimia." What is dangerous is insulin omission to keep weight under control. Box 15.7 shows warning signs to consider. Personalized care and referral to a mental health professional are needed.

TEACHING TOOL

Sick Day Guidelines

The following guidelines have been used with patients with diabetes who have brief illness, only during that emergency or for a maximum of 3 days:

1. Monitor blood glucose at least four times a day (before each meal and at bedtime). If you are too ill, have someone else check it for you. Write your levels down in case you need to discuss them with your doctor.
2. Test urine for ketones (if blood glucose is $\geq$250 mg/dL). Write down these levels.
3. Stick to a normal meal plan if possible.
4. Drink lots of sugar-free liquid (water, broth, tea) to prevent dehydration.
5. Call the physician if any of the following occurs:
   - Vomiting or diarrhea for more than 2 hours
   - Fever of 100.0° F or higher
   - Blood glucose levels 250 mg/dL or higher after two checks, or if levels do not go down after extra insulin
   - Spilling of moderate or large amounts of ketones in the urine
6. If you cannot tolerate regular foods, replace carbohydrates in the meal plan with liquid, semiliquid, or soft foods. A general rule is to consume approximately 15 g carbohydrates every 1 to 2 hours; the following list has good suggestions.

Foods Containing 15 g Carbohydrates

½ cup orange or grapefruit juice
⅓ cup grape or apple juice
½ cup ice cream
½ cup cooked cereal
¼ cup sherbet
⅓ cup regularly sweetened gelatin
1 cup broth-based soups (reconstituted with water)
1 cup cream soup
¾ cup regular soft drink (ginger ale, cola)
¼ cup milkshake
1½ cups milk
½ cup eggnog (commercial)
⅓ cup tapioca pudding
½ cup custard
1 cup plain yogurt
1 slice toast
6 saltine crackers

(Modified from Joslin Diabetes Center: *Stay healthy with diabetes: sick days.* Accessed 1 September, 2020, from https://www.joslin.org/patient-care/diabetes-education/diabetes-learning-center/advice-when-you-are-sick.)

BOX 15.6 Making Lifestyle Changes: Tips for Enhancing Conviction and Confidence

Enhancing Conviction

If conviction is very low, emphasize patient autonomy. "Perhaps now is not the right time to talk about this… I don't want to push you into a decision, it's clearly up to you. I suggest you take time to think about it…"

If conviction is very low, ask permission to provide new information. Avoid giving the same old lecture—vary the message.

Expand on limited conviction. "You said it was somewhat important that you change this behavior. Why did you score a 4 and not a 1? What would have to happen to move you up to a 6 or 7?"

Identify ambivalence. Avoid hard confrontation, which causes the patient to defend the attacked position. Identifying ambivalence helps the patient believe you understand their perspective: "So, you have considered this before, but you do not like people telling you what to do."

Identify barriers to considering change. Brainstorm replacements: "Watching television seems to help you relax. What else have you noticed helps you relax? How might you combine your goals of relaxing and improving physical fitness?"

Brainstorm around obstacles. "What will make it hard to increase your activity level?"

Address stated worries directly. "Because you are uncomfortable exercising in public, let's think of some other ways to increase your physical activity."

Discuss pros and cons. Have the patient list the benefits and costs of no change versus change. Start with benefits of no change—there are obviously benefits to the patient or they would not be continuing that behavior. Summarize and let the patient draw conclusions.

Help the patient take a hypothetical look "over the fence." "So you're not too sure about changing your diet. Imagine for a moment that you did make this change. How would that make you feel?"

Enhancing Confidence

Review previous change successes, praising positive steps and exploring obstacles. "Have you tried this before? How long did you continue that effort? What helped you succeed for that long? What do you think will work for you now? What obstacles were there? What might help with those obstacles now? Tell me about some of the things you have successfully changed in the past."

Expand on limited confidence. "You said you had some confidence that you could change this. Why did you score a 4 and not a 1? What would have to happen to move you up to a 6 or 7?"

Brainstorm solutions, coaching patient to select small, easy steps based on patient's previous experiences and preferences.

Facilitate the shift from success or failure to a stage model. "Most people have partial success several times before they succeed for good. Previous attempts to change increase the odds of success. People go through a period of not wanting to think about it, thinking about it, considering options, deciding to change, struggling to change, struggling with temptations or slips, and finally feeling like it's behind them. Sometimes people cycle through all or parts of that process several times before changing for good."

Address relapse prevention. Discuss "slips" rather than failures; brainstorm ways to break any pattern of slips that leads to a sense of failure; anticipate triggers and plan solutions.

(Modified with permission from American Academy of Family Physicians: Facilitating Treatment Adherence with Lifestyle Changes in Diabetes, 2004. Available at https://www.aafp.org/afp/2004/0115/p309.html. Accessed 2 September, 2020.)

Sick Days Medication List

- Opiates
- Sulfonylureas
- Angiotensin enzyme inhibitors
- Diuretics
- Metformin
- Angiotensin receptor blockers
- Nonsteroidal antiinflammatory agents
- Sodium Glucose Linked Transport 2 inhibitors

Fig. 15.8 Sick days medication list. (Modified from Sick days off – a simple strategy to prevent acute kidney injury and other adverse drug reactions, *Pharm J*, 2017. Accessed 2 September, 2020).

Metabolic Syndrome

Disproportionate abdominal fat deposition leads to excessive secretion of cytokines. Chronic low-grade inflammation in adipose tissue contributes to T2DM, cardiovascular diseases, and the metabolic syndrome. See Box 15.8 for further information on risks and management.

DIABETES MANAGEMENT THROUGH THE LIFE SPAN

Nutrition therapy is crucial for optimal blood glucose control and will be affected by various life stages: growth and development in children, growth spurts in teens, pregnancy, even the chronic conditions of aging.

Pregnancy

The risk of fetal abnormalities and mortality is increased in the presence of hyperglycemia, so every effort should be made to control blood glucose levels. Diabetes has reached epidemic proportions in indigenous populations around the globe, and there is an urgent need to improve the health of pregnant women with diabetes through timely and appropriate strategies (Harris et al., 2017).

Changes that take place during pregnancy greatly affect diabetes control and insulin use. Some hormones and enzymes produced by the placenta are antagonistic to insulin, thus reducing its effectiveness. Maternal insulin does not cross the placenta, but glucose does. The fetal pancreas increases insulin production if blood glucose levels get too high. The increased production of insulin causes macrosomia, the "large for gestational age (LGA)" infant. LGA newborns may experience respiratory difficulties, hypocalcemia, hypoglycemia, hypokalemia, or jaundice.

Individualization of nutrition therapy is contingent on maternal weight and height. Adequate calories and nutrients must meet the needs of the pregnancy and should be consistent with established maternal blood glucose goals (Table 15.6).

Blood glucose monitoring provides information about the impact of food on blood glucose levels. At the start, minimal SMBG four times a day should be planned (fasting and 1 or 2 hours after each meal), but it is not uncommon for pregnant women with diabetes to test blood glucose levels eight times per day. Blood glucose goals during pregnancy are as follows:

- Fasting: 95 mg/dL or less
- 1 hour postprandial: 140 mg/dL or less
- 2 hours postprandial: 120 mg/dL or less

There are no unique weight gain recommendations for women with diabetes. Desired weight gain goals are based on prepregnancy BMI and should be steady and progressive. Thin women should gain more weight than overweight or obese women. For an overweight or obese woman, an average weight gain of 15 pounds (6.8 kg) can be recommended.

No calorie adjustments are needed for the first trimester. During the second and third trimesters, an increased energy intake of approximately 100 to 300 kcal/day is recommended. High-quality protein should be increased by 10 g/day and can be supplied easily with one or two extra glasses of low-fat or skim milk or 1 to 2 ounces of meat or meat substitute. As with any pregnancy, 400 μg/day of folic acid is recommended for prevention of neural tube defects and other congenital abnormalities. Alcohol should not be consumed in any amount.

Energy restriction must be cautious. A minimum of 1700 to 1800 kcal/day of carefully selected foods has been found to prevent ketosis. Intakes less than this level are not advised.

Preexisting Diabetes and Pregnancy

A successful pregnancy for a woman who has diabetes requires planning and commitment. Because most fetal malformations occur during the first trimester of pregnancy, achieving and maintaining excellent glycemic control before conception and during early pregnancy are essential. Women with preexisting diabetes who become pregnant are vulnerable; fetal complications and compromised maternal health are risks.

The optimal period of care for a woman with diabetes is before conception. Ideally, preconception counseling should begin during puberty and continue through the childbearing years. Glycosylated hemoglobin levels should be normal or as close to normal as possible before conception is attempted. Insulin requirements rise during the second and third trimesters because of higher blood glucose levels caused by increased production of pregnancy-associated hormones that are insulin antagonists. Successful preconception care programs have used the following goals:

Before meals: Capillary whole-blood glucose 70 to 100 mg/dL or capillary plasma glucose 80 to 110 mg/dL

2 hours postprandial: Capillary whole-blood glucose less than 140 mg/dL or capillary plasma glucose less than 155 g/dL

Indeed, pregnancy will require greater attention to nutrition on a day-to-day basis. Guidance during early pregnancy should address food cravings and nausea. The meal

BOX 15.7 Warning Signs and Symptoms of Diabulimia

Emotional and behavioral

- Increasing neglect of diabetes management
- Secrecy about diabetes management
- Avoiding diabetes-related appointments
- Fear of low blood sugars
- Fear that "insulin makes me fat"
- Extreme increase or decrease in diet
- Extreme anxiety about body image
- Restricting certain food or food groups to lower insulin dosages
- Avoiding eating with family or in public
- Discomfort testing/injecting in front of others
- Overly strict food rules
- Preoccupation with food, weight, and/or calories
- Excessive and/or rigid exercise
- Increase in sleep pattern
- Withdrawal from friends and/or family activities
- Depression and/or anxiety
- Infrequently filled prescriptions

Physical

- A_{1c} of ≥9.0 on a continuous basis
- A_{1c} inconsistent with meter readings
- Unexplained weight loss
- Constant bouts of nausea and/or vomiting
- Persistent thirst and frequent urination
- Multiple diabetic ketoacidosis (DKA) or near DKA episodes
- Low sodium and/or potassium
- Frequent bladder and/or yeast infections
- Irregular or lack of menstruation
- Deteriorating or blurry vision
- Fatigue or lethargy
- Dry hair and skin

(Source: National Eating Disorders Association. Diabulimia. From https://www.nationaleatingdisorders.org/diabulimia-5. Accessed 2 September, 2020.)

BOX 15.8 Metabolic Syndrome

Metabolic syndrome (MetS) is a cluster of metabolic abnormalities along with chronic low-grade inflammation and oxidative stress. Criteria for MetS consist of the presence of any three of the following:

Component	Clinical Cutoff Values
Waist circumference	≥102 cm in men ≥88 cm in women
Triglycerides	≥150 mg/dL
HDL cholesterol	<40 mg/dL in men <50 mg/dL in women
Blood pressure (BP)	≥130 mm Hg systolic BP or ≥85 mm Hg diastolic BP
Fasting glucose	≥100 mg/dL
Diagnosis	Any 3 of the 5 features above

(Data from National Heart, Blood and Lung Institute (NHLBI): *What is metabolic syndrome?* Accessed 22 July, 2017, from https://www.nhlbi.nih.gov/health/health-topics/topics/ms.)

plan should be individualized, evolving throughout the pregnancy to meet changing nutritional needs and insulin requirements. Three meals and three snacks are usually recommended. Use of frequent home blood glucose monitoring is necessary to help the patient maintain normal fasting and postprandial glucose levels and avoid frequent or severe hypoglycemic reactions.

Gestational Diabetes

Gestational diabetes develops after about 24 weeks of pregnancy and occurs more often among Native American, Black American, and Hispanic/Latina American women (Daneshmand et al., 2019). Women in whom GDM develops are often obese, but weight reduction should not be attempted during the pregnancy.

Good glucose control is usually accomplished by individualization of intake and graphing of weight gain. Often, insulin may be prescribed in addition to MNT to reduce the risks of fetal macrosomia, neonatal hyperglycemia, and perinatal mortality. Treatment options can include oral antidiabetic pharmacologic therapies (Brown et al., 2017).

Glucose levels usually revert to normal after delivery, but there is an increased risk for later development of T2DM. Because significant differences are noted in the prevalence of T2DM among races, screening recommendations vary accordingly. Asian Americans should be screened for T2DM at a lower body mass index (BMI 23 kg/m²) than other racial groups (Choby, 2017). If compared with White Americans, using standardized BMI criteria to screen for risks may result in a large proportion of racial and ethnic minority groups being overlooked (Gujral et al, 2018).

T2D in the Young

Incidence and prevalence of T2DM in children, especially ethnic minority populations, have increased 30-fold over the past 20 years, causing the term epidemic to be used to describe the phenomenon. What has promoted this epidemic of T2DM in children? The answer is childhood obesity. The burden of diabetes and its accompanying complications affects many individuals, putting an enormous drain on health care resources. More young Americans will be taking potent medications for the rest of their lives.

Obesity is the most prominent clinical risk factor for T2DM in children and adolescents. About one third of children with T2DM have BMIs greater than 40, indicating morbid obesity, and 17% have BMIs greater than 45 (normal BMI range for the pediatric population is 35 to 39). Children and adolescents diagnosed with T2DM are generally between 10 and 19 years old, are obese, have a strong family history for T2DM, and have insulin resistance. Clinical signs that may indicate risk for T2DM include the following:

- Acanthosis nigricans (hyperpigmentation and thickening of the skin into velvety irregular folds in the neck and flexural areas), which reflects chronic hyperinsulinemia
- Polycystic ovary syndrome (PCOS), which is usually associated with insulin resistance and obesity (Box 15.9)
- Hypertension, which may occur in 20% to 30% of patients with T2DM

Girls are more susceptible than boys to T2DM, regardless of ethnicity. In addition, adolescents with T2DM generally have obese parents who also have insulin resistance or overt T2DM. Reasonable T2DM screening recommendations for children or adolescents are outlined in Box 15.10.

Generally, children and adolescents with T2DM have poor glycemic control. As with T2DM in adults, the ideal treatment goal is normalization of blood glucose values and A_1c. Successful control of hypertension and hyperlipidemia is also important. The key is to decrease the risk and slow the onset of the complications associated with diabetes.

The initial treatment depends on clinical symptoms. The range of disease at diagnosis varies from asymptomatic hyperglycemia to DKA and hyperosmolar HHNS. Both DKA and HHNS are associated with high morbidity and mortality in children. Nutrition therapy and exercise are obvious first-line treatments, but most children diagnosed with T2DM will also require drug therapy. Although insulin is the only FDA-approved drug for the treatment of diabetes in children, oral agents are most often used for children with T2DM.

BOX 15.9 Polycystic Ovary Syndrome

Polycystic ovary syndrome (PCOS) is the most common hormonal reproductive problem a woman of reproductive age can have. It can affect her menstrual cycle, fertility, hormones, insulin production, heart, blood vessels, and appearance. Clinical features include the following:

- Acanthosis nigricans
- Adult acne
- Dyslipidemia
- High level of male hormones (hyperandrogenism)
- Hirsutism
- Hyperinsulinemia or diabetes
- Infertility or recurrent pregnancy loss
- Luteinizing hormone hypersecretion
- Menstrual dysfunction or anovulation
- Possible development of small cysts in ovaries
- Sleep apnea
- Weight gain or obesity with upper body fat distribution
- Approximately 10% of women in the United States have PCOS. Obesity is present in half, and approximately 10% of this group will have T2DM by age 40 years. PCOS increases the risk for endometrial hyperplasia or cancer, diabetes, and heart disease. There is no single test to diagnose PCOS, and there is no cure. Treatment is based on an individual's symptoms.

(Data from Women's Health: *Polycystic ovary syndrome (PCOS).* Accessed 2 September, 2020 from https://www.womenshealth.gov/a-z-topics/polycystic-ovary-syndrome.)

BOX 15.10 Criteria for T2D Mellitus or Prediabetes in Children Under Age 18 Years

Consider screening for T2DM or prediabetes for all children who are overweight[a] and have two or more of the following risk factors:

Having a family member with T2D.

Being born to a mother with gestational diabetes (diabetes while pregnant).

Being Black American, Hispanic/Latino, Native American/Alaska Native, Asian Black, or Pacific Islander. Having signs of insulin resistance or conditions associated with insulin resistance (acanthosis nigricans, hypertension, dyslipidemia, polycystic ovarian syndrome, or small for gestational age birth weight). Blood glucose testing typically begins at 10 years old or when puberty starts, whichever is first, and is repeated every 3 years.

[a]Overweight (body mass index >85th percentile for age and gender; weight for height >85th percentile; or weight >120% of ideal for height)

(Data from CDC: Prevent T2D in Kids. From https://www.cdc.gov/diabetes/prevent-type-2/type-2-kids.html. Accessed 2 September, 2020.)

All children with T2DM should receive comprehensive self-management education, including SMBG, referral to a registered dietitian with knowledge and experience in nutritional management of children with diabetes, behavior modification strategies for lifestyle changes, increased daily physical activity, and decreased sedentary activity (e.g., TV viewing and computer use). There are many clever tools for teaching children, one of which is the traffic signal method (green for best choice foods, yellow for caution, red for foods to avoid). Other tools include smartphone applications (apps) for carbohydrate counting and glucose monitoring.

T2D in Older Adults

Older adults with diabetes are at risk for the development of macrovascular and microvascular complications, with higher overall risk for cardiovascular disease. They also are more likely to have issues that complicate diabetes management: frailty, depression, urinary incontinence, dementia, impaired vision, altered kidney function, and tendencies for recurrent hypoglycemia.

Key factors to consider are as follows (The Diabetes Council, 2020):

- Older patients with diabetes who are capable of activities of daily living without assistance and who have no cognitive impairment should have A_1c and blood sugar goals similar to those of a younger person.
- Avoiding low blood sugar is of paramount importance, and A_1c and blood sugar goals should be adjusted, along with careful pharmaceutical management.
- A_1c and blood sugar goals can be relaxed, but steps to avoid acute problems related to high blood sugars should be avoided (e.g., DKA).
- Avoid complications that lead to decreased functional capacity.

- Treat cardiovascular factors, such as high blood pressure or increased lipids; treat with aspirin if not contraindicated.
- Depression screening is important because elderly patients with diabetes experience more isolation, less support, and more feeling of hopelessness.

MISCELLANEOUS ISSUES: FASTING, BARIATRIC SURGERY, KETOGENIC DIETS

Some other issues pose a challenge for individuals who have diabetes. For example, fasting can be a problem for Muslims, especially during the long month of Ramadan. Concerns include possible hypoglycemia, hyperglycemia or diabetic ketoacidosis, and dehydration. Pregnant women, children, and the elderly who have diabetes should not be expected to fast.

Morbidly obese individuals who have prediabetes or T2DM may elect to have bariatric surgery. It is a valid option to treat T2DM, improving hyperglycemia and cardiovascular risk factors in adults. In adolescents, T2DM is a severe progressive form of diabetes with complications; in these patients, bariatric surgery is controversial but may improve outcomes (Khattab & Sperling, 2019).

Ketogenic diets, which are very low in carbohydrates and high in fats or proteins, have become popular. These diets are not totally safe and may be associated with nonalcoholic fatty liver disease or insulin resistance (Koskinski & Jornayvaz, 2017). Because results are controversial and improvements seem to be short term, ketogenic diets are not recommended for diabetes management.

SUMMARY

- Diabetes mellitus is a group of conditions characterized by either a relative or complete lack of insulin secretion by the beta cells of the pancreas or defects of cell insulin receptors, which results in disturbances of carbohydrate, protein, and lipid metabolism and hyperglycemia.
- Vitamin D deficiency plays a role in the onset of diabetes and metabolic syndrome.
- The two primary categories of glucose intolerance are T1D mellitus (T1DM) and T2D mellitus (T2DM).
- T1DM symptoms appear suddenly and include polyphagia, polyuria, polydipsia, and weight loss.
- Everyone with T1DM requires exogenous insulin to maintain normal blood glucose levels.
- The primary metabolic problem in T2DM is insulin resistance.
- Family history, ethnicity and obesity are the main risk factors for T2DM.
- The gradually occurring symptoms of T2DM are polyuria, polydipsia, fatigue, and frequent infections.
- Some individuals with T2DM may require insulin to optimize blood glucose control.
- Long-term complications of diabetes often lead to disability or premature death.
- Complications may be related to the level and frequency of hyperglycemia experiences throughout the life span in addition to genetic and environmental factors.
- Other forms of disturbed glucose metabolism include gestational diabetes mellitus and impaired glucose tolerance.
- Related disorders include hypoglycemia, diabetic ketoacidosis, hyperglycemic hyperosmolar nonketotic syndrome, and eating disorders.
- Control of blood glucose levels is the cornerstone of diabetes management.
- Maintenance of glucose homeostasis may require the use of insulin or other medicines, nutrition therapy, and exercise.
- Blood glucose can be monitored several ways: (1) fasting blood glucose, (2) glycosylated hemoglobin reported by reputable laboratories, and (3) self-monitoring with standardized devices.
- Nutrition therapy is an essential component of successful diabetes management, and its complexity requires a team approach.
- The diabetes management team should include a registered nurse, a physician or primary health care provider, a registered dietitian, and the person with diabetes.
- Family members should be included in education and counseling sessions when possible.
- For successful nutrition therapy, the team conducts thorough assessments, encourages the patient's role in goal setting, implements nutrition intervention, monitors results, and regularly evaluates the nutrition care plan.
- Guidelines include (1) planning for near normal blood glucose levels and optimal lipid levels; (2) individualizing diet plans; (3) having the patient reach a reasonable weight; and (4) if desired, enabling the patient to consume some foods that contain sugar if they are occasionally used instead of other carbohydrate foods.
- Nutrition recommendations for saturated fat, fiber, vitamins, and minerals are the same for individuals with diabetes as for the general population.
- Carbohydrates, sucrose, and alcohol are controlled because of the relationship of insulin to carbohydrate metabolism or to prevent or control complications.
- The Mediterranean diet can help to manage diabetes as well as the metabolic syndrome.
- Special care is needed for diabetes management during pregnancy, childhood, adolescence and aging. Individualized goals include efforts to preserve quality of life, manage hyperglycemia, avoid hypoglycemia, and prevent complications.
- Bariatric surgery is an effective solution for T2DM and should be suggested for the morbidly obese patient. Caution is advised for its use with children and teens.

THE NURSING APPROACH

Clinical Judgment and Next-Generation NCLEX® Examination-Style Questions

Case Study 1

T1D Mellitus

Jason, age 15 years, has come to diabetes camp this summer for the first time. Diagnosed with T1D mellitus (T1DM) 2 years ago, he is the only one in his family who has diabetes. He lives with his parents, a younger brother, and a younger sister. The camp nurse assessed Jason's situation and created a successful plan of care.

Assessment/Recognize Cues

Subjective (Information Told Directly to the Camp Nurse)

- "My blood sugar has been bouncing all over the place."
- "The nurse practitioner suggested that I come to diabetes camp. I want to control my blood sugar so I can feel better."
- "I have been thinking about getting an insulin pump. I hate checking my blood sugar and giving myself shots. I take four shots a day now. I'd like a pump that will measure my blood sugar and give me insulin automatically."
- "I want to be the same as my friends. They can eat whatever they want whenever they want. I don't want to be different."

Objective (Information from his Camp Admission Record)

- Blood glucose level 180 mg/dL
- Jason injects Lantus insulin (long acting) at bedtime and Humalog insulin (rapid acting) immediately before meals.
- He has not seen a dietitian since he was first diagnosed and does not follow any special meal plan.
- Last hemoglobin A_1c value was 8% (normal 4.4%–6.7%).Diagnoses (Nursing)/ Analyze Cues

1. Hyperglycemia related to inadequate blood glucose levels as evidenced by blood glucose 180 mg/dL and hemoglobin A_1c 8%
2. Need for health teaching as evidenced by "My blood sugar has been bouncing all over the place" and "I'd like a pump that will measure my blood sugar and give insulin automatically."

Planning

Patient Outcomes/Prioritize hypotheses

Short term (by the end of day 2 at camp):

- Jason will follow camp rules and participate fully in all activities and education sessions.
- He will have few or no episodes of hypoglycemia.
- He will observe how some campers use insulin pumps and will express interest in learning more.

Long term (by the end of camp in 5 days):

- He will make friends and express the desire to return to camp next summer.
- He will set a goal to continue at home to follow his meal plan and to check his blood glucose and give himself insulin before each meal and at bedtime.
- He will have few or no episodes of hypoglycemia.
- He will recognize that an insulin pump does not measure blood glucose and is not automatic.

Nursing Interventions/Generate Solutions

1. Set rules for camp and participate with campers in activities.
2. Give a presentation during an education session.
3. Be a role model by following a meal plan.
4. Be on call for emergencies.

Implementation/Take Action

1. Established the following rules for diabetic campers. Each camper will do the following:
   - Demonstrate to a counselor the correct technique for injecting insulin and using the camper's personal blood glucose meter.
   - Check and record blood glucose before each meal and at bedtime.
   - Follow the meal plan established by the camp dietitian.
   - Follow the prescription for insulin determined by the camp doctor, and meet with the camp doctor and nurse daily to discuss possible insulin adjustments.
   - Report any blood glucose level below 60 mg/dL to a counselor or the camp nurse, and consume crackers and juice as needed.
   - Participate in all planned group activities and education sessions.
   - Seek treatment for illness and injuries at the camp medical cabin.

   Rules are set to create order, safety, and a learning environment.
2. Accompanied campers to activities: swimming, boating, hiking, dancing, singing, and skits.

   Activities provide fun and opportunities for campers to make friends. Campers learn how to recognize and treat hypoglycemia that may occur following exercise. The nurse is present to treat emergencies and mingle socially with the campers.
3. Taught classes regarding sick-day management and recognition and treatment of hypoglycemia.

   Camp provides practical diabetes education and prepares campers to recognize and report problems of hyperglycemia and hypoglycemia.
4. Wore a fanny pack containing blood glucose testing equipment, glucose tablets, glucagon, and glucose for intravenous administration.

   Quick action is needed to treat hypoglycemia, as follows:
   - If a camper's blood glucose results are below 60 mg/dL and the camper is alert, they can eat glucose tablets or food containing 15 g of carbohydrate. After waiting 15 minutes, the camper should recheck the blood glucose level. If it is still low, the camper should again eat 15 g of food.
   - When a camper is not responsive enough to take glucose, glucagon can be given subcutaneously.
   - If necessary, a needle can be inserted into a vein for immediate injection of concentrated glucose.
5. Was on call for emergencies each night.

   Many episodes of hypoglycemia occur during the night. Sometimes a camper may fall from their bed with severe hypoglycemia, and this occurrence awakens counselors or other campers so they can seek help.
6. Served as a role model, following a meal plan established by the camp dietitian. Selected foods according to serving sizes and number of carbohydrates in an individualized meal plan.

   Measured foods, using measuring cups and spoons. Campers need good role models. They learn serving sizes by measuring foods.

Evaluation (by the Camp Nurse)/Evaluate Outcomes

Short term (at the end of 2 days):

- Jason had made friends and was having fun at activities.
- He checked his blood glucose level four times a day, followed his meal plan, and gave himself insulin before each meal and at bedtime, based on his doctor's prescription.
- He had no episodes of hypoglycemia.
- Jason expressed interest in learning more about insulin pumps.

Goals met.

Long term (at the end of camp on day 5):

- Jason stated he wanted to keep in touch with friends from camp and return to camp next summer.
- He said he wanted to continue measuring his blood glucose four times a day, follow his meal plan, and give insulin four times a day at home.
- He learned a lot about insulin pumps from friends at camp. He recognized that a pump does not measure blood glucose and is not automatic. He said he wants to learn more about carbohydrate counting and insulin pumps.

Continued

THE NURSING APPROACH—cont'd

- He had one episode of hypoglycemia late at night after hiking and swimming, and he treated it successfully with juice, crackers, and cheese.

Goals met.

Discussion Questions

Potential for hypoglycemia is another patient problem that could be added to Jason's care plan. Jason witnessed the nurse giving one of the campers a glucagon injection when the camper's blood glucose level was low and he was not alert enough to eat anything.

1. What are the signs and symptoms of hypoglycemia?
2. How does a glucagon injection raise blood glucose? After a client becomes more alert, what food should be given? Why?

Case Study 2

T2D Mellitus

Juanita, age 47 years, is from Mexico and has been newly diagnosed with T2D mellitus (T2DM). She speaks only a few words in English. Juanita's daughter, Maria, has accompanied her to the health clinic because she is bilingual and can act as an interpreter. Maria works as an accountant and is computer literate. Juanita was given a nutrition instruction sheet by the doctor; however, she could not read the English words, so she came to the clinic to learn what she should eat. Because the dietitian would not be available to meet with Juanita until 2 weeks later, the nurse gave initial instructions to Juanita and Maria.

Assessment/Recognize Cues

Subjective (Directly from Juanita or interpreted by her daughter)

- "My daughter told me what the instruction sheet said, but it doesn't have any of the foods I usually eat. Do I have to change everything I eat?"
- "The doctor said I shouldn't eat sugar anymore."
- "If I eat right, I don't need to take any diabetes medicine."
- "I usually cook tacos or enchiladas or burritos for my family. Can't I just eat what they eat?"
- "I don't go walking very often. I usually stay home."

Objective (From Physical Examination and Juanita's Medical Record)

- Height 5 feet, weight 135 pounds
- Blood glucose 160 mg/dL today 1 hour after eating lunch
- The doctor diagnosed diabetes after treating Juanita for a vaginal yeast infection and obtaining laboratory blood work needed for a diagnosis of diabetes.
- No diabetes medicine was prescribed.

Diagnoses (Nursing)/Analyze Cues

1. Need for health teaching related to new diabetes diagnosis as evidenced by desire to know what to eat, "Do I have to change everything I eat?" and "The doctor said I shouldn't eat sugar anymore."
2. Weight gain related to excess food and inadequate exercise as evidenced by 135% ideal body weight

Planning/Prioritize Hypotheses

Patient Outcomes

Short term (by the end of this visit):

- Juanita will understand and verbalize that the main dietary focuses are healthy food choices and weight loss.
- She will agree to read the Spanish resources about diabetes.
- She and her daughter will make an appointment to meet with the dietitian as soon as possible.

Nursing Interventions/Generate Solutions

1. Stress the importance of healthy food choices and weight loss.
2. Provide resources about diabetes in Spanish.

Implementation/Take Action

1. Told Juanita that she could still eat foods she prepares for her family, although it would be healthy for all to limit fat and sugar and salt.

   Meal plans are designed for individuals on the basis of usual eating patterns and preferences. Healthy food choices are applicable to the entire family.
2. Explained that Juanita should focus on small serving sizes to lose weight, which would improve diabetes control and general health.

   When an overweight or obese person with T2DM loses weight, glucose resistance is reduced and cardiovascular health is improved.
3. Gave Juanita a Spanish pamphlet on meal planning from the American Diabetes Association.

   This guide is a good introduction to healthy eating for people with diabetes, preparing the patient to meet with a dietitian. Brochures are generally helpful when written in the patient's language.
4. Informed Maria that the American Diabetes Association has Spanish educational materials.

   Authoritative resources are available for Hispanic/Latino patients who are newly diagnosed with diabetes. Many resources at American Diabetes Association are free, and cooking books for Latinos may be purchased.
5. Wrote down government websites for Spanish pamphlets about diabetes:
   - National Diabetes Education Program at www.ndep.nih.gov.
   - National Institute of Diabetes and Digestive and Kidney Diseases at www.diabetes.niddk.nih.gov.

   Many free Spanish resources are available from the government to help patients understand diabetes and what to eat.
6. Encouraged Juanita and her daughter to make an appointment to meet with the dietitian as soon as possible.

   The dietitian can design an individualized meal plan for the patient.
7. Suggested that Juanita make an appointment with the doctor for follow-up diabetes management and to ask about safe exercise, such as walking.

   Regular visits to the doctor are important to good diabetes management. The level of exercise should be determined by the doctor who knows about the patient's medical condition.

Evaluation/Evaluate Outcomes

Short term (at the end of the visit):

- Juanita and her daughter identified healthy food choices and weight loss as the main focuses for eating.
- They agreed to read the Spanish version of the meal planning guide.
- Maria indicated that she would visit the websites suggested.
- They made appointments with the dietitian and the doctor.

Goals met.

Discussion Questions

1. How could you help Maria explain the importance of appropriate serving sizes?
2. Compare and contrast the Plate Method for diabetes meal management and MyPlate (refer to Chapter 2 or www.ChooseMyPlate.com).

Continued

THE NURSING APPROACH—cont'd

Case Study 3

A registered nurse is assessing a 22-year-old obese Native American female who comes to the clinic with complaints of frequent pain and burning when she urinates for the last 6 months. She says that during this time she has been voiding a lot and has feelings of extreme thirst. She denies taking any prescribed medications. The patient states she gave birth to a three-week preterm 9-pound baby a year ago. She is not employed and likes to watch television. The patient denies any significant medical history except she tires easily. The only medical problem she ever had was some form of diabetes when she was pregnant. She tells the nurse that her mother and sister have diabetes and "take some pills for it." The nurse documents the following assessment findings: weight = 187 lbs., height = 5 feet 5 inches, body mass index (BMI) >31, pulse = 96 beats per minute, blood pressure = 136/88 mm Hg.

Highlight the information missing from the statement below by selecting from the list of options provided.

The nurse recognizes that the assessment findings that might suggest T2D mellitus (T2DM) include: ____________, ____________, ____________, ____________, ____________, ____________, and ____________.

Options

Alert and oriented	Family history of diabetes	Frequent urinary infections
BMI>31	Caring for infant	Excessive voiding
Easily fatigued	Polydipsia	Gestational diabetes

CRITICAL THINKING

Clinical Applications

Alan, aged 75 years, is a White man admitted to the hospital after a cerebrovascular accident. He has a history of T2D mellitus (T2DM), hypertension, moderate obesity, and possible alcohol abuse. Medications on admission are furosemide (Lasix), hydrochlorothiazide, propranolol (Inderal), and chlorpropamide (Diabinese) 500 mg bid. Alan comes to the clinic regularly, and at his last visit, he complained of blurred vision, polydipsia, polyuria, and a weight loss of 8 pounds in the past 2 weeks. He was admitted to the hospital with a diagnosis of urinary tract infection and hyperglycemic hyperosmolar nonketotic (HHNS) syndrome. Physical examination revealed the following:

- Height: 5 feet 11 inches
- Weight: 215 pounds
- Blood pressure: 160/82 mm Hg
- Cholesterol: 380 mg/dL
- Triglycerides: 300 mg/dL
- Blood sugar: 750 mg/dL
- Family history: Sister has had T2DM for 10 years

1. Explain how Alan's blood glucose level could become so high without producing ketones.
2. If this patient's HHNS is not treated, how would you expect his disease to progress?
3. What are Alan's blood glucose and lipid goals?
4. What is the purpose of the prescribed medications? Are there any possible drug-nutrient interactions?
5. How frequently should blood glucose levels be monitored?
6. What are possible complications if his T2DM remains uncontrolled?

WEBSITES OF INTEREST

American Association of Diabetes Educators (AADE)
https://www.diabeteseducator.org/
The American Association for Diabetes Educators (AADE) supports diabetes educators as they lead clients to self-management of diabetes and related chronic conditions.

American Diabetes Association (ADA)
www.diabetes.org
Educates and sponsors community services and research to prevent, cure, and manage diabetes.

National Diabetes Information Clearinghouse (NDIC)
www.diabetes.niddk.nih.gov
Functions as a diabetes information dissemination service of the National Institute of Diabetes and Digestive and Kidney Diseases (NIDDK), National Institutes of Health (NIH).

REFERENCES

Brown. J., et al. (2017). Oral anti-diabetic pharmacological therapies for the treatment of women with gestational diabetes. *Cochrane Database of Systematic Reviews (Online), 1*, CD011967.

Centers for Disease Control and Prevention (CDC) 2020: *Prediabetes*. From <https://www.cdc.gov/diabetes/basics/prediabetes.html>. Accessed 01.09.20.

Choby. B. (2017). Diabetes update: risk factors, screening, diagnosis, and prevention of T2D. *FP Essent, 456*, 20–26.

Daneshmand. S. S., et al. (2019). Bridging gaps and understanding disparities in gestational diabetes mellitus to improve perinatal outcomes. *Diabetes Spectrum, 32*, 317–323.

Gujral. U. P., et al. (2018). Ethnic differences in the prevalence of diabetes in underweight and normal weight individuals: The CARRS and NHANES studies. *Diabetes Res Clin Pract, 146*, 34–40.

Harris. S. B., et al. (2017). Call to action: a new path for improving diabetes care for indigenous peoples, a global review. *Diabetes Research and Clinical Practice, 123*, 120–133.

Heckert. J., et al. (2016). Gastric electric stimulation for refractory gastroparesis: a prospective analysis of 151 patients at a single center. *Digestive Diseases and Sciences, 61*, 168–175.

Khattab, A., & Sperling, M. A. (2019). Obesity in adolescents and youth: the case for and against bariatric surgery. *The Journal of Pediatrics, 207*, 18–22.

Koskinski, C., & Jornayvaz, F. R. (2017). Effects of ketogenic diets on cardiovascular risk factors: evidence from animal and human studies. *Nutrients, 9* pii: E517.

Lau, D. C., & Teoh, H. (2017). Current and emerging pharmacotherapies for weight management in prediabetes and diabetes. *Canadian Journal of Diabetes, 39*, S134–S141.

Mayo Clinic 2020: *T2D Overview*. From <https://www.mayoclinic.org/diseases-conditions/type-2-diabetes/symptoms-causes/syc-20351193>. Accessed 01.09.20.

Mirabelli. M., et al. (2020). Mediterranean diet nutrients to turn the tide against insulin resistance and related diseases. *Nutrients, 12,* 1066.

Reddy. M. A., et al. (2015). Epigenetic mechanisms in diabetic complications and metabolic memory. *Diabetologia, 58,* 443–455.

Savastio, S., et al. (2016). Vitamin D Deficiency and Glycemic Status in Children and Adolescents with T1D Mellitus. *PLoS One. Sep, 8;*11(9):e0162554

Singh. S. K., et al. (2020). Vitamin D deficiency in patients with diabetes and COVID- 19 infection. *Diabetes Metab Syndr, 14,* 1033–1035.

Sun. R., et al. (2019). Use of a patient portal for engaging patients with T2D: patterns and prediction. *Diabetes Technology & Therapeutics, 21,* 546–556. tandfonline.com/doi/abs/10.1080/14767058.2019.1566310. Accessed 01.08.2019.

The Diabetes Council 2020. *The elderly and diabetes: Everything you need to know.* From <https://www.thediabetescouncil.com/the-elderly-and-diabetes-everything-you-need-to-know/>. Accessed 01.09.20.

Wimalawansa. S. J. (2018). Associations of vitamin D with insulin resistance, obesity, T2D, and metabolic syndrome. *Journal of Steroid Biochemistry and Molecular Biology, 175,* 177–189.

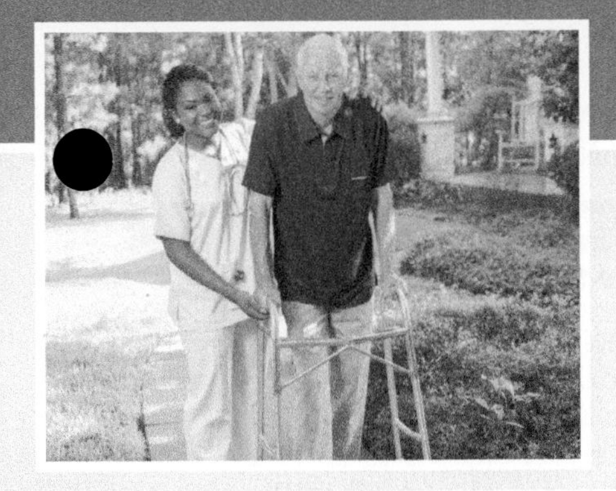

16

Nutrition in Metabolic Stress: Burns, Trauma, and Surgery

The patient with burns, trauma, sepsis, or major surgery has increased energy and nutrient demands. The stress response to injury and any preexisting malnutrition alter the healing rate and may lead to severe morbidity. A decrease in lean body mass is of concern as this component is responsible for all protein synthesis necessary for healing. Nutrition assessment and support need to be well orchestrated and precise.

RH Demling

http://evolve.elsevier.com/GRODNER/FOUNDATIONS

LEARNING OBJECTIVES

- Outline the responses of the body to starvation.
- Explain metabolic changes in uncomplicated stress and in hypermetabolic state of stress.
- Discuss the relationships among function of the immune system, nutritional status, and metabolic stress.
- List nutrients that are required for immune system functions.
- Describe systemic inflammatory response syndrome (SIRS), and identify conditions under which SIRS may occur.
- Define multiple organ dysfunction syndrome (MODS), including the rationale for close monitoring of nutrition support.

METABOLIC RESPONSE TO STRESS

It is important for nurses to understand that metabolic changes occur as a reaction to stress. Uncomplicated stress is present when patients are at nutritional risk, and severe stress is brought about by trauma, disease and some types of surgeries.

IMMUNE SYSTEM

When metabolic stress develops, hormonal and metabolic changes subdue the immune system's ability to protect the body. This activity is further depressed if nutritional status is impaired. A deadly cycle may develop: depressed immunity leads to increased risk of disease, disease impairs nutritional status, and compromised nutritional status further impairs immunity. Recovery requires that this cycle be broken.

Nutrition, Microbiota, and Immunity

A principal function of the gut microbiota is to protect the host from harmful bacteria and to prevent bacterial imbalance and gut dysbiosis (Kim et al., 2016). For optimal immunity, adequate nutrients must be available (Fig. 16.1). A well-nourished body is not ravaged by infections the way a poorly nourished body is.

Compromised nutritional status makes it difficult for the body to mount both a stress response and an immune response when confronted with a metabolic stressor such as a virus, surgery, or trauma.

Malnutrition affects each part of the immune system. Integrity of the skin and mucous membranes are compromised, and wound healing is slowed. In the gastrointestinal (GI) tract, microvilli become flat, reducing nutrient absorption. Damage to the GI tract increases the risk that infection-causing bacteria will spread outside the intestinal system (bacterial translocation). T-lymphocyte (T-cell) distribution is depressed. More time is needed for phagocytosis kill-time and lymphocyte activation. Finally, antibodies are fewer in number and less effective.

Several nutrients affect immune system functioning. Omega-3 fatty acids, vitamins A and C, and zinc each play a significant role. Table 16.1A outlines how specific nutrient deficiencies affect the immune system; Table 16.1B further defines the roles of micronutrients in immunity.

It is difficult to determine which exact nutrient deficiency results in symptoms when a patient is malnourished because of overlapping nutrient deficiencies, illness, weakness, anorexia, and infection. In addition, an unbalanced ratio of saturated to unsaturated fatty acids changes cell membrane composition and fluidity, contributing to allergic, autoimmune, and metabolic responses (Radzikowska et al., 2019).

In addition, inadequate protein and energy intake is a concern. It is known that gut microbiota diversity is decreased in old age and low prealbumin is an independent risk factor of in-hospital mortality, especially in infectious diseases like COVID-19 (Zuo et al., 2020). Personalized nutrition and supplementation known to improve immunity should be part of the medical treatment plan.

Globalization

Noncommunicable diseases (NCDs) such as obesity are a modern epidemic. Genetics, epigenetic factors, and the microbiota influence how individuals respond to diet and physical activity (Kubota, 2018). Changes in diet, nutrient content and quality, urbanization, more processing of foods, the marketing of unhealthy foods, and other factors have affected many populations. With globalization in developing countries comes an acceleration of urbanization, with an influx of people well beyond the capacity of cities to absorb them (Food and Agriculture Organization, 2020). In cities, food must be purchased and home gardens are rare. These global changes have affected household food security, the nutritional status of individuals, and food safety. The Cultural Diversity and Nutrition box Globalization and the Changing Food Supply provides a perspective on globalization.

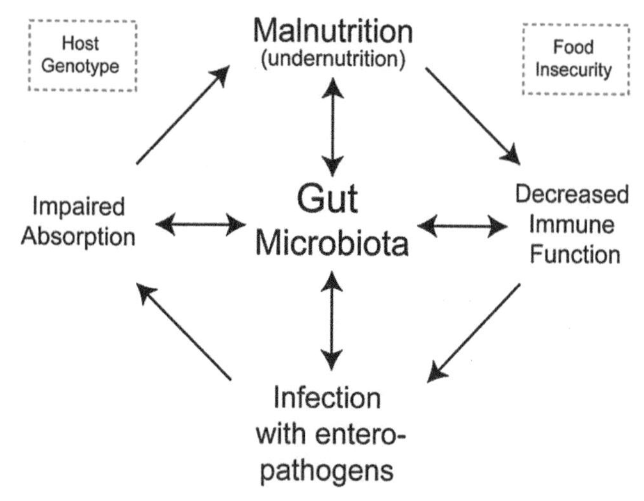

Fig. 16.1 Gut microbiota serve as a barrier to enteropathogenic infections; the barrier may be disrupted by malnutrition. (From Kau AL, et al: Human nutrition, the gut microbiome and the immune system, *Nature* 474:327–336, 2011.)

CULTURAL DIVERSITY AND NUTRITION

Globalization and the Changing Food Supply

Globalization and technology have brought better, more immediate communication throughout the world. These have also brought increased trade, greater food transport, more foodborne illnesses, new viruses (such as COVID-19), altered marketing, and other consequences. Although greater accessibility has promoted cultural fusion, there are disadvantages as well. The demands on natural resources are greater than ever to meet the needs of growing populations. Large food companies and restaurant chains have expanded their reach across the world; traditional foods are often in competition with "Westernized" diets. In many families, dining away from home means a less nutritious diet overall.

Culture includes religion, customs, language, traditions, ideas, and how we form our identity. With increased migration, the world is a more hybridized society than ever before. Local cultures are merging into one global identity and the more powerful nations tend to dominate. Economic globalization is here, but for some countries this means loss of their own distinctiveness.

Application to Nursing

Food safety is a concern. Some imported foods and foods brought from home to a hospital or long-term care setting may be contaminated. Microbial adaptation, changes in food production, and the introduction of pathogens into new geographic areas are emerging issues from globalization. Awareness of the risks of food safety must be a priority. These risks are accelerated for the patient undergoing the stressors of surgery, trauma, or burns.

THE STRESS RESPONSE

The body's response to metabolic stress depends on the magnitude and duration of the stress. Stress sets up a chain reaction involving hormones and the central nervous system that affects the entire body. Hormones altered by stress include the following:

- Aldosterone—corticosteroid that causes renal sodium retention
- Antidiuretic hormone (ADH)—stimulates renal tubular water absorption to conserve water and salt to support circulating blood volume.

TABLE 16.1A Role of Nutrients and Nutritional Status on Immune System Components

Immune System Component	Effects of Malnutrition	Vital Nutrients
Mucus	Decreased antibody secretions	Vitamin B_{12}, biotin, vitamins B_6 and C
Gastrointestinal tract	Flat microvilli, increased risk of bacterial spread to outside gastrointestinal tract	Arginine, omega-3 fatty acids
Skin	Integrity compromised, density reduced, wound healing slowed	Protein, vitamins A and C, niacin, zinc, copper, linoleic acid, vitamin B_{12}
T lymphocytes	Depressed T-cell distribution	Protein; arginine; omega-3 fatty acids; vitamins A, B_{12}, and B_6; folic acid; thiamine; riboflavin; niacin; pantothenic acid; zinc; iron
Macrophages and granulocytes	Longer time for phagocytosis kill time and lymphocyte activation	Protein; vitamins A, C, B_{12}, and B_6; folic acid; thiamine; riboflavin; niacin; zinc; iron
Antibodies	Reduced antibody response	Protein; vitamins A, C, B_{12}, and B_6; folic acid; thiamine; biotin; riboflavin; niacin

Table 16.1B Key Roles of Select Micronutrients in the Immune System

Micronutrient/ Role	Innate Immunity	Adaptive Immunity
Vitamin C	Effective antioxidant that protects against ROS and RNS produced when pathogens are killed by immune cells Regenerates other important antioxidants such as glutathione and vitamin E to their active state Promotes collagen synthesis, thereby supporting the integrity of epithelial barriers Stimulates production, function and movement of leukocytes (e.g., neutrophils, lymphocytes, phagocytes) Increases serum levels of complement proteins Has roles in antimicrobial and NK cell activities and chemotaxis Involved in apoptosis and clearance of spent neutrophils from sites of infection by macrophages	Can increase serum levels of antibodies Has roles in lymphocyte differentiation and proliferation
Vitamin D	Vitamin D receptor expressed in innate immune cells (e.g., monocytes, macrophages, dendritic cells) Increases the differentiation of monocytes to macrophages Stimulates immune cell proliferation and cytokine production and helps protect against infection caused by pathogens 1,25-dihydroxyvitamin D_3, the active form of vitamin D, regulates the antimicrobial proteins cathelicidin and defensin, which can directly kill pathogens, especially bacteria	Mainly inhibitory effect in adaptive immunity; for example, 1,25-dihydroxyvitamin D_3 suppresses antibody production by B cells and inhibits T cell proliferation
Vitamin A	Helps maintain structural and functional integrity of mucosal cells in innate barriers (e.g., skin, respiratory tract, etc.) Important for normal functioning of innate immune cells (e.g., NK cells, macrophages, neutrophils)	Necessary for proper functioning of T and B lymphocytes, and thus for generation of antibody responses to antigen Involved in development and differentiation of Th1 and Th2 cells and supports Th2 antiinflammatory response
Vitamin E	An important fat-soluble antioxidant Protects the integrity of cell membranes from damage caused by free radicals Enhances IL-2 production and NK cell cytotoxic activity	Enhances T cell-mediated functions and lymphocyte proliferation Optimizes and enhances Th1 and suppresses Th2 response
Vitamin B_6	Helps regulate inflammation Has roles in cytokine production and NK cell activity	Required in the endogenous synthesis and metabolism of amino acids, the building blocks of cytokines and antibodies Has roles in lymphocyte proliferation, differentiation and maturation Maintains Th1 immune response Has roles in antibody production
Vitamin B_{12}	Has roles in NK cell functions	May act as an immunomodulator for cellular immunity, especially with effects on cytotoxic cells (NK cells, $CD8^+$ T-cells) Facilitates production of T lymphocytes Involved in humoral and cellular immunity and one-carbon metabolism (interactions with folate)
Folate	Maintains innate immunity (NK cells)	Has roles in cell-mediated immunity Important for sufficient antibody response to antigens Supports Th 1-mediated immune response
Zinc	Antioxidant effects protect against ROS and RNS Helps modulate cytokine release and induces proliferation of $CD8^+$ T cells Helps maintain skin and mucosal membrane integrity	Central role in cellular growth and differentiation of immune cells that have a rapid differentiation and turnover Essential for intracellular binding of tyrosine kinase to T cell receptors, required for T lymphocyte development and activation Supports Th1 response
Iron	Involved in regulation of cytokine production and action Forms highly-toxic hydroxyl radicals, thus involved in the process of killing bacteria by neutrophils Important in the generation of ROS that kill pathogens	Important in the differentiation and proliferation of T lymphocytes Essential for cell differentiation and growth, component of enzymes critical for functioning of immune cells (e.g., ribonucleotide reductase involved in DNA synthesis)
Copper	Free-radical scavenger Antimicrobial properties Accumulates at sites of inflammation, important for IL-2 production and response May play a role in the innate immune response to bacterial infections	Has roles in T cell proliferation Has roles in antibody production and cellular immunity
Selenium	Essential for the function of selenium-dependent enzymes (selenoproteins) that can act as redox regulators and cellular antioxidants, potentially counteracting ROS Selenoproteins are important for the antioxidant host defense system affecting leukocyte and NK cell function	Involved in T lymphocyte proliferation Has roles in the humoral system (e.g., immunoglobulin production)

IL, interleukin; *NK*, natural killer; *RNS*, reactive nitrogen species; *ROS*, reactive oxygen species; *Th*, helper T cell.
(From Maggini, S., et al. Immune function and micronutrient requirements change over the life course, *Nutrients* 10: 1531, 2018.)

- Adrenocorticotropic hormone (ACTH)—acts on adrenal cortex to release cortisol (mobilizes amino acids from skeletal muscles)
- Catecholamines—epinephrine and norepinephrine from renal medulla stimulate hepatic glycogenolysis, fat mobilization, gluconeogenesis

Whether stress is uncomplicated (from altered food intake or activity level) or complicated by trauma or disease, metabolic changes take place throughout the body. The metabolic response to stress differs from the metabolic response to starvation and it is important to recognize the difference.

Effects of Stress on Nutrient Metabolism

The body's constant response to minor changes brought about by needs or environment was first called the "fight or flight" response, or general adaptation syndrome (GAS). The body constantly adapts to these minor environmental changes to maintain homeostasis. The stress response involves an integrated series of actions that involve the hypothalamus and hypophysis, sympathetic nervous system, adrenal medulla, and adrenal cortex. Significant effects of this response to stress are outlined in Table 16.2. These responses to stress produce multiple changes in metabolic processes throughout the body (Fig. 16.2).

Effects of Starvation

If we involuntarily go without food, this state is described as starvation. If we withhold food from ourselves for a time, that state is fasting. Whatever the reason for inadequate food intake and nourishment, results are the same. After a brief period of going without food or an interval of nutrient intake below metabolic needs, the body extracts stored carbohydrate and fat, as well as protein from muscles and organs, to meet energy demands.

Liver glycogen is used first to maintain normal blood glucose levels and to provide energy for brain and red blood cells. This source of energy is limited; glycogen stores are usually depleted in 24 hours. Unlike glycogen stores, lipid (triglyceride) stores may be substantial, and the body also begins to mobilize this energy source. As the amount of liver glycogen decreases, mobilization of free fatty acids from adipose tissue increases to provide energy needed by the nervous system. After approximately 24 hours without intake (especially carbohydrates), the prime source of glucose is from gluconeogenesis.

Brain cells use glucose for energy. During early starvation (~2 to 3 days), the brain uses glucose produced from muscle protein. As muscle protein is broken down for energy, the levels of branched-chain amino acids (BCAAs), consisting of

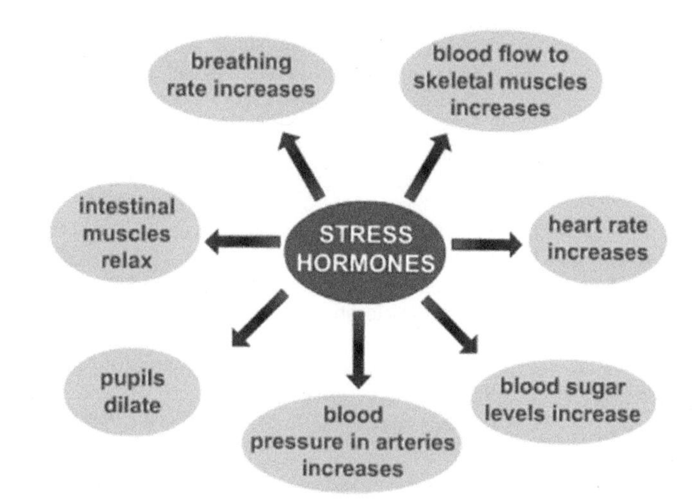

Fig. 16.2 The body changes that occur with the initial response to stress.

TABLE 16.2 Effects of the Stress Response

Target Organ	Hormonal Response	Physiologic Response	Signs/Symptoms
Sympathetic nervous system and adrenal medulla	Norepinephrine	Vasoconstriction	Pallor, decreased glomerular filtration rate, nausea, elevated blood pressure
Adrenal medulla	Epinephrine	Vasoconstriction	See above
		Increased heart rate	Elevated blood pressure
		Vasodilation	Increased skeletal muscle function
		Central nervous system (CNS) stimulation	More alert, increased muscle tone
		Bronchodilation	Increased O_2
		Glycogenolysis, lipolysis, gluconeogenesis	Increased blood glucose
Adrenal pituitary and cortex	Cortisol/glucocorticoids	CNS stimulation	Increased blood glucose, increased serum amino acids, delayed wound healing
		Protein catabolism, gluconeogenesis	
		Stabilize cardiovascular system	Enhance catecholamine action
		Gastric secretion	Ulcers
		Inflammatory response decreased	Decreased white blood cells (WBCs)
		Allergic response decreased	
		Immune response decreased	
	Aldosterone/mineralocorticoid	Increased blood pressure	Retained sodium and water, increased blood volume
Posterior pituitary	Antidiuretic hormone (vasopressin) and aldosterone	Water reabsorbed, increased blood volume, increased blood pressure	

(Data from Hubert, R.J., VanMeter, K.C. *Gould's pathophysiology for the health-related professions*, ed 5, Philadelphia, 2017, Elsevier.)

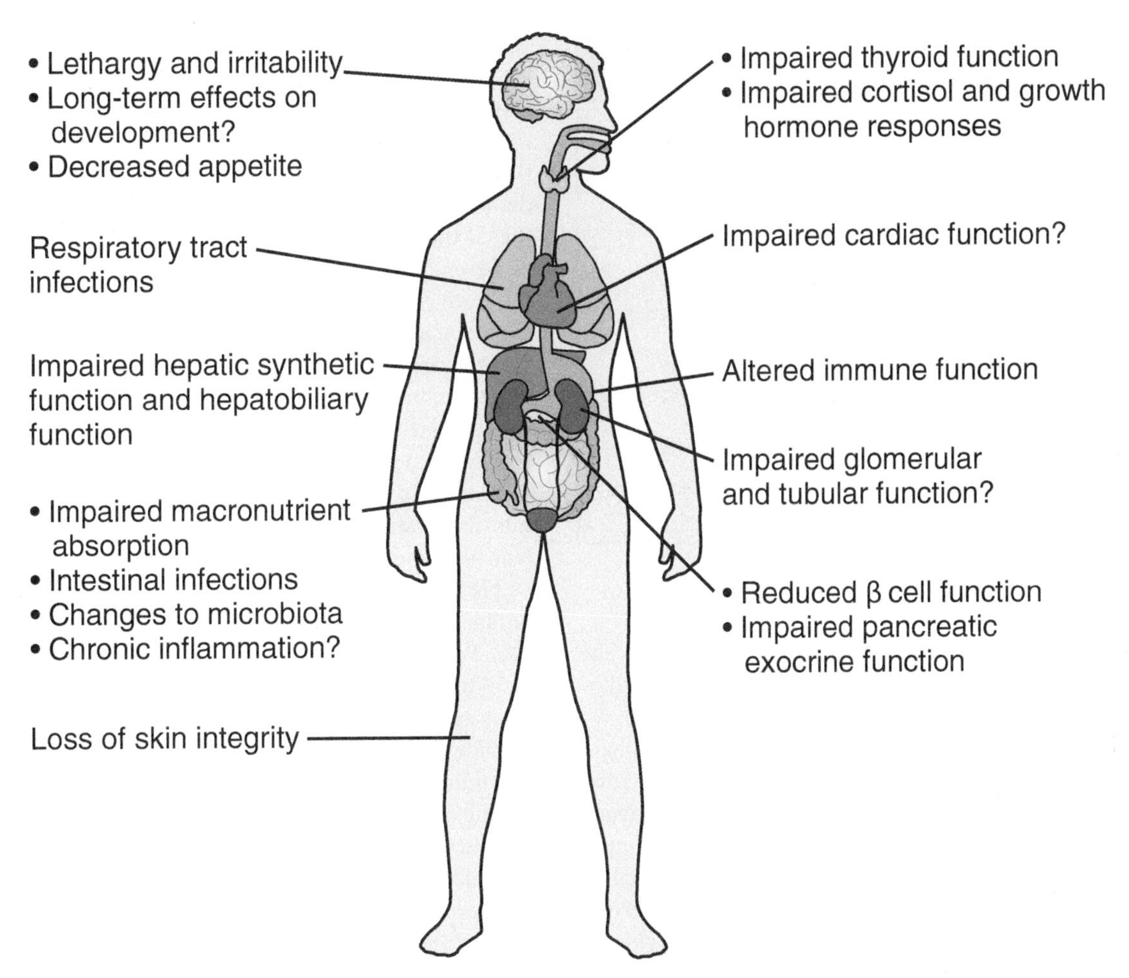

Fig. 16.3 Metabolic changes in starvation. (From Hoffer, L.J. Clinical nutrition: Protein-energy malnutrition in the inpatient, *CMAJ* 165:1345–1349, 2001. Accessed 6 September, 2020, from www.cmaj.ca/content/165/10/1345.figures-only.)

leucine, isoleucine, and valine, increase in circulation, although BCAAs are primarily metabolized directly inside muscle.

The body does not store any amino acids as it does glucose and triglycerides. The only internal sources of amino acids are lean body mass (muscle tissue), vital organs including heart muscle, and other protein-based constituents such as enzymes, hormones, immune system components, and blood proteins. By the second or third day of starvation, approximately 75 g of muscle protein is catabolized each day, a level inadequate to supply full energy needs of the brain. At this point, other sources of energy become more available. Fatty acids are hydrolyzed from the glycerol molecule, and both free fatty acids and glycerol are released into the bloodstream. Free fatty acids are used; glycerol can be used by the liver to generate glucose (gluconeogenesis).

If starvation is prolonged, the body preserves proteins by mobilizing more fat for energy. Production of ketone bodies from fatty acids is accelerated, and the body's demand for glucose decreases. Although some glucose is still vital for brain cells and red blood cells, these and other body tissues start to obtain the major proportion of their energy from ketone bodies. Muscle protein is still being catabolized but at a much lower rate, which prolongs survival.

An additional defense mechanism of the body to conserve energy is to slow its metabolic rate, thereby decreasing energy demands. With declining metabolic rate, body temperature drops, activity decreases, and sleep periods increase—all to allow the body to preserve energy. If starvation continues, intercostal muscles necessary for respiration are depleted, leading to pneumonia and respiratory failure. Starvation will continue until adipose stores are exhausted. Fig. 16.3 shows the phases.

Severe Stress

Whether stress is accidental (broken bones, trauma, or burns) or planned (surgery), the body reacts to it as well. During starvation, the body's metabolic rate slows, becoming hypometabolic. During severe stress, the body's metabolic rate rises profoundly, thus becoming hypermetabolic. This response to stress involves most metabolic pathways, with accelerated metabolism of lean body mass, negative nitrogen balance, and muscle wasting. Once the systemic response is activated, the physiologic and metabolic changes that follow may lead to septic shock.

The body's response to stress occurs in two phases. During the immediate postinjury (ebb) phase, decreased oxygen consumption, tissue hypoxia, decreased cardiac output, hypothermia (lowered body temperature), and lethargy occur (Table 16.3).

TABLE 16.3 Metabolic Responses to Severe Stress

Initial Injury (Ebb) Phase	Recovery (Flow) Phase
↓ Oxygen consumption	↑ Oxygen consumption
↓ Cardiac output	↑ Cardiac output
↓ Plasma volume	↑ Plasma volume
Hypothermia	Hyperthermia
	↑ Nitrogen excretion
↓ Insulin levels	Normal or elevated insulin levels
Hyperglycemia	Hyperglycemia
Hypovolemia	Normal volume
Hypotension	Usual blood pressure
↑ Lactate	Normal lactate
↑ Free fatty acids	↑ Free fatty acids
↑ Catecholamines, glucagon, cortisol	↑ Catecholamines, glucagon, cortisol
Insulin resistance	↑ Insulin resistance

↑, Increased; ↓, decreased.

Insulin levels drop because the glucagon level is elevated. The major medical concern during this time is to maintain cardiovascular effectiveness and tissue perfusion.

As the body responds to injury, the recovery (flow) phase begins, about 36 to 48 hours after injury. This phase follows fluid resuscitation and is characterized by increased oxygen consumption, hyperthermia (increased body temperature), increased cardiac output, and nitrogen excretion, as well as expedited catabolism of carbohydrate, protein, and triglycerides to meet the higher metabolic demands. Marked rises in glucose production, free fatty acids, and circulating hormones (insulin/glucagon/cortisol) occur. Recovery will last for days, weeks, or months, until the injury is healed.

Multiple stresses result in increased catabolism and even greater loss of body proteins. If the patient is in poor nutritional status before the stress of surgery, they are at greater risk for development of pneumonia or a wound infection accompanied by fever. As in starvation, energy requirements will be met from endogenous sources (within the body) if exogenous sources (food, outside the body) are not available or adequate. Intercostal muscles may be depleted, leading to pneumonia, or inadequate amino acid levels will impair antibody production and the immune response to infection. Both conditions have a negative impact on metabolic demands.

Food and Nutrition Therapies

Nutrients affected by hypermetabolic stress include protein, vitamins, and minerals. There are also concerns about total energy and fluid intake. During moderate metabolic stress, protein requirements have been reported to increase from 0.8 g/kg body weight (normal recommendation for an average healthy adult) to 1 to 1.5 g/kg body weight. In severe stress (e.g., thermal injuries exceeding 20% total body surface area [TBSA] or deep pressure ulcers), protein requirements may rise to 1.5 to 2 g/kg body weight. These levels allow for protein synthesis if sufficient energy is provided from carbohydrate and fat; extra fluid may also be needed.

Requirements of vitamins and minerals all increase during stress. Tissue repair especially depends on adequate intakes of vitamin C, zinc, calcium, magnesium, manganese, and copper. At the least, Dietary Reference Intake (DRI) levels of nutrients should be consumed, preferably from foods or tube feeding rather than from supplemental forms. Achieving requirements through food provides sufficient energy to meet increased demands during critical illness and maintains the integrity of the GI tract and its microbiota.

Several calculation formulas have been used to determine the resting metabolic rate (RMR) and energy needs of patients experiencing hypermetabolic stress. Handheld (Medgem) calorimeters are more accurate than predictive equations. Registered dietitians, in collaboration with the medical team, use these tools or formulas to determine energy requirements. Note that indirect calorimetry is the standard for determination of RMR in critically ill patients because actual measurement is more accurate than estimation using predictive equations (Academy of Nutrition and Dietetics, Evidence Analysis Library [EAL], 2020).

Fluid requirements during hypermetabolic stress are based on age, reflecting age-related modifications of body composition. For adults younger than 55 years, fluid needs are calculated at 35 to 40 mL/kg body weight. Adults between ages 55 and 65 years require a lower amount, 30 mL/kg body weight. Box 16.1 provides some general guidelines used in determining nutrition and fluid needs in metabolic stress.

The objectives for optimal metabolic and nutritional support in injury, trauma, burns, and sepsis are to do the following:

- Detect and correct preexisting malnutrition.
- Prevent progressive protein-calorie malnutrition.
- Optimize patient's metabolic state by managing fluid and electrolytes.
- Initiate specialized nutrition support (SNS) when it is anticipated that the critically ill patient will be unable to meet nutrient needs orally for a period of 5 to 10 days.
- Use enteral nutrition as the preferred route of feeding over parenteral nutrition whenever possible.

Because overfeeding is more problematic than underfeeding, some clinicians use an adjusted calculation of 20 to 21 kcal/kg actual body weight in obese patients. Clinical judgment must play a major role in the decision to begin or continue nutrition support.

Effects of Stress on Nutrient Metabolism

Protein Metabolism

Even if adequate carbohydrate and fat are available, skeletal muscle protein is mobilized for energy (amino acids are converted to glucose in the liver). There is decreased uptake of amino acids by muscle tissue and increased urinary excretion of nitrogen (Fig. 16.4).

In highly stressed patients, 1.5 to 2.0 g/kg/day is given to start. Close monitoring is needed to end negative nitrogen balance and its detrimental effects. To date, no studies have demonstrated a significant difference in infection, length of stay, or mortality rates based on the level of protein intake or method of protein delivery (EAL, 2020).

Some nonessential amino acids become "conditionally essential" during metabolic stress. Arginine, cysteine, glutamine, glycine, proline, serine and tyrosine fall into this category.

BOX 16.1 Nutrition Therapy for Metabolically Stressed Patients

Energy requirements are highly individual and may vary widely from person to person. Total kcal requirements depend on the basal energy expenditure (BEE) plus the presence of trauma, surgery, infection, sepsis, and other factors. The most accurate method to determine energy needs is indirect calorimetry. When indirect calorimetry cannot be performed, use of predictive formulas is necessary. The formulas with the best prediction accuracy for critically ill patients are the Ireton-Jones energy equations. Other formulas do not have adequate prediction accuracy because they were developed for the healthy population.

Ireton-Jones Energy Equations (IJEEs)

Spontaneously breathing (s) = 629 − 11(A) + 25(W) − 609(O)

Ventilator dependent IJEE (v) = 1925 − 10(A) + 5(W) + 281(S) + 292(T) + 851(B)

Age (A) in years; body weight (W) in kilograms (kg); sex (S, male = 1, female = 0); diagnosis of trauma (T, present = 1, absent = 0); diagnosis of burn (B, present = 1, absent = 0); obesity more than 30% above initial body weight from body mass index >27 (present = 1, absent = 0).

Protein Requirements

Additional protein is required to synthesize the proteins necessary for defense and recovery, to spare lean body mass, and to reduce the amount of endogenous protein catabolism for gluconeogenesis.

Vitamin/Mineral Needs

Needs for most vitamins and minerals increase in metabolic stress; however, no specific guidelines exist for provision of vitamins, minerals, and trace elements.

It is commonly believed that if the increased kcal requirements are met, adequate amounts of most vitamins and minerals are usually provided. In spite of this belief, vitamin C, vitamin A or beta carotene, and zinc may need special attention.

Fluid Needs

Fluid status can affect interpretation of biochemical measurements, as well as anthropometry and physical examination. Fluid requirements can be estimated using several different methods.

Micronutrient Supplementation

Vitamin C: 500 to 1000 mg/day in divided doses

Vitamin A: 1 multivitamin tablet containing vitamin A, one to four times daily

Zinc sulfate: 220 mg, one to three times daily

Fluid requirements based on:		Water (mL)
Weight		100 mL/kg for first 10 kg
		40 mL/kg/day
Age and weight	16–30 years (active)	35 mL/kg/day
	30–55 years	30 mL/kg/day
	55–75 years	25 mL/kg/day
	>75 years	
Energy needs	1 mL/kcal	
Fluid balance	Urine output + 500 mL/day	

(Data from Academy of Nutrition and Dietetics, Evidence Analysis Library: *Critical illness evidence-based nutrition practice guideline.* Accessed 27 July, 2017, from www.andevidencelibrary.com.)

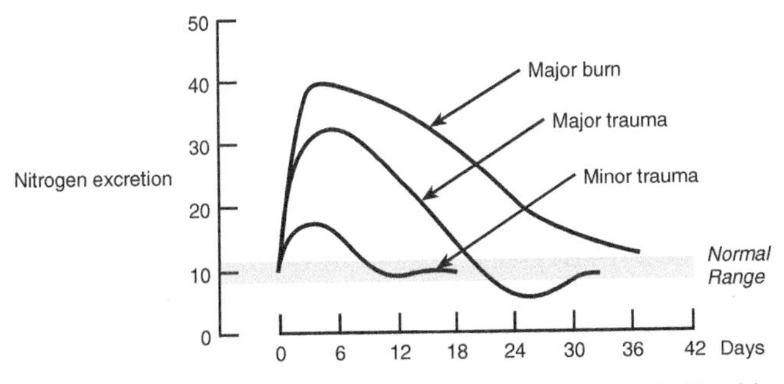

Fig. 16.4 Nitrogen excretion. (From Kinney, J.M., et al. *Nutrition and metabolism in patient care*, Philadelphia, 1988, Saunders.)

One of the more studied amino acids is glutamine, and many formulas now contain added glutamine.

During stress, glutamine is mobilized in large quantities from skeletal muscle and lung to be used directly as a fuel source by intestinal cells. Glutamine also plays a significant role in maintaining intestinal immune function and enhancing wound repair by supporting lymphocyte and macrophage proliferation, hepatic gluconeogenesis, and fibroblast function; see Fig. 16.5.

The clinician must recognize that not all patients can tolerate glutamine additives; they are contraindicated in severe liver disorders.

Carbohydrate Metabolism

Hepatic glucose production is increased and disseminated to peripheral tissues, although proteins and fats are being used for energy. Insulin levels and glucose use will increase, but hyperglycemia occurs that is not necessarily resolved by using exogenous insulin. It appears, to some extent, to be driven by an elevated glucagon-to-insulin ratio.

In general, carbohydrate should provide 60% to 70% of total calories. If carbohydrate is given parenterally, note that the maximum rate of glucose oxidation is 5 to 7 mg/kg/min or 7 g/kg/day. Overfeeding should not occur. Blood glucose levels should be monitored, with adjusted nutrition and insulin regimens to keep the serum glucose level less than 150 mg/dL.

Fat Metabolism

To support hypermetabolism and increased gluconeogenesis, fat is mobilized from adipose stores (through lipolysis) to provide energy. Lipolysis results from elevations of catecholamines, with a concurrent decrease in insulin production. If hypermetabolic patients are not fed during this period, fat stores and proteins are rapidly depleted. This malnutrition increases susceptibility to infection and may contribute to multiple organ dysfunction syndrome (MODS), sepsis, and death.

Fat administration should suffice to prevent essential fatty acid (EFA) deficiency and to provide extra energy. In general, fat should provide 15% to 40% of total calories. However, in stressed patients, feedings high in long-chain fatty acids may cause immunosuppression. Formulas should include more omega-3 fatty acids.

Hydration/Fluid Status

Increased fluid losses can result from fever, increases in perspiration or urine output, diarrhea, draining wounds, or diuretic

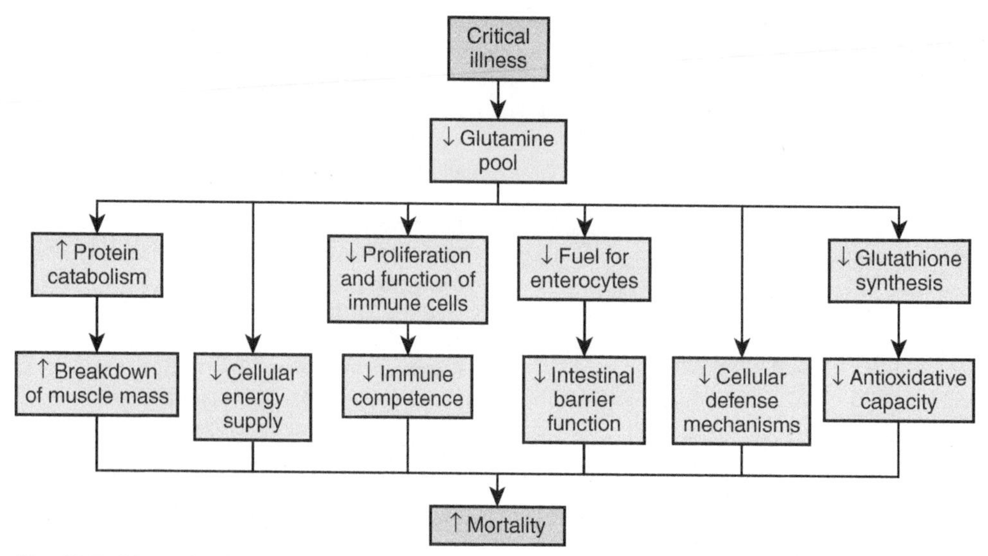

Fig. 16.5 Glutamine in critical illness. (Modified from Stehle, P., Sun, K.S. Glutamine: an obligatory parenteral nutrition substrate in critical care therapy, *Biomed Res Int* 2015:545467, 2015.)

therapy. An average calculation is 1 to 1.5 mL/kcal expended, or 30 to 40 mL/kg of body weight. Requirements may be decreased in the presence of heart, renal, or liver failure. Accurate intake and output (I&O) records are essential.

Vitamins and Minerals

When energy needs increase, vitamins and minerals must also be increased. Special attention should be given to vitamins A and C and zinc. Vitamin C is crucial for the collagen formation and wound healing. Supplements of 500 to 1000 mg/day are recommended. Vitamin A and beta carotene (the vitamin A precursor) play an important role in the healing process and as antioxidants.

Zinc increases the tensile strength (force required to separate the edges) of a healing wound. Supplements of 220 mg/day zinc sulfate (orally) may be used when the patient is stabilized. Additional zinc may be necessary with large intestinal losses, as in ileostomy drainage. It should not be used for longer than 2 weeks at a time; excessive amounts of zinc will suppress immunity.

Sepsis and septic shock cause a dramatic response to infection and life-threatening organ dysfunction (Strnad et al., 2017). The liver plays a central role in managing the immune defense system at that time. Thus, patients with cirrhosis are at high risk for organ failure or death when they are admitted with acute bacterial infections or hepatitis. Immune-enhancing formulas may be needed to reduce infectious complications in critically ill patients (EAL, 2020).

SURGERY AND TRAUMA

In a perfect world, all patients undergoing surgery would be at optimal nutritional status to tolerate the stress of the surgery and temporary starvation that follows. But all too often, surgical patients are malnourished secondary to the condition requiring surgery. They may experience anorexia, nausea, or vomiting, decreasing their oral intake. Fever may increase their metabolic rate, or nutritional needs may not be met because of malabsorption.

For surgery to be successful, patients who are malnourished must be identified early so corrective action may be arranged. Undernutrition can lead to decreased protein synthesis, weakness, organ failure (MODS), or even death.

Once admitted for surgery, patients are typically held at NPO (nothing by mouth) status for 8 hours before the operation. Oral intake is generally resumed within a day after surgery. The postoperative diet is "diet as tolerated" for most patients. Some people prefer a liquid diet, but it is no longer mandatory or recommended.

Special Considerations

Bariatric Surgery

Bariatric surgery is generally scheduled for patients with a body mass index (BMI) greater than 40 or for those individuals with a BMI greater than 35 if they have comorbidities. The surgical procedures cause weight loss by restricting the amount of food the stomach can hold, causing malabsorption of nutrients, or by a combination of both gastric restriction and malabsorption (American Society for Metabolic and Bariatric Surgery, 2017).

The most common bariatric surgery procedures are gastric bypass, sleeve gastrectomy, adjustable gastric band, and biliopancreatic diversion with duodenal switch (BPD/DS). Each surgery has its own advantages and disadvantages. Most bariatric surgeries are performed using minimally invasive laparoscopic surgery.

The Roux-en-Y gastric bypass (RYGB) resolves T2D in morbidly obese patients. Diabetes improves after gastric bypass surgery via several mechanisms, one of which is related to expression of angiopoietin-like protein 8 (ANGPTL8) and betatrophin in adipose tissue (Ejarque et al., 2017). The RYGB produces long-term weight loss of about 60% to 80% of excess weight and restricts the amount of food that can be consumed. Malabsorption or dumping syndrome can occur after this procedure from deficient oral dietary intake, lack of gastric secretions, and exclusion of proximal duodenum and jejunum.

Long-term vitamin and mineral deficiencies of vitamin B_{12}, iron, calcium, and folate are common.

The laparoscopic sleeve gastrectomy removes approximately 80% of the stomach. Rapid weight loss and vitamin and mineral deficiencies can become problematic. It is a nonreversible procedure.

The adjustable gastric band places an inflatable band around the upper portion of the stomach, creating a small stomach pouch above the band. It has the lowest rate of early postoperative complications and mortality and the lowest risk for vitamin and mineral deficiencies among bariatric procedures. It is adjustable and reversible. Mechanical problems can occur because there is a foreign object in the body. The procedure requires strict adherence to the postoperative diet and follow-up visits. Weight loss is slower and not as great as with the other surgeries.

The BPD/DS creates a smaller, tubular stomach pouch by removing a portion of the stomach; then a large portion of the small intestine is bypassed. The procedure results in 60% to 70% weight loss (60%–70% of excess weight loss or greater at 5-year follow-up). The BPD/DS has a greater potential to cause protein deficiencies and long-term deficiencies in iron, calcium, zinc, vitamin D, and the other fat-soluble vitamins. Strict dietary control with regular follow-up is needed.

For any of these procedures, a preoperative multidisciplinary effort is required. The team generally includes the dietitian, exercise physiologist, psychologist, and bariatric nurse coordinator. The best patient outcomes are achieved in a comprehensive, accredited facility or Center of Excellence (Azagury & Morton, 2016). After the procedure, discharge teaching is important (Table 16.4).

Other Gastrointestinal Surgeries

Poor preoperative nutritional status in GI patients has been linked to increased postoperative complications and poorer surgical outcome. When possible, preoperative nutrition support should be administered to malnourished patients for 7 to 14 days if the operation can be safely postponed. Carbohydrate loading or nutritional supplements can be administered before surgery.

Early enteral feeding is possible after most surgeries and helps to preserve integrity of the GI tract and its microbiota. In general, the European guideline for clinical nutrition and Enhanced Recovery After Surgery (ERAS) principles (Weimann et al., 2017) include:

- Integration of nutrition into the overall management of the patient
- Avoidance of long periods of preoperative fasting
- Re-establishment of oral feeding as early as possible after surgery
- Start of nutritional therapy early, as soon as a nutritional risk becomes apparent
- Metabolic control (e.g., of blood glucose)
- Reduction of factors which exacerbate stress-related catabolism or impair gastrointestinal function
- Minimized time on paralytic agents for ventilator management in the postoperative period
- Early mobilization to facilitate protein synthesis and muscle function.

TABLE 16.4 Dietary Sequence After Bariatric Surgery

Diet Order	Timing
Clear liquids (no more than ½ cup total)	1–2 days after surgery
Full liquids (gradually increase to no more than ¾ cup total)	Days 3–21
Pureed foods (gradually increase to no more than 1 cup total)	3–6 weeks after surgery
Regular (small meals and snacks with no more than 1 cup total; 2 oz total meat)	6 weeks on

High-Risk Surgical Procedures

Hip replacement, coronary artery bypass graft (CABG), any brain incision, and prostatectomy are examples of high-risk procedures. Although functional, cognitive, and psychological status are known to be crucial components of health in older persons, they are not often used in assessing the risk of adverse postoperative outcomes (Tang et al., 2020). Malnourished older patients who undergo these procedures have significantly longer lengths of hospital stay and mortality rates than well-nourished patients. Thus, preoperative nutrition and postoperative nutrition must be carefully planned and managed (Weimann et al., 2017).

Traumatic Brain and Spinal Cord Injuries

A traumatic brain injury (TBI) can occur with a concussion or other type of accident. The more severe the head injury, the greater the release of catecholamines (norepinephrine and epinephrine) and cortisol and the greater the hypermetabolic response. Thus, patients will be severely hypermetabolic and catabolic. Figure 16.6 shows the effects of a TBI.

The primary phase of injury occurs at impact; the mechanical forces can disrupt the brain parenchyma and integrity of the

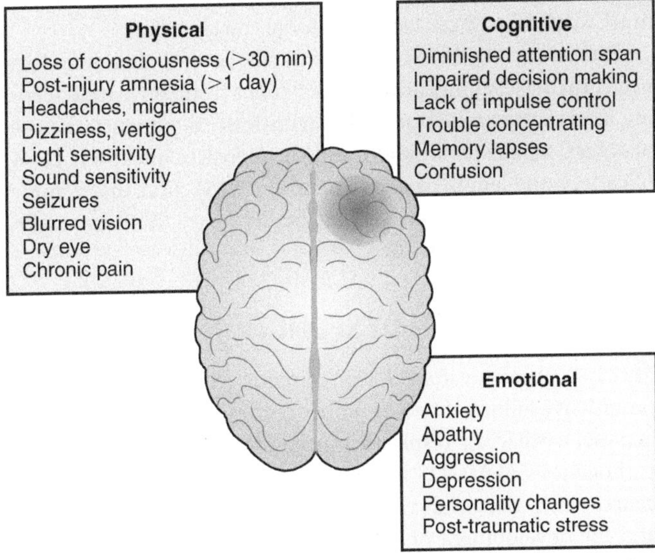

Fig. 16.6 Moderate or severe traumatic brain injury. (*TBI*) (Modified from TheraSpecs. Symptoms of moderate or severe TBI. https://www.theraspecs.com/blog/symptoms-moderate-severe-traumatic-brain-injury-tbi/n Accessed 3 September, 2020.)

blood–brain barrier (Bennett et al., 2016). This is followed by a secondary phase over the next hours, days, or months with a systemic and neuroinflammatory response of cytokines, growth factors, and activation of a complex network of pathways (Bennett et al., 2016). TBI causes primary brain damage and activates glial cells and immune and inflammatory cells, including mast cells in the brain associated with neuroinflammatory responses that cause secondary brain damage (Kempuraj et al., 2020). To reduce the hypermetabolic response and inflammation, an enteral tube feeding may be needed. As the patient progresses, a swallowing evaluation is needed before oral feeding to determine safety and risk of aspiration.

Spinal cord injuries (SCIs) result in lifelong disability. The initial mechanical trauma is followed by a damaging secondary injury cascade, like the patient with a traumatic brain injury (Ahuja & Fehlings, 2016). Many neuroprotective therapies are being tested. Long term, the patient with SCI will be at risk for cardiovascular disease, and a nutritional intervention may be needed (Bigford & Nash, 2017).

Patients with multiple traumas in addition to SCI have high nutritional demands. The SCI patient is at risk for malnutrition and should be monitored closely. Gradually, with recovery, patients with either TBI or SCI need a lower calorie intake to prevent excessive weight gain.

SYSTEMIC INFLAMMATORY RESPONSE SYNDROME

Systemic inflammatory response syndrome (SIRS) describes the inflammatory response and tissue injury that occurs in infection, pancreatitis, ischemia, burns, multiple traumas, shock, and organ injury. For diagnosis, the site of infection must be established, and at least two of the following are present: body temperature over 38° C or under 36° C; heart rate greater than 90 beats per minute; respiratory rate more than 20 breaths per minute (tachypnea); $PaCO_2$ under 32 mm Hg (hyperventilation); or white blood cell (WBC) count over 12,000/mm^3 or under 4000/mm^3. SIRS may be caused by bacterial translocation.

Patients with SIRS are hypermetabolic and their nutrient needs increase significantly. They benefit from early tube feeding intervention when possible. In critically ill patients, the use of enteral versus parenteral nutrition decreases infectious complications and length of stay (Elke et al., 2016). Note that volume and total energy restrictions may be necessary. With hyperglycemia, insulin is usually needed.

MULTIPLE ORGAN DYSFUNCTION SYNDROME

Multiple organ dysfunction syndrome (MODS) involves the progressive failure of two or more organ systems (e.g., the renal, hepatic, cardiac, or respiratory systems) at the same time. The pathogenesis of MODS is complex. Gut barrier failure is associated with bacterial translocation, systemic inflammation, and the development of MODS (Piton & Capellier, 2016). The uncontrolled inflammatory response leads to lung failure, followed by failure of the liver, intestine, and kidney. Myocardial failure generally manifests later, but central nervous system changes can occur at any time.

Higher levels of calories and protein are necessary to meet increased metabolic demands. Early enteral feedings (see Chapter 12) appear to maintain gut mucosal mass and barrier function and to promote normal enterocytic growth in the gut. These achievements are not possible with fasting or with parenteral feedings (Table 16.5).

Unfortunately, chronic critical illness (CCI) is an epidemic in intensive care unit survivors, with a persistent dysregulated immune response that causes a persistent inflammation, immunosuppression, and catabolism syndrome (PICS). Elderly patients are especially vulnerable to this illness (Rosenthal et al., 2018). More research is needed to address this condition effectively.

Refeeding Syndrome

Refeeding syndrome summarizes the physiologic and metabolic complications associated with reintroducing nutrition too rapidly in a malnourished person. These complications include glucose and electrolyte shifts that lead to cardiac insufficiency, heart failure, respiratory distress, convulsions, coma, or even death. Many conditions can lead to refeeding syndrome (see Box 16.2).

Overfeeding a patient with protein-energy malnutrition can result in many complications or death if not initiated correctly. Introduction of excess carbohydrate can overload various

TABLE 16.5 Nutritional Concerns in Multiple Organ Dysfunction Syndrome

System	Effects
Pulmonary	Acute respiratory distress syndrome (ARDS): patients requiring ventilator support may need higher lipid content in their diets (even with cardiac failure)
Gastrointestinal	Abdominal distention and ascites Intolerance to internal feedings Paralytic ileus Diarrhea Ischemic colitis Mucosal ulceration Bacterial overgrowth in stool
Liver	Increased serum ammonia level Hepatic encephalopathy
Hypermetabolism	Decreased lean body mass Muscle wasting Severe weight loss Negative nitrogen balance Hyperglycemia
Central nervous system	Lethargy Altered level of consciousness
Immune	Fever: increased energy needs Infection: increased energy needs Decreased lymphocyte count Anergy
Gallbladder	Abdominal distention Unexplained fever: increased kcal needs Decreased bowel sounds

(Data from Escott-Stump, S. *Nutrition and diagnosis-related care*, ed 8, Baltimore, 2016, Wolters-Kluwer Health.)

BOX 16.2 Populations Potentially at Risk for Refeeding Syndrome

- Alcohol and substance-use disorders
- Anorexia nervosa
- Bariatric surgery and bowel resections
- Child abuse and starvation
- Critical illness
- Extreme exercise (athletes, military recruits)
- Malabsorption (such as celiac disease)
- Malignancy
- Mental health disorders
- Patients in the emergency room
- Renal failure/hemodialysis
- Starvation during protest, famine, and migration

(From Da Silva, J.S.V., et al. ASPEN consensus recommendations for refeeding syndrome. *Nutrition in Clin Pract* 35:178–192, 2020.)

enzymatic and physiologic functions that were adapted during malnutrition. As feeding is initiated, rapid changes occur in thyroid and endocrine function, increasing oxygen consumption, cardiac output, insulin secretion, and energy expenditure. Electrolyte shifts are the most dangerous changes. Metabolic changes are described here.

Phosphorus

During starvation, total phosphorus is greatly reduced. With feeding, increased cellular influx of phosphorus occurs, leading to severe extracellular hypophosphatemia. This will occur in enteral and parenteral feeding but can be prevented by a slower rate of nutrient infusion. Cardiac decompensation occurs when sodium shifts also play a role. In addition, hypophosphatemia can lead to tissue hypoxia and, subsequently, altered tissue function.

Potassium

Potassium is greatly reduced in tissues. During feeding, extracellular fluid levels fall (hypokalemia), possibly leading to life-threatening arrhythmias.

Magnesium

Magnesium is also greatly reduced in tissues. With the anabolic condition of feeding, extracellular fluid levels drop (hypomagnesemia), leading to cardiac depression, arrhythmias, neuromuscular weakness, irritability, and hyporeflexia.

Glucose Metabolism

When high-glucose feedings are given, the starved patient loses the stimulus for gluconeogenesis (an important adaptive mechanism during nutritional depletion). Suppression of gluconeogenic glucose production leads to a corresponding decrease in amino acid use and negative nitrogen balance. Hyperglycemia can precipitate osmotic diuresis, dehydration, hypotension, hyperosmolar nonketotic coma, ketoacidosis, and metabolic acidosis (see Chapter 15).

Fluid Intolerance

Refeeding with carbohydrate results in sodium and water excretion. With concurrent sodium ingestion, such excretion can lead to a rapid expansion of extracellular fluid volume, fluid retention, and subsequent weight gain. This enhanced fluid retention may in turn be exacerbated by the loss of tissue mass resulting from starvation.

Nutrients must be reintroduced to the malnourished patient while medical and metabolic status is closely monitored. Careful estimation of energy requirements should be made through a complete nutritional assessment. Weight and fluid balance should be monitored daily to assess the rate of weight regain. Care should be taken to minimize fluid retention (weight gain >1 kg/wk) and to provide daily repletion of phosphorus, potassium, and magnesium.

Refeeding syndromes are associated more often with parenteral nutrition than enteral feeding (see Chapter 12). Before feedings are initiated, serum levels of potassium, magnesium and phosphorus should be checked. Initiate with 100 to 150 of dextrose or 10 to 20 kcal/kg body weight during the first day, progressing by 33% of goal for several days to reach desired intake levels (da Silva et al., 2020). It is also important to evaluate vital signs and cardiorespiratory monitoring during the initiation phase of calorie replacement.

After 1 week, intake of kcal, fluid, and sodium can be liberalized without fear of consequences because the various metabolic equilibrations should have taken place. Thus, common sense and discretion are of key importance in the feeding of semi-starved and chronically ill patients.

BURNS (THERMAL INJURY)

Burns produce tissue destruction that results in circulatory and metabolic alterations requiring the compensatory response to injury. Major body burns have significant effects on nutritional status because of the stress response that causes prolonged hypermetabolism and muscle wasting (Ogunbileje et al., 2016).

Thermal burns are usually characterized as contact (hot solid object), flame (direct contact with flames), or scald (heated liquid) injuries. Nonthermal causes include chemical, electrical, and radioactive sources. Burns are also classified by physical appearance, symptoms associated with the affected skin, and percent of body surface burned (Table 16.6). First-degree burns (or partial-thickness injury) involve only the epidermis, resulting in simple reddening of the area, with no injury to underlying dermal or subcutaneous tissue. Sunburns are an example of first-degree burns caused by ultraviolet radiation damage to skin; these burns heal within 3 to 5 days without scarring.

Second-degree burns (superficial partial-thickness injury and deep partial-thickness injury) involve two categories of burn depth. Superficial partial-thickness burns are characterized by redness and blistering that affects the epidermis and some dermis. Deep partial-thickness burns are characterized by destruction of epidermis and dermis (resulting in a waxy, white, mottled appearance), leaving only skin appendages such as hair follicles and sweat glands. Second-degree burns take weeks to months to heal.

Third-degree burns (full-thickness injury) are characterized by destruction of the entire epidermis, dermis, and often, the underlying subcutaneous tissue. Occasionally, muscle or bone

TABLE 16.6 Burn Injury Classification

Classification of Burns by Depth

Burn Thickness	Deepest Skin Structure Involved	Appearance	Pain	Prognosis (Without Surgical Intervention)
Superficial (first-degree)	Epidermis	Dry, blanching erythema	Painful	Heals without scarring, 5–10 days
Superficial partial-thickness (second-degree)	Upper dermis	Blisters; wet, blanching erythema	Painful	Heals without scarring, <3 weeks
Deep partial-thickness (second-degree)	Lower dermis	Yellow or white, dry, nonblanching	Decreased sensation	Heals in 3–8 weeks; likely to scar if healing >3 weeks
Full-thickness (third-degree)	Subcutaneous structures	White or black/brown, nonblanching	Decreased sensation	Heals by contracture >8 weeks; will scar

(Modified from Haines E, Fairbrother H: Optimizing emergency management to reduce morbidity in pediatric burn patients, *Pediatric Emergency Medicine Practice* 12:5, 1–23 ©2015 EB Medicine. Used with permission. www.ebmedicine.net.)

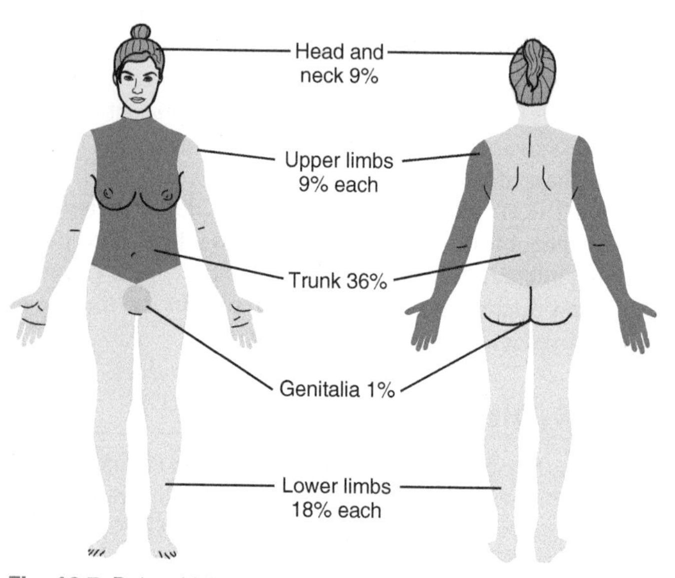

Fig. 16.7 Rule of Nines. An assessment tool with estimates of the percentages (in multiples of nine) of the total body surface area burned. (Modified from Lumen Learning. Injuries of the skin. https://courses.lumenlearning.com/wm-biology2/chapter/injuries-of-skin/. Accessed 6 September, 2020.)

tissue may be destroyed. The burn site may look white, or blackened and charred. Fourth-degree burns go through both layers of the skin and underlying tissue as well as deeper tissue, possibly involving muscle and bone. There is no feeling in the area because the nerve endings are destroyed. Third-degree and fourth-degree burns cannot heal independently and require skin grafts.

In addition to pain and infection management and wound care, nutrition support is one of the most significant considerations. The first 24 to 48 hours of treatment for such patients are dedicated to replacement of fluid and electrolytes. Fluid needs are based on the patient's age and weight, and the extent of the burn. Total body surface area (TBSA), used to estimate the extent of the burn, can be estimated using the "rule of nines" (Fig. 16.7).

Burn wounds heal only when the patient is in an anabolic (building up muscle) state. Therefore, feeding should be initiated as soon as the patient has been hydrated. Enteral feedings should be initiated within a day after injury to prevent ileus, stress

TABLE 16.7 Nutritional Goals for Burned Patients

Goal	Action(s)
Support role of skin as a barrier against bacteria and viruses	Control environmental temperature Monitor fluid and electrolyte balance Control pain and anxiety Cover wounds early
Meet accelerated nutritional needs	Provide adequate calories and maintain preburn weight within 5%–10% Provide adequate protein to achieve positive nitrogen balance Replete visceral proteins and maintain lean body muscle mass
Prevent micronutrient deficiency	Provide nutrition enterally within 6–18 hours after burn injury. Use parenteral nutrition only if the gut is not working.
Prevent Curling's ulcer in large burns over 30% body surface area	Provide antacids or continuous enteral feedings
Manage hyperglycemia	Use exogenous insulin as needed

ulceration, and the effects of catabolism. Placement of the feeding tube in the small bowel should be considered when patient is in supine position or under heavy sedation. Anabolic steroids (oxandrolone) are prescribed to stimulate appetite and appear to benefit anabolic protein production. (Dobbe et al., 2019).

Nutritional goals for patients with burns are outlined in Table 16.7. Early enteral nutrition (EN) may allow the following objectives to be achieved:

- Nutrient needs satisfied
- Improved feeding tolerance
- Decreased incidence of bacterial translocation
- Decreased number of infectious episodes
- Decreased antibiotic therapy
- Improved nitrogen balance
- Reduced urinary catecholamines
- Diminished serum glucagon
- Suppressed hypermetabolic response
- Enhanced visceral protein status

Energy needs vary according to the size of the burn. Several methods may be used to estimate energy and protein needs in burned patients when indirect calorimetry is not available. One of the simplest and easiest to use is the Curreri formula (adults), as follows:

- (25 kcal × kg of body weight) + (40 kcal × %TBSA)
- 16 to 18 kcal × kg of body weight if patient more than 125% regular body weight
- Burns more than 50%: use a maximum value of 50% TBSA.

Note that estimates using the Curreri formula may exceed actual energy needs, but it is not uncommon for a patient to need 4000 to 5000 calories per day.

After a severe burn, protein is lost through urine, the wound, and increased gluconeogenesis. Calories from protein are generally not calculated into total energy needs. Carbohydrates and fats provide protein-sparing and are nonprotein energy sources. Whether a patient receives adequate amounts of energy or protein is evaluated by wound healing rate, graft "take," and basic nutritional assessment parameters.

It is assumed that the rate of sepsis is reduced in burn patients who are supported by early enteral nutrition (within 48 hours). However, more randomized clinical trials are needed to measure outcomes such as mortality rates, feeding intolerance, GI complications, duration of mechanical ventilation, or pneumonia (Fuentes Padilla et al., 2019).

In conjunction with increased energy demands, vitamin and mineral needs are increased in burn patients, but exact requirements have not been identified. Most patients will be given vitamins higher than the usual recommended intake because of the high calories. Special consideration is given to vitamin C (collagen synthesis, immune function) and vitamin A (immune function and epithelialization). Supplements are commonly recommended.

Regardless of nutritional interventions, the outcome of a burn injury affects the whole family. See the *Personal Perspectives* box Eight Ways to Care for Caregivers.

Nursing Approach

In fluid-resuscitated, critically ill patients, EN started within 24 to 48 hours after injury or admission to the intensive care unit (ICU) reduces the incidence of infectious complications (EAL, 2020). Nurses can alert the registered dietitian to ensure adequate energy provision when the patient's status changes, as with new fever or skin breakdown.

It is important to closely monitor blood glucose levels. Hyperglycemia is associated with infection, morbidity, even mortality. The goal is to keep blood glucose between 140 and 180 mg/dL (McMahon, 2013). Insulin drip and sliding scale should be used, with conversion to subcutaneous insulin as possible.

Weight may be difficult to obtain and inaccurate owing to fluid shifts and dressings. Scales must be recalibrated on a schedule to ensure accuracy. Regular documentation of weights and I&O records becomes essential because many complications arise during the recovery process.

Evaluating patient position should be part of the monitoring plan for tube-fed patients, and aspiration precautions are needed. To decrease the incidence of aspiration pneumonia and reflux of gastric contents into the esophagus and pharynx, a 45-degree head of bed elevation should be used when not contraindicated.

Evaluating gastric residual volume (GRV) in critically ill patients is another part of a monitoring plan to assess tolerance of EN. Blue dye should never be used to detect aspiration. EN should be withheld when a GRV is 250 mL or over is documented on two or more consecutive occasions. Note that holding EN when GRV is less than 250 mL is associated with delivery of less EN than prescribed. Above all, responses to a feeding include evaluations of intake and output (fluid intake and stooling), tolerance of feeding regimen, and the actual amount of nutrition delivered.

PERSONAL PERSPECTIVES

Eight Ways to Care for Caregivers

Carly Bowers is the wife of a burn survivor and founder of Bowers Ministry. Her husband, David, was severely burned in an oxygen flash fire in 1999 and was not expected to survive his injuries. This is her story.

Growing up, my life was neat and tidy. So many things were clear-cut and simple. For so long, I was a student, a daughter, and a friend. I played those roles when the time called for it, and it seemed easy to me. Then I became a mom and suddenly was thrust into a world in which I was everything to my precious girl. I wasn't just her mom; I was her chef, nurse, chauffer, teacher, disciplinarian, friend, and number one fan. Then my husband, David, suffered a severe burn injury, and the roles swirled and melded more than they ever had in my life. I was now a mom, with all the responsibilities that role brings; a wife, with all the responsibilities that role brings; and a caregiver. This was uncharted territory for me, and adjusting to this new role was one of the hardest things I've ever done. Juggling all these roles was exhausting!

Most people who are called to care for a family member are not trained professional caregivers—we are just thrown into this role because of life's unexpected twists and turns. We try to do our best, but sometimes feel like we aren't doing it well, or because we don't have the necessary tools, we burn out because of the stress and exhaustion. Here are some helpful hints on how to take care of yourself when you're caring for a loved one. I hope to share some practical ways to care for yourself if you are a caregiver or offer ways to help a friend or family member who has taken on the daunting responsibility of being a caregiver.

- Learn as much as you can so you can be your loved one's advocate.
- Get rest, eat, and get some fresh air every day.
- Take care of yourself physically, emotionally and spiritually. Meditate. Pray. Take up yoga. Watch an inspiring movie each week. Pick what works for YOU.
- Help your loved one maintain as much independence as possible.
- You don't have to do it all. Ask for help from family and friends. And better yet, be willing to accept help!
- Get support from counseling or support groups. It is difficult to effectively care for your loved one if you are suffering emotionally and physically too.
- It's okay to have feelings of anxiety/worry, anger, guilt, fear, despair... Don't try to hide or suppress your true feelings. Deal with your feelings. Grieve over what you've lost.
- Try to stay connected to your friends and life outside of taking care of your loved one. It's okay to take a break, as hard as it might seem.

Carly Bowers
Southeast Texas

(Modified from Bowers, C. *8 ways to care for caregivers.* Grand Rapids, MI, 2014, The Phoenix Society. Accessed 6 September, 2020, from https://www.phoenix-society.org/resources/7-ways-to-care-for-caregivers.)

SUMMARY

- The stress response of the body also affects nutritional status.
- Whether the stress response is caused by physiologic or psychologic determinants, the entire body is affected.
- Starvation leads to decreased energy expenditure, use of alternative fuels, decreased protein wasting, and use of stored glycogen in 24 hours.
- In late starvation, fatty acids, ketones, and glycerol provide energy for all tissues except brain, nervous system, and red blood cells.
- Metabolic changes occur in uncomplicated stress, which is present when patients are at nutritional risk, or in severe stress caused by trauma or disease.
- In a hypermetabolic state, stress causes accelerated energy expenditure, glucose production, and glucose cycling in liver and muscle. Hyperglycemia can occur from either insulin resistance or excess glucose production via gluconeogenesis. Muscle breakdown is also accelerated.
- Many hormone levels are altered by stress.
- The functioning of the immune system is affected by the hormonal and metabolic changes that occur. The immune system cannot protect the body when impaired nutritional status accompanies metabolic stress.
- Nutrients that affect the immune system include omega-3 fatty acids, vitamins A and C, and zinc.
- Systemic inflammatory response syndrome (SIRS) describes the inflammatory response that occurs in infection, pancreatitis, ischemia, burns, multiple traumas, shock, and organ injury. Patients with SIRS are hypermetabolic.
- Multiple organ dysfunction syndrome (MODS) results from direct injury, trauma, or disease or as a response to inflammation; the response is usually in an organ distant from the original site of infection or injury.
- Refeeding syndrome can occur when a malnourished patient is fed too many calories too quickly. In critical care, begin with slow feeding methods and progress to desired levels as tolerated.
- Severely burned patients have profound hypermetabolism and require high-energy, low-volume feedings.

THE NURSING APPROACH

Clinical Judgment and Next-Generation NCLEX® Examination-Style Questions

Case Study 1

Nutritional Needs During Physical Stress

Daniel, age 65 years, had pneumonia 2 days after his left hip replacement. He is receiving physical therapy, intravenous (IV) antibiotics, supplemental oxygen, and a high-kcal, high-protein diet. The hospital dietitian met with Daniel to individualize his diet on the basis of his Orthodox Jewish religion.

Assessment/Recognize Cues

Subjective (From Patient Statements)

- "The muscles in my chest ache from coughing, and my hip hurts."
- Pain rating: 3 of 10
- "I don't feel like eating, but if I have to eat, I want to observe dietary laws for an Orthodox Jew."
- "I feel tired and sometimes short of breath."

Objective (From Physical Examination)

- Eats small amounts of food, then pushes the food tray away
- Drinks about 1200 mL of fluid per day (mostly water)
- Tympanic temperature 101.2° F
- Crackles in lungs bilaterally
- O_2 saturation 90% with oxygen at 6 L via nasal cannula
- White blood count 14,000/mm^3
- Productive cough, with thick yellow sputum
- Surgical wound on left hip intact without redness or drainage

Diagnosis (Nursing)/Analyze Cues

1. Potential for weight loss related to inadequate food intake (secondary to shortness of breath and discomfort) and increased metabolic stresses (surgery, infection, and fever), as evidenced by "I don't feel like eating," eats small amounts then pushes meal tray away, drinks about 1200 mL of fluid per day
2. Decreased gas exchange related to pneumonia as evidenced by O_2 saturation 90% on 6 L via nasal cannula

Planning/Prioritize Hypotheses

Patient Outcomes

Short term (by discharge to a rehabilitation center in 5 days):

- Eating moderate amounts of food, especially protein-rich and nutrient-dense foods
- Drinking at least 2000 mL per day
- No weight loss
- No shortness of breath, O_2 saturation 95% without supplemental oxygen
- Afebrile (no fever)
- White blood cell (WBC) count less than 10,000/mm^3
- Decrease or absence of crackles in lungs
- No signs of infection of surgical wound on left hip

Nursing Interventions/Generate Solutions

1. Provide high-kcal, high-protein diet.
2. Maintain dietary intake according to Orthodox Jewish kosher dietary laws.

Implementation/Take Action

1. Asked Daniel's family to bring in kosher ground meat and special serving dishes.
   Ground meat provides high protein and requires little energy for chewing. If the hospital does not have a kosher kitchen, kosher meals may be ordered from special suppliers. Family members may be able to obtain kosher food and reassure the patient that it is truly kosher. Meat (no pork or shellfish) must be properly slaughtered, blessed by a rabbi, and cooked in a kosher kitchen. Dishes reserved for meat must be separated from dishes for milk, and meat cannot be served in the same meal as milk.
2. Asked Daniel and his family to inform nursing or dietary staff about special dietary needs, particularly for upcoming holidays and the Sabbath.
   Culturally sensitive staff will ask individuals and families how they can meet special dietary needs.

THE NURSING APPROACH—cont'd

3. Provided rest periods and oral care before meals, and gave pain medicine as needed.
   Rest helps increase patient energy, and a fresh mouth promotes appetite. Patients eat more food when comfortable.
4. Pointed out the high-protein and nutrient-dense foods on meal trays and encouraged Daniel to eat them first.
   When patients can eat only small amounts of food, nourishment is better if they choose nutrient-dense foods.
5. Conferred with the dietitian and physician concerning high-kcal, high-protein snacks between meals.
   Increased kcal are needed to compensate for metabolic stresses, and additional protein is needed for healing and building up immunity. Frequent small meals are easier to consume than large meals when the patient is short of breath. Some doctors prefer to limit milk products for patients with respiratory problems because of potential phlegm. Milk-based supplements must be served several hours before or after meats, according to Jewish dietary laws.
6. Provided a vitamin/mineral supplement, as prescribed by the physician.
   Bone healing requires adequate calcium and vitamin D. Vitamins A and C help promote wound healing. B vitamins are needed in stressful conditions.
7. Offered water frequently between meals and encouraged drinking 2000 mL of fluid per day.
   Fluid intake is needed to replace fluids lost during fever. Additional fluids help thin sputum, making it easier for the patient to cough up the sputum. Liquids during meals should be minimized if patient feels full after eating little food.
8. Recorded intake and output and weighed the patient daily.
   Records can help show balance or imbalance of fluid intake (by mouth and by intravenous fluid) and fluid output (urine). Adequate nutrition is needed to prevent weight loss.
9. Encouraged Daniel to get a pneumonia shot this year and a flu shot every year.
   Serious respiratory infections may be prevented by immunizations. Generally, only one pneumonia shot is given, preferably when an adult becomes 65 years old. Influenza shots must be received by the patient annually, usually in the fall. Health promotion is an important nursing responsibility.

Evaluation/Evaluate Outcomes

Short term (at discharge to the rehabilitation center on the fifth day):

- Daniel was eating moderate amounts of food.
- He was drinking 2000 mL of fluids per day.
- No weight loss.
- No shortness of breath, O_2 saturation 95% without supplemental oxygen.
- Tympanic temperature 99° F.
- WBC 9500/mm^3.
- Decreased crackles in lungs.
- No signs of infection of surgical wound on left hip.

Goals met.

Discussion Questions

1. How would Daniel's diet plan be different if he did not request a kosher diet?
2. Compare and contrast a diet for a patient with pneumonia versus a patient with severe burns.

Case Study 2
SIRS Conditions

The nurse is caring for a patient diagnosed with systemic inflammatory response syndrome (SIRS). The nurse knows that to diagnose this condition as SIRS, the site of infection must be identified and that at least two of the following conditions must be present.

Place an X in the boxes of the conditions that define SIRS

1. Body temperature >38° C or <36° C
2. BP <100/60
3. Respiratory rate >16 breaths/min
4. Hypoglycemia
5. White blood cell (WBC) count >12,000/mm^3 or <4000/mm^3
6. $Paco_2$ <32 mm Hg (hyperventilation)
7. Heart rate >100 beats/minute
8. Red blood cell (RBC) count 4.5 million to 5.9 million cells per microliter (mcL)

Patients with SIRS are hypermetabolic and their nutrient needs increase significantly. They benefit from early tube feeding intervention when possible. In critically ill patients, the use of enteral versus parenteral nutrition decreases infectious complications and length of stay (Elke et al., 2016). Note that volume and total energy restrictions may be necessary. With hyperglycemia, insulin is usually needed.

CRITICAL THINKING

Clinical Applications

Kristin, aged 19 years, is a member of her college's cheerleading team and was involved in a serious motor vehicle accident when the team was returning from a game. She was admitted through the emergency department of your hospital suffering from multiple fractures and contusions. Kristin is 5 feet 5 inches tall and weighed 120 pounds before the accident. Because she is young, looked healthy, and is somewhat muscular from being a cheerleader, the physician did not request a consult for the dietitian to evaluate Kristin's nutritional status. After she had been in intensive care 2 weeks, pneumonia developed. The nurse learned that before the automobile accident, Kristin had been using a commercial weight loss product and was consuming approximately 400 kcal/day for 3 months before the accident in an attempt to "make weight" so that she could remain on the cheerleading team.

1. How did the very low-calorie diet (VLCD) affect Kristin's nutritional status?
2. Why did pneumonia develop?
3. Describe the variety of stresses Kristin experienced.
4. Could the pneumonia have been prevented? How?

WEBSITES OF INTEREST

American Society for Enteral and Parenteral Nutrition
http://www.nutritioncare.org/
A key resource for tips on enteral and parenteral nutrition for the critically ill patient.

Burnsurgery.org
www.burnsurgery.org
Offers up-to-date educational tools on burn care and treatment for health professionals.

REFERENCES

Academy of Nutrition and Dietetics, Evidence Analysis Library: *Critical illness evidence-based nutrition practice guideline*. From: www.andevidencelibrary.com. (Accessed 6 September, 2020).

Ahuja, C. S., & Fehlings, M. (2016). Concise review: bridging the gap: novel neuroregenerative and neuroprotective strategies in spinal cord injury. *Stem Cells Translational Medicine*, *5*, 914–924.

American Society for Metabolic and Bariatric Surgery: *Bariatric surgery procedures*. From: https://asmbs.org/patients/bariatric-surgery-procedures. (Accessed 6 September, 2020).

Azagury, D. E., & Morton, J. M. (2016). Patient safety and quality improvement initiatives in contemporary metabolic and bariatric surgical practice. *The Surgical Clinics of North America*, *96*, 733–742.

Bennett, E. R., et al. (2016). Genetic influences in traumatic brain injury, Chapter 9. In D. Laskowitz & G. Grant (Eds.), *Translational research in traumatic brain injury*. Boca Raton (FL): CRC Press/ Taylor and Francis Group.

Bigford, G., & Nash, S. (2017). Nutritional Health Considerations for Persons with Spinal Cord Injury. *Topics in spinal cord injury rehabilitation*, *23*, 188–206.

Da Silva, J. S. V., et al. (2020). ASPEN Consensus Recommendations for Refeeding Syndrome. *Nutrition in Clin Pract*, *35*, 178–192.

Dobbe, L., et al. (2019). Assessment of the impact of oxandrolone on outcomes in burn injured patients. *Burns*, *45*, 841–848.

EAL (Evidence Analysis Library). *Academy of Nutrition and Dietetics*, available at: https://www.andeal.org/topic.cfm?menu=5302. Accessed 12/1/2020.

Ejarque, M., et al. (2017). Angiopoietin-like protein 8/betatrophin as a new determinant of type 2 diabetes remission after bariatric surgery. *Translational Research: The Journal of Laboratory and Clinical Medicine*, *84*, 35–44.

Elke, G., et al. (2016). Enteral versus parenteral nutrition in critically ill patients: an updated systematic review and meta-analysis of randomized controlled trials. *Critical care (London, England)*, *20*, 117.

Food and Agriculture Organization: Globalization of food systems and nutrition. From: http://www.fao.org/ag/agn/nutrition/urban_globalization_en.stm. (Accessed 6 September, 2020).

Fuentes Padilla, P., et al. (2019). Early enteral nutrition (within 48 hours) versus delayed enteral nutrition (after 48 hours) with or without supplemental parenteral nutrition in critically ill adults. *Cochrane Database of Systematic Reviews*, *10*, CD012340. 31 October, 2019.

Kempuraj, D., et al. (2020). Mast cell activation, neuroinflammation, and tight junction protein derangement in acute traumatic brain injury. *Mediators of Inflammation*, *2020*, 4243953.

Kim, D., et al. (2016). Gut microbiota in autoimmunity: potential for clinical applications. *Archives of Pharmacal Research*, *39*, 1565–1576.

Kubota, T. (2018). Preemptive epigenetic medicine based on fetal programming. *Advances in Experimental Medicine and Biology*, *1012*, 85–95.

McMahon, M. M. (2013). A.S.P.E.N. clinical guidelines: Nutrition support of adult patients with hyperglycemia. *J Parenteral and Enteral Nut*, *37*, 23–36.

Ogunbileje, J. O., et al. (2016). Hypermetabolism and hypercatabolism of skeletal muscle accompany mitochondrial stress following severe burn trauma. *American Journal of Physiology. Endocrinology and Metabolism*, *311*, 436–448.

Piton, G., & Capellier, G. (2016). Biomarkers of gut barrier failure in the ICU. *Current Opinion in Critical Care*, *22*, 152–160.

Radzikowska, U., et al. (2019). The influence of dietary fatty acids on immune responses. *Nutrients*, *11*, 2990.

Rosenthal, M. D., et al. (2018). Chronic critical illness: application of what we know. *Nutr in Clin Pract*, *33*, 39–45.

Tang, V. L., et al. (2020). Association of functional, cognitive, and psychological measures with 1-year mortality in patients undergoing major surgery. *JAMA Surg*, *155*, 412–418.

Weimann, A., et al. (2017). ESPEN guideline: Clinical nutrition in surgery. *Clinical Nutr*, *36*, 623–650.

Zuo, P., et al. (2020). Decreased prealbumin level is associated with increased risk for mortality in elderly hospitalized patients with COVID-19. *Nutrition*, *78*, 110930.

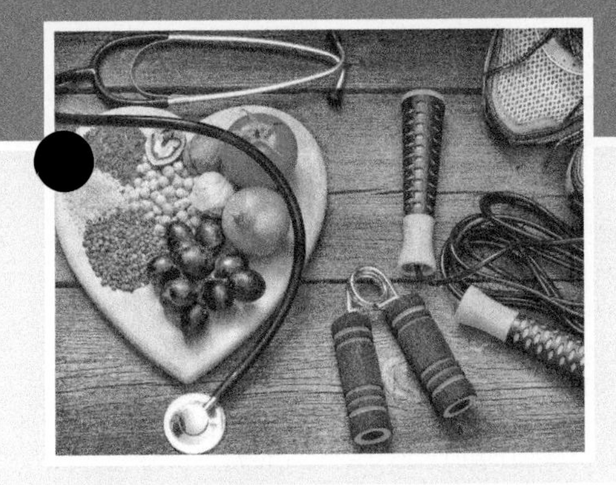

17

Nutrition for Cardiopulmonary Diseases

Some people think plant-based, whole foods diet is extreme. Half a million people a year will have their chests opened and a vein taken from their leg and sewn onto their coronary artery. Some people would call that extreme.

Caldwell Esselstyn

http://evolve.elsevier.com/GRODNER/FOUNDATIONS

LEARNING OBJECTIVES

- List the diseases and conditions that constitute cardiovascular disease (CVD).
- Identify the CVD risk factors that are controllable, noncontrollable, and predisposing.
- Discuss the goals of nutrition therapy for CVD.
- Describe hypertension (HTN) and its treatment regimens.
- Explain the focus of nutrition therapy to reduce risk of myocardial infarctions (MIs) and heart failure (HF).
- Identify the main categories of pulmonary disorders and the importance of nutritional status.
- Describe the goal of nutrition therapy for chronic obstructive pulmonary disease (COPD), asthma, respiratory failure and tuberculosis (TB).

HEART AND LUNG HEALTH

The physical health dimension is affected because cardiovascular disease (CVD) affects the heart, an essential organ; this disease impairs functioning of many other body systems. Determining one's own risk factors and devising a program to reduce the effects will depend on intellectual health. Emotional health is stressed when client denial occurs; many individuals view heart problems as something that happens only to other people! Because of increased education through the work of health associations and health departments, many restaurants and resorts serve "heart healthy" entrées; with careful selections, social health can continue. Spiritual health is manifested through the optimistic attitude that taking care of our bodies is a sacred task. Environmental health affects health status by increasing risk of chronic bronchitis, asthma, and emphysema when air is polluted or if smoking damages the body.

CARDIOVASCULAR DISEASES

Coronary Artery Disease

Cardiovascular disease (CVD) encompasses a group of diseases and conditions that affect the heart and blood vessels: coronary artery disease (CAD) (also called coronary heart disease [CHD]), hypertension (HTN), peripheral artery disease, heart failure, and congenital heart diseases. CVD continues to be the leading cause of death for American men and women in all ethnic and racial groups. Although death rates from CVD have declined, the burden of the disease remains high; Box 17.1 lists facts that everyone should know about heart disease.

Many people who have heart attacks die before they ever reach a hospital for treatment, a situation that emphasizes the need for prevention of heart disease. Health professionals cannot assume that patients newly diagnosed with CAD, regardless of education or socioeconomic level, are knowledgeable about the disorder and relevant treatments.

Three types of preventive strategies are in place. Primary prevention is a public health effort. Secondary prevention behaviors reduce the effects of heart disease. Tertiary prevention is designed to minimize further complications or to restore health. For CVD, these efforts may involve significant lifestyle changes combined with medication. Learning more about the disorder is a goal for patients and their families (see the *Personal Perspectives box Go Red for Women* and Fig. 17.1).

BOX 17.1 Things to Know About Heart Disease and Stroke

Cardiovascular disease is the leading global cause of death, accounting for more than 17.3 million deaths per year, a number that is expected to grow to more than 23.6 million by 2030.

Cardiovascular diseases claim more lives than all forms of cancer combined.

About 85.6 million Americans are living with some form of cardiovascular disease or the aftereffects of stroke.

Nearly half of all Black American adults have some form of cardiovascular disease—48% of women and 46% of men.

Heart disease is the leading cause of death for people of most ethnicities in the United States, including Black, Hispanic, and White Americans.

Heart attacks have several major warning signs and symptoms: chest pain or discomfort; upper body pain or discomfort in the arms, back, neck, jaw, or upper stomach; shortness of breath; or nausea, lightheadedness, or cold sweats.

(Modified from American Heart Association: *Heart and stroke facts*, Dallas, 2017, Author. Accessed 6 September, 2020, from https://www.heart.org/idc/groups/ahamah-public/@wcm/@sop/@smd/documents/downloadable/ucm_480086.pdf; and Centers for Disease Control and Prevention: *Heart disease facts*, Atlanta, 2020, Author. Accessed 6 September, 2020, from https://www.cdc.gov/heartdisease/facts.htm.)

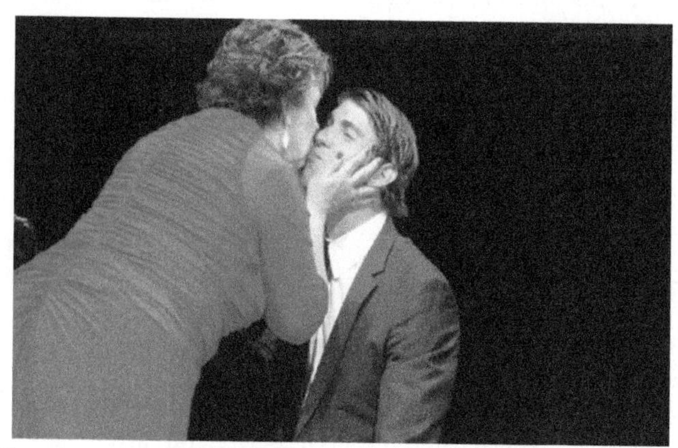

Fig. 17.1 Debbie Phelps kissing her son, Olympic medalist Michael Phelps, at the Red Dress Event, New York City, 2012. (Photo courtesy S. Escott-Stump.)

Atherosclerosis

Atherosclerosis is the chronic inflammatory process in which damage to the arterial wall can lead to coronary artery disease, stroke, and peripheral artery disease (Fig. 17.2). This condition begins early in life. Vitamin D deficiency has been consistently associated with elevated levels of C-reactive protein (CRP) and increased risk for CVD (Li et al., 2019). Vitamin D supplements are inexpensive, simple, and safe when taken in daily doses that do not exceed the established tolerable upper intake level (UL) of the National Academy of Sciences.

The development of lesions in coronary arteries causes chest pain (angina pectoris) if blood flow is partially occluded. If blood flow to the heart is completely occluded, a heart attack myocardial infarction (MI) occurs. If a clot (thrombosis) occurs in a cerebral artery, a stroke cerebrovascular accident (CVA) occurs. Peripheral artery disease (PAD) develops when atherosclerosis in the abdominal aorta, iliac arteries, and femoral arteries produces temporary insufficient blood flow in the arteries on exertion (intermittent claudication) or ischemic necrosis of the extremities, which may lead to gangrene.

PERSONAL PERSPECTIVES

Go Red for Women

Go Red for Women is a national campaign of the American Heart Association. The movement encourages women to engage in heart-healthy activities to reduce their personal risk of heart disease, the number one killer of women. The message of the movement, Love Your Heart, spreads awareness that prevention is possible—one heart at a time through the empowerment of women. Go Red for Women local events take place in most communities. National Wear Red Day, the major event of the campaign, asks everyone to wear something red in February to highlight ways to reduce risks by simple acts such as the following:

- Seeing a health care provider
- Consuming a healthier diet
- Being more physically active
- Educating others about heart disease

When you wear red blouses, dresses, ties, lipstick, shoes, or jackets, think "I love my heart!" For more information, check out the American Heart Association Go Red for Women webpage at www.goredforwomen.org.

The Coca-Cola Company and the National Heart Lung and Blood Institute (NHLBI) have partnered on behalf of women and heart disease. In February, they sponsor a Heart Truth Red Dress Event at the beginning of Fashion Week in New York City. Movie stars and media personalities are invited to participate in a runway event, all wearing designer red dresses. Fig. 17.1 shows a kiss between Debbie Phelps and her son, Olympic hero Michael. Their presence at this event sent a great message to all women: take care of your hearts for family and loved ones! For the "Heart Truth" information, go to https://www.nhlbi.nih.gov/health-topics/education-and-awareness/heart-truth/about.

Sylvia Escott-Stump
Winterville, NC

Cholesterol and Dyslipidemia

Cholesterol is an essential component of cell membranes and a precursor of bile acids, steroid hormones, and vitamin D. Cholesterol is a not actually a lipid, but it travels in the bloodstream in lipoprotein spheres, made of lipids and proteins. Plasma lipoproteins are usually measured after fasting (Table 17.1). They include very low-density lipoproteins (VLDLs), low-density lipoproteins (LDLs), and high-density lipoproteins (HDLs). LDLs make up 60% to 70% of total serum cholesterol (TC) and HDLs make up the remainder. When LDL and HDL ratios are unbalanced, the condition is called dyslipidemia. Low HDL is a level less than 40 mg/dL in men and 50 mg/dL in women.

VLDLs are largely composed of triglycerides, the most common type of fat found in the bloodstream. The body gets triglyceride directly from foods and produces more in the liver. Normal serum triglyceride levels range from about 50 to 250 mg/dL. Factors that may elevate triglycerides include long-term and excessive alcohol intake, obesity and physical inactivity, diabetes, chronic kidney disease, nephrotic syndrome, and genetics.

Apolipoprotein C-III (ApoC-III) is a key regulator of triglyceride metabolism and is linked to CAD risk (van Capelleveen et al., 2017). Intermittent hypoxemia from obstructive sleep apnea (OSA) is another trigger of dyslipidemia. The TG/HDL-C ratio

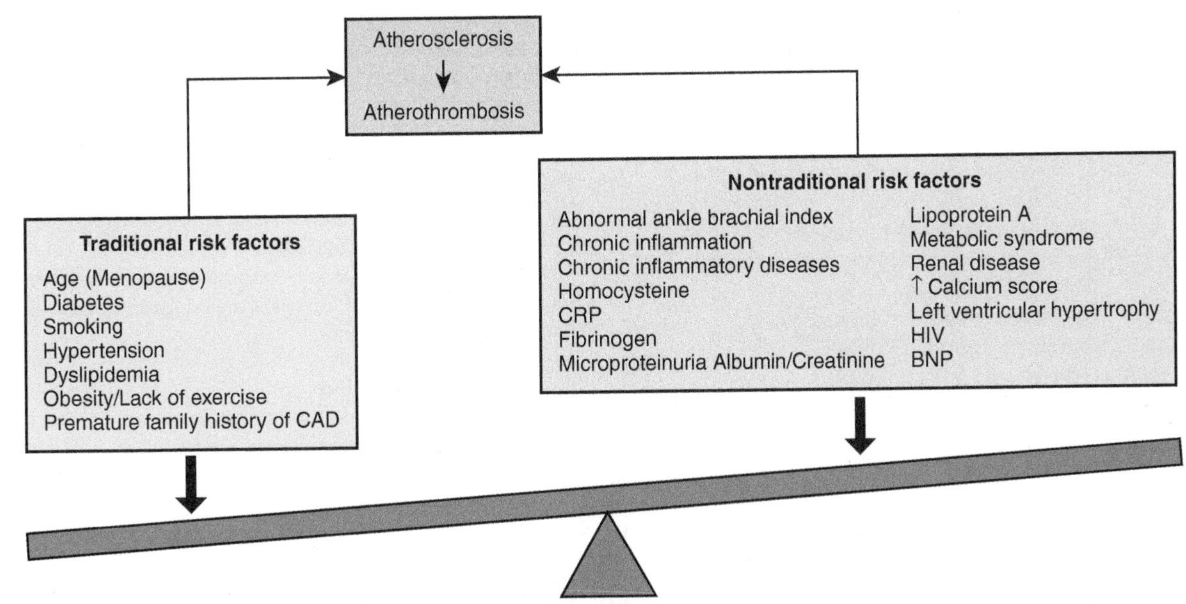

Fig. 17.2 Risk factors for coronary artery disease (*CAD*).Traditional versus nontraditional risk factors for CAD. The expanding list of nontraditional biomarkers is outweighed by the standard risk factors for predicting future cardiovascular events and adds only moderately to standard risk factors. *BNP*, B-type natriuretic peptide; *BP*, blood pressure; *CRP*, C-reactive protein; *HDL*, high-density lipoprotein cholesterol; *HIV*, human immunodeficiency virus infection. (Modified from Boudi, F.P. risk factors for coronary artery disease. From https://emedicine.medscape.com/article/164163-overview. Accessed 8 September, 2020.)

TABLE 17.1 Classification of Serum Lipid Values

CHOLESTEROL AND TRIGLYCERIDE LEVELS IN ADULTS				
	Total	High-Density Lipoprotein	Low-Density Lipoprotein	Triglicerides
High	≥240	n/a	≥160	≥200
Borderline	200–239	n/a	130–159	150–199
Good	<200	≥40	<100	<150
Low	n/a	<40	n/a	n/a

(U.S. Department of Health and Human Services, Mayo Clinic, and Cleveland Clinic. Modified from National Cholesterol Education Program (NCEP): *Third report of the NCEP expert panel on detection, evaluation, and treatment of high blood cholesterol in adults (Adult Treatment Panel III)*, Washington, DC, 2001, National Institutes of Health, National Heart, Lung, and Blood Institute. The Adult Treatment Panel III (ATP III) is the summation of several decades of research on the relation of atherogenic lipoproteins to atherosclerotic cardiovascular disease.)

tends to be high, suggesting that it might be a marker of a detrimental metabolic profile in patients with OSA (Silva et al., 2018).

High intakes of saturated fatty acids (SFAs) affect the size of low-density lipoprotein cholesterol (LDL-C) particles, but there do not seem to be significant associations between dietary fat intake and lipoprotein levels (Alaghehband et al., 2017). The body makes 70% of its own cholesterol, so dietary cholesterol is no longer a risk factor in heart disease. The hypothesis that high TC or LDL-C causes atherosclerosis and CVD has been shown to be false (Ravnskov et al., 2018). Thus, nutrition advice has shifted to the promotion of healthy fat choices through the Mediterranean diet.

Genetic Influences

Plasma lipid levels have a strong heritability factor. Genetic studies show a relationship between lifelong elevations in triglyceride-rich lipoprotein cholesterol (TRL-C) and CVD (Bittencourt et al., 2017). Genetic mutations, such as apolipoprotein E (ApoE) polymorphisms, also contribute to CAD. A person's APOE genotype alters the inflammatory effect of obesity, which is why some obese individuals are spared coronary events and others are not.

Elevated plasma lipoprotein(a) (Lp[a]) level is another genetically determined risk factor (Orso & Schmitz, 2017). High Lp(a) occurs in all ethnic groups but is more common among African Americans and South Asians. Blood tests for Lp(a) are not included in standard lipid panels. A heart attack or stroke at an early age (younger than age 55 for men, younger than age 65 for women) signifies the need for family members to be tested. High LDL-C levels even while taking statins or other LDL-lowering medications may be another reason to be tested.

Other Risk Factors

Fixed risk factors cannot be modified; these include increasing age, male gender, genes, and family history of premature CHD.

TABLE 17.2 Risk Factors in Cardiovascular Disease

Noncontrollable	Age and gender (men >45 years, women after menopause) Elevated lipoprotein (a), inherited Ethnicity (Black Americans, Mexican Americans, Native Americans, Native Hawaiians, some Asian Americans) Family history of coronary heart disease Sex (all men, but women mostly after menopause)
Mostly controllable	Diabetes and prediabetes High blood cholesterol and triglyceride levels High blood pressure Lack of physical activity Obstructive sleep apnea Overweight and obesity Smoking Stress Unhealthy diet
Predisposing	Elevated homocysteine levels Elevated C-reactive protein High fibrinogen levels

(Data from Mayo Clinic: *Diseases and conditions: coronary artery disease*, n.d. Accessed 8 September, 2020, from http://www.mayoclinic.org/diseases-conditions/coronary-artery-disease/symptoms-causes/dxc-20165314; and National Heart, lung and Blood Institute: *What are coronary heart disease risk factors?* 2016. Accessed 8 September, 2020, from www.nhlbi.nih.gov/health/health-topics/topics/hd/.)

Modifiable nonlipid risk factors include HTN, cigarette smoking, diabetes, obesity, physical inactivity, and atherogenic diet. Table 17.2 provides a summary.

Coronary artery calcification (CAC) has been noted as a risk, but it is usually correlated with other factors. Elevated inflammatory markers C-reactive protein and fibrinogen are associated with CAC and atherosclerosis, especially in men (Nagasawa et al., 2015).

Vitamin D deficiency is linked to cardiovascular disease, obesity, insulin resistance, HTN, dyslipidemia, and T2D. More research is needed to identify proper interventions needed for cardiovascular health (Trehan et al., 2017).

Physical Activity

Obesity (especially abdominal obesity), insulin resistance, and physical inactivity are detrimental to cardiac health. The heart is a muscle and requires exercise. Thus, lifestyle modifications such as weight control and increased physical activity are primary interventions. A variety of activities can be used. (See the *Cultural Diversity and Nutrition* box Using T'ai Chi to Reduce Cardiovascular Risk.)

Food and Nutrition Therapies

The *Dietary Guidelines for Americans* provide an excellent resource for planning healthy meals. Goals include intake of better types of fats, plant-based proteins, and plenty of fiber. Weight loss may also be needed (Box 17.2). Patients with or at risk for CHD should be referred to registered dietitians for complicated nutrition therapy.

Dietary factors have an additive effect. A Mediterranean diet is cardioprotective (Box 17.3).

CULTURAL DIVERSITY AND NUTRITION

Using T'ai Chi to Reduce Cardiovascular Risk

Interventions that are age and culturally appropriate for physical activity can reduce cardiac risks and enhance quality of life. In China, t'ai chi is a form of exercise favored by older adults. T'ai chi is a mind-body practice that began as a martial art. One moves slowly while focusing on breathing deeply and clearing the mind of distracting thoughts. In Western societies, t'ai chi is part of health practices associated with traditional, complementary, and alternative medicine (TCAM). T'ai chi exercise is a good option for heart patients with limited exercise tolerance.

Application to Nursing

T'ai chi has Chinese origins but is an appropriate exercise for adults of any background. Yoga is another effective complementary treatment. Programs such as cardiac rehabilitation should include exercises and activities adapted from a variety of cultures.

BOX 17.2 Ten Heart-Healthy Diet and Lifestyle Recommendations

1. Use up at least as many calories as you take in. Start by knowing how many calories you should eat and drink to maintain your weight.
2. Increase the amount and intensity of your physical activity to match the number of calories you take in. Aim for at least 150 minutes of moderate physical activity or 75 minutes of vigorous physical activity—or an equal combination of both—each week.
3. Follow the Mediterranean or DASH (Dietary Approaches to Stop Hypertension) eating plan. Eat a variety of nutritious foods from all the food groups, and focus on the following:
   - A variety of fruits and vegetables
   - Fiber-rich whole grains
   - Low-fat dairy products
   - Skinless poultry and fish, prepared in healthy ways
   - Nuts and legumes
   - Olive oil and non-tropical vegetable oils
4. Eat fewer nutrient-poor foods: saturated fats, *trans* fat, sodium, red meat, sweets, and sugar-sweetened beverages.
5. Eat a variety of fresh, frozen, and canned vegetables and fruits without high-calorie sauces or added salt and sugars. Replace high-calorie foods with fruits and vegetables.
6. Eat fish at least twice a week, especially sources of omega-3 fatty acids (salmon, etc.).
7. Select fat-free (skim) and low-fat (1%) dairy products.
8. Avoid foods containing partially hydrogenated vegetable oils.
9. Choose foods with less sodium and prepare foods with little or no salt.
10. Use alcohol in moderation: one drink per day (women) and no more than two drinks per day (men). Red wine contains resveratrol, a protective substance.

(American Heart Association. From: https://www.heart.org/en/healthy-living/healthy-eating/eat-smart/nutrition-basics/aha-diet-and-lifestyle-recommendations. Accessed 8 September, 2020.) Reprinted with permission © 2020 American Heart Association, Inc.

Substitute monounsaturated fat for saturated fats; choose more almonds, walnuts, pistachios, extra-virgin olive oil, and canola oil. Liquid vegetable oils, semiliquid margarines, and margarines low in *trans* fatty acids are good choices. The best diet also includes many fruits and vegetables, and whole grains.

Daily intakes of 2 to 3 g of plant stanols or sterol esters (isolated from soybean and tall pine tree oils) are an additional therapeutic option. Products on the market that contain stanols include some brands of orange juice, cereals, and spreads such as Take Control and Benecol.

Substitute plant-based proteins for animal proteins. Plant-based protein foods (e.g., legumes, dry beans, nuts, whole grains, and vegetables) contain no saturated fat. Healthy animal proteins include fat-free or low-fat dairy products, egg whites, fish, skinless poultry, and lean cuts of beef and pork.

Drug Therapy

The major drugs used to treat dyslipidemia are statins. If statins are not tolerated, there are some other alternatives (Table 17.3).

MYOCARDIAL INFARCTION

Heart attacks (myocardial infarctions) are the single largest killer of adult men and women in the United States. An American suffers a heart attack every 20 seconds, and someone dies from one every minute. Disability or death can result after an MI, depending on how much heart muscle is damaged.

BOX 17.3 Principles of the Mediterranean Diet

Daily

- Eat plant-based foods: fruits and vegetables, whole grains, nuts, beans, soy, and legumes.
- Include healthy dairy choices: cheese and yogurt.
- Replace butter with healthy fats such as olive oil and canola oil.
- Use herbs and spices instead of salt to flavor foods.
- Relax and enjoy meals with family and friends.
- Get plenty of exercise.

At Least Twice a Week

- Eat eggs, fish, and poultry.
- Drink red wine in moderation (optional).

Monthly

- Limit red meat to no more than a few times a month.
- Limit sweets.

Food and Nutrition Therapies

The purpose of nutrition therapy for patients suffering from an MI is to reduce the workload of the heart. Sodium, saturated fats, fluid, and calories are controlled according to the patient's needs. Small, frequent meals are better than three large meals. Large meals raise myocardial oxygen demand by increasing splanchnic (visceral) blood flow.

This is also a good time to initiate education about the Mediterranean diet to prevent further coronary events (Booth et al., 2014). Omega-3 fatty acids appear to reduce the risk of blood clots, but their beneficial effects are reduced if the overall diet is atherogenic (Singh et al., 2016). Suggest tuna, salmon, halibut, sardines, mackerel, and lake trout to replace red meats for meals several times a week. Whole-grain intake also lowers the risk for future heart attacks. Rye and oats are especially beneficial (Helnaes et al., 2016). It is important to avoid gluten-free diets unless medically prescribed for celiac disease.

Caffeine-containing beverages may be temporarily restricted to avoid myocardial stimulation. During the rehabilitation phase, coffee and other caffeine-containing foods may be consumed in moderation.

Peripheral Artery Disease

Peripheral artery disease (PAD) causes blockages in the lower legs and prevents healthy blood flow back to the heart. It can lead to a heart attack or stroke. PAD is common after age 60 years and is found in 12% to 20% of older individuals.

A healthy diet to prevent PAD includes unsaturated fats like fish, nuts, and seeds and excludes saturated fats (red meat, butter, and whole milk). Because sodium is another concern, cut back on intake of processed meats, fast food, and convenience

TABLE 17.3 Major Drugs Used to Treat Dyslipidemia

Category	LDL-C	Non-HDL-C	TG	HDL-C	Major drug name
Statin	↓↓~↓↓↓	↓↓~↓↓↓	↓	~↑	Pravastatin, Simvastatin, Fluvastatin, Atorvastatin, Pitavastatin, Rosuvastatin
Intestinal cholesterol transporter inhibitor (Cholesterol absorption inhibitor)	↓↓	↓↓	↓	↑	Ezetimibe
Anion exchange resin	↓↓	↓↓	↑	↑	Colestimide, Cholestyramine
Probucol	↓	↓		↓↓	Probucol
PCSK9 inhibitor	↓↓↓↓	↓↓↓↓	↓↓~↓↓	~↑	Evolocumab, Alirocumab
MTP inhibitor	↓↓↓	↓↓↓	↓↓↓	↓	Lomitapide
Fibrate	↑~↓	↓	↓↓↓	↑↑	Bezafibrate, Fenofibrate, Clinofibrate, Clofibrate
Selective peroxisome proliferator-activated receptor *a* modulator (SPPARM*a*)	↑~↓	↓	↓↓↓	↑↑	Pemafibrate
Nicotinic acid derivative	↓	↓	↓↓	↑	Niceritrol, Nicomol, Tocopheryl nicotinate
N-3 polyunsaturated fatty acid			↓		Ethyl icosapentate, Omega-3-acid ethyl ester

HDL, High-density lipoprotein; *LDL*, low-density lipoprotein.
(Modified from Yamashita, et al. Clinical applications of a novel selective PPARα modulator, pemafibrate, in dyslipidemia and metabolic diseases 26:389–402, 2019. Available from https://www.researchgate.net/figure/Classification-of-Medications-Used-to-Treat-Dyslipidemia-According-to-Their-Efficacytbl1332088648. Accessed 10 September, 2020.)

foods like frozen dinners, canned soup, and processed cheese. Guidelines also emphasize careful management of hyperglycemia and smoking cessation (Gerhard-Herman et al., 2016).

HYPERTENSION

Hypertension (HTN) is a major risk factor for stroke, myocardial infarction, vascular disease, and chronic kidney disease. Nearly 1 out of 2 adults in the United States has hypertension (108 million); many are recommended lifestyle modifications only (Million Hearts, 2020).

In about 95% of cases of HTN, the cause is not evident; this condition is called essential or primary hypertension. Genetic factors are involved; see (Fig. 17.3). For some individuals, an overactive hormonal renin-angiotensin-aldosterone system plays a part. Indeed, primary hypertension is being considered a syndrome and not a disease (Manosroi & Williams, 2019).

Secondary hypertension is the term used when a specific cause of elevated blood pressure can be identified. Examples include Cushing's syndrome, polycystic kidney disease, diabetic nephropathy, thyroid disorders, or primary aldosteronism. Classifications of blood pressure are shown in Figure 17.4.

Although sometimes called a "silent killer," HTN is easily detected and usually controllable. Prescribed treatment regimens for HTN are individualized and vary because the disease differs in degree of severity. Medications may include thiazide diuretics, beta blockers, angiotensin-converting enzyme (ACE) inhibitors, calcium channel blockers, and several others.

Food and Nutrition Therapies

Weight loss is the most effective means of lowering blood pressure. Weight reduction facilitates lower blood pressure even when it is only a loss of 10 to 15 pounds. Weight reduction and sodium restriction also augment the effects of antihypertensive medications. Diet for weight loss and control should include an energy restriction and an aerobic exercise prescription, such as for walking or swimming.

Other lifestyle modifications are decreasing alcohol consumption, increasing physical activity if one is sedentary, smoking cessation, decreasing sodium intake, and increasing intake of potassium, magnesium, and calcium. Box 17.4 summarizes the lifestyle modifications that help reduce high blood pressure and overall cardiovascular risk.

The estimated dietary intake of salt is about 9 to 12 g per day, significantly above the World Health Organization recommended level of less than 5 g salt per day (Rust & Ekmekcioglu, 2017). Most comes from sodium added during the processing of foods. The other main source is discretionary use of table salt (sodium chloride). A small portion of dietary sodium also comes from natural sodium content of foods.

The U.S. National High Blood Pressure Education Program recommends trying lifestyle modifications for 3 to 6 months in patient with mild to moderate HTN. Eating a diet that is rich in whole grains, fruits, vegetables, and low-fat dairy products and skimps on saturated fat can lower blood pressure by up to 11 mm Hg; the eating plan is known as the Dietary Approaches to Stop Hypertension (DASH) plan (Mayo Clinic, 2020).

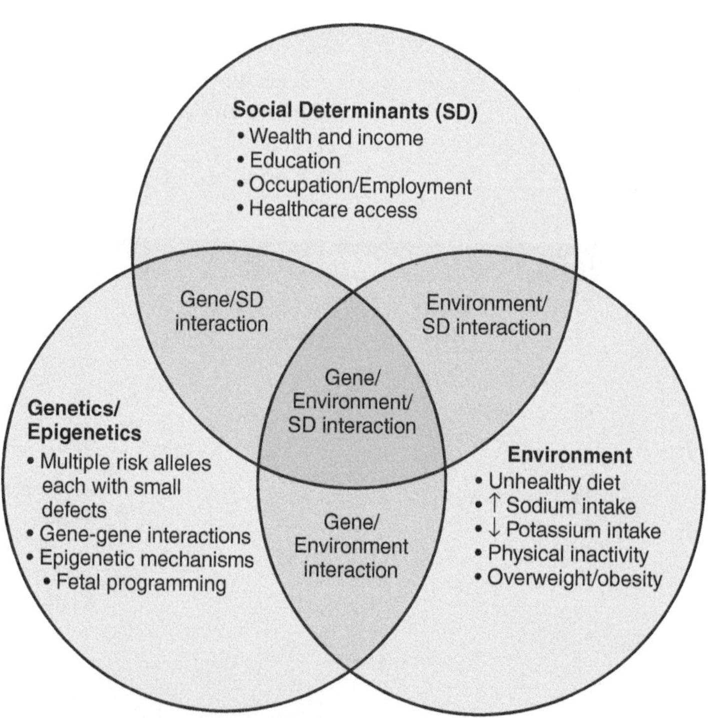

Fig. 17.3 Major determinants of blood pressure (BP) in primary hypertension and their interactions in adults. Genetic/epigenetic, environmental, and social determinants interact to increase BP in virtually all hypertensive individuals and populations. *SD*, Social determinants. (Modified from Carey, R.M., et al. Prevention and control of hypertension: *JACC* Health Promotion Series. *J Am Coll Cardiol* 72: 1278–1293, 2018.)

If diet is an issue, the DASH diet will lower blood pressure within 2 weeks. Research suggests that high intakes of cruciferous vegetables (e.g., broccoli, cabbage, cauliflower) may be especially beneficial (Connolly et al., 2020). The DASH eating plan is described in Table 17.4. The number of daily servings from each group can be modified according to individual energy needs (see the *Teaching Tool* box Strategies for Adopting DASH).

		Other risk factors (RF), asymptomatic organ damage (OD) or disease				
		No other RF	1–2 RF	≥3 RF	OD, CKD stage 3 or diabetes	Symptomatic CVD, CKD stage ≥4 or diabetes with OD/RFs
Blood Pressure (mmHg)	High normal SBP 130–139 or DBP 85–89		Low risk	Low to moderate risk	Moderate to high risk	Very high risk
	Grade 1 HT SBP 140–159 or DBP 90–99	Low risk	Moderate risk	Moderate to high risk	High risk	Very high risk
	Grade 2 HT SBP 160–179 or DBP 100–109	Moderate risk	Moderate to high risk	High risk	High risk	Very high risk
	Grade 3 HT SBP ≥180 or DBP ≥110	High risk	High risk	High risk	High to very high risk	Very high risk

Fig. 17.4 Classification of hypertension in adults. (America Heart Association. Blood Pressure. From https://www.heart.org/en/health-topics/high-blood-pressure. Accessed 8 September 2020. *CKD*, chronic kidney disease; *CVD*, cardiovascular disease; *DBP, SBP*)

TEACHING TOOL

Strategies for Adopting DASH

Dietary changes are best achieved through small changes in food selections. Use this list of tips to initiate discussion and encourage dietary compliance.

Change gradually:

- If you now eat one or two vegetables a day, add a serving at lunch and another at dinner.
- If you do not eat whole fruit now, or have only juice at breakfast, add a serving to your meals or have it as a snack.
- Gradually increase your use of fat-free and low-fat dairy products to three servings a day. For example, drink milk with lunch or dinner instead of soda, sugar-sweetened tea, or alcohol. Choose low-fat (1%) or fat-free (skim) dairy products to reduce your intake of saturated fat, total fat, cholesterol, and kcal.
- Read food labels on margarines and salad dressings and choose those lowest in saturated fat. Processed foods must now be *trans*-fat free.

Treat meat as one part of the whole meal, instead of the focus:

- Limit meat to 6 ounces a day (two servings)—all that is needed. A serving of 3 to 4 ounces is about the size of a deck of cards.
- If you currently eat large portions of meat, cut portion sizes back gradually—by half or a third at each meal.
- Include two or more vegetarian-style (meatless) meals each week, such as beans or legumes.
- Increase servings of vegetables, rice, pasta, and dry beans in meals. Try casseroles, pasta, and stir-fry dishes, which have less meat and more vegetables, grains, and dry beans.

Use fruit or other foods low in saturated fat, cholesterol, and kcal as desserts and snacks:

- Fruits and other low-fat foods offer great taste and variety. Use fruits canned in their own juice. Fresh fruits require little or no preparation. Dried fruits are a good choice to carry with you.
- Try these snacks ideas: unsalted pretzels or nuts mixed with raisins; graham crackers; low-fat, fat-free, or frozen yogurt; popcorn with no salt or butter added; and raw vegetables.

Try the following other tips:

- Choose whole-grain breads, cereals, and pasta to get added nutrients, such as minerals and fiber.
- If you have trouble digesting dairy products, try taking lactase enzyme pills or drops (available at drugstores and groceries) before eating dairy foods, or buy lactose-free milk or milk with lactase enzyme added to it.
- Use fresh, frozen, or sodium-free canned vegetables.

(Modified from Mayo Clinic: *Nutrition and healthy eating.* Accessed 2 July, 2018 from NHLBI. https://www.nhlbi.nih.gov/health-topics/dash-eating-plan.)

BOX 17.4 Lifestyle Tips for Hypertension

Eat a Healthy Diet

Choose healthy meal and snack options to help you avoid high blood pressure and its complications. Be sure to eat plenty of fresh fruits and vegetables.

Talk with your health care team about eating a variety of foods rich in potassium, fiber, and protein and lower in sodium and saturated fat. For many people, making these healthy changes can help keep blood pressure low and protect against heart disease and stroke.

Keep Yourself at a Healthy Weight

Being overweight or obese increases your risk for high blood pressure. To determine whether your weight is in a healthy range, doctors often calculate your body mass index (BMI). Doctors sometimes also use waist and hip measurements to assess body fat.

Talk with your health care team about ways to reach a healthy weight, including choosing healthy foods and getting regular physical activity.

Be Physically Active

Physical activity can help keep you at a healthy weight and lower your blood pressure. Get at least 2 hours and 30 minutes of moderate-intensity exercise, such as brisk walking or bicycling, every week; that's about 30 minutes a day, 5 days a week. Children and adolescents should get 1 hour of physical activity every day.

Do Not Smoke

Smoking raises your blood pressure and puts you at higher risk for heart attack and stroke. If you do not smoke, do not start. If you do smoke, quitting will lower your risk for heart disease. Your doctor can suggest ways to help you quit.

Limit How Much Alcohol You Drink

Do not drink too much alcohol, which can raise your blood pressure. Men should have no more than 2 alcoholic drinks per day, and women should have no more than 1 alcoholic drink per day.

Get Enough Sleep

Not getting enough sleep on a regular basis is linked to an increased risk of heart disease, high blood pressure, and stroke.

(Data from Centers for Disease Control and Prevention. *Prevent High Blood Pressure.* https://www.cdc.gov/bloodpressure/prevent_manage.htm. Accessed 10 September, 2020. https://www.cdc.gov/bloodpressure/.)

TABLE 17.4 Dietary Approaches to Stop Hypertension Diet Pattern[a]

Food Group	Daily Serving(s) (Except Where Noted)	Serving Sizes	Examples and Notes	Significance to the Dietary Approaches to Stop Hypertension Diet Pattern
Grains and grain products	7–8	1 slice bread 1-ounce dry cereal[b] ½ cup cooked rice, pasta, or cereal	Whole-wheat bread, English muffin, pita bread, bagel; cereals; grits; oatmeal	Major source of energy and fiber
Vegetables	4–5	1 cup raw, leafy vegetables ½ cup cooked vegetables 6 ounces vegetable juice	Tomatoes, potatoes, carrots, peas, squash, broccoli, turnip greens, collards, kale, spinach, artichokes, beans, sweet potatoes	Rich sources of potassium, magnesium, and fiber
Fruits	4–5	6 ounces fruit juice 1 medium fruit ¼ cup dried fruit ½ cup fresh, frozen, or canned fruit	Apricots, bananas, dates, grapes, oranges, orange juice, tangerines, strawberries, mangoes, melons, peaches, pineapple, prunes, raisins	Important sources of potassium, magnesium, and fiber
Low-fat or free dairy foods	2–3	8 ounces milk 1 cup yogurt 1½ ounces cheese	Fat-free or 1% milk, fat-free or low-fat buttermilk; nonfat or low-fat yogurt; part-skim mozzarella cheese, nonfat cheese	Major sources of calcium and protein
Meats, poultry, and fish	≥2	3 ounces cooked meats, poultry, or fish	Select only lean meats; trim away visible fats; broil, roast, or boil, instead of frying; remove skin from chicken	Rich sources of protein and magnesium
Nuts, seeds, and legumes	4–5 per week	1½ ounces or ½ cup nuts ½ ounce or 2 tablespoons seeds ½ cup cooked legumes	Almonds, filberts, mixed nuts, peanuts, walnuts, sunflower seeds, kidney beans, lentils	Rich sources of energy, magnesium, potassium, protein, and fiber
Fats and oils[c]	2–3	1 teaspoon soft margarine 1 tablespoon low-fat mayonnaise or salad dressing 2 tablespoons light salad dressing 1 teaspoon vegetable oil	Soft margarine, low-fat mayonnaise, light salad dressing, vegetable oil (e.g., olive, corn, canola, or safflower)	DASH has 27% of kcal as fat, including that in or added to foods
Sweets	5 per week	1 tablespoon sugar 1 tablespoon jelly or jam ½ ounce jelly beans 8 ounces lemonade	Maple syrup, sugar, jelly, jam, fruit-flavored gelatin, jelly beans, fruit punch, sorbet, ices, hard candy	Sweets should be low in fat

[a]This diet is based on 2000 kcal/day. This table indicates the number of recommended daily servings from each food group with examples of food choices. The number of servings may increase or decrease, depending on individual calorie needs.

[b]Equals ½ to 1¼ cups depending on cereal type. Check the product's nutrition label.

[c]Fat content changes serving counts for fats and oils. For example, 1 tablespoon of regular salad dressing equals 1 serving; 1 tablespoon of low-fat dressing equals ½ serving; 1 tablespoon of fat-free dressing equals 0 servings.

(From National Institutes of Health, National Heart, Lung, and Blood Institute: DASH Eating Plan. From https://www.nhlbi.nih.gov/health/health-topics/topics/dash/followdash. Accessed 8 September, 2020.)

BOX 17.5 Patient Tips for Lowering Sodium

Know your sodium limit

Ask your doctor how much sodium is okay for you. The general guidance is:

Healthy adults and teens age 14 and older need to limit their sodium intake to no more than 2,300 mg a day.

For people with high blood pressure – and people with blood pressure that's between normal and high – limiting sodium to 1,500 mg a day may be helpful.

Children under age 14 need no more than 1,500 to 2,200 mg a day of sodium, depending on how old they are.

Shop for low-sodium foods

Most of the sodium we eat doesn't come from our salt shakers. Sodium is in almost all the processed and prepared foods we buy – even foods that don't taste salty, like bread or tortillas.

When you are shopping, limit these items that are high in sodium:

Processed meats, poultry, and seafood – like deli meats, sausages, and sardines

Sauces, dressings, and condiments

Instant foods, like flavored rice or noodles.

At the grocery store

Check the label. Use the Nutrition Facts label to check the amount of sodium in foods and compare different options.

Try to choose products with ≤5% daily value (DV). A sodium content of ≥20% DV is high.

Look for foods labeled "low sodium," "reduced sodium," or "no salt added." But keep in mind that some low-sodium foods don't have those labels. Check the Nutrition Facts label to be sure!

Make healthy changes

Swap out foods that are higher in sodium for healthier options. You can:

Snack on unsalted nuts instead of salted pretzels or chips.

Choose skinless chicken and turkey, lean meats, or seafood instead of deli meats or sausages.

Go for vegetables that are fresh, frozen, or canned. Pick frozen vegetables without sauce and canned vegetables with the least amount of sodium.

Cook more at home

Making your own meals is a great way to eat less sodium, because you are in control of what goes into your food.

If you use canned foods, rinse them before eating or cooking with them. This will wash away some of the salt.

Use condiments and spreads that are unsalted or lower in sodium. If you use regular spreads, use less.

Don't add salt to the water when you cook pasta or rice.

Try different herbs and spices to flavor your food, like ginger or garlic, instead of salt.

Take the salt shaker off your table.

Get less salt when you eat away from home

Ask if there are any lower-sodium dishes on the menu.

When you order, ask that salt not be added to your food.

Get dressings and sauces on the side so you can add only as much as you need.

Add more potassium to your diet

Replace high-sodium foods with high-potassium foods. Eating foods with potassium can help lower your blood pressure.

Good sources of potassium include potatoes, cantaloupe, bananas, beans, milk, and yogurt.

(From My Healthfinder. Eat Less Sodium – Quick Tips. Accessed 8 September, 2020 from https://health.gov/myhealthfinder/topics/health-conditions/heart-health/eat-less-sodium-quick-tips#.)

An even larger drop in blood pressure is seen when the DASH eating plan is combined with sodium restriction (Box 17.5). The largest reduction in blood pressure is seen in those using the DASH eating plan with the sodium intake level of 1500 mg/day, a moderately severe restriction (Box 17.5 and Table 17.5).

Maintaining sodium consumption at a low level is a challenge, given the amount of sodium added to foods during processing and manufacturing. Salt adds its own salty flavor to foods, alters other tastes and flavors, and conceals bitterness without necessarily causing the foods to taste salty. As a result, when salt is reduced or removed from a food, the saltiness and other flavors of that food are changed. Although there is currently no acceptable substitute for salt that provides similar taste satisfaction, a salt substitute may be prescribed for some patients. The *Teaching Tool box Seven Sneaky Sodium Stowaways* gives tips on helping patients recognize foods potentially high in sodium.

TEACHING TOOL

Seven Sneaky Sodium Stowaways

Provide patients with an easy way to remember categories of foods that may be high in sodium. Label reading is often an absolute necessity. Sodium hides in seven categories of foods in the form of salt or as part of an added ingredient. These are the seven sneaky categories of sodium stowaways:

*S*nack foods (corn chips, potato chips, pretzels, peanuts, certain crackers)

*S*easonings and nonnutritive sweeteners (onion or garlic salt, monosodium glutamate, sodium saccharin)

*S*oups (canned and dried mixes)

*S*auces (dried mixes and bottled, including ketchup)

*S*moked meats and fish (preserved ham and lox)

*S*auerkraut and other pickled foods (pickles, relishes, pickled herring)

*S*odium-processed luncheon meats (bologna, salami, ham, corned beef).

HEART FAILURE

Heart failure (HF) is a form of cardiac decompensation. Left ventricle failure produces pulmonary congestion, whereas right ventricular failure results in systemic congestion that causes poor perfusion to all organ systems.

Hypertensive heart disease leads to the development of diastolic dysfunction, left ventricular hypertrophy, and heart failure; thus, the treatment of hypertension can prevent the development of HF (Sorrentino, 2019). HF affects an estimated 5.7 million Americans, and about 670,000 people are diagnosed with HF each year. There is an expanding prevalence of HF after myocardial infarction, as well as increasing numbers of people who have diabetes, chronic kidney disease, and obesity (McCullough et al., 2016). Lifestyle modification with exercise and weight loss can improve diastolic function and reduce the risk for heart failure (Sorrentino, 2019).

TABLE 17.5 Dietary Approaches to Stop Hypertension: A Sample Menu With Less Salt

This sample menu provides five fruit servings, five vegetable servings, and four dairy servings

2300-mg Sodium Menu	Sodium (mg)	Substitutions to Reduce Sodium to 1500 Mg	Sodium (mg)
Breakfast			
¾ cup bran flakes	220	¾ cup shredded wheat cereal	1
1 slice whole-wheat bread	149	½ cup fruit yogurt, fat free, no sugar added	86
1 cup low-fat milk	107		
1 teaspoon soft (tub) margarine	26	1 teaspoon soft (tub) margarine, unsalted	0
Lunch			
¾ cup chicken salad	179	Omit salt from recipe	120
2 slices whole-wheat bread	299		
1 tablespoon Dijon mustard	373	1 tablespoon regular mustard	175
½ cup fruit cocktail, juice pack	5		
Salad:			
½ cup fresh cucumber slices	1		
½ cup tomato wedges	5		
1 tablespoon sunflower seeds	0		
1 teaspoon Italian dressing, reduced calorie	43		
Dinner			
3 ounces spicy baked fish	50	Omit salt from recipe	
1 cup green beans, cooked from frozen, without salt	12		
1 small baked potato	14		
2 tablespoons fat-free sour cream	21		
1 tablespoon chopped scallions	1		
2 tablespoons grated cheddar cheese, natural, reduced fat	67	2 tablespoons cheddar cheese, natural, reduced fat, low sodium	1
1 small whole-wheat roll	148		
1 teaspoon soft margarine	26	1 teaspoon soft margarine, unsalted	0
1 medium peach	0		
1 cup low-fat milk	107		
Snack			
1 cup orange juice	5		
⅓ cup almonds, unsalted	0		
¼ cup raisins	4		
1 cup fruit yogurt, fat free with no sugar added	173		

Spicy Seasoning Mix

Mix together the following ingredients and store in airtight container: 1½ teaspoons white pepper, ½ teaspoon cayenne pepper, ½ teaspoon black pepper, 1 teaspoon onion powder, 1¼ teaspoons garlic powder, 1 tablespoon dried basil, 1½ teaspoons dried thyme.

(From National Institutes of Health, National Heart, Lung, and Blood Institute: *Description of the DASH eating plan*, Bethesda, MD, n.d., Author. Accessed 10 September, 2020, from https://www.nhlbi.nih.gov/health-topics/dash-eating-plan.)

Food and Nutrition Therapies

Chronic HF is a multisystem disease with important comorbidities such as anemia, insulin resistance, and cardiac cachexia. If the HF is caused by valve failure, most dietary measures will not be effective. If excessive sodium intake has been part of the etiology, then nutrition therapy focuses on restricting dietary sodium.

Patients with mild to moderate HF are often prescribed a sodium restriction of 3000 mg/day. People whose disease is unresponsive to this level or who have severe HF are more likely to benefit from sodium restriction to 2000 mg/day.

Fluid restriction of 1 to 2 L is sometimes indicated with low serum sodium. Fluid requirements in HF depend on medical status and the use of diuretics. Because thirst is a problem when fluid is limited, chewing gum or use of a saliva substitute may be helpful.

Include high-fiber foods such as cooked dried peas and beans (legumes), whole-grain foods, bran, cereals, pasta, rice and fresh fruit. High-fiber foods contain antioxidants that are cardioprotective. Another protective factor is omega-3 fatty acid (eicosapentaenoic acid [EPA] + docosahexaenoic acid [DHA]) in the form of fish oil or intake of salmon, tuna, herring and other choices.

With an anticoagulant like warfarin (Coumadin), foods high in vitamin K can alter the drug's metabolism. Veggies with vitamin K include Brussels sprouts, cabbage, collard greens, kale, mustard greens, spinach, and turnip greens. Note that convenience foods and mixed dishes may also contain vitamin K (Harshman et al., 2017). Monitor use of multivitamins; if used, they should be taken daily so protein levels can be regulated accordingly. Keep the amount of vitamin K from food and supplements about the same from day to day.

If medical therapies are limited by tolerability, hypotension, electrolyte disturbances, and renal dysfunction, coenzyme Q10 (CoQ10) may be useful (Sharma et al., 2016). CoQ10 is chemically similar to vitamin K and helps transport energy (adenosine triphosphate [ATP]) across cell membranes.

Cardiac Cachexia

In the elderly, frailty is often accompanied by HF and sarcopenia, a systemic skeletal muscle disease that also impairs the function of respiratory muscles. Early satiety, anorexia, nausea, gastrointestinal (GI) congestion, and shortness of breath lead to cardiac cachexia. Unless managed, micro- and macronutrient deficiencies and sarcopenia lead to severe malnutrition, hospitalizations, or death (McCullough et al., 2016).

Energy requirements are 20% to 30% greater than basal needs because of increased cardiac and pulmonary energy demands and metabolic rate. Protein and energy intake should be sufficient to maintain body weight. Use volume-concentrated formulas if fluid restriction is necessary. Meeting these increased nutrient and energy requirements is problematic; use caution so as not to overfeed the patient.

Calorie-dense (1.5 kcal/mL) nutritional supplements help to increase energy and protein intake. If needs cannot be met orally, consider enteral or parenteral nutrition. When enteral nutrition is used, continuous rather than bolus feedings are favored because they reduce myocardial oxygen consumption.

ROLE OF NURSING

A multidisciplinary approach is beneficial for HF patients; muscular training and nutritional interventions are important. Although dietitians are responsible for developing the medical nutrition plan and for in-depth counseling, nurses reinforce those concepts and answer any additional questions of patients and their families.

Nurses play a major role in teaching people how to reduce cardiovascular risk factors, including reinforcement of dietary modifications. The emphasis has shifted away from standardized information sheets toward an individualized, tailored approach. Thus, familiarity with key dietary principles will make the discussions easier.

Family Education

Modifications in lifestyle are easier to follow when the entire family is supportive and compliant. Dietary education should include individuals who buy and prepare meals or snacks for the patient. By including all family members in the educative process, not only is the health of the individual with CAD enhanced but primary risk factors for younger family members can be lessened. Lists of health associations, community hospitals, and other organizations offering cooking courses and of bookstores or public libraries with available heart-healthy cookbooks are excellent adjuncts for nutrition counseling. Lifelong health promotion habits that develop early can benefit everyone.

Demystifying Labels

Label reading is an important skill for everyone but is especially so for someone with diet-related illnesses, including HTN and CVD. Educating patients about use of food label information helps demystify the process of limiting dietary fat and sodium. Food labels may display two types of messages about packaged food: nutrient content claims and health claims. Federal regulations formulated by the U.S. Food and Drug Administration (FDA) control how certain terms can be used in labeling. Table 17.6 defines terms related to nutrients of concern for patients with CVD.

PULMONARY DISEASES

Disorders of the pulmonary system are classified into two categories. The first consists of disorders that result in chronic long-term changes in pulmonary function, such as chronic obstructive pulmonary disease (COPD), a collective phrase for chronic bronchitis, asthma, or emphysema. COPD is the second leading cause of disability in the United States.

The second category contains disorders that cause acute changes in pulmonary function, such as respiratory distress syndrome (RDS) and acute respiratory failure (ARF). These disorders can develop in patients who are critically ill, in shock, severely injured or septic. For ARF and RDS, the purpose of nutrition therapy is to inhibit tissue destruction by providing extra nutrients for hypermetabolic conditions without contributing to the decline in pulmonary function.

Chronic Obstructive Pulmonary Disease

Smoking, exposure to fumes or secondhand smoke, and genetics play a role in the onset of COPD. In early stages, it can progress silently, without noticeable shortness of breath. Gradually, symptoms include increased breathlessness, frequent coughing (with and without sputum), wheezing, and tightness in the chest.

Energy required for breathing is something most of us often take for granted. High energy demands, however, occur in patients with COPD while they are just breathing. These patients therefore have an increased likelihood of malnutrition. It is common to see significant weight loss from both fat stores and muscle mass.

Muscle wasting is most evident in the diaphragm and respiratory muscles. Thus, the presence of malnutrition contributes to the patient's decline. The goal of nutrition therapy for this category is to maintain respiratory muscle strength and function and to prevent or correct malnutrition.

Food and Nutrition Therapies

Malnutrition of individuals with COPD is multifactorial. Contributing factors include altered taste because of chronic

TABLE 17.6 Nutrient Content Claims

Claim	Requirements
"High," "rich in," or "excellent source of"	Contains ≥20% of the daily value (DV). May be used on meals or main dishes to indicate that the product contains a food that meets the definition but may not be used to describe the meal.
"Good source," "contains," or "provides"	Contains 10%–19% of the DV. These terms may be used on meals or main dishes to indicate that the product contains a food that meets the definition but may not be used to describe the meal.
"More," "fortified," "enriched," "added," "extra," or "plus"	Contains ≥10% of the DV than an appropriate reference food. May only be used for vitamins, minerals, protein, dietary fiber, and potassium.
"Lean"	On seafood or game meat products that contain <10 g total fat, 4.5 g or less saturated fat, and <95 mg cholesterol per 100 g (for meals and main dishes, meets criteria per 100 g and per labeled serving). On mixed dishes, not measurable with a cup, that contain <8 g total fat, 3.5 g or less saturated fat, and <80 mg cholesterol.
"Extra lean"	On seafood or game meat products that contains <5 g total fat, <2 g saturated fat and <95 mg cholesterol per 100 g (for meals and main dishes, meets criteria per 100 g and per labeled serving).
"High potency"	May be used on foods to describe individual vitamins or minerals that are present at 100% or more of the recommended dietary allowance (RDA) on a multi-ingredient food product that contains ≥100% of the RDA for at least two-thirds of the vitamins and minerals with RDAs and that are present in the product at ≥2% of the RDA (e.g., "High potency multivitamin, multimineral dietary supplement tablet").
"Modified"	May be used in statement of identity of a food that bears a relative claim (e.g., "Modified fat cheesecake, contains 35% less fat than our regular cheesecake.")
"Fiber" claims	If a fiber claim is made and the food is not low in total fat, then the label must disclose the level of total fat per labeled serving.
Claims using the term "antioxidant"	For claims characterizing the level of antioxidant nutrients in a food, an RDA must be established for each of the nutrients that are the subject of the claim. Each nutrient must have existing scientific evidence of antioxidant activity. The level of each nutrient must be sufficient to meet the definition for "high," "good source," or "more." Beta carotene may be the subject of an antioxidant claim when the level of vitamin A present as beta carotene in the food is sufficient to qualify for the claim. Name(s) of nutrient(s) that is (are) the subject of the claim is (are) included as part of the claim (e.g., high in antioxidant vitamins C and E).

(Data from U.S. Food and Drug Administration: *Food labeling guide: guidance for industry*, Washington, DC, Author. Accessed on 8 September, 2020, from https://www.fda.gov/Food/GuidanceRegulation/GuidanceDocumentsRegulatoryInformation/LabelingNutrition/ucm2006828.htm.)

BOX 17.6 Maximizing Food Intake in Chronic Obstructive Pulmonary Disease

Here are ideas to make mealtimes easier and more nutritious by increasing energy and protein without increasing the amount of food eaten.

Feeding the Patient With Chronic Obstructive Pulmonary Disease

- Suggest that patients consume small, frequent meals.
- Encourage patients to eat the most when well rested, such as the first meal of the day.
- Encourage the use of high-calorie, high-protein supplements.
- Teach patients to swallow as little air as possible when eating.
- Encourage the use of easily prepared or convenience foods to decrease any fatigue.

In Clinical and Home Health Care Settings

- Eat high-calorie foods first.
- Try more frequent meals and snacks.
- Add margarine, butter, mayonnaise, sauces, gravies, and peanut butter to foods.
- Limit liquids at mealtimes.
- Try cold foods, which can give less sense of fullness than hot foods.
- Rest before meals.

At Home

- Keep favorite foods and snacks on hand.
- Keep ready-prepared meals available for periods of increased shortness of breath.
- Eat larger meals when you are not as tired.
- Avoid foods that you know cause gas.
- Add skim milk powder (2 tablespoons) to regular milk (8 oz) to add protein and kcal.
- Use milk or half-and-half instead of water when making soups, cereals, instant puddings, cocoa, or canned soups.
- Add grated cheese to sauces, vegetables, soups, and casseroles.
- Choose dessert recipes that contain egg, such as sponge cake, angel food cake, egg custard, bread pudding, and rice pudding.

mouth breathing and excessive sputum production, fatigue, anxiety, depression, increased energy requirements, frequent infections, and the side effects of multiple medications. Preventing malnutrition will not only help preserve muscle strength needed for pulmonary function but also maintain the integrity of the immune system. The first step in this prevention is to provide adequate nutrition. Anorexia, early satiety, nausea, and vomiting are all common in these patients. Box 17.6 discusses tips for maximizing food intake in COPD.

Energy expenditure is usually elevated, but it will vary according to a person's level of physical activity. Moreover, energy balance and nitrogen balance go hand in hand; visceral and somatic proteins can only be conserved if optimal energy balance is maintained. Indirect calorimetry is the most accurate method of determining energy expenditure for hospitalized patients with COPD.

Adequate protein stimulates the ventilatory drive. Patients may require 1.2 to 1.9 g protein per kg of body weight for

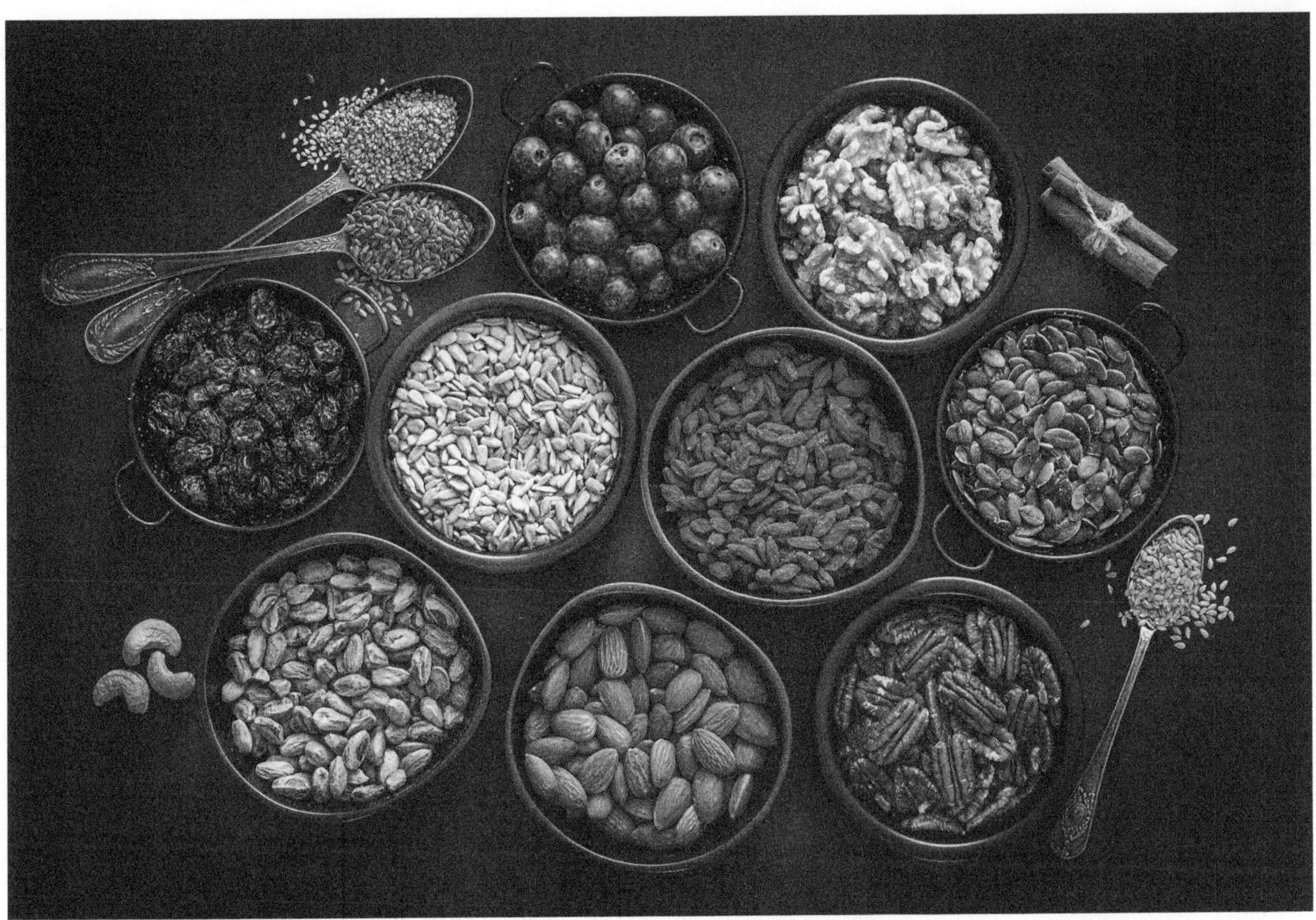

Fig. 17.5 Antioxidant rich foods include fruit, vegetables, whole grains and nuts. (From © iStock photo; Credit: fcafotodigital.)

maintenance and 1.6 to 2.5 g/kg for repletion. Offer foods such as milk, eggs, cheese, meat, fish, poultry, nuts, beans, and legumes. The perception that milk is not well tolerated is an old wives' tale and should be dismissed.

Higher intake of iron favors oxidative stress; use caution with supplements. However, it is prudent to include dietary sources of vitamin D and the other antioxidants (vitamins C and E and selenium); see Fig. 17.5. COPD patients with hypoxemia will benefit from a lycopene-enriched diet (Kentson et al., 2018).

Offer 4 to 6 small meals a day and reduce sodium intake. Too much sodium may cause edema and discomfort. Ask the registered dietitian about the use of spices and herbs for seasoning foods.

Respiratory Quotient

The respiratory quotient (RQ) is the ratio of carbon dioxide produced to the amount of oxygen consumed. Carbohydrate metabolism produces the greatest amount of carbon dioxide and therefore has the highest RQ. The physiologic range for RQ is 0.67 to 1.3. Fat metabolism produces the least amount of carbon dioxide and has the lowest RQ (0.7). An RQ greater than 1 may indicate that carbohydrate is the primary energy source, and it is evidence of accumulating carbon dioxide, making respiration that much more difficult for a patient with COPD.

Providing nutrients in proper combination is important to reduce production of carbon dioxide and maintain pulmonary function. High fat and low carbohydrate ratios are recommended. This issue is particularly crucial when weaning the ventilator-dependent patient.

When each type of macronutrient is metabolized, carbon dioxide and water are produced. The important issue is to provide adequate nutrition without overfeeding the patient. Overfeeding also produces an excessive amount of carbon dioxide, reflected in an RQ greater than 1.

Cystic Fibrosis

Cystic fibrosis (CF) is an autosomal recessive inherited disease of the mucus-producing exocrine glands. CF is characterized by high levels of sodium and chloride in saliva, tears, and sweat and highly viscous secretions in the pancreas, bronchi, bile ducts, and small intestine that may be obstructive. CF occurs in about 1 of every 3300 live births of Caucasian infants and 1 in every 15,300 non-White births. Physical signs such as growth retardation, failure to gain weight, abdominal protuberance, lack of subcutaneous fat, and poor muscle tone are common findings. Frequent pulmonary infections, pancreatic insufficiency, and GI malabsorption put individuals with CF at great nutritional risk.

The average survival for a patient with CF in the United States is 37 years. Death most often results from malnutrition, bronchopneumonia, lung collapse, and cor pulmonale (see the *Personal Perspectives* box Two Brothers: Ways of Coping.)

PERSONAL PERSPECTIVES

Two Brothers: Ways of Coping

My oldest son, Nathan, was 18 years old when he was finally diagnosed with cystic fibrosis (CF).

Although we both had been waiting a long time to get an answer to what had been plaguing him, I'd been hoping and praying that he'd escape the CF sentence. The diagnosis, however, did not come as a surprise because exactly 35 days earlier, my younger son, Caleb, at 14 years, had already been diagnosed with CF.

Caleb's Story

Somehow, Caleb had maintained his composure upon receiving the news. He graciously thanked the doctors and office staff in the same way that Nathan would a month later. But his reaction was remarkably more relaxed than his older brother's. As we drove home, Caleb occupied himself by texting his friends. "Do you want to talk about it, Caleb?" I asked gently. "No, Ma," he replied without looking up from his phone, "I'm talking to my friends right now."

And as soon as we got into our apartment, Caleb busted out into a rap and dance: "Cystic fibrosis ain't got nuttin' on me. Cystic fibrosis ain't got nuttin' on me. Cystic fibrosis ain't got nuttin' on me ..." For the next few months, Caleb took his new diagnosis in stride, although getting him to take his medications consistently was initially difficult. Caleb pushed himself and his body. He rocked CF and he rocked it hard. He participated in basketball, running, weight training, pull-ups, push-ups, and sit-ups every day.

By the time the summer rolled around, he looked, and must have felt, indestructible. And as he got better physically, he improved in consistency with his meds. Or maybe it was the other way around. Regardless, mentally he chose to be in a good place and it showed in his overall health status. Soon he had off-the-charts lung function to prove it. I remember his doctor showing his readings to other doctors and staff with unrivaled excitement and celebration.

Nathan's Story

Nathan's diagnosis story is different. His brother had already been diagnosed so we knew what we were dealing with. While Caleb was starting to adjust to life with CF, Nathan was finishing his freshman year at New York University. He had already done the research on his brother's disease: a disease whose symptoms looked like his own. By the time he sat in the doctor's chair and waited for the results from the blood work, he already knew the life expectancy statistics, the progression of the disease, how you can be fine one day and then suddenly worse the next.

Upon receiving his diagnosis, Nathan expressed those concerns, along with a few others, to the doctor. "What about insurance when I'm not covered under my parent's plan? How will I afford the mounting health care costs?" He knew, even before his diagnosis, that his theater degree would not necessarily sustain him financially. He shared those fears as well and was told that he should consider transferring to the Stern School of Business at NYU. But to Nathan—and most people, I imagine—the thought of giving up his dreams to accommodate the progressive nature of a disease that he didn't ask for was something that he couldn't comprehend.

Nathan spent the following days wondering what this illness meant for his career and his life. He questioned if he would be able to pursue his passions in theater and art when his meds would cost significantly more than the average person's. He thought about whether he would have to settle for an office job that would provide him with health coverage but would not allow him to pursue his dreams.

Like Caleb, Nathan also struggled with adapting to the CF therapy regimen. A year later, he was still inconsistent. But participating in a clinical trial prompted a steadiness and routine with his meds that has persisted. Around this time, Caleb also took a serious interest in learning more about CF. Although their reactions to the initial diagnosis were very different, they ended up on the same path. They are both still learning how to live their lives without letting CF take over. Today they strive to live in the present—not the past or the future—because worrying about both is a waste of time.

Michelle Patrovani
Broward County, Florida

(Modified from Patrovani, M. *Late CF diagnosis: two brothers, two stories*, Bethesda, MD, 2016, Cystic Fibrosis Foundation. Accessed on 8 September, 2020 from https://www.cff.org/CF-Community-Blog/Authors/Michelle-Patrovani.)

Food and Nutrition Therapies

Nutrition is of prime importance in the treatment of CF. Nutritional requirements vary depending on the age of the patient and severity of disease. Poor nutritional status because of undernutrition contributes to poor growth, pulmonary complications, and susceptibility to infection. There are also links between intestinal inflammation and dysbiosis (an imbalance in intestinal microbial populations) in CF (Garg & Ooi, 2017).

The primary goal of nutritional therapy for patients with CF is to exceed the Dietary Reference Intakes (DRIs) for kcal and all other nutrients by 1.2 to 2 times. Dietitians estimate individual energy requirements based on basal metabolic rate, activity level, lung function, and fat absorption.

Improvements in pancreatic enzyme replacement therapy now allow higher amounts of dietary fat intake in patients with CF, which were previously prohibited. Because fat provides such a concentrated source of energy, it does not need to be restricted if pancreatic enzyme replacement therapy is individualized and sufficient.

Although sodium requirements may be considerably higher for patients with CF, routine sodium supplementation appears unnecessary because the average American diet contains an overabundance. However, multivitamin supplements should be prescribed. Fat-soluble vitamins may be prescribed in a water-miscible form if fat malabsorption is severe.

Probiotics may be beneficial, as gut dysbiosis is associated with GI symptoms. Probiotics can significantly reduce fecal calprotectin (a marker of intestinal inflammation) in children and adults with CF (Coffey et al, 2020). More clinical trials are needed to identify the best type and dosage.

Infants. Since initiation of universal newborn screening for CF, significant improvement has occurred in nutritional status, with normalization of weight in the first year of life, but length stunting remains common (Leung, 2017). Pancreatic enzyme replacement therapy should be used along with all types of milk products, including breast milk, in infants with CF. Supplemental fat or carbohydrate may be necessary for some infants to increase calorie density to more than 20 kcal/ounce. Introduction of solid food is the same as that for infants without CF.

Childhood to adulthood. Nutritional adequacy of the diet, compliance with pancreatic enzymes, and growth patterns should be closely monitored because, as the child with CF becomes older and more independent, compliance may become questionable. Reevaluation of the patient's diet is important to ascertain if recommendations are adequate to support growth and maintain nutritional status.

As changes occur in the disease process and growth continues, nutritional needs also change. Weight gain, linear growth, and level of pancreatic enzyme replacement therapy should also be closely monitored and assessed during this time. The young adult with CF will continue to require pancreatic enzymes and extra calories and micronutrients.

Regular evaluation by a registered dietitian should be scheduled. Poor clinical outcomes are often associated with undernutrition. Complicated clinical situations that directly affect nutrition include lung transplantation, cystic fibrosis–related diabetes, and bone health.

Acute Respiratory Failure and Respiratory Distress Syndrome

The recent coronavirus disease (COVID-19) pandemic has led to many cases of acute respiratory distress and failure. The virus is highly infectious. Patients may develop an acute respiratory distress syndrome, then multiorgan failure (Matera et al., 2020). Most patients with ARF require mechanical ventilation, so in such cases, nutrition support may be provided via enteral or parenteral nutrition.

Patients with ARF may suffer from malnutrition, which impairs recovery and prolongs weaning from mechanical ventilation. A diet that minimizes carbon dioxide production while maintaining good nutrition is recommended.

Food and Nutrition Therapies

Malnutrition and the method of feeding will influence the outcome in respiratory disease or failure. Nutrition therapy is important to maintain or replenish nutritional status and can positively or negatively influence weaning from mechanical ventilation. Because a significant number of patients with pulmonary disease or respiratory failure have clinically relevant malnutrition, nurses and other health care professionals caring for them should always be alert to alterations in nutritional status.

Nutrition support should be initiated as soon as possible. Caution is needed to avoid overfeeding in the first week; high calorie feedings are beneficial after that time (Peterson et al., 2018). Goals are similar to those for COPD: high calorie, high protein, moderate to high (50% nonprotein kcal) fat, with moderate (50% nonprotein kcal) carbohydrate.

Enteral nutrition. Early enteral nutrition is recommended in several guidelines for mechanically ventilated patients, especially children (Srinivasan et al., 2020). Commercial formulas that provide 40% to 50% of total kcal from fat are available. Higher caloric density formulas may be necessary when fluid is restricted. The use of immune-enhancing products is not yet supported by evidence.

Low-osmolality feedings are started slowly to avoid gastric retention and diarrhea. Continuous administration is recommended unless otherwise contraindicated. Because of the risk for aspiration, special precautions are suggested, such as elevating the head of the bed or using a tube placed into the duodenum or jejunum.

Parenteral nutrition. Parenteral nutrition may be needed for acute respiratory failure. High glucose concentrations can lead to excess carbon dioxide production, making weaning from the ventilator more difficult; therefore, they should be avoided. The optimal parenteral solution should provide adequate protein to maintain nitrogen balance and 1 to 2 g of lipid per kilogram of body weight. Remaining caloric needs can then be met by carbohydrates. It is additionally recommended to infuse nutrition support for these clients over the whole 24-hour period, not just intermittently.

Nutrition status monitoring in the critically ill is best managed by qualified team members. Daily calorie counts, daily weights, and biochemical parameters are necessary to assess response to nutrition support. A comparison of nutritional

TABLE 17.7 Antioxidant-Rich Foods

Food	Antioxidant Nutrients
Acorn squash, pumpkin, winter squash	Beta carotene
Apples	Catechins
Apricots, cantaloupe, peaches	Beta carotene
Beans	Catechins, vitamin E
Beets	Anthocyanins
Bell peppers	Beta carotene, vitamin C
Berries	Anthocyanins, catechins, ellagic acid (in raspberries and strawberries), resveratrol (in blueberries), vitamin C
Broccoli, greens, spinach	Beta carotene, lutein, vitamin C
Brown rice	Selenium
Carrots	Beta carotene
Chicken	Selenium
Citrus fruits	Vitamin C
Corn	Lutein
Egg	Lutein (in yolks); selenium, vitamin A
Eggplant	Anthocyanins
Garlic and onions	Selenium
Grapefruit, pink	Lycopene, vitamin C
Grapes, red wine	Anthocyanins (in red and purple grapes), resveratrol
Mango and papaya	Beta carotene, vitamin C
Milk	Vitamin A
Nuts, nut butters, oils, seeds	Vitamin E
Oatmeal	Selenium
Peanuts	Resveratrol
Prunes	Anthocyanins
Salmon, tuna, seafood	Selenium
Sweet potatoes	Beta carotene, vitamin C
Tea, black or green	Catechins
Tomatoes (canned)	Lycopene, vitamin C
Watermelon	Lycopene, vitamin C
Wheat germ, whole grains	Selenium, vitamin E

(Copyright 2010 Academy of Nutrition and Dietetics. Used with permission.)

intake with indirect calorimetry provides useful guidance to monitor the adequacy of nutrition support. Collaboration with clinical dietitians is best to monitor transition from parenteral to enteral feedings to conventional feeding.

Asthma

Prenatal and postnatal exposure to air pollution and various allergens can trigger asthma in children. Occupational exposures and oxidative stress play a role for adults. A healthy diet and avoidance of obesity during pregnancy, childhood, and aging may reduce asthma exacerbations.

Antioxidant dietary approaches are suggested (see Table 17.7). A variety of fruits, vegetables, and whole grains provide natural sources of dietary fiber, iron, magnesium, and phosphorus. Vitamins C and D and omega-3 fatty acids (such as in fish oil) are important nutrients to emphasize. Manipulation of the gut microbiome through prebiotic foods is a strategy to influence the immunopathology of asthma (Williams et al., 2016). Fig. 17.6 shows prebiotic foods.

Tuberculosis

Tuberculosis (TB) has been declared a global health emergency by the World Health Organization. Nearly one-third of the world's population is infected. With international travel and immigration, more individuals will be exposed. The prevalence of HIV/AIDS is another health threat for the immunocompromised population.

Nutrition support should be initiated as soon as possible in the patient with TB to prevent or correct weight loss and malnutrition. Multiple medications are necessary, and strict adherence to scheduled administration will help resolve the disease. However, compliance is often a challenge.

Obesity and T2D are risk factors for TB (Pavan Kumar et al., 2016). Chronic inflammation undermines the body's immune system. Vitamin D may also play a role; low serum levels should be corrected in patients with T2D to protect against TB infection.

Although there is no special diet for TB, a high-calorie, high-protein, nutrient-rich meal plan is suggested with small, frequent feedings.

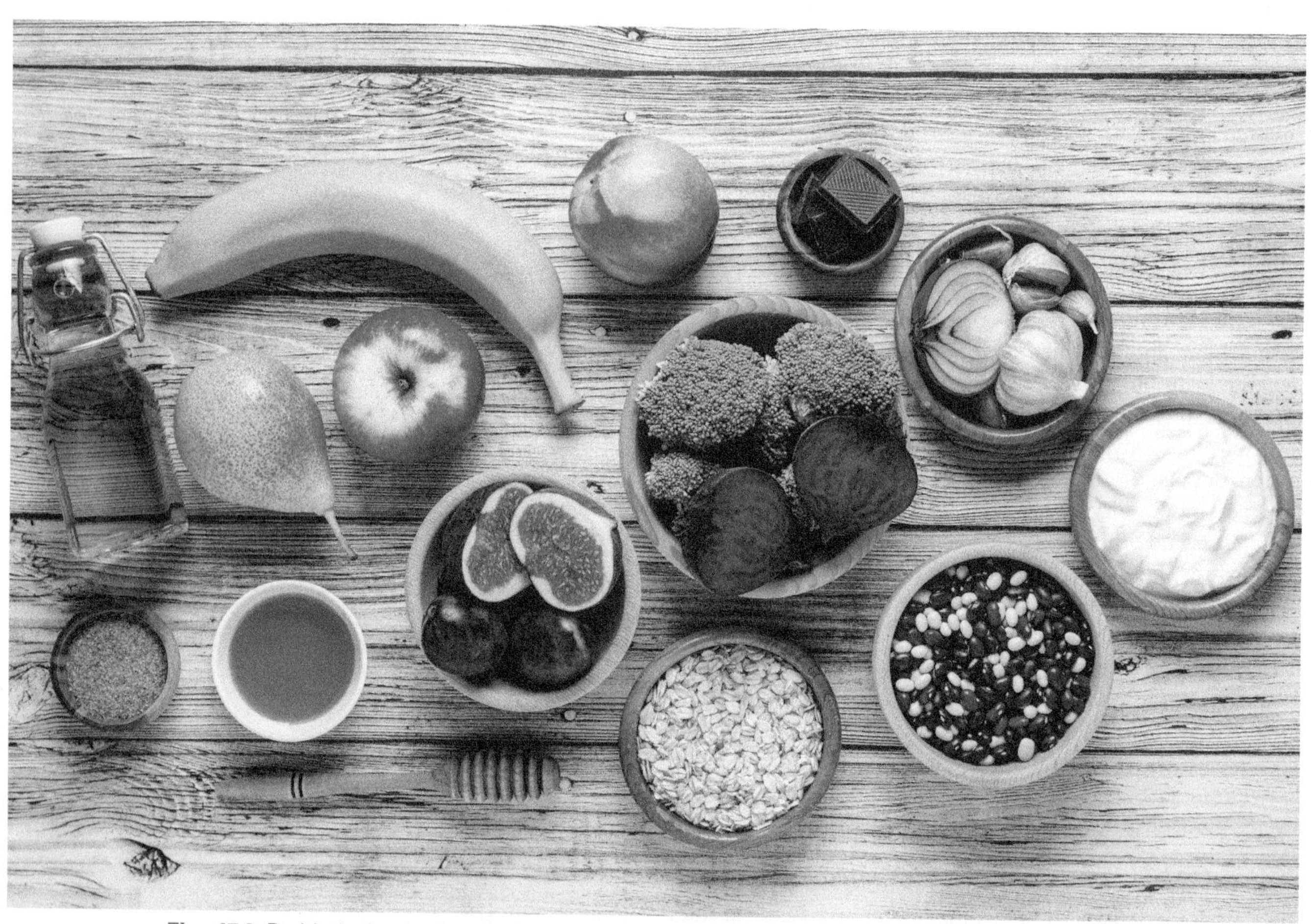

Fig. 17.6 Prebiotic foods that support a healthy microbiome include onions, garlic, Jerusalem artichokes, bananas, asparagus, buckwheat groats, fennel, cabbage, dandelion greens, and oats. (From © iStock photo; Credit: tbralnina.)

SUMMARY

- Cardiovascular disease (CVD) consists of a group of diseases and conditions that affect the heart and blood vessels. They include coronary artery disease (CAD, also known as coronary heart disease [CHD]), hypertension (HTN), peripheral artery disease (PAD), and heart failure (HF).
- CVD risk factors are categorized as controllable, noncontrollable, or predisposing.
- Controllable or lifestyle factors include tobacco use, diet, and physical inactivity. Noncontrollable factors are gender, age, and family history.
- Predisposing conditions may be diabetes mellitus, hypertension (HTN), obesity, and dyslipidemia.
- Atherosclerosis is the chronic inflammatory development of lesions in coronary arteries that can lead to arteriosclerosis, angina pectoris, or myocardial infarction.
- If thrombosis occurs in a cerebral artery, a cerebrovascular accident or hemorrhagic stroke occurs.
- CAD risk is assessed through measurement of inflammatory markers and the proportions of different lipoproteins in the bloodstream.
- Plasma lipoproteins are synthesized in the liver. They contain varying amounts of triglycerides, cholesterol, phospholipids, and proteins.
- Plasma lipoproteins are classified according to composition and density: chylomicrons, high-density lipoproteins (HDLs), low-density lipoproteins (LDLs), and very low-density lipoproteins (VLDLs).
- Dietary interventions for heart disease include weight loss, following the DASH diet, and decreasing alcohol intake.
- Goals of nutrition therapy are to reduce saturated fat and *trans* fatty acid intake while increasing monounsaturated fats (such as extra-virgin olive oil).
- HTN for which the cause is not known is called primary or essential HTN. Genetics play an important role.
- In secondary HTN, the cause of elevated blood pressure can be identified.
- Prescribed treatment regimens for HTN are individualized and vary because the disease differs in its degree of severity.
- First-line HTN treatment is usually nonpharmacologic, focused on lifestyle modifications.
- Weight reduction and sodium restriction augment the use of antihypertensive medications.
- Myocardial infarction (MI) is the single largest killer of adults in the United States. The purpose of nutrition therapy in patients with MI is to reduce the workload of the heart.
- CAD, lung disease, complications of hypothyroidism, or damage to the myocardial or cardiac muscle can cause heart failure (HF).
- HF is characterized by decreased blood flow to the kidneys and retention of sodium and fluid. Patients with HF often experience edema of the feet and ankles and shortness of breath.
- To lessen the workload of the heart in HF, nutrition therapy focuses on restricting dietary sodium.
- Pulmonary disease is characterized by wasting and malnutrition, largely because of the disorder itself or the secondary consequences of treatment on the gastrointestinal tract.
- Two categories of pulmonary disorders cause either chronic changes in pulmonary function, such as chronic obstructive pulmonary disease (COPD) and cystic fibrosis, or acute changes in pulmonary function, such as respiratory distress syndrome (RDS) and acute respiratory failure (ARF).
- The goal of nutrition therapy for COPD is to maintain respiratory muscle strength and function while preventing or treating existing malnutrition.
- As pulmonary disorders progress, nutritional status tends to decline and malnutrition exacerbates, reducing respiratory muscle function and ventilatory drive.
- Acute respiratory failure or distress may develop in patients who are critically ill, in shock, severely injured, have COVID-19 or sepsis.
- For ARF and RDS, nutrition therapy is designed to inhibit tissue destruction by providing the extra nutrients required for hypermetabolic conditions.
- Malnutrition and the method of refeeding influence the outcome in pulmonary disease or respiratory failure.

Note that cystic fibrosis, tuberculosis, asthma, and related pulmonary disorders warrant regularly scheduled contact with a registered dietitian, especially patients at high risk for malnutrition and those with multiple disorders.

THE NURSING APPROACH

Clinical Judgment and Next-Generation NCLEX® Examination-Style Questions

Case Study 1

Hypertension and Heart Failure

The home health nurse visited Reba, a 70-year-old Black American woman who had been diagnosed with heart failure and hypertension. Laboratory tests revealed elevated triglycerides, cholesterol, and low-density lipoprotein (LDL) cholesterol. The nurse had first become acquainted with Reba when Reba was discharged from the hospital after an acute episode of pulmonary edema. The physician advised Reba to begin a walking program, starting slowly. The physician prescribed a 2-gram-sodium, low-fat, low-calorie diet. Several medications had been prescribed, including an angiotensin-converting enzyme (ACE) inhibitor, a statin, and a diuretic. In a previous visit, the nurse instructed Reba to monitor her pulse and blood pressure daily and to weigh herself daily. The purpose of this follow-up visit was to determine the patient's compliance with the treatment plan and to assess her current health status.

Assessment/Recognize Cues

Subjective (From Patient Statements)

- "Sometimes I forget whether I have taken my medicines."
- "I've kept a record of my pulse, blood pressure, and weight almost every day."
- "Today I weighed 2 pounds more than I did when I was in the hospital."
- "I feel really tired. I get short of breath when I climb stairs [dyspnea]. I haven't been going for walks."
- "I have trouble breathing when I lie down at night" [orthopnea].
- "I usually warm up a can of soup or a frozen dinner because I am too tired to cook. I like it when my granddaughter brings me cake and doughnuts."

Objective (From Physical Examination)

- Height 5 feet 8 inches, weight 182 pounds with truncal obesity
- Blood pressure 162/85 mm Hg; temperature 98° F; pulse 92, irregular; respirations 18, unlabored
- Lung sounds clear
- Pitting edema in ankles
- Jugular venous distention

Diagnoses (Nursing)/Analyze Cues

1. Fluid overload related to decreased cardiac output and excess sodium intake as evidenced by blood pressure 162/85, pitting edema of ankles, jugular venous distention, weight 2 pounds higher than during hospitalization
2. Heart failure related to hypertension, weakened cardiac muscles, and obesity as evidenced by pulse 92 irregular, fatigue, shortness of breath with activity, and orthopnea

Planning/Prioritize Hypotheses

Patient Outcomes

Short term (at the end of this visit):

- Reba will agree to meet with a dietitian to learn about an individualized nutrition plan and healthy food choices.
- She will commit to read labels and choose foods lower in sodium and fat.
- She will plan to obtain a small medicine organizer.

Long term (at follow-up visit in 1 month):

- Weight 178 pounds; blood pressure 140/85
- Edema absent or nonpitting, lungs clear
- Reports less fatigue; walking short distances regularly
- Electrolyte values within normal range and lipid levels reduced

Nursing Interventions/Generate Solutions

1. Check Reba's home records of blood pressure, pulse, and weight.
2. Teach her about general dietary measures to reduce her edema.
3. Set up an appointment with a dietitian for an individualized plan.
4. Review her medications and teach her when to notify the doctor.

Implementation/Take Actions

1. Measured vital signs, reviewed the log that Reba had recorded, and praised Reba for her conscientious efforts.
   Vital signs help determine the effectiveness of treatments for heart failure and hypertension. Praise often motivates a patient to continue positive behaviors.
   a. Asked Reba to demonstrate how she takes her pulse and blood pressure, using her home blood pressure monitoring equipment.
   b. Compared Reba's results with the nurse's.
   To look for valid trends in results, accuracy of measurement technique is needed.
2. Reviewed Reba's record of daily weights and explained how weight increases with excessive sodium intake.
   a. Taught Reba that sodium causes the body to retain fluid, contributing to weight gain, edema, and dyspnea (difficulty breathing).
   b. Showed Reba how to read labels and choose soups and frozen dinners that are lower in sodium.
   c. Gave her a list of foods that are high in sodium and thus should be limited or avoided.
   d. Told her about herbs that can be used in place of salt to flavor food.
   Patients are more likely to comply with nutrition therapy if they understand the reasons for restrictions and are given practical suggestions as to how to adhere to guidelines.
3. Taught Reba guidelines for making healthy food choices based on fat and calories.
   a. Recommended eating fish and chicken instead of red meat, as well as increasing whole grains, fruits and vegetables, and skim milk (with lactase if needed).
   Omega-3 fatty acids from fish may reduce clot formation, reducing the risk of coronary occlusion. Red meat is a source of cholesterol. Soluble fiber can help reduce LDL cholesterol levels. Lactase additives can be added to milk if necessary because many Black Americans have lactose intolerance.
   b. Explained that the type of fats are more important than low fat or low cholesterol in the diet.
   Replace saturated fats with extra virgin olive oil or canola oil for meal choices.
   c. Recommended nutritious low-calorie foods to help Reba lose weight and thus decrease the workload of the heart.
   Obesity increases peripheral resistance and cardiac workload. Reducing high-fat desserts can help with weight loss and reduction of lipid levels.
   d. Recommended small, frequent meals rather than large meals, with rest periods before meal preparation and eating.
   Small meals require less energy for eating and digesting food. Rest periods can reduce oxygen consumption, relieve shortness of breath and fatigue, and help increase appetite.
4. Asked Reba to show the nurse her medications and recommended placing medications in a small weekly organizer.
   Small medicine holders may designate the days of the week, alerting the patient to whether medicine has been taken on a particular day.
5. Asked Reba to tell the nurse the purpose of each medicine and when each should be taken.
   Verifying a patient's understanding of prescribed medications is important for safety and effectiveness.

Continued

THE NURSING APPROACH—cont'd

6. Informed Reba about side effects and special precautions needed when taking her medications.
   ACE inhibitors reduce blood pressure by causing vasodilation. ACE inhibitors decrease peripheral resistance or afterload, but they can produce orthostatic hypotension. Patients should be advised to rise slowly from bed to avoid becoming dizzy. ACE inhibitors can increase serum potassium levels so patients on this medication should have labs drawn to monitor serum potassium. Another common side effect of ACE inhibitors is a persistent cough, which may take up to a month or longer to subside.
   Statins, or 3-hydroxy-3-methylglutaryl coenzyme A (HMG-CoA) reductase inhibitors, increase high-density lipoprotein (HDL) cholesterol while decreasing LDL cholesterol and total cholesterol synthesis. Unexplained muscle pain should be reported immediately because statins can cause rhabdomyolysis (a serious condition that causes injury or death of muscle tissue). Liver function tests should be drawn frequently because statins can cause serious liver damage. Depending on the statin, grapefruit juice should be avoided because it interacts with the enzymes that break down this medication, causing the medication to accumulate in large amounts in the body.
   Diuretics promote loss of sodium and water from the body. Some diuretics waste potassium, but other medicines may conserve potassium. Frequent laboratory tests are necessary to monitor serum potassium levels because there is danger of death if the potassium levels are too high or too low.
7. Instructed Reba regarding when to call the doctor—for example, when she gains 3 pounds or more in 2 days, when she has difficulty breathing, and when edema gets worse. Also, she should call if her blood pressure is 180/90 or higher and/or her pulse is less than 60.
   A gain of 1 kg of weight (2.2 pounds) could indicate retention of 1 L of fluid. Hypertension may lead to a stroke, so medications may need to be adjusted.
8. Set up an appointment with a dietitian for an individualized nutrition plan.
   Because the diet combines several components, it could be confusing to the patient.
9. Encouraged her to begin a walking program for 10 minutes each day, as approved by the doctor.
   Regular exercise strengthens cardiac muscle and increases peripheral vascular blood flow. It also helps with weight reduction.

Evaluation/Evaluate Outcomes

Short term (at the end of the visit):

- Reba agreed to meet with a dietitian.
- She said she would read labels and choose foods lower in sodium and fat.
- She planned to ask her granddaughter to buy a small medicine organizer at the drugstore for her.
- Reba made an appointment with the nurse for a visit in 1 month.

Goals met.

Discussion Questions

1. Compare and contrast the basic principles of the Mediterranean diet and the DASH diet.
2. *Trans* fats increase LDL levels and decrease HDL cholesterol levels, so they should be restricted. Which foods are likely to contain *trans* fats and thus should be avoided?

Case Study 2

Myocardial Infarction Symptoms

The intensive care unit nurse is caring for a patient admitted with a myocardial infarction (heart attack). The nurse reviews the patient's record and expects to note what signs/symptoms of heart attack the patient probably had upon admission.

Place an X in the boxes of the symptoms of myocardial infarction.

1. Upper body pain
2. Warm sweats
3. Family history of coronary heart disease (CHD)
4. Chest pain/discomfor
5. Lightheadedness
6. Discomfort in the arms, back, neck, or upper stomach
7. Nausea
8. Vomiting

CRITICAL THINKING

Clinical Applications

Kevin, age 69 years, is admitted to the coronary care unit of your hospital. He is 6 feet tall, has a medium frame, and weighs 210 pounds. He has gained 30 pounds since he retired 4 years ago, which he attributes to boredom and lack of exercise. Three months before admission, Kevin began to experience chest pain that radiated up his neck and down to his stomach. He has a history of hypertension and elevated serum cholesterol levels. After admission to the hospital, Kevin is diagnosed with having had an acute myocardial infarction.

Test results for serum lipids are as follows:

Cholesterol: 300 mg/dL
LDL-C: 200 mg/dL
HDL-C: 30 mg/dL
Triglycerides: 600 mg/dL

Medications prescribed after admission: atenolol (Tenormin), diltiazem (Cardizem), nitroglycerin

Diet order: Mediterranean diet

1. What are Kevin's risk factors for cardiovascular disease?
2. Define the term myocardial infarction and describe what happens when a myocardial infarction occurs.
3. What specific guidelines are included in the Mediterranean diet recommendations?

While caring for Kevin you learn that he snacks on high-fat cheeses, ice cream, potato chips, corn chips, peanuts, and crackers. He also drinks whole milk and eats a lot of butter on his bread at every meal.

1. What characteristics of Kevin's intake contradict the Mediterranean diet recommendations?
2. What are some alternative foods that are appealing to Kevin that he could eat for snacks?

HDL-C, High-density lipoprotein cholesterol; *LDL-C*, low-density lipoprotein cholesterol.

WEBSITES OF INTEREST

American Heart Association (AHA)

www.americanheart.org

Contains resources, interactive educational materials, and everyday strategies and support for prevention and treatment of heart disease and stroke.

American Lung Association

http://www.lung.org/

Leading organization working to improve lung health and prevent lung disease. Many resources and research studies are available.

World Hypertension League (WHL)

http://www.whleague.org/

Advocates for the detection, prevention, and treatment of HTN in populations globally through association with the World Health Organization.

REFERENCES

Alaghehband, F. R., et al. (2017). Dietary fatty acids were not independently associated with lipoprotein subclasses in elderly women. *Nutrition Research, 43*, 60–68.

Bittencourt, M. S., et al. (2017). Relation of fasting triglyceride-rich lipoprotein cholesterol to coronary artery calcium score (from the ELSA-Brazil Study). *The American Journal of Cardiology, 119*, 1352–1358.

Booth, J. N., et al. (2014). Effect of sustaining lifestyle modifications (nonsmoking, weight reduction, physical activity, and Mediterranean diet) after healing of myocardial infarction, percutaneous intervention, or coronary bypass (from the Reasons for Geographic and Racial Differences in Stroke Study). *The American Journal of Cardiology, 113*, 1933–1940.

Coffey, M. J., et al. (2020 Jan 22). Probiotics for people with cystic fibrosis. *Cochrane Database of Systematic Reviews, 1*(1), CD012949.

Connolly, E. L., et al. (2020). A randomized controlled crossover trial investigating the short-term effects of different types of vegetables on vascular and metabolic function in middle-aged and older adults with mildly elevated blood pressure: The VEgetableS for vascular hEaLth (VESSEL) study protocol. *Nutrition Journal, 19*, 41.

Garg, M., & Ooi, C. Y. (2017). The enigmatic gut in cystic fibrosis: linking inflammation, dysbiosis, and the increased risk of malignancy. *Current Gastroenterology Reports, 19*, 6.

Gerhard-Herman. M. D., et al. (2016). AHA/ACC Guideline on the management of patients with lower extremity peripheral artery disease: executive summary: a report of the American College of Cardiology/American Heart Association Task Force on Clinical Practice Guidelines. *Circulation, 135*, e686–e785. 2017.

Helnaes, A., et al. (2016). Intake of whole grains is associated with lower risk of myocardial infarction: the Danish Diet, Cancer and Health Cohort. *The American Journal of Clinical Nutrition, 103*, 999–1007.

Kentson, M., et al. (2018). Oxidant status, iron homeostasis, and carotenoid levels of COPD patients with advanced disease and LTOT. *European Clinical Respiratory Journal, 5*, 1447221.

Leung, D. H. (2017). Effects of diagnosis by newborn screening for cystic fibrosis on weight and length in the first year of life. *JAMA Pediatr, 171*, 546–554.

Li, Q., et al. (2019). Association of C-reactive protein and vitamin D deficiency with cardiovascular disease: A nationwide cross-sectional study from National Health and Nutrition Examination Survey 2007 to 2008. *Clinical Cardiology, 42*, 663–669.

Manosroi, W., & Williams, G. H. (2019). Genetics of human primary hypertension: Focus on hormonal mechanisms. *Endocrine Reviews, 40*, 825–856.

Matera, M. G., et al. (2020). Pharmacological management of COVID-19 patients with ARDS (CARDS): A narrative review. *Respiratory Medicine, 171*, 106114.

Mayo Clinic: 10 ways to control high blood pressure without medication. From https://www.mayoclinic.org/diseases-conditions/high-blood-pressure/in-depth/high-blood-pressure/art-20046974. Accessed 8 September, 2020.

McCullough, P. A., et al. (2016). Nutritional deficiencies and sarcopenia in heart failure: a therapeutic opportunity to reduce hospitalization and death. *Reviews in Cardiovascular Medicine, 17*, S30–S39.

Million Hearts: Estimated hypertension prevalence, treatment, and control among U.S. adults. From: https://millionhearts.hhs.gov/data-reports/hypertension-prevalence.html. Accessed 8 September, 2020.

Nagasawa, S. Y., et al. (2015). Associations between inflammatory markers and subclinical atherosclerosis in middle-aged white, Japanese-American and Japanese men: the ERA-JUMP study. *Journal of Atherosclerosis and Thrombosis, 22*, 590–598.

National Institutes of Health, National Heart, Lung, and Blood Institute: DASH eating plan: lower your blood pressure (NIH Publ. 06-4082). From: www.nhlbi.nih.gov/health/public/heart/hbp/dash/new_dash.pdf. Accessed 8 September, 2020.

Orso, E., & Schmitz, G. (2017). Lipoprotein(a) and its role in inflammation, atherosclerosis and malignancies. *Clin Res Cardiol Suppl, 12*, S31–S37.

Pavan Kumar, N., et al. (2016). Type 2 diabetes mellitus coincident with pulmonary or latent tuberculosis results in modulation of adipocytokines. *Cytokine, 79*, 74–81.

Peterson, S. J., et al. (2018). Early exposure to recommended calorie delivery in the intensive care unit is associated with increased mortality in patients with acute respiratory distress syndrome. *JPEN J Parented Enteral Nutr, 42*, 739–747.

Ravnskov, U., et al. (2018). LDL-C does not cause cardiovascular disease: a comprehensive review of the current literature. *Expert Review of Clinical Pharmacology, 11*, 959–970.

Rust, P., & Ekmekcioglu, C. (2017). Impact of salt intake on the pathogenesis and treatment of hypertension. *Advances in Experimental Medicine and Biology, 956*, 61–84.

Sharma, A., et al. (2016). Coenzyme Q10 and heart failure: a state-of-the-art review. *Circ Heart Fail, 9*, e002639.

Singh, S., et al. (2016). Eicosapentaenoic acid versus docosahexaenoic acid as options for vascular risk prevention: a fish story. *American Journal of Therapeutics, 23*, 905–910.

Silva, L. O. E., et al. (2018). Metabolic profile in patients with mild obstructive sleep apnea. *Metabolic syndrome and related disorders, 16*, 6–12.

Sorrentino, M. J. (2019). The evolution from hypertension to heart failure. *Heart failure clinics, 15*, 447–453.

Srinivasan, V., et al. (2020). Early enteral nutrition is associated with improved clinical outcomes in critically ill children: A secondary analysis of nutrition support in the heart and lung failure-pediatric insulin titration trial. *Pediatric critical care medicine: a journal of the Society of Critical Care Medicine and the World Federation of Pediatric Intensive and Critical Care Societies, 21*, 213–221.

Trehan, N., et al. (2017). Vitamin D deficiency, supplementation, and cardiovascular health. *Crit Pathw Cardio, 16*, 109–118.

van Capelleveen, J. C., et al. (2017). Apolipoprotein C-III levels and incident coronary artery disease risk: the EPIC-Norfolk prospective population study. *Arteriosclerosis, Thrombosis, and Vascular Biology, 37*, 1206–1212.

Williams, N. C., et al. (2016). A prebiotic galactooligosaccharide mixture reduces severity of hyperpnoea-induced bronchoconstriction and markers of airway inflammation. *The British Journal of Nutrition, 116*, 798–804.

18

Nutrition for Diseases of the Kidneys

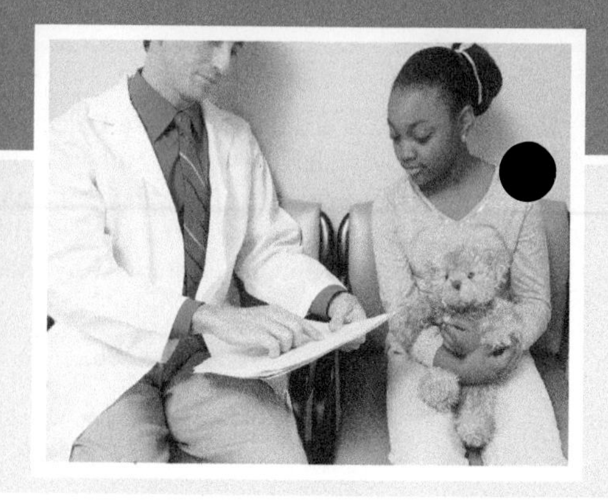

Kidney transplants seem so routine now. But the first one was like Lindbergh's flight across the ocean.

Joseph Murray

http://evolve.elsevier.com/GRODNER/FOUNDATIONS

LEARNING OBJECTIVES

- State the primary function of the kidneys.
- Discuss the causes and results of nephrotic syndrome.
- Identify determinants of nutrition needs in acute renal failure (ARF).
- Describe chronic kidney disease (CKD) and the focus of nutrition management.
- Discuss the different nutrition therapies for dialysis patients.
- Summarize the objectives to be considered in the implementation of the National Renal Diet.
- Explain the composition of renal calculi and ways to reduce risk of stone formation.

THE KIDNEY IN HEALTH

Although often taken for granted, our kidneys filter approximately 1 L of blood per minute to remove excess fluid and more than 200 waste products from the body. They also perform vital metabolic and hormonal functions. Because kidneys play so many roles in wellness, kidney disease has serious consequences. The nutritional needs of patients with kidney disease are complex, ever-changing, and demanding. These factors present a challenge to the patient, family members, doctors, nurses, dietitians, and other health care team members.

Functions of the kidneys affect total physical well-being. Nutrition therapy is essential for enhancing the physical health dimension. Intellectual health requires clients to understand their own anatomy and physiology, to fully comprehend their kidney disorder, and to follow a complicated diet. The chronic nature and potentially life-threatening aspects of kidney disorders may be emotionally draining. Social health is also strained. Significant others are worn down by the responsibility of caring for loved ones with renal disorders. Dialysis disrupts normal routines and social relationships. Healthy spirituality may lower blood pressure and enhance the physical response to treatment. Environmental health may be affected by the presence of excessive amounts of sodium and other minerals in the water supply.

KIDNEY FUNCTION

The chief life-preserving function of the kidneys is to maintain chemical homeostasis in the body. They process components within the blood to maintain fluid, electrolyte, and acid-base balance by eliminating wastes in the urine. Each kidney has approximately 1 million microscopic "workhorses" called nephrons (Fig. 18.1).

Each nephron filters and resorbs essential blood constituents, secretes ions to maintain acid-base balance, and excretes fluid and other substances as urine. Other important functions of kidneys are manufacturing hormones to regulate blood pressure (renin), stimulating production of red blood cells (erythropoietin), and regulating calcium and phosphorus metabolism in the final step of vitamin D synthesis. Kidneys also detoxify some drugs and poisons (Box 18.1).

Both congenital and adult renal diseases have a gene-environment component, which involves alterations to the epigenetic information imprinted during development (Hilliard & El-Dahr, 2016). There is a clear association between prematurity, low birth weight and chronic kidney disease (CKD), caused by decreased nephron mass at birth, leading to CKD, hypertension and albuminuria in adolescence or adulthood (Starr & Hingorani, 2018). This reduction in nephron number (renal hypoplasia) is a predisposing factor.

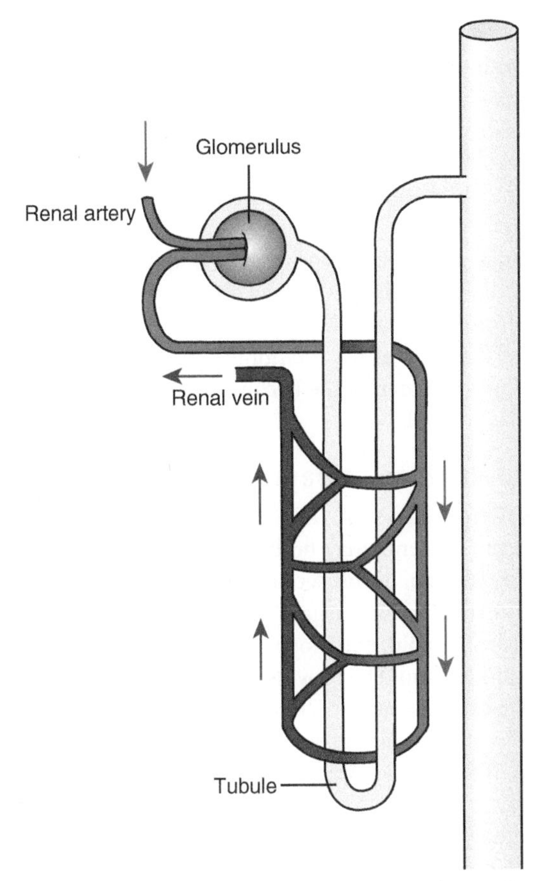

Fig. 18.1 The nephron. Each nephron has a glomerulus to filter blood and a tubule that returns needed substances to the blood and pulls out additional wastes. Wastes and extra water become urine. (Modified from National Institute of Diabetes and Digestive and Kidney Diseases. Your kidneys & how they work. https://www.niddk.nih.gov/health-information/kidney-disease/kidneys-how-they-work. Accessed 15 September, 2020.)

BOX 18.1 Major Functions of the Kidney

Regulation of blood pressure (renin-angiotensin system)
Regulation of extracellular fluid volume
Regulation of osmolarity
Regulation of ion concentrations
Regulation of pH for acid-base balance
Excretion of waste products, toxins, drugs
Stimulation of red blood cell production (erythropoietin)
Regulation of calcium, phosphorus, vitamin D_3 metabolism

Congenital abnormalities of the kidney and urinary tract (CAKUT), inflammatory, obstructive, and degenerative diseases affect kidneys in different ways. These disorders interfere with nephron regulation of the products of metabolism. Ultimately, kidney failure leads to homeostatic failure and, if not relieved, death.

Worldwide, CKD is a health crisis. 10% of the population worldwide is affected by CKD, and millions die each year because they do not have access to affordable treatment (National Kidney Foundation, 2020). Also, in people aged 65 through 74 years worldwide, it is estimated that one in five men, and one in four women, have CKD.

NEPHROTIC SYNDROME

Nephrotic syndrome describes a complex of symptoms that can occur after damage to the capillary walls of the glomerulus. Glomerular damage results in increased urinary excretion of protein (proteinuria, $\geq$40 mg/m^2/hour), which leads to decreased serum levels of albumin (hypoalbuminemia, (<25 g/L)), and edema (Downie et al., 2017).

Nephrotic syndrome often results from primary glomerular disease (glomerulonephritis), nephropathy secondary to amyloidosis (accumulation of waxy starchlike glycoprotein), diabetes mellitus, infectious disease, or systemic lupus erythematosus (SLE) a chronic inflammatory disease.

Treating nephrotic syndrome includes addressing the underlying cause as well as taking steps to reduce high blood pressure, edema, high cholesterol, and infection (National Institute of Diabetes and Digestive and Kidney Diseases, 2017). In some children, diminished proteinuria results from eliminating cow's milk and the use of a gluten-free diet (Uy et al., 2015).

The syndrome may be treated with corticosteroids and statins. Immunosuppressive medications are used to prevent relapses and treat corticosteroid-resistant disease (Wang & Greenbaum, 2019). When it is resistant to treatment, the condition may progress to renal failure.

Food and Nutrition Therapies

Primary goals are to control hypertension, minimize edema, decrease urinary albumin losses, prevent protein malnutrition and muscle catabolism, supply adequate energy, and slow the progression of renal disease. Patients need to consume adequate amounts of protein (1 g/kg/day) and energy (35 kcal/kg/day) to prevent malnutrition from catabolism of lean body tissue. Good sources of protein are lean meats, well-trimmed poultry, eggs (limit 2 per week), fish, shellfish, beans, and nuts.

Complex carbohydrates, fruits, and vegetables should be the basis of the diet because protein may have to be limited. If a gluten-free diet leads to clinical improvement, enabling reduction or discontinuation in steroid dosage, wheat, rye, and barley would be restricted (Lemley et al., 2016).

Because elevated lipids can be a problem, use healthy oils such as olive, canola, coconut, or sunflower. Limit use of whole-fat dairy products and avoid the partially hydrogenated oils found in processed and fast food (*trans* fats).

A high dietary sodium intake is detrimental to the nephron. Sodium intake may be limited to control hypertension and edema. Commercial preparation of processed meats and foods adds substantial amounts of sodium (see Chapter 17). Intake of cheese, canned foods, dried pasta and rice mixes, and canned or dried soups should be controlled. For more specific sodium content of foods, consult the Food Composition Table on the Evolve website.

Role of Nursing

The nurse and dietitian often develop the care plan together. They partner in educating patients about dietary advice, including foods high in sodium (Box 18.2). It is essential for nursing personnel to monitor and document patient weights. Intake and output (I&O) should be recorded at least every shift.

BOX 18.2 Foods High in Sodium

Condiments
Pickles, olives (black and green), salted nuts, meat tenderizers, commercial salad dressings, monosodium glutamate (MSG, Accent), steak sauce, ketchup, soy sauce, Worcestershire sauce, horseradish sauce, chili sauce, commercial mustard, salt, seasoned salts (onion, garlic, celery), butter salt

Breads/Starches
Salted crackers, potato chips, corn chips, popcorn, pretzels, dehydrated potatoes

Meats/Meat Substitutes
Cured, smoked, and processed meats (ham, bacon, corned beef, chipped beef, hot dogs, luncheon meats, bologna, salt pork, canned salmon, and tuna); all cheeses except low-sodium and cottage cheese; convenience foods (microwave and TV dinners); peanut butter

Beverages
Commercial buttermilk, instant hot cocoa mixes

Soups
Canned soups, dehydrated soups, bouillon

Vegetables
Sauerkraut, hominy, pork and beans, canned tomato and vegetable juices

https://www.dietaryguidelines.gov/food-sources-potassium

BOX 18.3 Hidden Sources of Sodium

- Baking powder
- Drinking and cooking water
- Medications:
  - Antacids
  - Antibiotics
  - Cough medicines
  - Laxatives
  - Pain relievers
  - Sedatives
- Mouthwash
- Toothpaste

Hidden sources of salt may be found in the water supply, medications, even oral hygiene products. Because toothpaste and mouthwash often contain a significant amount of sodium, patients should be instructed not to swallow them (Box 18.3).

ACUTE RENAL FAILURE

Acute renal failure (ARF) is characterized by an abrupt loss of renal function that may or may not be accompanied by oliguria or anuria. The most common cause of ARF is either acute tubular necrosis (ATN), which is injury after a decreased blood supply, or a nephrotoxic cause, such as certain medications. Although a few patients do not experience any reduction in urine output, some experience the following three stages:

1. Oliguric phase (24–48 hours after initial injury; lasts 1–3 weeks): Retention of excessive amounts of nitrogenous compounds in the blood, acidosis, high serum potassium and phosphorus levels, hypertension, anorexia, edema, and risk of water intoxication (indicated by low sodium levels).
2. Diuretic phase (lasts 2–3 weeks): Urinary output is gradually increased.
3. Recovery phase (lasts 3–12 months): Kidney function gradually improves, but there may be some residual permanent damage.

Note that most patients with ARF require at least a short period of dialysis. Dialysis allows diffusion of waste particles to move from an area of high to one of lower concentration, osmosis of fluid across the membrane, and movement of fluid (urine) across the membrane because of the artificially created pressure differential.

Food and Nutrition Therapies

The underlying cause of the ARF will determine nutrient requirements. Patients may be hypermetabolic if renal failure is caused by trauma, burns, septicemia, or infection. These conditions and renal failure negate the patient's appetite, increasing the risk for rapid nutritional decline. Nonprotein calories (30–40 kcal/kg) should be provided for weight maintenance and to meet the extra demands. Fats, oils, simple carbohydrates, and low-protein starches are given. If dialysis is not necessary for treatment, 0.6 g to 0.8 g of protein per kg body weight is often prescribed.

When dialysis is used as part of the medical treatment, protein intake can be liberalized to 1.0 to 1.4 g/kg. In either situation, high-quality proteins (animal sources such as milk, eggs, meat, poultry, fish) are recommended. Diets containing less than 60 g/day of protein may be deficient in niacin, riboflavin, thiamine, calcium, iron, vitamin B_{12}, and zinc; these nutrients may be supplemented during convalescence.

During the oliguric phase, sodium is restricted to 1000 to 2000 mg/day and potassium to 1000 mg/day. Both sodium and potassium, the principal electrolytes, may be lost during the diuretic phase or during dialysis. Therefore, losses should be replaced as needed, depending on urinary volume, serum levels, and frequency of dialysis. Box 18.4 lists foods high in potassium.

Over time, diets that are not controlled for phosphorus, potassium, and protein-energy malnutrition are associated with a greater risk for bone and heart diseases. High phosphorus intake disrupts the hormonal regulation of phosphate, calcium, and vitamin D. High phosphorus and calcium levels also lead to dangerous calcium deposits in blood vessels, lungs, eyes, and heart, even leading to increased risk of heart attack, stroke or death (National Kidney Foundation, 2020).

Role of Nursing

During the oliguric phase, fluids are restricted to the amount of the patient's output (urine, vomitus, and diarrhea) plus 500 mL. During the diuretic phase, large amounts of fluid may be needed to replace losses. Close monitoring of I&O is essential. Constipation can occur from restricted intake of fluids and fresh fruits (most are high in potassium), bed rest, and the effects of medication.

Nurses help coordinate patient and family education with the renal dietitian. Complex nutrition education often involves

BOX 18.4 Foods High in Potassium

Food	Standard Portion Size	Potassium in Standard Portion (mg)[a]
Potato, baked, flesh and skin	1 medium	941
Prune juice, canned	1 cup	707
Carrot juice, canned	1 cup	689
Passion-fruit juice, yellow or purple	1 cup	687
Beet greens, cooked from fresh	½ cup	654
White beans, canned	½ cup	595
Plain yogurt, nonfat	1 cup	579
Sweet potato, baked in skin	1 medium	542
Salmon, Atlantic, wild, cooked	3 ounces	534
Clams, canned	3 ounces	534
Pomegranate juice	1 cup	533
Tomato juice, canned	1 cup	527
Orange juice, fresh	1 cup	496
Soybeans, green, cooked	½ cup	485
Chard, swiss, cooked	½ cup	481
Lima beans, cooked	½ cup	478
Vegetable juice, canned	1 cup	468
Chili with beans, canned	½ cup	467
Yam, cooked	½ cup	456
Halibut, cooked	3 ounces	449
Tuna, yellowfin, cooked	3 ounces	448
Acorn squash, cooked	½ cup	448
Soybeans, mature, cooked	½ cup	443
Chocolate milk (1%, 2% and whole)	1 cup	418–425
Banana	1 medium	422
Spinach, cooked from fresh or canned	½ cup	370–419
Peaches, dried, uncooked	¼ cup	399
Prunes, stewed	½ cup	398
Skim milk (nonfat)	1 cup	382
Refried beans, canned, traditional	½ cup	380
Apricots, dried, uncooked	¼ cup	378
Lentils, cooked	½ cup	365
Avocado	½ cup	364
Tomato sauce, canned	½ cup	364
Kidney beans, cooked	½ cup	357
Navy beans, cooked	½ cup	354

(From U.S. Department of Agriculture (USDA). Appendix 10 – Foods High in Potassium. https://health.gov/our-work/food-nutrition/2015-2020-dietary-gu Accessed 15 September, 2020.)

reduced protein, sodium, potassium, phosphorus, and fluid intake. Avoidance of highly processed foods, fast foods, and convenience foods may be needed.

Adherence is better when both diet and education efforts are individualized to each patient and adapted over time (Beto et al., 2016). The Food Composition Table on the Evolve website lists the specific protein, sodium, potassium and phosphorus content of foods. More guidance on nutrition advisement can be found at https://www.kidney.org/nutrition.

CHRONIC KIDNEY DISEASE

Chronic kidney disease involves progressive, irreversible loss of kidney function over days, months, or years. Common causes are glomerulonephritis, nephrosclerosis (necrosis of the renal arterioles from hypertension), obstructive diseases (kidney stones, tumors, congenital birth defects of kidneys and urinary tract), diabetes mellitus, SLE, and illicit use of analgesics or street drugs. Regardless of the cause, retention of nitrogenous waste products and fluid and electrolyte imbalances affect all body systems.

Use of beta blockers, renin-angiotensin blockers, diuretics, statins, and aspirin is helpful in the early stages of CKD (Liu et al., 2014). Before dialysis is required, management focuses on slowing the progression and minimizing complications. Once CKD reaches end-stage renal disease (ESRD), management centers on reducing uremia (excessive amounts of urea and other nitrogenous waste products in the blood) by various renal replacement treatments: hemodialysis, peritoneal dialysis (PD), or renal transplantation.

Diabetic kidney disease is the leading cause of chronic and end-stage kidney disease in the United States and worldwide (Afkarian et al., 2016). Mortality among the patients with CKD and ESRD remains high because of the very high incidence of coronary artery disease, cardiac hypertrophy, and heart failure (Niizuma et al., 2017). Although CVD and kidney disease are closely related, nontraditional factors such as disturbed mineral and vitamin D metabolism play a larger role than traditional hypertension and dyslipidemia (Liu et al., 2014).

Food and Nutrition Therapies

Medical nutrition therapy (MNT) is a legal term regulated by the federal government that allows Medicare recipients to have "pre-end-stage renal disease" nutrition counseling from a qualified renal dietitian. The goal is to slow or prevent the progression to the need for dialysis.

Ideally all individuals at risk for renal failure should be given personalized nutrition counseling and advice a year before dialysis is needed. The renal dietitian evaluates the results of laboratory assessments (blood urea nitrogen [BUN], creatinine, sodium, potassium, phosphorus, glucose). The next step is to determine current versus ideal intakes of fluid, energy, protein, lipid, phosphorus, potassium, sodium, vitamin, and mineral from meals or nutrition support.

Nutritional management depends on method of treatment in addition to medical and nutritional status of the patient. Table 18.1

TABLE 18.1 Treatments and Major Concerns for Pre–End-Stage Renal Disease, Hemodialysis, and Peritoneal Dialysis

	Pre-End-Stage Renal Disease	Hemodialysis	Peritoneal Dialysis
Treatment modalities	Diet + medication	Diet + medication + hemodialysis Dialysis using vascular access for waste product and fluid removal	Diet + medication + peritoneal dialysis Dialysis using peritoneal membrane for waste product and fluid removal
Duration concerns	Indefinite	3–4 hours 3 days/week	3–5 exchanges 7 days/week
	Hypertension, glycemic control in patients with diabetes mellitus	Bone disease, hypertension	Bone disease, weight gain, hyperlipidemia, glycemic control in patients with diabetes mellitus
	Glomerular hyperfiltration, rise in blood urea nitrogen, bone disease	Amino acid loss, interdialytic electrolyte and fluid changes	Protein loss into dialysate, glucose absorption from dialysate
	Anemia, cardiovascular disease	Anemia, cardiovascular disease	Anemia, cardiovascular disease

(Data from Academy of Nutrition and Dietetics: *Chronic kidney disease nutrition management module 1—Chronic kidney disease basics: epidemiology, identification and monitoring and medical nutrition therapy*, Chicago, 2013, Author.)

TABLE 18.2 Nutrition Guidelines for Chronic Renal Failure Without Dialysis, Chronic Renal Failure With Hemodialysis, or Peritoneal Dialysis

Nutrient	Chronic Renal Failure Without Dialysis	Hemodialysis	Peritoneal Dialysis	Comments
Energy	30–35 kcal/kg ideal body weight (IBW)	35 kcal/kg IBW if <age 60; 30–35 kcal/kg sIBW if >age 60	30–35 kcal/kg IBW	
Protein	0.6–1.0 g/kg IBW	1.2 g/kg IBW	1.2–1.3 g/kg IBW	At least 50% from high biologic value animal plant sources
Sodium	Individualized, 2–3 g/day	2–3 g/day	2–4 g/day	
Potassium	Individualized to cover losses with diuretics	2–3 g/day	3–4 g/day	
Phosphorus	8–12 mg/kg IBW or 0.8–1.2 g/day	0.8–1.2 g/day or <17 mg/kg IBW	0.8–1.2 g/day	May require phosphate binder
Fluid	As desired	750–1000 mL + urine output/day	Unrestricted if weight and blood pressure controlled and residual renal function is 2–3 L/day	
Vitamin/mineral supplementation	As appropriate	As appropriate	As appropriate	Supplements designed specially for patients undergoing dialysis are available; supplements of vitamin C should not exceed 100 mg/day to prevent hyperoxalemia; vitamin A supplementation is not recommended; in patients receiving recombinant human erythropoietin (rHuEPO), iron supplementation is almost always required; zinc supplementation may be helpful for patients with impaired taste

(Data from National Kidney Foundation, Kidney Dialysis Outcomes Quality Initiative: *KDOQI clinical practice guidelines for nutrition in chronic renal failure*, Bethesda, MD, 2000, Author. Accessed 15 September, 2020 from https://www.kidney.org/sites/default/files/docs/kdoqi2000nutritiongl.pdf.)

provides a comparison of the treatment methods and concerns. The Kidney Disease Outcomes Quality Initiative (KDOQI) of the National Kidney Foundation has multiple guidelines; see https://www.kidney.org/professionals/guidelines.

Dietary modifications should start as early as possible to minimize uremic toxicity, delay progression of renal disease, and prevent wasting and malnutrition. Goals are to limit foods with metabolic byproducts and to provide sufficient calories to prevent body tissue catabolism (Table 18.2).

It is important to design appropriate food combinations that the patient will accept and enjoy. This task is complicated, but there are renal dietitian specialists who are credentialed as board-certified specialists in renal nutrition (CSRs) and enjoy the challenge. High biologic value proteins are the preferred protein sources for patients with renal disease. Some protein foods in vegan diets are of low biologic value. Ovo-vegetarian and ovo-lacto vegetarian diets include high biologic value protein sources, but they also tend to be high in phosphorus. Thus,

BOX 18.5 Sample Renal Diet Menu

The National Renal Diet is often used to develop diet guidelines and meal plans. The tool is useful and provides visual indicators, such as shown in the following table:

High phosphorus
High sodium—each serving counts as 1 starch choice and 1 salt choice
High sodium—each serving counts as 1 vegetable choice and 2 salt choices
High sodium—each serving counts as 1 vegetable choice and 3 salt choices

Examples of a diet within these renal guidelines might include the following pattern, with some portions increased for individuals needing more kcal. Intake of some foods cannot be increased because of their phosphorus content; thus, the renal dietitian must individualize the plan.

Breakfast

½ cup milk (whole)—4 g protein, 120 kcal, 80 mg sodium, 100 mg phosphorus
⅓ cup cooked oatmeal—2 g protein, 90 kcal, 80 mg sodium, 35 mg phosphorus
1 poached egg—7 g protein, 65 kcal, 25 mg sodium, 65 mg phosphorus
1 small bagel—4 g protein, 180 kcal, 160 mg sodium, 70 mg phosphorus
1 tsp margarine—trace protein, 45 kcal, 55 mg sodium, 5 mg phosphorus
2 jelly packs
Coffee
Nondairy creamer, 1 Tbsp
2 sugar or sugar substitute packets

Lunch

¼ cup cottage cheese—7 g protein, 65 kcal, 25 mg sodium, 65 mg phosphorus
1 oz canned tuna (canned without salt)—7 g protein, 65 kcal, 25 mg sodium, 65 mg phosphorus
1 cup salad with lettuce, cabbage, shredded carrots, cucumbers—2 g protein, 50 kcal, 30 mg sodium, 40 mg phosphorus
Balsamic vinegar + 1 Tbsp olive oil—trace protein, 45 kcal, 55 mg sodium, 5 mg phosphorus
1 small dinner roll—2 g protein, 90 kcal, 80 mg sodium, 35 mg phosphorus
1 tsp margarine—trace protein, 45 kcal, 55 mg sodium, 5 mg phosphorus
2 jelly packs
1 medium tangerine—0.5 g protein, 70 kcal, 15 mg phosphorus
Hot tea
2 sugar or sugar substitute packets

Dinner

2 oz chicken, shredded for tacos—14 g protein, 130 kcal, 50 mg sodium, 130 mg phosphorus
1 flour tortilla (6-inch diameter)—2 g protein, 90 kcal, 80 mg sodium, 35 mg phosphorus
¾ cup shredded lettuce, 2 tbsp chopped onion
¼ cup salsa—1 g protein, 25 kcal, 15 mg sodium, 20 mg phosphorus
½ cup peas, cooked and prepared without salt—1 g protein, 25 kcal, 15 mg sodium, 20 mg phosphorus
Plain muffin, 1 small—2 g protein, 90 kcal, 80 mg sodium, 35 mg phosphorus
Angel food cake, 1 oz—2 g protein, 90 kcal, 80 mg sodium, 35 mg phosphorus
Sliced peaches (½ medium)—0.5 g protein, 70 kcal, 15 mg phosphorus
1 tsp margarine—trace protein, 45 kcal, 55 mg sodium, 5 mg phosphorus
1 cup lemonade—trace protein, 100 kcal, 15 mg sodium, 5 mg phosphorus

Snacks

10 pretzel sticks—2 g protein, 90 kcal, 80 mg sodium, 35 mg phosphorus
1 cup plain popcorn—2 g protein, 90 kcal, 80 mg sodium, 35 mg phosphorus
1 apple—0.5 g protein, 70 kcal, 15 mg phosphorus
1 cup cranberry juice cocktail—trace protein, 100 kcal, 15 mg sodium, 5 mg phosphorus

For more information, handouts and tips, see:

1. Academy of Nutrition and Dietetics. National Kidney Diet: Dish Up a Kidney-Friendly Meal. https://www.eatrightstore.org/product-type/brochures-handouts/dish-up-a-kidney-friendly-meal
2. National Kidney Foundation. Nutrition and Kidney Disease Stages I–IV. https://www.kidney.org/nutrition/Kidney-Disease-Stages-1-4
3. NIDDK. Eating Right for Chronic Kidney Disease https://www.niddk.nih.gov/health-information/kidney-disease/chronic-kidney-disease-ckd/eating-nutrition

careful planning is required. Box 18.5 provides a sample menu based on the National Renal Diet.

Because malnutrition is so clearly associated with mortality in renal failure, continuing assessment of nutritional status and dietary compliance will be important. One point of emphasis is that the renal guidelines and food lists are only a starting point for individualized meal plans and education. Patient compliance is enhanced by designing meal plans to meet the specific needs of each patient.

Role of Nursing

Patients often find the renal diet difficult to follow for a long period. Motivation, support, and encouragement are crucial. Nurses play an important role in helping patients maintain good nutritional status, weight, morale, and appetite by reinforcing the nutrition education. Through formal and informal teaching, nurses can help patients appreciate the need for the stringent diet.

There is a direct relationship between adherence to the diet and symptoms that reduce quality of life. Because patients may find that foods "don't taste like they used to," nurses can encourage the use of spices such as garlic, onions, and oregano to enhance the flavor of allowed foods. They should discuss any patient concerns with the renal dietitian so they can be resolved.

HEMODIALYSIS

During hemodialysis, blood is shunted from the patient's body by way of a special vascular access or shunt (usually in the nondominant forearm), thinned with heparin, cleansed of excess fluid and waste products through a semipermeable membrane, and then returned to the patient's circulation (Fig. 18.2). The dialysate (dialysis solution) is an electrolyte solution similar in composition to normal plasma. Each solution will vary by patient's needs; the most common variable is potassium.

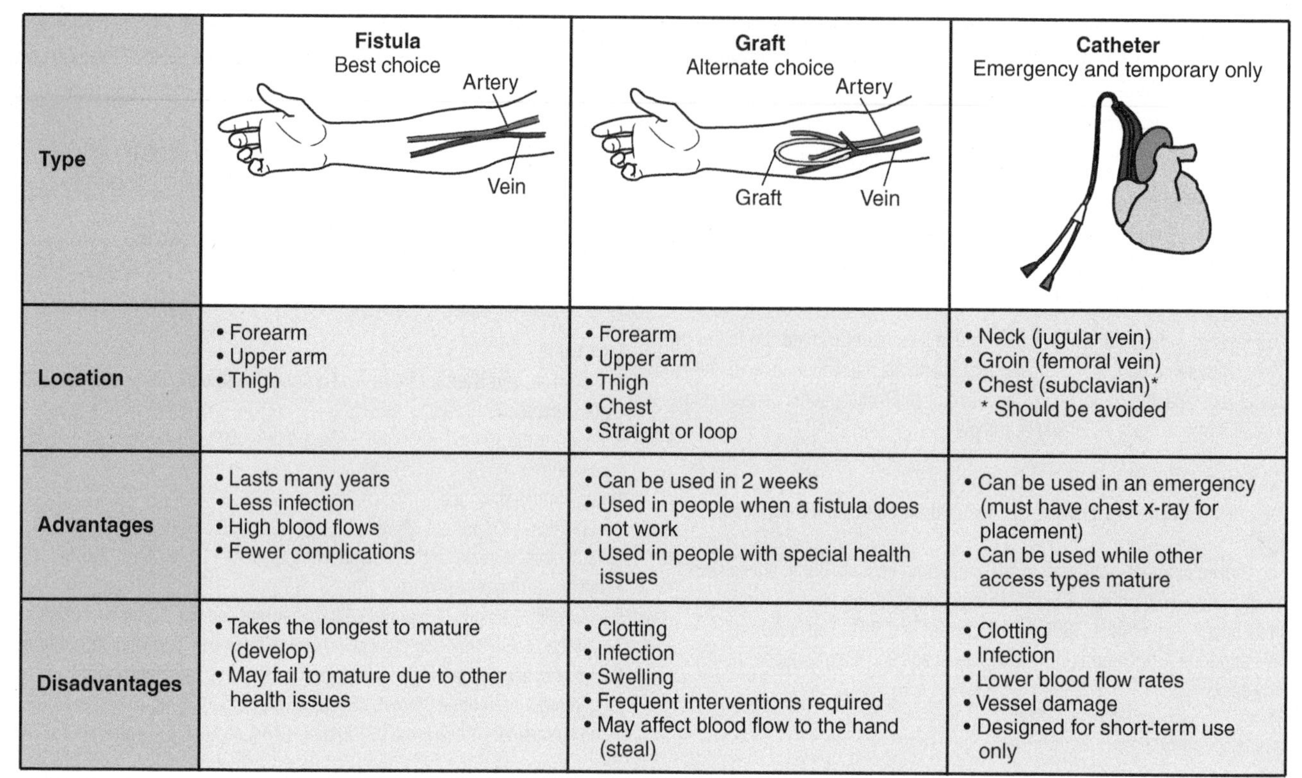

Type	Fistula Best choice Artery Vein	Graft Alternate choice Artery Graft Vein	Catheter Emergency and temporary only
Location	• Forearm • Upper arm • Thigh	• Forearm • Upper arm • Thigh • Chest • Straight or loop	• Neck (jugular vein) • Groin (femoral vein) • Chest (subclavian)* * Should be avoided
Advantages	• Lasts many years • Less infection • High blood flows • Fewer complications	• Can be used in 2 weeks • Used in people when a fistula does not work • Used in people with special health issues	• Can be used in an emergency (must have chest x-ray for placement) • Can be used while other access types mature
Disadvantages	• Takes the longest to mature (develop) • May fail to mature due to other health issues	• Clotting • Infection • Swelling • Frequent interventions required • May affect blood flow to the hand (steal)	• Clotting • Infection • Lower blood flow rates • Vessel damage • Designed for short-term use only

Fig. 18.2 Types of vascular access in hemodialysis and their advantages or disadvantages. From northwest kidney center. hemodialysis vascular access types. (Modified from https://nwrn.org/patients-a-family/ptedres/treatop/vapt/acctypes.html. Accessed 15 September, 2020.)

The average treatment lasts 3 to 6 hours and is usually performed three times per week. Hemodialysis is performed in a dialysis unit by trained staff. Patients who have received special training may assist in their own treatment.

Food and Nutrition Therapies

Individual diet prescriptions (see Table 18.2) are determined by residual kidney function, dialysate components, duration of dialysis, and rate of blood flow through the artificial kidney. The meal plan is designed, monitored, and reevaluated by the renal dietitian. Objectives are to attain or maintain good nutritional status, prevent excessive accumulation of waste products and fluid between treatments, and minimize the effects of metabolic disorders that occur.

Protein

Recommendations for protein are intended to counteract losses from dialysis, abnormalities in protein metabolism, altered albumin turnover, increased amino acid degradation, inflammation, and infection. The recommended protein intake for patients receiving hemodialysis is 1.2 g protein per kilogram standard body weight per day with at least 50% of the dietary protein being of high biologic value (animal sources).

Energy

Energy expenditure in patients undergoing hemodialysis is similar to that in healthy individuals. For adult patients younger than 60 years, daily energy intake of 35 kcal/kg of standard body weight is recommended. Obese individuals and adults older than age 60 years may benefit from 30 kcal/kg.

Fat

Patients receiving hemodialysis are at risk for lipid disorders. As such, saturated fat is limited and *trans* fats should be avoided. It is beneficial to use fish oils and olive oil because they reduce damage from inflammatory cytokines.

Sodium and Fluid

Sodium and fluid restrictions should be individualized to manage weight gain between dialysis procedures, blood pressure, and residual renal function. Foods that are liquid at room temperature (beverages, milk, creamer, juices, soups, ice chips, ice cubes) contain water, as do foods like gelatin, pudding, and ice cream. Some fruits and vegetables contain a high percentage of water, such as melons, grapes, apples, oranges, tomatoes, lettuce, and celery. When you count the amount of fluid per day, be sure to count these foods.

The recommended fluid gain between dialysis treatments is less than 5% of the patient's dry (nonedematous) weight. Corresponding sodium and fluid restrictions are as follows:

- Fluid output >1 L (1000 mL) per day: 2 to 4 g/day sodium and 2 L/day fluid
- Fluid output <1 L (1000 mL) per day: 2 g/day sodium and 1 to 1.5 L/day (1000–1500 mL) fluid
- Anuria: 2 g/day sodium and 1 L/day (1000 mL) fluid

Helping patients manage their fluid intake includes identifying measurements correctly (see Box 18.6).

BOX 18.6 Patient Tips for Managing Fluid Restrictions

Use a measuring cup to find out the amount of liquid of a favorite glass or mug.
Keep track of the amount of liquid each day on a sheet of paper or in a notebook:
- 1 ounce of fluid = 30 mL or 30 cc
- ½ cup or 4 ounces of fluid = 120 mL or 120 cc
- 1 cup or 8 ounces of fluid = 240 mL or 240 cc
- 2 cups or 16 ounces of fluid = 480 mL or 480 cc
- 1 quart or 32 ounces = 4 cups of fluid = 960 cc = about 1 L

Use a small glass to drink from and drink only when thirsty.
Take pills with applesauce or pureed fruits.
Use sour candy or gum to moisten the mouth.
Add some lemon juice to water or ice; the sour taste lessens thirst.
Swish mouth with mouthwash but do not swallow.
Freeze 20 grapes and eat throughout the day as 1 fruit serving.
Suck on frozen blueberries, strawberries, pineapple tidbits, fruit cocktail, or sliced peaches.
Use a breath spray.
Chew sugar-free gum.
Use a room humidifier or vaporizer to moisten the air.
Avoid carbonated beverages; sip ice water instead to quench thirst.
Avoid salty and spicy foods, which tend to increase thirst.
Keep blood glucose levels under control with diabetes.

Potassium

Dietary potassium restriction varies depending on urine output. Excretion of potassium increases as glomerular filtration rate declines. Generally, 2.5 g/day of potassium is well tolerated. On the other hand, patients with anuria or constipation may experience hyperkalemia. Patients with insulin deficiency or metabolic acidosis, those in a hypercatabolic state, and those being treated with beta blockers or aldosterone antagonists may require a stricter potassium restriction.

Phosphorus and Calcium

Phosphorus is routinely restricted in patients receiving hemodialysis. High serum levels contribute to secondary hyperparathyroidism and raise the calcium-phosphorus product in the plasma. Although an intake of 12 mg/kg/day is a typical recommendation, this restriction often must be liberalized to meet protein needs. Foods high in phosphorus, such as milk, milk products, cheese, beef liver, chocolate, nuts, and legumes, are usually severely limited. Fig. 18.3 shows a food pyramid for renal patients.

Iron and Trace Minerals

Anemia results from decreased renal production of erythropoietin, the hormone that stimulates bone marrow to produce red blood cells. An adequate available iron supply is necessary for normal erythropoiesis to take place. Supplementation of trace minerals is not necessary unless a deficiency is suspected or documented. Serum levels of chromium, magnesium, and other minerals should be measured several times a year.

Vitamin D

In renal failure, kidneys lose their endocrine function of producing calcitriol, the active form of vitamin D. Although many forms of vitamin D are available for supplementation, it is the active form (D_3) that helps prevent bone disease. The active form is available in oral form as calcitriol (Rocaltrol) and in an intravenous (IV) form for use during hemodialysis as calcitriol (Calcijex), paricalcitol (Zemplar), or doxercalciferol (Hectorol).

Other Vitamins

Patients treated with hemodialysis are at risk for deficiencies of water-soluble vitamins, particularly vitamin B_6 and folic acid. The reason is twofold: poor intake and loss of the nutrients during dialysis. Supplementation of the fat-soluble vitamins A, E, and K is usually not necessary. In fact, patients treated with hemodialysis have been reported to experience vitamin A toxicity.

Role of Nursing

Phosphate binders are medications used to control serum phosphorus levels; they are given with meals. The medications of choice are calcium carbonate (Tums), calcium acetate, and sevelamer hydrochloride (Renagel).

Recombinant erythropoietin (EPO), given as epoetin alfa (Epogen), may be given intravenously during dialysis or subcutaneously just after dialysis treatment. Oral or IV iron supplementation is often necessary before EPO to replenish iron stores.

Patients who have inadequate oral intake are at risk for nutrient deficiencies and poor nutritional status. Anorexia, nausea, vomiting, dietary restrictions, and changes in taste acuity or food preferences (especially red meat and sweets) are common complaints. When patients experience changes in taste, it may be useful to offer foods with sharp, distinct flavors to stimulate appetite (Box 18.7).

Almost half of individuals with CKD have diabetes and cardiovascular disease; one third of patients requiring hemodialysis have diabetes. These patients should maintain consistent carbohydrate content as well as renal modifications.

PERITONEAL DIALYSIS

Peritoneal dialysis (PD) removes excess fluid and waste products from the blood by using the lining of the abdominal cavity (peritoneum) as the dialysis membrane (Fig. 18.4). Dialysate is instilled and removed through a catheter that has been surgically placed into the peritoneal cavity. Waste products cross the membrane passively from the peritoneal capillaries into the dialysate.

The dialysate contains dextrose, which increases osmolality of the solution and facilitates removal of excess fluid. As the fluid moves from vascular space into the peritoneal cavity, osmolality of the solutions becomes equal. Toxins and excess fluids collected in the peritoneal cavity are then drained through the catheter and discarded. An advantage of PD is that it is usually performed in the home.

Intermittent Peritoneal Dialysis

Intermittent peritoneal dialysis (IPD) involves infusion of approximately 2 L of dialysate over 20 to 30 minutes. Dialysate is then drained by gravity, and the process is repeated over an 8- to

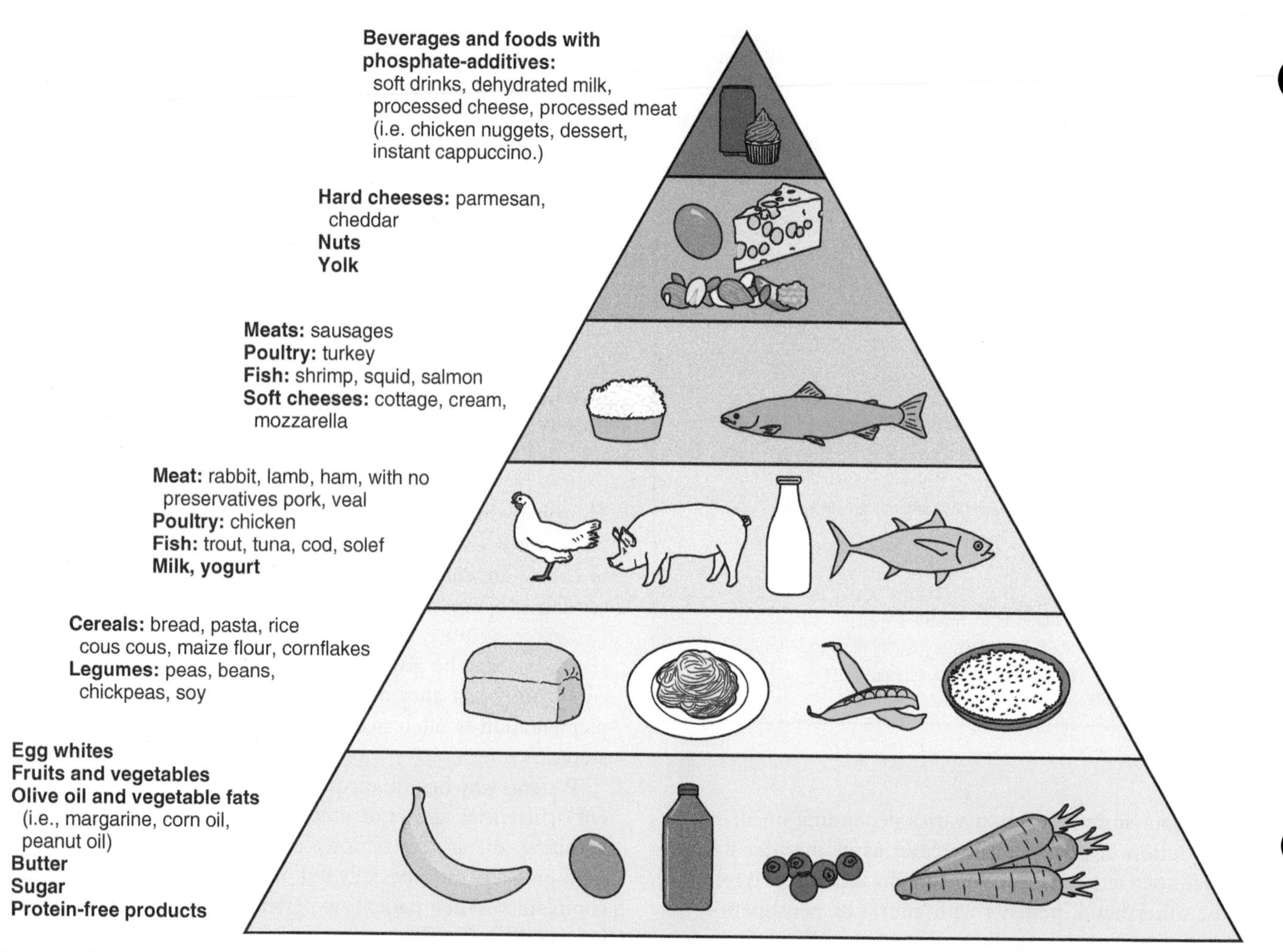

Fig. 18.3 Phosphorus pyramid for renal patients. Foods are distributed on six levels for their phosphorus content, phosphorus to protein ratio and phosphorus bioavailability. Each level has a colored edge (from green to red) that corresponds to recommended consumption frequency, highest at the base (unrestricted intake) and the lowest at the top (avoid as much as possible). Fruits and vegetables must be used with caution in dialysis patients to avoid excessive potassium load. Fats must be limited in overweight or obese patients to avoid excessive energy intake. Sugar must be avoided in diabetic or obese patients. Protein-free products are shown for patients not on dialysis therapy and who need protein restriction but a high energy intake. (Modified from D'Alessandro C et al: The "phosphorus pyramid": a visual tool for dietary phosphate management in dialysis and CKD patients, *BMC Nephrol* 16:9, 2015.)

10-hour period. IPD can be performed manually or mechanically four or five times per week. During the time of dialysis, patients are restricted to a chair or bed. This method is not commonly used as a long-term treatment modality because of the time involvement.

Continuous Ambulatory Peritoneal Dialysis

Continuous ambulatory peritoneal dialysis (CAPD) entails infusion of dialysate in four or five "exchanges" into the peritoneum over 24 hours. A specific volume of dialysate is infused and allowed to dwell for approximately 4 hours. At the end of the designated time, dialysate containing waste and excess fluid is drained by gravity, and a new exchange begins. Dialysate is present 24 hours per day in the peritoneum, except for the 20- to 30-minute exchange when dwelling dialysate is drained and fresh dialysate is instilled. Dialysis exchanges are done continuously, 7 days a week. CAPD is a reasonable procedure for adults who work outside the home and can complete the procedure discreetly while at work.

Continuous Cycling Peritoneal Dialysis

Continuous cycling peritoneal dialysis (CCPD) is a combination of IPD and CAPD. At night, a mechanical cycler performs three dialysate exchanges. During the day, a fourth exchange is infused throughout the day. At bedtime, the fourth exchange is drained, and the process is started again. Although restricted to bed during nighttime infusions, patients are ambulatory during the day. Thus, CCPD is another reasonable option for working adults.

Food and Nutrition Therapies

Objectives for PD are to (1) maintain good nutritional status while replacing albumin lost in the dialysate, (2) minimize complications of fluid imbalance, (3) minimize symptoms of

BOX 18.7 Suggestions for Patients With Altered Sense of Taste

- Brush teeth and tongue six to eight times per day.
- Rinse mouth with a chilled mouthwash (commercial product, or water mixed with lemon juice); or try cool black or green tea, lightly salted water, or baking soda and water before eating.
- Chew gum.
- Before meals, drink water with lemon, suck a lemon wedge or hard candy before meals.
- Prepare foods with a variety of colors and textures. Cold foods may not have as much flavor.
- Use aromatic herbs and hot spices to add more flavor; however, avoid adding more sugar or salt to foods.
- Try different or unusual flavors such as basil, oregano, rosemary, tarragon, mustard, catsup, and mint.
- If diet permits, add small amounts of cheese, bacon bits, butter, olive oil, or toasted nuts on vegetables.
- Avoid combination dishes, such as casseroles, that can hide individual flavors and dilute taste.
- For metallic taste, try using plastic utensils instead of regular silverware.

(Modified from National Institute on Deafness and Other Communication Disorders. Taste Disorders. https://www.nidcd.nih.gov/health/taste-disorders, Accessed 15 September, 2020.)

uremic toxicity, and (4) minimize secondary metabolic disorders. As with hemodialysis, patients treated with PD are at risk for deficiencies of water-soluble vitamins and minerals. A daily multivitamin supplement that includes folic acid and vitamin D is also recommended. In addition, some patients receive recombinant EPO for correction of anemia and need an iron supplement to maximize the effectiveness of the drug.

Energy requirements for patients treated with PD are usually lower than for HD because 60% of the dialysate is absorbed. Dextrose is used as an osmotic agent in PD dialysate and must be taken into consideration when energy needs are calculated, especially when the patient has diabetes.

Protein losses during PD range from 20 to 30 g/day and are reflected in slightly higher dietary protein recommendations (see Table 18.2). Serum BUN and creatinine, uremic symptoms, and weight should be monitored as indicators of sufficient protein intake, and the diet should be adjusted accordingly.

During PD, sodium, potassium, and fluid are continually removed, making severe dietary restrictions unnecessary. However, it is important to remember that nutrient needs vary among patients, so individualized recommendations are still necessary. Many sodium tips and guidelines are available (University of San Francisco Medical Center, 2020).

Restriction of dietary phosphorus is critical to prevent development of **osteodystrophy** (defective bone development). Unfortunately, higher protein requirements for PD consequently provide high amounts of phosphorus. Therefore, restricting or eliminating dairy products will be necessary to control phosphorus intake. Phosphorus is also controlled by prescribed phosphate binders. Calcium supplementation is usually prescribed.

Other minerals must be checked regularly. Magnesium (Mg) inhibits vascular calcification; coronary artery calcification is highly prevalent among dialysis patients (Molnar et al., 2017). Low serum magnesium (Mg) is associated with increased cardiovascular mortality in PD patients (Cai et al., 2016).

Role of Nursing

All forms of PD require special training of the patient and caregiver. Anorexia, nausea, and vomiting are common signs of uremia and inadequate dialysis. Consequently, nutritional status is an important measure. The National Kidney Foundation suggests regular and ongoing nutritional assessment of patients undergoing PD by a renal dietitian and other team members.

Excessive weight gain and other factors should be carefully reviewed with each visit. The absorption of glucose from PD dialysate presents a special challenge for patients with diabetes. Weight gain is caused by the increased calorie load of the dialysate. Blood glucose levels and hyperlipidemia become more difficult to control. Dehydration is another concern when there is excessive fluid removal and extracellular fluid volume deficits. Thus, careful monitoring of blood glucose, I&O, and weights are preventive measures in this patient population.

KIDNEY TRANSPLANTATION

Kidney transplantation is the best renal replacement option for people with ESRD. Unfortunately, the waiting time is often prolonged for many years. Waiting lists continue to grow across the world despite remarkable advances in the transplantation process (Maciel et al., 2017). Even with public engagement campaigns, there is a shortage of donors (see the *Cultural Diversity and Nutrition* box Barriers to Organ Donations).

CULTURAL DIVERSITY AND NUTRITION

Barriers to Organ Donations

Different beliefs and cultures reflect diverse legislations and donation practices among different countries, creating a challenge for individuals waiting for transplant (Maciel et al., 2017). In the United States, there is a shortage of organ donations from members of minority groups. This is a concern because successful organ transplantation requires some matching of genetic characteristics.

Efforts of the DC Organ Donor Program, the Dow Take Initiative Program, and the National Minority Organ Tissues Transplant Education Program have succeeded; African Americans now rank above Caucasian and Hispanic Americans in numbers of organ donors per million in the United States (Callender et al, 2016). Culturally appropriate interventions can be used to engage and educate minority groups. Key recommendations include the following: (1) simplify educational materials that are culturally sensitive, with the appropriate reading level and available in multiple languages, (2) invite transplant patients and donors to advisory panels, digital storytelling, and patient-reported outcomes, and (3) train all members of the health team to understand their role as advocates (Waterman et al, 2020).

(Data from Callender CO, et al: Organ donation in the United States: the tale of the African-American journey of moving from the bottom to the top, *Transplant Proc* 48:2392–2395, 2016; Maciel CB, et al: Organ donation protocols, *Handb Clin Neurol* 140:409–439, 2017; and Waterman et al: Amplifying the patient voice: Key priorities and opportunities for improved transplant and living donor advocacy and outcomes during COVID-19 and beyond, *Curr Transplant Rep* 1:1–10, 2020.)

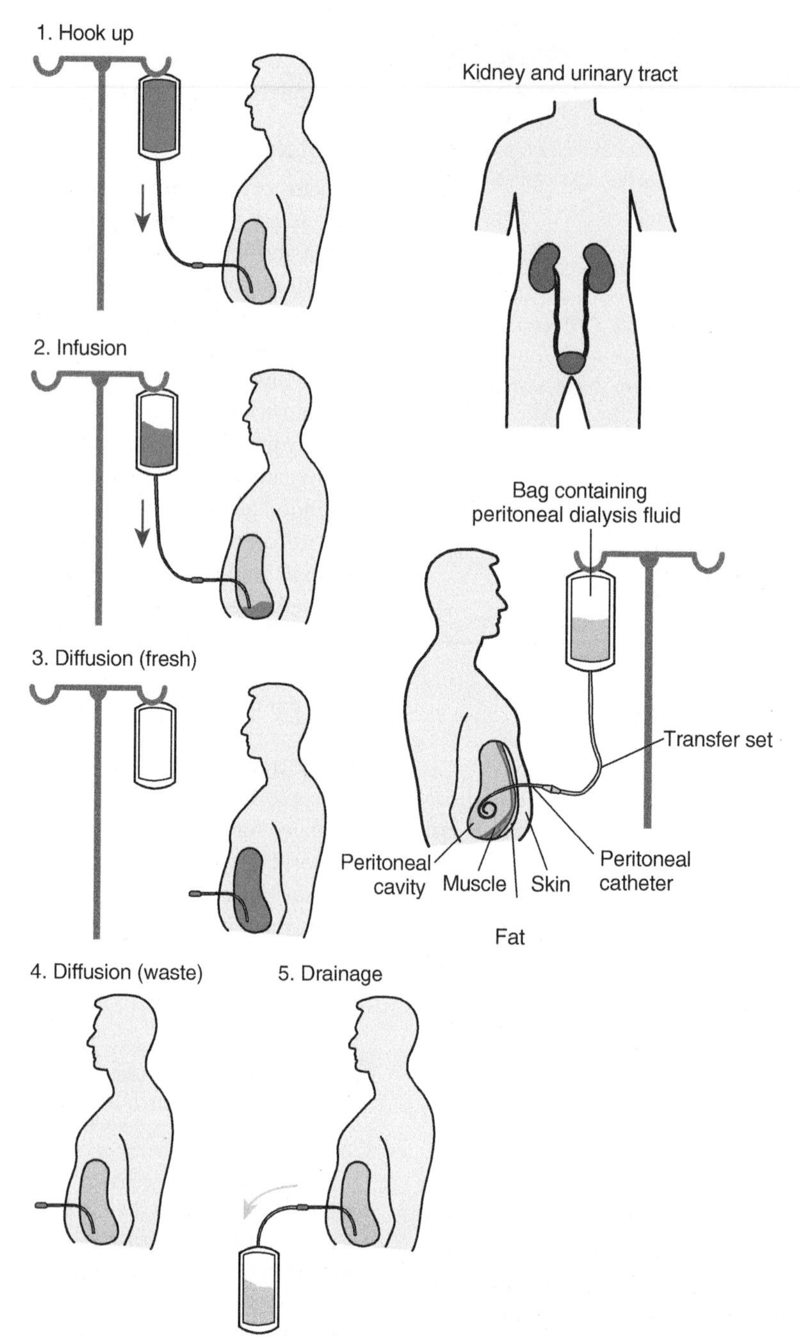

Fig. 18.4 Continuous ambulatory peritoneal dialysis; 20-minute exchanges usually are given four or five times a day every day. (Modified from Adobe Stock. Continuous ambulatory peritoneal dialysis CAPD. https://stock.adobe.com/images/continuous-ambulatory-peritoneal-dialysis-capd/207779105 Accessed 15 September, 2020.)

Food and Nutrition Therapies

Pretransplantation

Nutritional status is evaluated to identify and correct deficits before surgery. Poor nutritional status is caused by protein, blood, and nutrient loss during dialysis; the catabolism of chronic illness; anorexia and altered taste; suboptimal oral intake; and depression. Decreased visceral protein stores and body weight are common, as are deficiencies of vitamin B_6, folic acid, vitamins C and D, and iron. Nutrition therapy requires an individualized approach, as outlined in Table 18.2.

Immediately After Transplantation and Long Term

Energy needs in the immediate posttransplantation period are high (30–35 kcal/kg) because of stress from surgery and catabolism. These requirements decline approximately 6 to 8 weeks after transplantation, and intake should then be provided to achieve and maintain a desirable body weight. Restriction of dietary protein is not necessary. In fact, protein catabolism is increased as the result of surgery and the administration of corticosteroids for immunosuppression.

Steroid therapy may cause glucose intolerance and therefore necessitate control of total carbohydrate intake. Transplantation

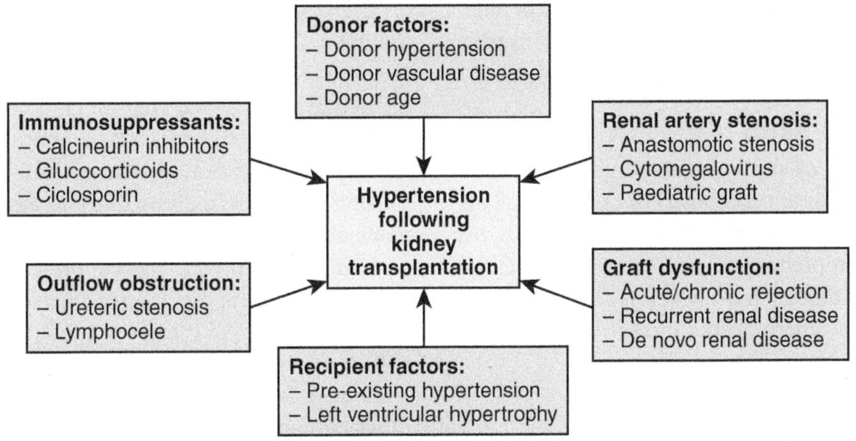

Fig. 18.5 Factors contributing to hypertension following kidney transplant. (Modified from Pugh D, et al: Management of Hypertension in Chronic Kidney Disease, *Drugs* 79:365–379, 2019.)

is often complicated by worsening or new-onset diabetes (Lo et al., 2017). Saturated fats are limited if dyslipidemia occurs, whereas foods rich in omega-3 fatty acids may improve plasma lipid patterns and decrease systemic inflammation.

Fluids are generally unrestricted and limited only by graft function. Because many drugs after transplantation influence nutritional needs and status, careful follow-up may prevent problems. For example, recommendations regarding sodium and potassium should be individualized for each patient, especially with hypertension; see Fig. 18.5.

Role of Nursing

Nutritional care of renal transplant recipients involves continual reassessment of nutritional goals and efficacy of therapy during the different phases of recovery. Nurses can be very helpful by discussing and reinforcing the measures that are needed. For example, the immunosuppressant drugs often cause weight gain and secondary diabetes as a long-term consequence after transplantation. Patients will need support and guidance on how to manage and cope after the procedure.

More than 80% of kidneys transplanted from cadavers still function well 1 year after surgery. Outcomes are even better for transplants from living donors. Nurses play an essential role for both sets of families and friends of the donor and the transplant recipient (see the *Personal Perspectives* box Organ Donation: Helping Families Cope).

KIDNEY STONES

Renal calculi are a common urologic condition. Kidney stone formation (urolithiasis) is more common among men than women, and approximately half of those in whom renal calculi develop have them again within a decade. They occur in children after diarrhea or infections, in hot climates, or with anatomic abnormalities.

Stone formation occurs with low urine volume from inadequate fluid intake; alkaline urinary pH; excessive urinary excretion of calcium, oxalate, uric acid, or a combination; and decreased substances in the urine that normally inhibit stone formation. Kidney stones can occur with obesity, dehydration, high-protein diets, gastric bypass surgery, inflammatory bowel

PERSONAL PERSPECTIVES

Organ Donation: Helping Families Cope

It was such a pleasure to watch my brother-in-law, David, marry his high school sweetheart, Carol. They had dated for years and finally made the marital plunge in June of 1987. Our 3-year-old son was the ringbearer, adorable in his little white tux, which matched that of his uncle. How joyful that day was for all!

Seven months later, on a clear, cold night in January, David was in a car accident. He had been playing cards with friends until the early morning hours. His drive home was unfamiliar, in an older part of the city where the highway was narrow and poorly marked for night driving. Evidently, he headed in the wrong direction. While making a U-turn on the highway, a woman on her way to work did not see him and crashed into the back of his car. David's car spun around, and he was thrown through the hatchback onto the pavement. Even though a medical helicopter was quickly called to transport him to a large tertiary care center, it was too late. He had already experienced massive brain trauma, with a closed-head injury and extensive swelling. Unlike soft tissue, the human cranium has no room to expand.

David was connected to a ventilator, and the many tests began. His family had been called, which included my husband. I stayed at home with our son until he called later that day. It was urgent for us to go to the hospital because signs did not promise any recovery. Because David was married, his wife was to make decisions for him, but the rest of us had opinions as well. His sister was a nursing supervisor, and I was a registered dietitian, so we had seen many head trauma cases. We were all ready to play a part in his recovery, however long that would take.

Unfortunately, David failed the Glasgow Coma Scale tests and was truly "brain dead." His doctors indicated that no family decision was necessary; they would automatically remove the life support. It was so sad to look at this beautiful young man with few signs of trauma, a newlywed less than a year. We realized that there would be no nieces or nephews to play with our children. No more holidays together, no more beach vacations or life event celebrations. No more David and Carol, no more intact family.

At some point that day, the nurses and chaplain helped us discuss organ donation. We were encouraged to touch David and say our goodbyes. Carol knew that David had signed up for organ donation. It was okay for organs other than his heart; that was where she "resided" in him. In this terrible and painful weekend, we all knew this was the right thing to do. His organs would give others the chance to live a healthy life, even if he could not do so.

Our minister was outstanding in his love and support, suggesting to grieve a little each day and not hurry to "get on with our lives." That advice and knowing that others had been given a second chance helped us accept that David's life had a courageous, if unplanned, purpose.

Sylvia Escott-Stump
Winterville, NC

disease, hyperparathyroidism, and strong family history of renal stones. Fortunately, most people require just minimally invasive surgery as treatment.

Food and Nutrition Therapies

Different causes and types of stones require individualization of diets. Most stones (≥60%) are composed of calcium oxalate. Only 8% to 9% are struvite, 10% are uric acid stones, and 1% are cystine stones. A comprehensive diet history is essential to identify the necessary dietary modifications (Box 18.8). All stone treatments require a generous fluid intake.

Calcium Oxalate Stones

Too much calcium in the urine (hypercalciuria) is the most common cause in 50% of people who form calcium stones. Stone formation is influenced more by oxalate than by calcium in the urinary tract. Oxalate is found primarily in foods of plant origin and is the end-product of ascorbic acid metabolism. Restriction of dietary oxalate intake has been used to reduce risk of recurrence. Box 18.9 provides guidance.

BOX 18.8 Dietary Recommendations for Kidney Stones

- Tailor diet to specific metabolic disturbance and individual dietary habits.
- Include a high fluid intake to produce at least 2 L/day of urine (2–3 L/day intake).
- Avoid severe dietary calcium restriction. Consume calcium-rich foods instead of supplements.
- Limit oxalate-rich foods: spinach, rhubarb, beets, nuts, chocolate, tea, wheat bran, and strawberries.
- Limit supplemental vitamins C and D to recommended dietary allowance (RDA) for gender and age.
- Choose plant-based proteins over animal proteins several times a week.
- Limit salt intake.
- Use 5 or more servings of fruits and vegetables per day for potassium sources.

BOX 18.9 Dietary Treatment for Hypercalciuria

Limit daily calcium intake to 600–800 mg/day unless otherwise instructed
Limit dietary oxalate, especially when calcium intake is reduced. High oxalate levels are found in strong teas, rhubarb, beets, okra, spinach, Swiss chard, sweet potatoes, nuts, tea, chocolate, black pepper, and soy products.
Avoid excessive purines and animal protein (<1.7 g/kg of body weight)
Reduce sodium (salt) and refined sugar to the minimum possible
Increase dietary fiber (12–24 g/day)
Limit alcohol and caffeine intake
Increase fluid intake, especially water (sufficient to produce at least 2 L of urine per day)

Modified content reproduced with permission from Medscape Drugs & Diseases (https://emedicine.medscape.com/), from Leslie SW, Fathallah-Shaykh S. Hypercalciuria. Medscape Drugs & Diseases. Updated Apr 23, 2019. Available at: https://emedicine.medscape.com/article/2182757-overview. Accessed 29 March 2021.)

High intake of fruits and vegetables with a balanced intake of low-fat dairy products carries the lowest risk for kidney stones (Ferraro et al., 2020). It is important to avoid large doses of supplemental calcium and vitamin D.

Low intake of potassium is another risk factor for stone development. Potassium reduces urinary calcium excretion by causing transient sodium diuresis and increased renal phosphate absorption. Diets high in potassium and lower in animal protein may help with prevention (Ferraro et al., 2016). Thus, the Mediterranean diet is a reasonable choice.

Uric Acid Stones

Uric acid is a metabolic product of purine metabolism (a nitrogen-containing compound in protein). Uric acid stones are associated with acidic urine (hyperuricosuria) and gout. Allopurinol (Zyloprim) is effective in reducing high levels of uric acid. The key therapy is weight loss. A balanced vegetarian diet with dairy products seems to be the most protective diet (Ferraro et al., 2020).

Cystine Stones

Cystine stones form in people with a hereditary disorder that causes the kidneys to excrete excessive amounts of the amino acid cystine (cystinuria). The goal of treatment is to reduce urinary cystine concentration. To do this, urine volume should be greater than 3 L/day, and urine should be alkalinized to a pH in the range of 6.5 to 7. Restrictions in animal protein and sodium are associated with reduced cystine production (Heilberg & Goldfarb, 2013).

Struvite Stones

Struvite stones are caused by urinary tract infections by bacteria that split urea into ammonium in urine. No specific diet is needed other than avoidance of dehydration. Surgery or lithotripsy is almost always performed.

Role of Nursing

Education is important in the prevention and treatment of renal calculi. Only a motivated and informed patient can be expected to maintain a long-term preventive program. For people with a history of kidney stones, doctors usually recommend passing about 2.6 quarts (2.5 L) of urine a day. Measuring urine output is an important task.

Helping patients manage their medications is another nursing role. To help prevent calcium stones from forming, a thiazide diuretic or a phosphate-containing preparation may be ordered. To prevent uric acid stones, allopurinol is used to reduce uric acid levels and to keep urine alkaline. To prevent struvite stones, long-term use of antibiotics in small doses can keep urine free of bacteria that cause infection.

Nurses can also help to correct misinformation. For example, caffeine-containing beverages as part of a normal lifestyle do not cause fluid loss greater than the volume ingested. They do have a mild diuretic effect, but they do not appear to increase the risk of dehydration. Thus, coffee and tea can be consumed as some of the required fluids each day to decrease stone formation.

SUMMARY

- The chief life-preserving function of the kidneys is to help maintain chemical homeostasis in the body.
- Various inflammatory, obstructive, and degenerative diseases affect the kidneys in different ways and interfere with normal functioning of nephrons that regulate products of metabolism.
- Because of glomerular damage, nephrotic syndrome results in increased urinary excretion of protein, decreased serum albumin levels, hyperlipidemia, and edema. Some individuals benefit from a gluten-free or allergy elimination diet.
- Nephrotic syndrome may resist treatment and progress to renal failure. The primary goals of medical nutrition therapy are to control hypertension, minimize edema, decrease urinary albumin losses, prevent protein malnutrition and muscle catabolism, supply adequate energy, and slow the progression of renal disease.
- Acute renal failure (ARF) is characterized by an abrupt loss of renal function that may or may not be accompanied by oliguria or anuria; common causes are trauma, hemorrhage, shock, nephrotoxic chemicals or drugs, septicemia, and streptococcal infection.
- Nutritional needs in ARF are determined by the underlying cause of the condition and whether dialysis is used for treatment. Patients may be hypermetabolic if the renal failure was caused by trauma, burns, septicemia, or infection.
- Chronic kidney disease (CKD) is the result of progressive, irreversible loss of kidney function. It can develop over days, months, or years. CKD always leads to retention of nitrogenous waste products and fluid and electrolyte imbalances that affect all body systems.
- Before end-stage renal failure, management focuses on slowing progression and minimizing complications of CKD. A prerenal failure intervention with a qualified dietitian is recommended.
- Once CKD progresses to renal failure, management focuses on reducing uremia with various treatment modalities: conservative management, hemodialysis, peritoneal dialysis, and renal transplantation.
- Planning renal diets requires skill in calibrating intakes of fluids, energy, protein, lipids, phosphorus, potassium, sodium, vitamins, and other minerals.
- The National Renal Diet can be used to develop diet guidelines and meal plans. Individual renal diet prescriptions are based on residual kidney function, dialysate components, duration of dialysis, and rate of blood flow through the artificial kidney.
- Objectives are to attain or maintain good nutritional status, prevent uremic toxicity and fluid imbalance between treatments, and minimize effects of metabolic disorders caused by CKD, hemodialysis, and peritoneal dialysis.
- Nutritional care of renal transplant recipients involves continual reassessment of nutritional goals and efficacy of therapy during the different phases of care.
- Renal calculi are a common, recurrent urologic condition. Most are composed of calcium oxalate or phosphorus, with a small proportion made up of cystine, uric acid, or struvite. Uric acid is a metabolic product of purines.
- Sufficient fluid intake has the most significant impact on reducing risk of stone formation. A high-potassium, low–animal protein intake may be beneficial, similar to the Mediterranean diet principles.
- Calcium oxalate stone formation is influenced more by the amount of oxalate in the urinary tract than by the amount of calcium. Oxalate is found primarily in plant foods and is the end-product of ascorbic acid metabolism.

THE NURSING APPROACH

Clinical Judgment and Next-Generation NCLEX® Examination-Style Questions

Case Study 1

Chronic Renal Failure

Ian, age 28, was diagnosed with end-stage renal disease (ESRD) a few months ago subsequent to glomerulonephritis. His kidneys produce very little urine or sometimes none at all, requiring Ian to receive hemodialysis treatments three times a week. He hopes for a kidney transplant, but the waiting list is long. The nurse wants to encourage him.

Assessment/Recognize Cues

Subjective (From Patient Statements)

- "I don't have any energy. I'm tired all of the time."
- "Food doesn't taste good anymore. I don't have any appetite."
- "I'm sick of trying to follow the diet the dietitian recommended. It's not worth it."
- "Why try? Dialysis will take care of any extra fluid and minerals."
- "I know what I am supposed to eat, but it's too hard. I just eat and drink what I like whenever I want to."

Objective (From Physical Examination)

- Generalized ashen skin color, pale conjunctivae, wasted appearance
- BP 162/105, pulse 92, respirations 20
- Low hemoglobin and hematocrit, high blood urea nitrogen (BUN) and creatinine
- Weight gain of 6 pounds since last hemodialysis 2 days ago
- Edema of ankles, crackles (sounds) in both lungs

Diagnoses (Nursing)/Analyze Cues

1. Fluid overload related to impaired renal function and excessive intake of fluid and sodium as evidenced by oliguria, weight gain of 6 pounds, ankle edema, crackles in both lungs, and BP 162/105.
2. Decreased adherence related to lack of motivation, as evidenced by "I'm sick of trying to follow the diet the dietitian recommended," "Why try? Dialysis will take care of any extra fluid and minerals," and "I know what I am supposed to eat, but it's too hard. I just eat and drink what I like whenever I want to."

Continued

THE NURSING APPROACH—cont'd

3. Fatigue related to anorexia secondary to impaired renal function as evidenced wasted appearance and by patient saying "I don't have any energy. I am tired all of the time."

Planning

Patient Outcomes

Short term (by the end of the nurse–patient interaction):

- Commits to meet with the renal dietitian to plan a diet he can follow
- Recognizes the connections among diet, effectiveness of dialysis, and feeling better
- Agrees to take charge of his health by continuing dialysis and taking prescribed medications

Long term (by 2 weeks):

- Says he is following the renal diet and feels more energetic
- No more than 1- to 2-pound weight gain per day between dialysis treatments
- BP 130/85, no ankle edema, lungs clear

Nursing Interventions/Generate Solutions

1. Refer Ian to the renal dietitian.
2. Try to motivate him to adhere to the medical plan, including medical nutrition therapy.
3. Discuss why following the renal diet is necessary and how it can help him feel better.

Implementation/Take Actions

1. Referred Ian to the renal dietitian.
   The renal dietitian can help individualize the complex diet according to the patient's lifestyle, health condition, and food preferences. The dietitian also can teach the patient how to apply general principles of the renal diet.
2. Explained the connections among pathophysiology, diet, and patient problems (signs and symptoms).
   A patient may be motivated to make healthy food choices if he can see a direct positive effect. Failed kidneys cannot remove fluids, electrolytes, and nitrogenous wastes. Restricting certain foods and some fluid intake can help alleviate signs and symptoms of uremia and fluid and electrolyte problems.
   a. Discussed the need to ingest adequate calories (including carbohydrates and unsaturated fats) and high biologic value proteins (soy, lean red meats, fish, chicken, eggs, and milk) to reduce urea formation.
      Nausea, anorexia, and metallic tastes may be reduced by decreasing urea production. Adequate intake of calories decreases protein catabolism, thus decreasing nitrogenous waste. High–biologic value proteins produce less urea than low–biologic value proteins (e.g., grains and cereals).
   b. Discussed the need to restrict fluids and sodium to reduce fluid retention.
      Hypertension, peripheral edema, and pulmonary edema may result from excessive fluid intake, accentuated by sodium retention. Because the heart has to work harder, heart failure may occur. Dialysis can remove some fluid, but it is more effective and better tolerated by the patient if large accumulations of fluid are not present.
   c. Discussed the need to restrict potassium to avoid problems in the heart.
      Too much potassium, resulting from decreased excretion by the kidneys, can cause deadly dysrhythmias. Foods high in potassium should be avoided or limited, such as bananas, oranges, potatoes, tomatoes, and milk. Milk is often limited to 12 cup per day because it is high in both potassium and phosphorus.
   d. Discussed the need to restrict phosphorus to avoid problems in the bones.
      Failed kidneys cannot remove phosphorus, and dialysis does not remove phosphorus well. Phosphorus concentration in the blood is inversely related to serum calcium level, so a high level of phosphorus causes decreased absorption of calcium from the intestines. The resultant hypocalcemia stimulates the parathyroid gland to keep the serum calcium level in a safe range, and it does so by pulling calcium from the bones. This puts the patient at risk for bone fractures. Foods high in phosphorus should be limited, such as milk, cheese, nuts, legumes, beef liver, and chocolate.
3. Helped Ian plan what he can do to improve his health and nutrition.
   Helping the patient take charge of his health provides a sense of control and empowerment.
   a. Choose foods from the National Renal Diet.
      Foods are grouped into choices by the amount of protein, calories, sodium, phosphorus, and potassium that the foods contain. The dietitian can specify the number of servings in each choice (group), allowing the patient to eat any food within the choice and still follow guidelines of medical nutrition therapy. Choices (groups) include protein, fruits and vegetables, dairy and phosphorus, bread/grains, fluid, and high-kcal foods and flavoring.
   b. Weigh and measure foods periodically to match recommended serving sizes.
      Accuracy is needed to obtain expected results.
   c. Eat small, frequent meals, spacing protein foods throughout the day.
      Small, frequent meals are usually better tolerated than large meals when the patient has nausea and anorexia. Spreading proteins throughout the day helps control the amount of urea that is in the patient's body at any one time.
   d. Brush teeth frequently and chew gum if desired.
      Good oral care makes the mouth feel fresher, improving the taste of food. Chewing gum improves taste in the mouth and can stimulate salivary glands, providing moisture in the mouth and possibly decreasing thirst.
   e. Set a target range of gaining no more than 1 to 2 pounds per day between hemodialysis treatments. Weigh self every morning, and adjust fluid and sodium intake to avoid exceeding the target.
      Working toward a goal can provide motivation. Daily fluid allotment is generally 500 to 1000 mL plus the amount of urine output.
   f. Make a plan for spacing out allowed fluids throughout the day, including foods that melt at room temperature or are high in water content.
      Spreading out fluid intake can help control thirst. Using smaller glasses and freezing some fluids to eat like ice pops may also reduce thirst.
4. Encouraged Ian to adhere to the medical plan, including both undergoing hemodialysis three times per week and taking medications.
   Hemodialysis involves circulating blood through a dialyzer (artificial kidney) to remove urea, metabolic waste products, toxins, and excess fluid. Failed kidneys cannot produce the hormone erythropoietin (necessary for red blood cell production), so anemia is common. Epoetin alfa (Epogen) is given to stimulate red blood cell synthesis. In addition, iron, B vitamins, and folic acid are usually prescribed to enhance the erythropoiesis. Failed kidneys cannot produce calcitriol (the active form of vitamin D), so it may be taken orally to promote absorption of calcium and subsequent bone formation. Usually phosphate binders (such as calcium carbonate) are prescribed by a physician and taken with each meal to facilitate fecal elimination of phosphorus.
5. Suggested involving his family and friends in meal planning.
   Family support is extremely helpful. A person with renal failure often lacks energy for grocery shopping and food preparation. Families can eat similar meals with the patient, though serving sizes will probably vary.
   a. Recommended purchasing a renal diet cookbook.
      Recipes from a renal diet cookbook can add variety to the family meal.
   b. Advised Ian to avoid salt and salt substitutes (usually potassium) and add spices such as garlic, onions, and oregano to food.
      Adding spices adds flavor to foods.
6. Helped Ian write some short-term goals.
   Achievement of small steps provides encouragement.

Continued

THE NURSING APPROACH—cont'd

a. Asked how Ian would reward himself when he achieved each goal.
Positive reinforcement helps establish desirable behaviors.
b. Reminded him that he must stay healthy to be prepared for a possible kidney transplant.
Kidney transplants succeed best when the patient is healthy. Patients are more likely to be considered for a kidney transplantation if they are healthy and taking charge of their health.

Evaluation/Evaluate Outcomes

Short term (by the end of the nurse–patient interaction):

- Ian stated he was willing to meet with the dietitian at the dialysis center and follow the dietitian's recommendations.
- Ian said he could see how eating the right foods and following the medical plan might make him feel better.
- He agreed to continue taking prescribed medications and getting hemodialysis.

Goals met.

The nurse planned to meet with Ian again in 2 weeks.

Discussion Questions

Ian met with the nurse for follow-up in 2 weeks. He kept a record of his weight, his urine output, and his fluid intake every day for the 2 weeks. He gained 1 to 2 pounds per day between dialysis treatments. He reported that he felt better during the days that he adhered closely to his fluid restrictions. The nurse praised him for his efforts.

1. When assessing Ian, what signs and symptoms would the nurse look for to validate improvement in fluid balance?
2. Ian said he had met with the dietitian but was still having a hard time maintaining his diet. How could the nurse motivate Ian and help him set some small, realistic goals?

Case Study 2

The nurse is caring for a patient admitted with kidney stones. The nurse knows that certain conditions are related to kidney stones.

Select all that apply.
Use an X to mark the conditions that are related to kidney stones.

Conditions Related to Kidney Stones

1. Strong family history of renal stones
2. Hypoparathyroidism
3. High-fat diet
4. Gastric bypass surgery
5. Fluid overload
6. Obesity
7. Inflammatory bowel disease
8. Cholecystitis

CRITICAL THINKING

Clinical Applications

Julia, aged 40 years, works full time in an office and has a sedentary lifestyle. She is 5 feet 6 inches tall, has a medium frame, and weighs 125 pounds (dry weight). Her usual body weight is 132 pounds. Her appetite has not been good for the past 3 months, but it is improving. She is on hemodialysis for 3 hours three times per week. Her urine output is approximately 500 mL/24 hours.

Her predialysis laboratory results include BUN 57 mg/dL; Na^+ 133 mEq/L; K^+ 4.7 mEq/L; Po_4 6.3 mg/dL; Ca^{2+} 9.5 mg/dL; serum albumin 3 g/dL; and ferritin 7 µg/L. Her diet prescription is 2200 kcal, 70 to 80 g protein, 2000 mg Na^+, 2000 mg K^+, 1000 mg Po_4, and 1500 mL fluid.

Julia's diet history indicates that she doesn't like meat but does like cheese and orange juice and will occasionally overindulge on these foods. She admits to having had too much cheese and orange juice when she came in for her last dialysis.

1. What is the purpose of hemodialysis?
2. How are metabolic waste products removed during dialysis?
3. Give two explanations why Julia's serum albumin levels are decreased.
4. Why is the serum ferritin often low in renal patients?
5. Why are high biologic value proteins recommended for patients on hemodialysis?

Julia is considering trying a type of peritoneal dialysis so she won't have to go to the kidney dialysis center three times each week.

1. Explain how peritoneal dialysis works.
2. What dietary changes might need to be made if Julia switches to peritoneal dialysis?

BUN, Bod urea nitrogen.
(Courtesy Kim Dittus, PhD, RD, Syracuse University, Syracuse, NY.)

WEBSITES OF INTEREST

Life Options Rehabilitation Program
www.lifeoptions.org
Helps individuals live well and long with kidney disease; includes Kidney School, an interactive, web-based kidney learning center.

National Kidney and Urological Diseases Information Clearinghouse (NKUDIC)
kidney.niddk.nih.gov
Functions as an information dissemination service of the National Institute of Diabetes and Digestive and Kidney Diseases (NIDDK).

National Kidney Foundation – Nutrition
https://www.kidney.org/nutrition
Tips for managing the diet in kidney diseases; includes recipes.

Renal Support Network (RSN)
http://www.rsnhope.org/
Provides nonmedical services to those affected by chronic kidney disease as a nonprofit, patient-focused, patient-run organization.

REFERENCES

Afkarian, M., et al. (2016). Clinical manifestations of kidney disease among us adults with diabetes, 1988–2014. *The Journal of the American Medical Association*, *316*, 602–610.

Beto, J. A., et al. (2016). Strategies to promote adherence to nutritional advice in patients with chronic kidney disease: a narrative review and commentary. *International Journal of Nephrology and Renovascular Disease*, *9*, 21–33.

Cai, K., et al. (2016). Hypomagnesemia is associated with increased mortality among peritoneal dialysis patients. *PLoS One*, *11*, e0152488.

Downie, M. L., et al. (2017). Nephrotic syndrome in infants and children: pathophysiology and management. *Paediatrics and International Child Health*, *37*, 248–258.

Ferraro, P. M., et al. (2016). Dietary protein and potassium, diet-dependent net acid load, and risk of incident kidney stones. *Clinical Journal of the American Society of Nephrology*, *11*, 1834–1844.

Ferraro, P. M., et al. (2020). Risk of kidney stones: influence of dietary factors, dietary patterns, and vegetarian-vegan diets. *Nutrients*. *12*, 779.

Heilberg, I. P., & Goldfarb, D. S. (2013). Optimum nutrition for kidney stone disease. *Advances in Chronic Kidney Disease*, *20*, 165–174.

Hilliard, S. A., & El-Dahr, S. S. (2016). Epigenetics of renal development and disease. *The Yale Journal of Biology and Medicine*, *89*, 565–573.

Lemley, K. V., et al. (2016). The effect of a gluten-free diet in children with difficult-to-manage nephrotic syndrome. *Pediatrics*, *138*(10), 1542.

Liu, M., et al. (2014). Cardiovascular disease and its relationship with chronic kidney disease. *European Review for Medical and Pharmacological Sciences*, *18*, 2918–2926.

Lo, C., et al. (2017). Glucose-lowering agents for treating pre-existing and new-onset diabetes in kidney transplant recipients. *Cochrane Database of Systematic Reviews (Online)*(2), CD009966.

Maciel, C. B., et al. (2017). Organ donation protocols. *Handbook of Clinical Neurology*, *140*, 409–439.

Molnar, A. O., et al. (2017). Lower serum magnesium is associated with vascular calcification in peritoneal dialysis patients: a cross sectional study. *BMC Nephrology*, *18*, 129.

National Kidney Foundation 2020. *Phosphorus and your diet*. From https://www.kidney.org/atoz/content/phosphorus. (Accessed 11 September, 2020).

National Kidney Foundation 2020: *Global Facts: About Kidney Disease*. From https://www.kidney.org/kidneydisease/global-facts-about-kidney-disease. (Accessed 10 September, 2020).

National Institute of Diabetes and Digestive and Kidney Diseases (NIDDK) 2017: *Nephrotic syndrome in adults*. From https://www.niddk.nih.gov/health-information/kidney-disease/nephrotic-syndrome-adults. (Accessed 14 September, 2020).

Niizuma, S., et al. (2017). Renocardiovascular biomarkers: from the perspective of managing chronic kidney disease and cardiovascular disease. *Frontiers in Cardiovascular Medicine*, *4*, 10.

Starr, M. C., & Hingorani, S. R. (2018). Prematurity and future kidney health: the growing risk of chronic kidney disease. *Current Opinion in Pediatrics*, *30*, 228–235.

University of California San Francisco Medical Center: Guidelines for a low sodium diet, n.d. From www.ucsfhealth.org/education/guidelines_for_a_low_sodium_diet/. (Accessed 14 September, 2020).

Uy, N., et al. (2015). Effects of gluten-free, dairy-free diet on childhood nephrotic syndrome and gut microbiota. *Pediatric Research*, *77*, 252–255.

Wang, C. S., & Greenbaum, L. A. (2019). Nephrotic Syndrome. *Pediatric Clinics of North America*, *66*, 73–85.

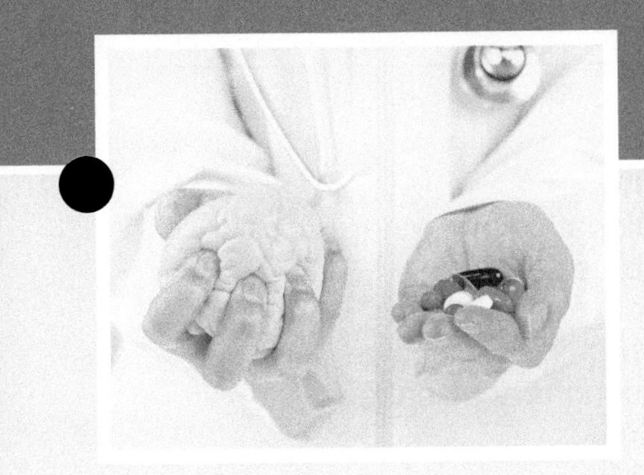

19

Nutrition for Neuro-Psychiatric Disorders

Changes in gut microbiota can modulate the peripheral and central nervous systems, resulting in altered brain functioning and suggesting the existence of a microbiota gut–brain axis. Diet can also change the profile of gut microbiota and, thereby, behavior. Effects of bacteria on the nervous system cannot be disassociated from effects on the immune system since the two are in constant bidirectional communication.

J. Bienenstock et al. (2015)

http://evolve.elsevier.com/GRODNER/FOUNDATIONS

LEARNING OBJECTIVES

- Explain the rationale for nutrition interventions that alter the microbiome for neurodegenerative disorders such as Alzheimer's disease (AD), Parkinson's disease (PD), and amyotrophic lateral sclerosis (ALS).
- Identify foodborne illnesses after which Guillain-Barré syndrome (GBS) may occur.
- Discuss the relationship of food-related triggers to migraine occurrence.
- List two neurologic disorders for which a plant-based or Mediterranean dietary pattern is suggested.
- Compare and contrast the eating disorders (EDs) anorexia nervosa (AN) and binge-eating disorder (BED).
- Assess the similarities of nutritional requirements for bipolar spectrum, depression, and schizophrenia.

NUTRITION IN BRAIN HEALTH

Transmission of maternal microbes to the offspring is critical for proper wiring of the gut–brain axis, immunity, and metabolic development. This transmission is altered by various factors such as Cesarean delivery, gestational age at birth, the use of antibiotics in early life, infant feeding, and hygiene practices. Inflammatory processes, infections, and host immune responses cause chronic neurologic damage. Psychiatric and metabolic disorders are also linked: diabetes, hypertension, insulin resistance, metabolic syndrome, obesity, attention deficit disorders, depression, psychosis, sleep apnea, inflammation, autism, and schizophrenia (SCZ) operate through common gut–brain pathways.

The brain requires a steady stream of glucose, has a lipoprotein membrane around each cell, and depends on amino acids to make neurotransmitters. Thus, a healthy nervous system and the blood–brain barrier need a varied diet with multiple nutrients to work properly.

Bioactive nutrients are modifiable factors capable of preserving a healthy brain status (Abate et al., 2017). Deficiencies of vitamins B_{12}, B_6, C, or E, folic acid, iron, selenium, and zinc imitate the effects of radiation on the body by damaging DNA. Insufficient dietary precursors (tryptophan, tyrosine, and choline) affect the functioning of nerves and neurotransmitters.

The **Maillard reaction** is another factor. It is a complex series of reactions that involve a spontaneous chemical reaction between carbohydrates and tissue proteins. The end-products are called **advanced glycation end-products (AGEs)** (Fig. 19.1). AGEs contribute to oxidative stress, causing aging and neurodegeneration in Alzheimer's disease as well as diabetes, cardiovascular disease, and other inflammatory conditions (Byun et al., 2017). To decrease the effects of AGEs, cook foods at low temperatures with water-based moisture (steaming, stewing, poaching, and braising) instead of frying.

Different pathogens directly trigger neurotoxic pathways and are risk factors for neurodegenerative disorders. For neurologic problems, team members must collaborate to discuss patient health status, medical therapies, prescribed medicines, herbs and alternative therapies, and appropriate nutrition treatments. Prevention of malnutrition, restoration of feeding abilities, and improved nutritional quality of life are priorities in these disorders.

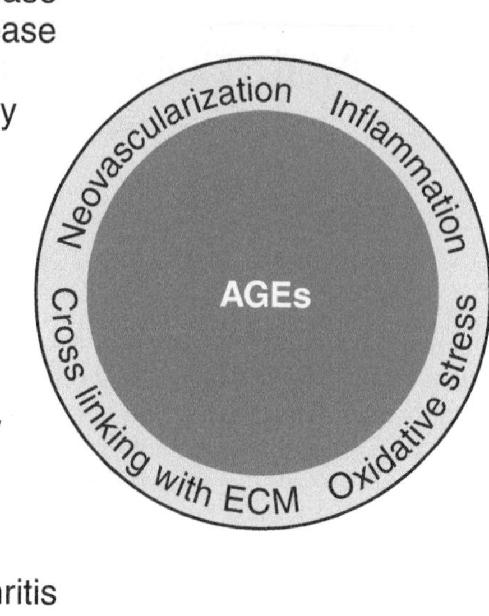

Fig. 19.1 Advanced glycation end-products (AGEs) and their effects. ECM, Extracellular matrix. (Modified from Byun, K., et al. Advanced glycation end-products produced systemically and by macrophages: A common contributor to inflammation and degenerative diseases, *Pharmacology & Therapeutics* 177:44–55, 2017.)

NEUROLOGIC DISORDERS

Alzheimer's Disease

Alzheimer's disease (AD) involves progressive deterioration of intellect, memory, personality, and self-care. It is the most common form of dementia. Early stages of AD manifest with memory loss and other cognitive changes (Box 19.1).

Neurodegeneration can occur from chronic oxidative stress. High levels of circulating lipids and glucose imbalances cause lipid peroxidation, diminish the antioxidant systems, and create neuronal damage and an insulin-resistant brain state (Rojas-Gutierrez et al., 2017). A diet rich in vitamins and polyphenols and low in saturated fatty acids is needed.

BOX 19.1 Ten Warning Signs of Alzheimer's Disease

- Memory loss that disrupts daily life
- Challenges in planning or solving problems
- Difficulty completing familiar tasks at home, at work, at leisure
- Confusion with time or place
- Trouble understanding visual images or spatial relationships
- New problems with words in speaking or writing
- Misplacing things and losing the ability to retrace steps
- Decreased or poor judgment
- Withdrawal from work or social activities
- Changes in mood or personality

(Data from Alzheimer's Association: *Know the 10 signs; early detection matters.* Accessed 19 September, 2020, from http://www.alz.org/national/documents/checklist_10signs.pdf.)

Food and Nutrition Therapies

Foods rich in vitamins B6 and B12 and folate help lower elevated total homocysteine (tHcy) levels, which can be a common problem. Many fruits, vegetables, spices, omega-3 fatty acids, marine products, and the Mediterranean diet (Fig. 19.2) are beneficial, as are natural sources of vitamins C and E, zinc, copper, and selenium.

Good sources of antioxidants with antiinflammatory properties should also be consumed. Blueberries, cranberries, kale, strawberries, spinach, and coffee intake may improve cognitive function. The flavone apigenin is abundantly present in common fruits, such as grapefruit, and vegetables, such as parsley, celery, onions, oranges, tea, chamomile, artichokes, and dried oregano. Finally, curcumin, the active ingredient in turmeric, has beneficial effects on brain health as an antioxidant and through its amyloid β-binding, antiinflammatory, tau inhibition, metal chelation, neurogenesis activity, and synaptogenesis promotion (Salehi et al., 2020). Whereas current formulations have been limited by poor bioavailability, new drugs are under study for use with Alzheimer's and other neurological conditions.

Application to nursing. Patients with AD are often malnourished; assessing nutrition status is essential to providing care. As the disease progresses, the ability to recognize hunger, thirst, and satiety is impaired and weight loss and dehydration are common. Because of forgetfulness, decreased appetite, and constant pacing, it is important to monitor intake, assist with feeding, provide nutrition supplements, and try to decrease mealtime distractions.

Another concern is caregiving. Depending on the stage, levels of care are more demanding. Of the seven stages of AD, stages 6 and 7 require the most assistance. Incontinence and dehydration can be concerns. Box 19.2 discusses other issues.

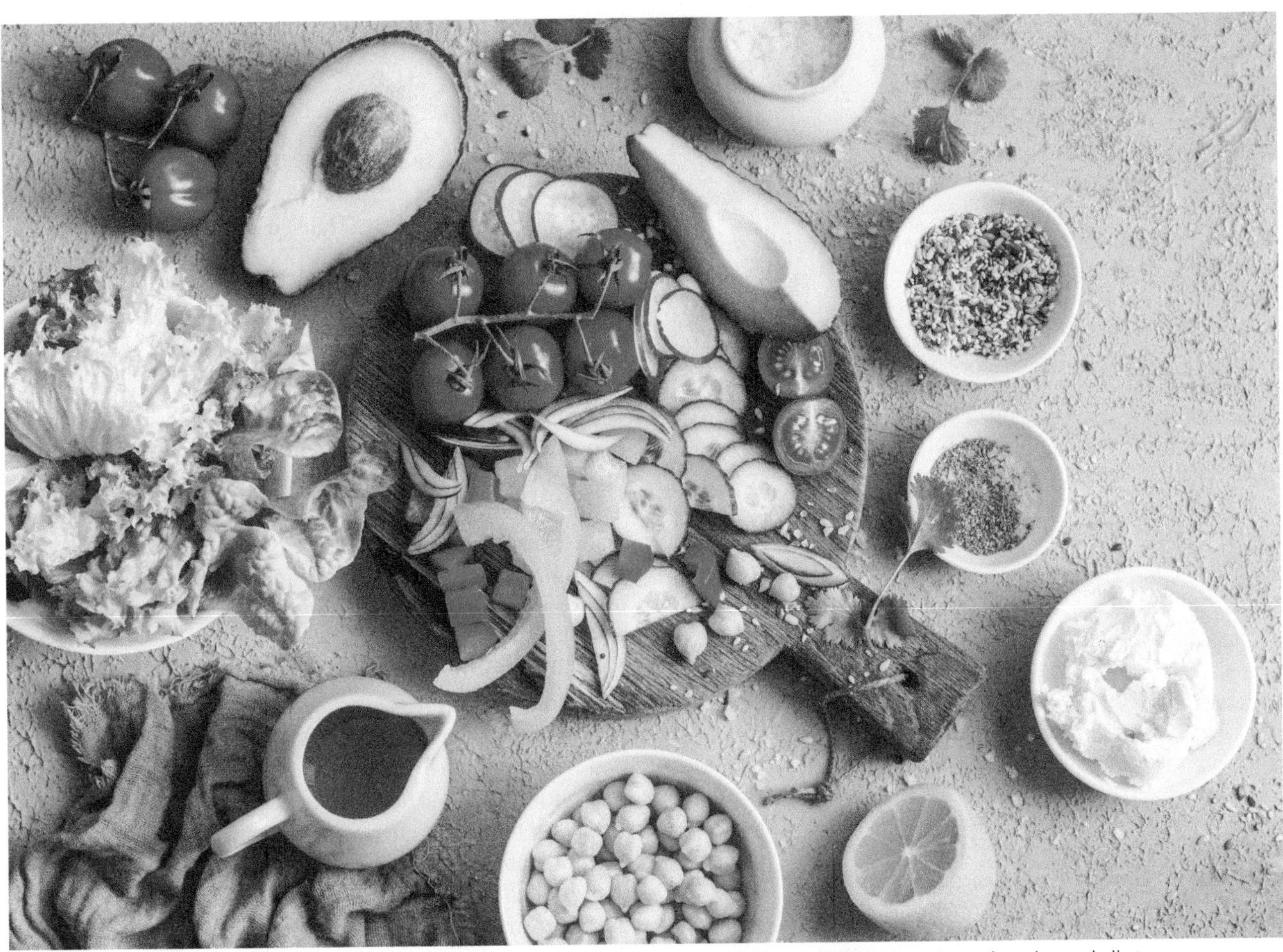

Fig. 19.2 Foods of the Mediterranean Diet. The Mediterranean diet promotes a plant-based diet with plenty of fruits, vegetables, bread and other grains, potatoes, beans, nuts and seeds; olive oil as a primary fat source; and dairy products, eggs, fish and poultry in low to moderate amounts. (From © iStock Photo; Credit: OksanaKiian.)

The *Cultural Diversity and Nutrition* box Inadequate Treatment in Dementia discusses cultural issues in relation to delayed recognition and treatment.

Amyotrophic Lateral Sclerosis

Amyotrophic lateral sclerosis (ALS), also known as Lou Gehrig's disease, is a progressive degenerative motor neuron disease that destroys nerve cells from the spinal cord to the muscle cells in adults. Persistent environmental pollutants, including pesticides, represent a modifiable risk factor involved in ALS (Sun et al., 2017). Symptoms of ALS include muscular wasting, atrophy, difficulty speaking, drooling, loss of reflexes, respiratory infections or failure, spastic gait, and weakness. Both upper and lower motor neurons are affected, with progressive paralysis and respiratory failure.

Food and Nutrition Therapies

ALS alters energy intake and expenditure. Respiratory failure occurs after loss of bulbar, cervical, and thoracic motor neurons. The inspiratory lung muscles are affected. Malnutrition occurs from elevated metabolic needs and swallowing dysfunction in the lower set of cranial nerves. This malnutrition produces neuromuscular weakness and adversely affects patients' quality of life.

Dysphagia, depression, cognitive impairment, difficulty with self-feeding and meal preparation, hypermetabolism, anxiety, respiratory insufficiency, and fatigue with meals increase the risk of malnutrition. With dysphagia, different types of thickening agents should be offered for better patient compliance (Burgos et al., 2017).

Early and frequent nutrition assessment and intervention are essential to prevent and manage malnutrition. Implementation of an adequate calorie diet, dietary texture modification, use of adaptive eating utensils, and placement of a percutaneous endoscopic gastrostomy (PEG) tube will be important considerations. PEG insertion is safe even with significant respiratory muscle weakness if performed by a qualified team (Kak et al., 2017).

Application to nursing. Mechanical ventilation is usually necessary. Strategies must be in place to position the patient to a maximal mechanical advantage, prevent aspiration pneumonia, reduce secretions, and provide noninvasive positive pressure ventilation.

In later stages, when PEG feeding is needed, it may not improve quality of life. Individuals have the right to refuse tube

BOX 19.2 Final Stages in Alzheimer's Disease

Stage 6: Severe Cognitive Decline

People with severe cognitive decline:

- Lose awareness of recent experiences as well as of their surroundings.
- Remember their own name but have difficulty with their personal history.
- Distinguish familiar and unfamiliar faces but have trouble remembering the name of a spouse or caregiver.
- Need help dressing properly and may, without supervision, make mistakes such as putting pajamas over daytime clothes or shoes on the wrong feet.
- Experience major changes in sleep patterns—sleeping during the day and becoming restless at night.
- Need help handling details of toileting (e.g., flushing the toilet, wiping or disposing of tissue properly).
- Have increasingly frequent trouble controlling their bladder or bowels.

Stage 7: Very Severe Cognitive Decline

People in stage 7 of Alzheimer's disease:

- Lose the ability to respond to their environment, to carry on a conversation and, eventually, to control movement; may still say words or phrases.
- Experience major personality and behavioral changes, including suspiciousness and delusions (such as believing that their caregiver is an impostor) and compulsive, repetitive behavior, like hand-wringing or tissue shredding.
- Tend to wander or become lost.
- Need help with much of their daily personal care, including eating and using the toilet.
- May also lose the ability to smile, to sit without support, and to hold their heads up.
- Have abnormal reflexes, and their muscles grow rigid.

(Data from Alzheimer's Association: *Late-stage caregiving.* Accessed 19 September, 2020, from www.alz.org/care/alzheimers-late-end-stage-caregiving.asp#food.)

CULTURAL DIVERSITY AND NUTRITION

Inadequate Treatment in Dementia

Patients of minority groups often receive a delayed diagnosis or inadequate treatment for dementia. Ethnic and racial differences in biologic risk factors, such as genetics and cardiovascular disease, may help to explain disparities in the incidence and prevalence of Alzheimer's disease (AD), whereas race-specific cultural factors affect diagnosis and treatment.

Cultural factors include differences in perceptions about what is normal aging and what is not, lack of adequate access to medical care, and issues of trust between minority groups and the medical establishment. For example, Native American and Alaska Natives are considered an "invisible minority" but are one of the nation's fastest growing populations (Garrett et al., 2015). In many cases, this group has hidden health care needs and delayed access to services. Racial biases are inherent in the cognitive screening tools widely used by clinicians. Controlling for literacy level can mitigate these biases.

To further characterize diverse populations, biomarker-based diagnostic tools are used. For example, there is evidence supporting vitamin D as a causal risk factor for AD. Different populations have single nucleotide polymorphisms (SNPs) that are strongly related to serum vitamin D levels (Mokry et al., 2017). As well, preventive measures (such as statin use) to reduce risk will vary in effectiveness across the different races and ethnicities (Zissimopoulos et al., 2017).

(Data from Garrett, M.D., et al. Mental health disorders among an invisible minority: depression and dementia among American Indian and Alaska native elders, *Gerontologist* 55:227–36, 2015; Mokry, L.E., et al. Genetically decreased vitamin D and risk of Alzheimer disease, *Neurology* 87:2567–2574, 2016; Zissimopoulos, J.M., et al. Sex and race differences in the association between statin use and the incidence of Alzheimer disease, *JAMA Neurol* 74:225–232, 2017.)

feeding and prefer not to prolong their suffering. The nurses can help family members accept the decisions of the patient.

Coma

Coma is the unconscious state in which the patient is unresponsive to verbal or painful stimuli. Impaired consciousness or coma can occur from a stroke, head injury, meningitis, encephalitis, sepsis, lack of oxygen, epileptic seizure, toxic effects of alcohol or drugs, liver or kidney failure, high or low blood glucose levels, or altered body temperature. The Glasgow Coma Scale (GCS) is used to assess level of consciousness; a score of 8 or less is usually indicative of coma.

A persistent vegetative state (PVS) is a deep state of unconsciousness. PVS is not brain death. The person is still alive but unable to move or react. A patient in PVS does not have the ability to request or refuse treatment. A person may enter a minimally conscious state (MCS) after being in a coma or vegetative state, either temporarily or permanently. The doctor must determine the patient's current diagnosis.

Food and Nutrition Therapies

Nutrition support is associated with improved survival, in patients with coma. Most patients are tube fed. Enteral nutrition with a standard, polymeric enteral formula should be initiated within 24 to 48 hours after admission. Comatose patients achieving the target energy intake can avoid malnutrition and immunodeficiency (Qi et al., 2016).

Application to nursing. Patients with coma or PVS will not be able to answer questions or respond to requests; thus, a family member or legal guardian must be the advocate and assist with informed consent. Understanding the patient's wishes allows the health team and family to make valid decisions about initiating, withholding, or withdrawing artificial nutrition and hydration. Family counseling is especially important as ethical or legal issues come into play.

Epilepsy and Seizure Disorders

A seizure is the result of uncontrolled excessive neuronal discharges in the brain. Epilepsy involves a disturbance of the nervous system with recurrent seizures, loss of consciousness, convulsions, motor activity, or behavioral abnormalities. Seizures are classified by their clinical manifestation. A grand mal seizure involves an aura, a tonic phase, and a clonic phase. A petit mal seizure involves a momentary loss of consciousness. Overall, a single seizure does not imply epilepsy. Indeed, there are many forms of epilepsy, each with its own symptoms.

Food and Nutrition Therapies

The ketogenic diet (KD) is a treatment that has been used for refractory epilepsy for nearly a century. This is a high-fat, low-carbohydrate diet, individualized for each patient. The typical long-chain triglyceride KD provides 3 to 4 g of fat for every 1 g of carbohydrate and protein. This high-fat diet produces ketone bodies, which boost energy production (adenosine triphosphate [ATP]) in brain tissue. In children this diet results in benefits in seizure control, comparable to that achieved with antiepileptic drugs.

Bone health, metabolism of vitamin D, and calcium absorption are impaired with antiepileptic drugs. Problems include

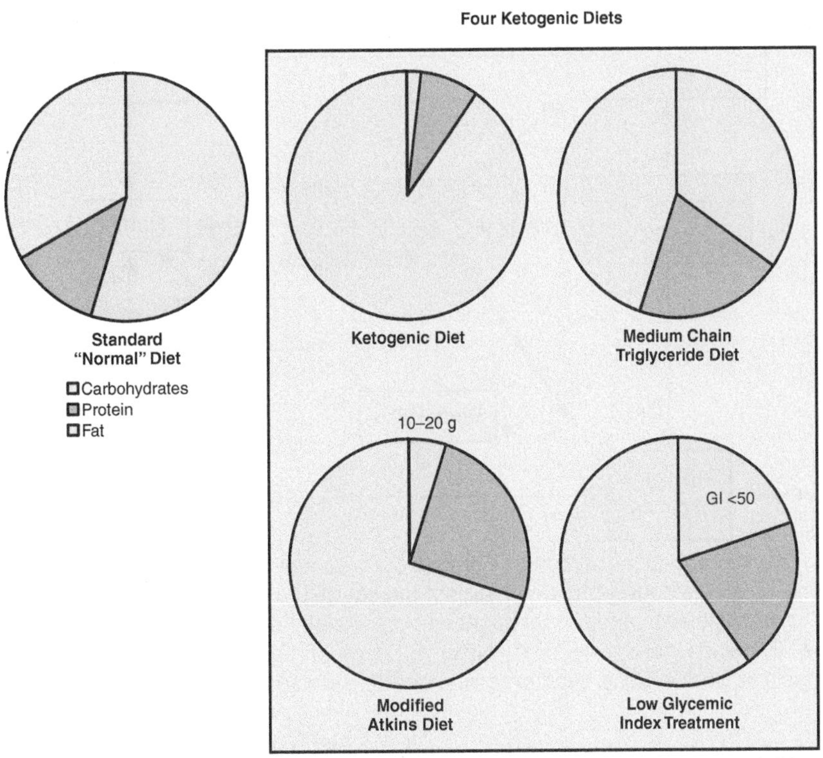

Four Ketogenic Diets

Standard "Normal" Diet

Carbohydrates
Protein
Fat

Ketogenic Diet

Medium Chain Triglyceride Diet

10–20 g

GI <50

Modified Atkins Diet

Low Glycemic Index Treatment

Fig. 19.3 Ketogenic diet comparisons. Four ketogenic diets are available, with variable effectiveness in seizure control. Individualization is the key. (From Regulatory Affairs Professionals Society. The Ketogenic Diet for Drug-Resistant Epileptic Patients. Modified from: https://www.raps.org/regulatory-focus%E2%84%A2/news-articles/2017/10/intractable-epilepsy-and-the-value-of-formulated-ketogenic-diet-products. Accessed 18 September, 2020.)

bone mineral density loss and double or triple the risk of fracture (Fraser et al., 2015). Low-dose vitamin D supplementation should be prescribed, and compliance followed up.

The KD is supervised by a dietitian who monitors the nutritional status and can teach what can and cannot be eaten. If patients find the diet difficult to tolerate, a medium-chain triglyceride (MCT) diet improves overall acceptance. MCTs are quickly digested and are more ketogenic than long-chain triglycerides. Although overall caloric restriction may improve the efficacy of the ketogenic diet, the diet may slow growth in children. An alternative diet that is not as strict uses a low–glycemic index treatment, with more liberal total carbohydrate intake. The modified Atkins diet can also promote seizure control (Martin-McGill et al., 2020). Fig. 19.3 shows the differences between a normal diet, the ketogenic diet and the modified Atkins diet.

Application to nursing. The KD can be challenging. There are side effects, such as dehydration, constipation, high serum cholesterol, and even kidney stones. The patient and family members will need a great deal of support and education. With children, the nurse can share ideas listed in the *Teaching Tool* box Tips for Parents About the Ketogenic Diet.

TEACHING TOOL

Tips for Parents About the Ketogenic Diet

- Most children handle the initial fasting surprisingly well because of the promise of fewer seizures.
- Getting into a routine when fixing meals should make things easier.
- Involve your child in measuring food by guiding the child while they place food on the gram scale.
- Your child may feel hungry (because the diet restricts calories) and may try to sneak food from the refrigerator, and even from the pet's dish. Using water with saccharin and splitting meals in half may help fight hunger pains.
- Use a salad plate to present each meal, because the smaller plate makes it look as if the child is getting more food.
- If your child loves dessert, always keep a stock of homemade ice cream pops in the freezer. These are then calculated into meal plans.
- Keep a few preprepared meals in small plastic containers in the fridge. Label them carefully for your older child's use if you are not home or your child goes to a friend's house.
- Cut foods into interesting shapes to make them more appealing.
- Check with your doctor about how to handle hot days when your child perspires more than usual.

(Data from Epilepsy Foundation: Ketogenic diet, n.d. Accessed 4 August, 2017, from http://www.epilepsy.com/learn/treating-seizures-and-epilepsy/dietary-therapies/ketogenic-diet.)

Guillain-Barré Syndrome

Guillain-Barré syndrome (GBS) is a rare, acute inflammatory demyelinating polyneuropathy with rapidly increasing weakness, numbness, pain, and paralysis of the legs, arms, trunk, face, and respiratory muscles. The exact cause is unknown, but it often occurs a few days or weeks after infection with a respiratory illness, influenza, or *Campylobacter jejuni.*

Campylobacter jejuni is a common trigger for GBS, igniting autoimmunity as a response (Ebrahim Soltani et al., 2019).

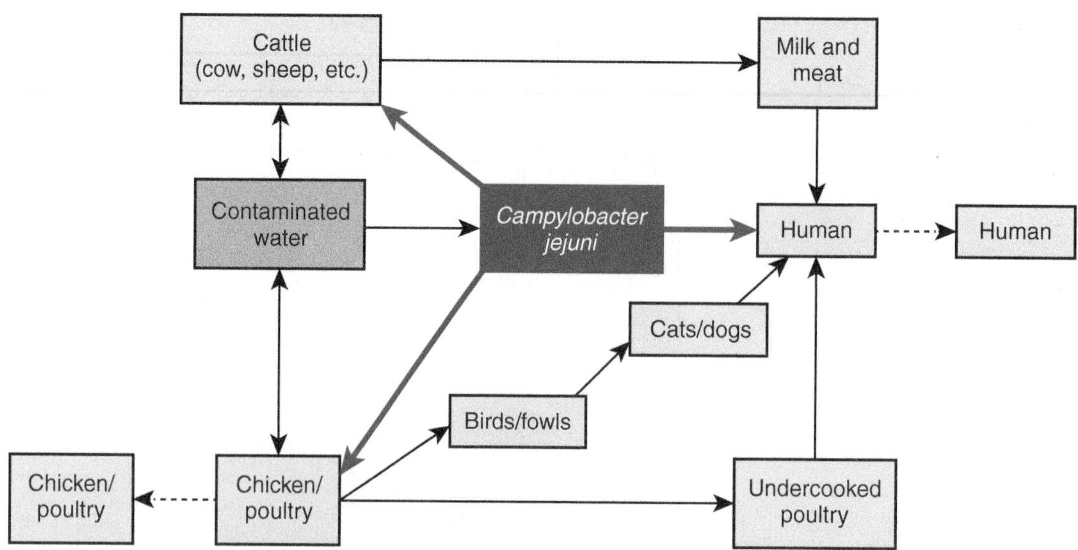

Fig. 19.4 Sources and transmission of *Campylobacter jejuni.* Chicken is a natural reservoir of *C. jejuni.* Sometimes antibodies produced against the bacterium mimic the host nerve gangliosides, resulting in demyelination and axonal degeneration of peripheral nerves that cause Guillain-Barré syndrome. (Modified from Nyati, K.K., Nyati, R., Role of *Campylobacter jejuni* infection in the pathogenesis of Guillain-Barré syndrome: an update, *Biomed Res Int* 2013:852195, 2013.)

Contaminated water, undercooked poultry, and unpasteurized milk are often sources (Fig. 19.4). The bacterium resides in the epithelial layer of the human gastrointestinal tract and causes bloody diarrhea, fever, cramping, and headache.

Older individuals are at greater risk. GBS may progress to respiratory failure, paralysis of lower extremities, or quadriplegia. Patients may experience unstable blood pressure, aspiration, impaired speech, muscular pain, low-grade fever, tachycardia, and chronic urinary tract infections. With proper care, most patients recover completely.

Food and Nutrition Therapies

In patients with GBS who have dysphagia and difficulty with chewing, tube feeding may be required. In later stages of the disease, weakness or paralysis may inhibit the patient's ability to self-feed, leading to weight loss and anorexia. Discussion about safe food handling is important for preventing reinfection, including proper cooking temperatures for chicken and the use of pasteurized milk products.

Application to nursing. Sometimes ventilatory assistance is needed. Although most people recover from GBS within a few weeks, some have residual effects for years. Some may need intensive care support followed by wheelchair assistance. No treatment has been totally effective. Patients and family members need support and education on how to manage care for GBS, especially when dysphagia and constipation occur.

Huntington's Disease

Huntington's disease (HD) is a genetic neurodegenerative disorder with symptoms that are linked to progressive dysfunction and neuronal death; the causative gene is mutated huntington (HTT) protein (Carroll et al., 2015). Prevalence is high in populations of European ancestry (Lee et al., 2015). HD generally develops between ages 30 and 50 years, with chorea, cerebral degeneration, cognitive decline, and speech difficulties. Weight loss, increased proinflammatory signaling, and behavioral changes begin years before the movement disorder. Unfortunately, there is no cure, and death is often a result of pneumonia, suicide, or a fall.

Food and Nutrition Therapies

Nutritional intake is an important consideration. Polyphenols play a beneficial role in the prevention and the progress of chronic diseases related to inflammation, including neurodegeneration (Yahfoufi et al., 2018). Thus, a diet rich in plant foods with citrus fruits, grapes, berries, cocoa, nuts, green tea, and coffee is recommended. Folic acid, coenzyme Q10, and unsaturated fatty acids are also important for neuroprotection. When diets of high glycemic index deliver sugar to the blood rapidly and exacerbate symptoms, carbohydrate control may be needed.

Because of dysphagia and the inability to self-feed, patients are at high risk for aspiration and malnutrition. Although stem cell transplantation shows promise, it is not yet available as a treatment modality.

Application to nursing. Remotivation therapy leads to increased self-awareness, greater self-esteem, and improved quality of life. Many people with HD require texture-modified diets (Moorhouse & Fisher, 2016). In later stages, tube feeding may be required. Eventually, there is complete dependency and the need for full-time care.

Migraine Headache

Migraine is a brain disorder resulting from altered sensory stimuli and trigeminal nerve dysfunction. Migraine headaches (migraines) affect millions of people in the United States. They often begin between the ages of 10 and 40 years and diminish after age 50 years; they are more common in women than in men.

Lack of food or sleep, exposure to light, anxiety, stress, fatigue, caffeine withdrawal, or hormonal irregularities can set off an attack. Nausea, vomiting, and acute sensitivity to light or sound may occur along with headache, vasospasm, and visual disturbances.

Medical management includes high-dose aspirin, in doses from 900 to 1300 mg, taken at the onset of symptoms as an effective and safe treatment option (Biglione et al., 2020). Acupuncture, massage, yoga, biofeedback, meditation, spinal manipulation, chiropractic care, some supplements and botanicals, diet alteration, and hydrotherapy are commonly suggested (Millstine et al., 2017).

Food and Nutrition Therapies

Food allergy is common in people with migraine. Food sensitivities often occur within 24 hours after consumption of the offending food or beverage. Egg white and cow's milk are foods that may trigger migraines in sensitive individuals. It is important that testing be done before nutrient-rich foods are eliminated from the patient's diet. Treatment begins with a headache-food diary and the selective avoidance of foods presumed to trigger attacks. Migraines may also be reduced with intake of fish oil and olive oil.

Application to nursing. Exercise, relaxation, massage therapy, biofeedback, and adequate sleep may reduce discomfort. Long-term prophylactic use of low-dose aspirin is effective for some individuals. Patients should improve their sleep habits, limit caffeine intake, pursue regular exercise, and identify triggers. People who are prone to migraines are at risk for stroke and should be monitored carefully. See the *Personal Perspectives* box Thank Goodness for Menopause!

> **PERSONAL PERSPECTIVES**
>
> ***Thank Goodness for Menopause!***
>
> It was always a nuisance, those monthly periods from age 13 years onward. However, the bigger nuisance involved migraine headaches, which would come insidiously and without warning! The migraines started in my teens and continued for nearly four decades. Often, I would come home from work with a pounding headache; I would sleep for an hour or two before dinner could be started. If I did not close my eyes, the migraine would just bring more misery. Gradually, in my fifties the headaches began to subside. I never thought I would say it, but thank goodness for menopause!
>
> **Sylvia Escott-Stump**
> *Winterville, NC*

Multiple Sclerosis

Multiple sclerosis (MS) is an autoimmune disease with complex genetic and environmental risk factors. Low serum levels of vitamin D, smoking, childhood obesity, and infection with the Epstein-Barr virus are likely triggers (Dobson & Giovannoni, 2019). Healthy gut bacteria and their products may protect against inflammation.

MS has a high incidence among Caucasians and affects women two to three times as often as men. The age at onset is between 20 and 40 years. MS leads to scarring and the loss of myelin sheath, the insulating material around nerve fibers. The disease causes progressive or episodic nerve degeneration and disability. Symptoms include tingling; numbness in arms, legs, trunk, or face; double vision; fatigue; weakness; clumsiness; tremor; stiffness; sensory impairment; loss of position sense; and respiratory problems. Dysphagia, spasticity, and bladder dysfunction are long-term consequences.

Food and Nutrition Therapies

There is insufficient evidence to determine whether supplementation with antioxidants or other dietary interventions have any impact on MS-related outcomes (Parks et al., 2020). Safe levels of vitamin D, food sources of omega-3 fatty acids, and an antioxidant-rich Mediterranean diet can certainly be promoted.

Application to nursing. Patients with MS may have periods of remission; others may experience a progressive decline. For some, full dependency for many activities of daily living or a wheelchair becomes necessary. Adaptations for dining, shopping, and cooking at home require interprofessional collaboration with the physical therapist, the occupational therapist, and the registered dietitian (Fig. 19.5).

Myasthenia Gravis

Myasthenia gravis (MG) is an autoimmune disorder caused by autoantibodies at the neuromuscular junction that attack acetylcholine receptors. The attack prevents acetylcholine from stimulating muscle contraction. The neuromuscular junction lies beyond the protection of the blood–brain barrier and is particularly vulnerable to antibody-mediated attack. MG involves the thymus gland. Initially the ocular muscles are affected, with intermittent drooping eyelids (**ptosis**) and double vision (**diplopia**). Weak voice, pneumonia or respiratory arrest, and sleep apnea are also commonly found.

A few forms of MG are congenital. Acquired neuromuscular junction disorders include botulism, autoimmune MG, and drug-induced MG. When MG is suspected, an edrophonium (Tensilon) test involves insertion of a small intravenous catheter through which the agent is given, blocking degradation of acetylcholine. The short-term availability of acetylcholine results in improved muscle function, often in the eye area.

Removal of the thymus gland works for some patients. For others, general immunosuppression becomes the primary treatment. Broad-based immunotherapies, such as corticosteroids, azathioprine, mycophenolate, tacrolimus, and cyclosporine, have been effective in controlling symptoms of myasthenia but have many side effects (Menon et al., 2020). New treatments include autologous stem cell transplantation and drugs that target specific immune cells.

Food and Nutrition Therapies

Dysphagia is a concern in patients with MG. Other concerns requiring nutritional intervention include diabetes and thyroid conditions for which dietary alterations will be necessary. The Mediterranean diet, antioxidant-rich foods, and

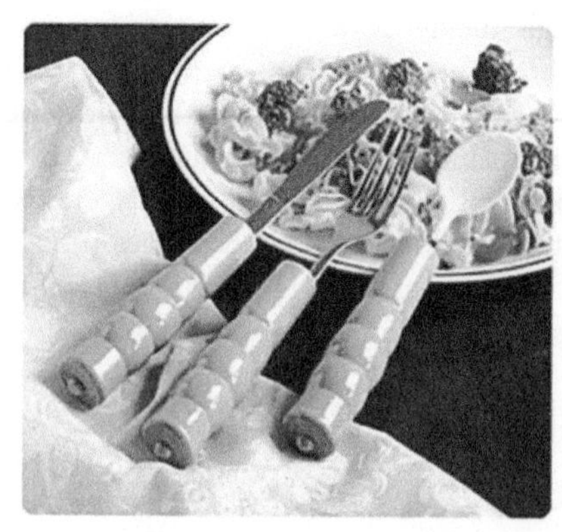
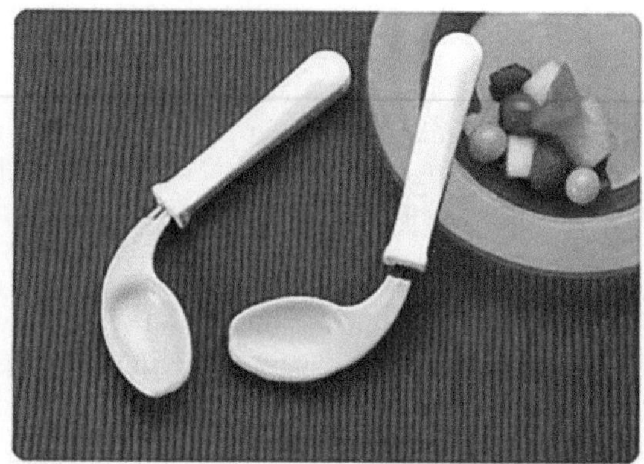
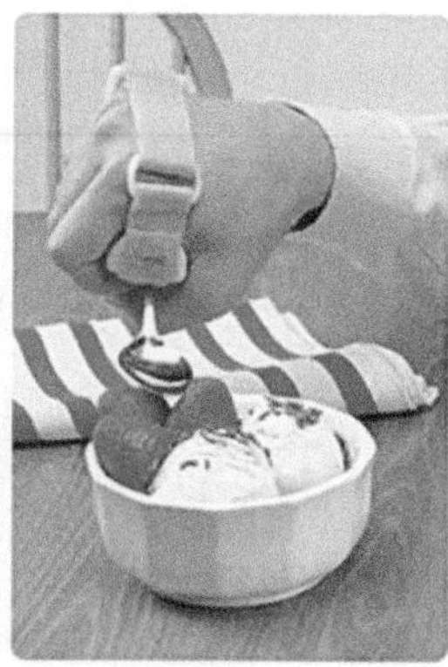

Fig. 19.5 Adaptive feeding devices. The person living with multiple sclerosis may benefit from adaptive feeding devices. The occupational therapist can help determine which tools are suitable. From Swallowing Disorder Foundation. Adaptive Feeding Devices. By: Debbie Zwiefelhofer, RDN, LD. Accessed 19 September 2020. https://swallowingdisorderfoundation.com/adaptive-feeding-devices/.

omega-3 fatty acids are healthy choices. Although vitamin D is a potential target for treating autoimmune diseases, large, double-blind, placebo-controlled, randomized studies are needed.

Application to nursing. Patients with MG present with fatigue and weakness. Assistance with feeding may be required. With immunosuppressive therapies, patients may experience nausea, vomiting, or diarrhea as well as higher risk for infections.

Parkinson's Disease

Parkinson's disease (PD) is a neurodegenerative disorder that affects 1% to 2% of persons 60 years and older. Losses of dopaminergic neurons occur in the brain. Genetics, exposure to pesticides and herbicides, traumatic brain injury, history of melanoma, and oxidative stress have all been implicated. Symptoms are shown in Box 19.3.

BOX 19.3 Symptoms of Parkinson's Disease

- Tremor of hands, arms, legs, jaw, and face
- Rigidity or stiffness of limbs and trunk
- Slowness of gait and movement (bradykinesia)
- Postural or coordination difficulty
- Problems with speech
- Depression and dementia-related symptoms

(Modified from Parkinson Disease Foundation: *What is Parkinson disease?* Accessed 19 September, 2020, from https://www.parkinson.org/Understanding-Parkinsons/What-is-Parkinsons/Stages-of-Parkinsons.)

Approaches such as deep brain stimulation and treatment with levodopa-carbidopa enteral suspension can help alleviate medication-resistant tremor and dyskinesias (Armstrong & Okun, 2020). Although levodopa is required, its long-term use is associated with potentially disabling motor complications. Patients with PD may also develop nonmotor symptoms such as psychosis, depression, cognitive impairment, autonomic disturbances, and sleep disturbances.

Nonpharmacologic approaches (such as exercise and physical, occupational, and speech therapies) are beneficial (Armstrong & Okun, 2020). Progressive resistance exercise and dance therapy are promising.

Food and Nutrition Therapies

Inflammation is part of the problem; thus, a healthy microbiome is important; see Fig. 19.6. Adherence to a Mediterranean diet is associated with slower cognitive decline. A low saturated fat intake is also desirable (Box 19.4). Vitamin D, fish sources of omega-3 fatty acids, whey proteins, caffeine, an antioxidant-rich diet, probiotics, prebiotics and symbiotic are being examined for their effects (Gazerani, 2019).

Weight loss is a common finding and should be addressed because PD patients are at a high risk of malnutrition. Factors affecting nutritional status are age, motor symptoms and stage severity, rigidity-dominant type, and thyroid hormone replacement therapy (Tomic et al., 2017).

Application to nursing. Unintentional weight loss is common in the patient with PD, from increased energy expenditure because of tremor, dyskinesias, and rigidity. Thus, most patients require either a longer time with meals, assistance, or dysphagic dietary adaptations. Extra calories and protein may also be needed.

Stroke

A stroke or cerebrovascular accident (CVA) involves damage to a portion of the brain resulting from loss of blood supply after a blood vessel spasm, clot, or rupture. Inflammation in the neural cells plays a central role in the pathogenesis of the disease.

Obesity, heavy or binge drinking, physical inactivity, smoking, or use of cocaine or methamphetamines are lifestyle risks that can be controlled. Other risk factors include hypertension, diabetes mellitus, high cholesterol, atrial fibrillation, heart failure, oral contraceptive or estrogen use, and obstructive sleep apnea. Men have a higher risk than women at a younger age, but women are more likely to die from strokes.

Sporadic strokes can occur, but most of those have a genetic component. Transient ischemic attacks (TIAs) are brief episodes of blood loss to the brain from a clot or an embolism; TIAs often precede a larger stroke.

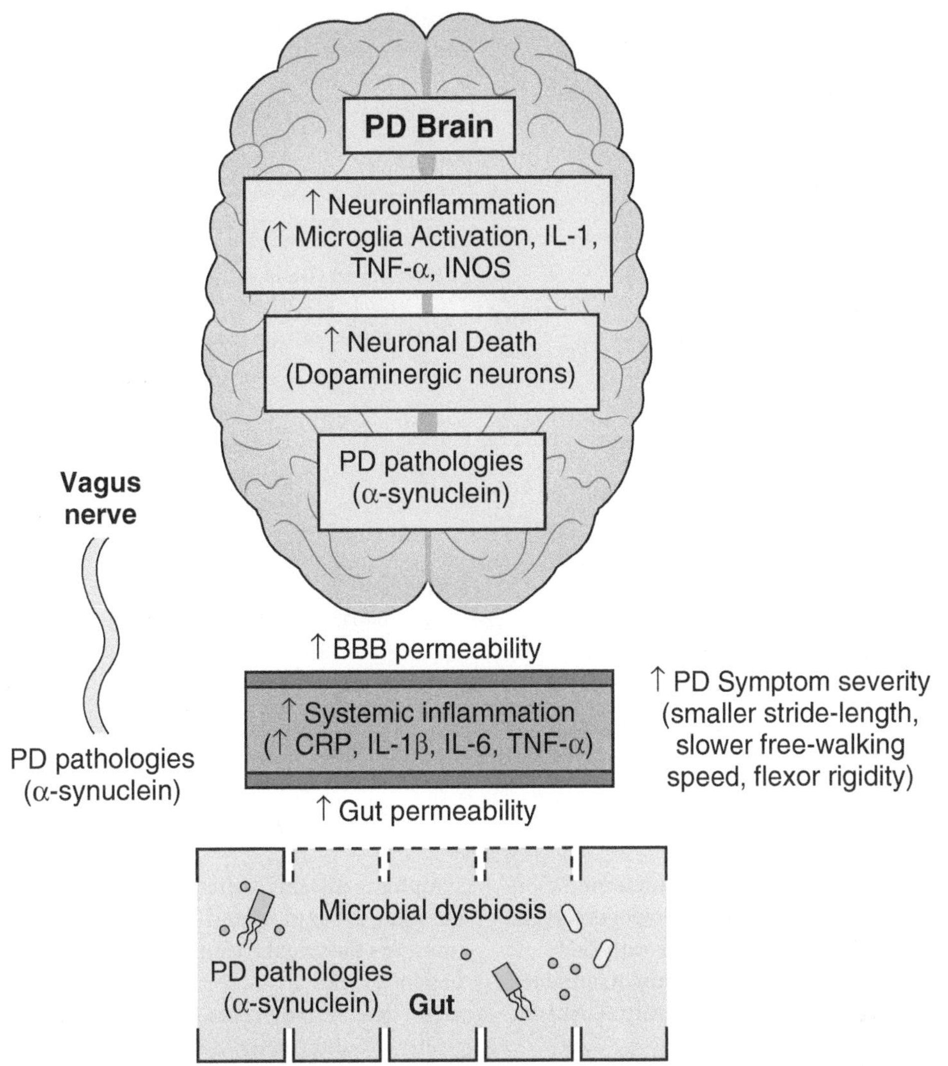

Fig. 19.6 Gut microbiota and Parkinson's disease. The role of gut microbiota in the pathogenesis of Parkinson's disease. *BBB*, blood brain barrier; *CRP*, C-reactive protein; *IL*, interleukin; *iNOS*, inducible nitric oxide synthase; *PD*, Parkinson's disease; *TNF*, tumor necrosis factor. (Modified from Gazerani, P. Probiotics for Parkinson's Disease. Int J Mol Sci. 20:4121, 2019.)

Food and Nutrition Therapies

Intake of red and processed meats, refined grains, sweets, and desserts should be limited. Instead, offer high quality protein; magnesium and potassium from cruciferous and green leafy vegetables; citrus fruits; and carotenoids should be used. Both fish and omega-3 fatty acids seem to prevent thrombotic strokes. Thus, a plant-based Mediterranean diet is recommended.

Application to nursing. The patient who has suffered a stroke needs medical treatment within 60 minutes. Left-sided CVA affects sight and hearing most commonly, including the ability to see where foods are placed on a plate or tray. Patients with a right-hemisphere, bilateral, or brainstem CVA have significant problems with self-feeding, swallowing, and speech.

Motor deficits may occur with muscle weakness of the tongue and lips. With nerve damage, lack of coordination and sensory deficits occur, including the inability to feel food in the mouth. Cognitive deficits include difficulty sustaining attention, poor short-term memory, visual field problems, impulsiveness, aphasia, and judgment problems such as not knowing how much food to take or what to do with the food once it reaches the mouth.

Each case is unique. The interprofessional treatment team may include the neurologist, a rehabilitation doctor (physiatrist), nurse, dietitian, physical therapist, occupational therapist, recreational therapist, speech therapist, social worker, case manager, psychologist, or psychiatrist.

PSYCHIATRIC CONDITIONS

Eating Disorders

Anorexia Nervosa and Avoidant/Restrictive Food Intake Disorder

Anorexia nervosa (AN) is an eating disorder in which the patient severely rejects food, causing extreme weight loss, low

BOX 19.4 Colorful Antioxidant-Rich Foods

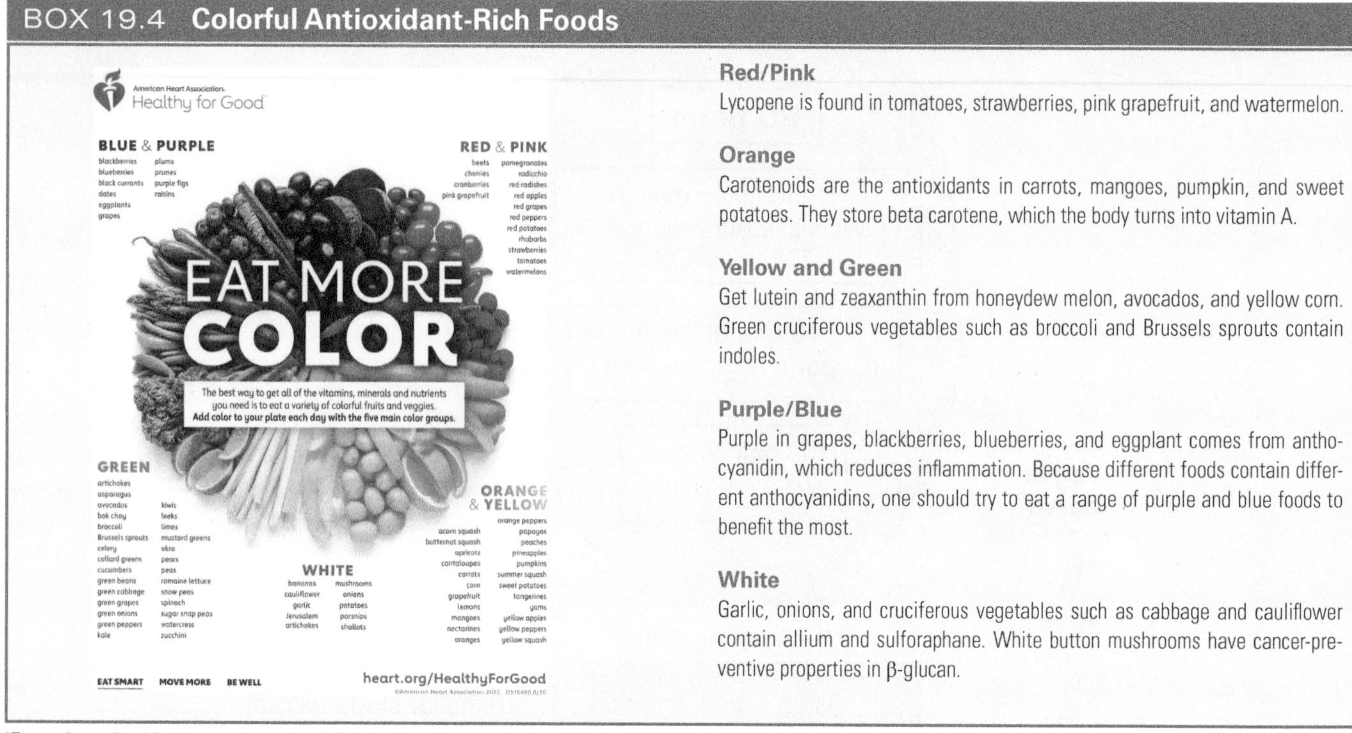

Red/Pink

Lycopene is found in tomatoes, strawberries, pink grapefruit, and watermelon.

Orange

Carotenoids are the antioxidants in carrots, mangoes, pumpkin, and sweet potatoes. They store beta carotene, which the body turns into vitamin A.

Yellow and Green

Get lutein and zeaxanthin from honeydew melon, avocados, and yellow corn. Green cruciferous vegetables such as broccoli and Brussels sprouts contain indoles.

Purple/Blue

Purple in grapes, blackberries, blueberries, and eggplant comes from anthocyanidin, which reduces inflammation. Because different foods contain different anthocyanidins, one should try to eat a range of purple and blue foods to benefit the most.

White

Garlic, onions, and cruciferous vegetables such as cabbage and cauliflower contain allium and sulforaphane. White button mushrooms have cancer-preventive properties in β-glucan.

(From America Heart Association. Eat More Color Infographic. Accessed 19 September, 2020 https://www.heart.org/en/healthy-living/healthy-eating/add-color/eat-more-color.). Reprinted with permission © 2020 American Heart Association, Inc.

basal metabolic rate, and exhaustion. The severe undernutrition causes adaptive endocrine changes including hypogonadism, growth hormone resistance, low insulin-like growth factor 1 (IGF-1) levels, hypercortisolemia, altered secretion of appetite-regulating hormones, and low bone mineral density (Baskaran et al., 2017).

The common age of onset is between ages 12 and 25 years, mostly in girls. However, 10% of cases occur in men (Johns Hopkins Medicine, 2017). Signs include relentless pursuit of thinness, misperception of body image, and restrained eating, binge eating, or purging. The intense fear of becoming fat is not diminished as weight loss progresses.

Anorexic individuals are perfectionistic, meticulous, sensitive to criticism, and socially insecure. Many dancers, gymnasts, wrestlers, models, and entertainers struggle with AN.

Some women with AN who present with social and flexibility difficulties may have an unrecognized autism spectrum disorder (Westwood et al., 2018). Obsessive-compulsive disorder (OCD), anxiety, depression and behavioral inflexibility may also be present.

Early detection and treatment are important. Oral symptoms, including mucosal, dental, and saliva abnormalities, are observed in the early stages. Weight is 85% or less of former weight at diagnosis, and women usually have amenorrhea and low bone density.

The main concern is inadequate energy intake, but diet alone will not solve the eating disorder (Hay et al., 2015). Teens often fake cooperation with treatment plans, delaying recovery and leading to malnutrition. Emotion acceptance behavior therapy (EABT) is a treatment that emphasizes management of anorexic symptoms by increasing awareness of emotions, decreasing emotion avoidance, and resuming valued activities and relationships outside the eating disorder (Wildes et al., 2014). Most patients make a full recovery with treatment. Without treatment, death often occurs from cardiac arrhythmia.

In **avoidant/restrictive food intake disorder (ARFID)** patients have restrictive eating related to emotional problems or gastrointestinal symptoms. They are distinct from those with AN or BN; there is no binge eating, purging, excessive exercise, body image problems, or functional dysphagia. They are often younger than anorexia patients, but ARFID can be found at any age (Strandjord et al., 2015). ARFID patients are not just "picky eaters"; they have a longer duration of illness and a greater likelihood of comorbid medical or psychiatric symptoms (Fisher et al., 2014).

Food and nutrition therapies. Specially qualified registered dietitians should be involved in all levels of care of patients with eating disorders, including individual and group treatment programs. Enteral nutrition is the preferred route of feeding; it can increase weight and improve cognitive and physical functioning. Weight gain that is too rapid may lead to refeeding syndrome, with severe fluid and electrolyte imbalances, cardiac dysrhythmias, or sudden death; 2 kg per week weight gain is sufficient. Thus far, no specific pharmacologic treatment is available.

Application to nursing. Nurses may identify physical signs and symptoms of AN, such as amenorrhea, headaches, irritability, constipation, syncope, dizziness, loss of muscle mass, dry skin, carotenoderma (yellowing skin), hair loss, or the presence of lanugo hair. Monitor vital signs for hypotension, bradycardia, hypothermia, and orthostatic changes. For constipation, assure adequate intake of fluids, fruits, vegetables, and whole grains.

Psychological counseling will be needed. Enlisting family support is important. To assist with other treatments (such as cognitive-behavioral therapy), nurses benefit from specialized training.

Patients with ARFID report high levels of anxiety, fear of vomiting or choking, and food texture issues. Treatment includes cognitive-behavioral therapy to counteract the sensory sensitivity, lack of interest in eating, and fear of aversive consequences.

Binge-Eating Disorder and Bulimia

Binge-eating disorder (BED) involves recurrent episodes of eating over a discrete period an amount of food larger than most people would eat in the same time, a sense of lack of control over the eating episodes, rapid or secretive eating, guilt, and shame. BED is the most prevalent eating disorder in the United States, affecting 2.8 million adults (Johns Hopkins, 2020; Binge Eating Disorders, 2020). Binge eating is a serious problem, with weight cycling and psychologic distress. Chronic dieting may predispose vulnerable individuals to binge eating, alcoholism, or drug abuse.

Obese individuals with BED demonstrate more impulsivity in response to food stimuli, with loss of control over eating, consumption of more calories, more guilt and negative emotions, and more psychopathology than nonobese individuals who have BED (Montano et al., 2016). Tailored approaches and emotional regulation are important for recovery.

Bulimia nervosa (BN) is an eating disorder in which food addiction is the primary coping mechanism. Criteria for diagnosis include recurrent episodes of binge eating, a sense of lack of control, self-evaluation unduly influenced by weight or body shape, and recurrent and inappropriate compensating behavior (vomiting, use of laxatives or diuretics, fasting, excessive exercise) two times weekly for 3 months or longer. When not bingeing, individuals with BN tend to be dieting; when hungry, they may binge and purge again. Their self-worth tends to be associated with thinness. Bulimic people use food as a coping mechanism. Because disturbances in neuronal systems modulate feeding, mood, and impulse control, altered serotonin levels contribute to the disordered eating.

Food and nutrition therapies. Mindfulness-based eating awareness training (MB-EAT) involves training in mindfulness meditation and guided practices that are designed to address the core issues. Mindfulness-based approaches address binge eating, emotional eating and eating in response to external cues. Patients can also be taught the skills of intuitive eating (Richards et al., 2017).

Application to nursing. The interprofessional team approach is best coordinated with the physician, the nurse, a qualified dietitian, and a mental health professional. An appropriate exercise program under the guidance of a physical therapist may also be offered.

The family members of people with an ED need much support. Nurses can help equip parents with skills, guidance, and techniques to be a support person in the recovery process. Therapeutic conversation is one type of beneficial training.

Bipolar Disorder

Bipolar affective disorder (BPAD) is a severe chronic mental illness that is separated into three types that involve clear changes in mood, energy, and activity levels. Abnormalities in brain biochemistry and circuits are responsible for the extreme shifts in mood, energy, and functioning.

Bipolar disorders often develop in the late teens or early adult years, usually before age 25 years. In general, the later the onset of an observable mood disorder, the less severe the case. The World Health Organization reports that BPAD is the sixth leading cause of years lived with disability worldwide. Outcomes are improved with earlier diagnosis and treatment.

The most effective long-term treatments are lithium and valproic acid. Biomarker and treatment studies of omega-3 fatty acids in bipolar disorder show promise as well. Medical comorbidities are common. They can be categorized as cardiometabolic (diabetes, stroke, hyperlipidemia, metabolic syndrome); noncardiovascular (seizures, asthma, migraine headache, cancer); and substance use disorders (Sylvia et al., 2015).

Food and Nutrition Therapies

Adults with bipolar disorders are at risk for many nutrient inadequacies, as well as occasional excesses. Many signaling pathways respond to hormones and nutrition. Because healthier diets protect mental health, individuals with mood disorders could benefit from nutritional interventions to improve diet quality. The Mediterranean diet and intake of omega-3 fatty acids (from salmon, herring, tuna, etc.) are good options to implement.

Application to nursing. Anxiety disorders, posttraumatic stress disorder (PTSD), social phobia, and attention-deficit/hyperactivity disorder (ADHD) may be comorbidities with BPAD. For “dual diagnoses,” both psychotherapy and appropriate medications are important. During the depressive phase of the illness, patients may try to self-medicate with alcohol or other substances, leading to problems with abuse or dependence. Painful physical symptoms are also common. Thus, treatment of both physical and emotional symptoms associated with mood disorders may increase a patient’s chance of achieving remission. Referral to a mental health subspecialist for initiation and management of drug treatment and resources for psychotherapy are important measures (Holder, 2017).

DEPRESSION

Depression involves changes in body chemistry (neurotransmitters) because of a mix of genetics and environmental stress. Depression most often develops between 25 and 44 years. With dysthymia, depression is expressed as poor appetite or overeating, insomnia or oversleeping, low energy, fatigue, irritability, and high stress. Children and teens who have dysthymia or depression may experience frequent headaches and absences from school.

Major depressive disorder (MDD) is quite disabling and has a high morbidity rate. Persons with MDD have had at least one major depressive episode for 14 days or longer, and such episodes may be recurrent throughout their lives. Men with MDD often mask signs of depression by working long hours or drinking too much. Women may experience depression during times of hormonal change: menstruation, pregnancy, miscarriage, the postpartum period, and menopause.

Postpartum depression (PPD) is distinctive from major depression in that it begins during pregnancy. This depression occurs in about 15% of pregnancies, negatively affecting both mother and child. Early detection and treatment are needed.

In late-life depression, older individuals experience depression along with a chronic disease such as heart disease, diabetes, or hypertension. In nursing homes, it is expected that about 50% of residents have some form of depression for which medication should be prescribed.

Food and Nutrition Therapies

Many persons with depression have a deficiency of brain serotonin. Painful physical symptoms are common in depressive disorders; abnormalities of serotonin and noradrenaline are strongly associated with pain perception. A mixed diet of protein and carbohydrate should provide adequate amounts of tryptophan, the precursor of serotonin. Include turkey, chicken, milk, potatoes, pumpkin, sunflower seeds, turnip and collard greens, and seaweed as food sources.

Monitoring of nutrition and physical health is important therapy. Antidepressants, omega-3 fatty acids, and physical activity enhance neuroplasticity. An antiinflammatory diet protects against depression, whereas a diet rich in highly processed, refined foods may promote it. A mixed diet containing magnesium, folic acid, calcium, selenium, zinc, omega-3s, and antioxidant foods improves the functions of brain receptors. Vitamin D is another consideration; supplementation, sunlight exposure, and light therapy are often beneficial.

Application to nursing. Often, nursing personnel are the first to note depressive symptoms. Diagnosis of depression is indicated by any four of the following symptoms: SIGECAPS (*s*leep changes, loss of *i*nterest, inappropriate *g*uilt (hopelessness), *e*nergy decline, *c*oncentration changes, *a*ppetite changes, *p*sychomotor changes, and *s*uicidal thoughts). Prolonged sadness and unexplained crying spells, chronic irritability and agitation or anxiety, chronic pessimism or indifference, indecisiveness, social withdrawal, and unexplained aches and pains may also be present.

Some of the medications used in depression can have undesirable side effects. Older forms of monoamine oxidase inhibitors (MAOIs) may cause a hypertensive crisis when taken with foods such as aged cheeses, Chianti wine, and other tyramine-containing foods.

Schizophrenia

Schizophrenia (SCZ) is a group of disorders manifested as disordered thinking, hallucinations, delusions, apathy, social withdrawal, and mood or behavioral disturbances (delusional, catatonic, or paranoid). Delusions may involve control, persecution, grandiosity, or abnormal fears. Hallucinations are perceptions of an external stimulus without a source in the external world. In the resulting psychosis, the individual loses contact with reality.

Less than 1% of the population experiences SCZ, with onset generally between ages 16 and 30 years (earlier in males). There is a strong genetic component (Fig. 19.7). There are many DNA variants in the brains of individuals with SCZ. Schizophrenia is triggered by interactions between genes and environmental factors, such as exposure to viruses, malnutrition before birth, problems during birth, and psychosocial factors.

SCZ can be either episodic or chronic. Patients often have problems with substance abuse, long-term unemployment, poverty, or homelessness. SCZ patients have markedly premature mortality, often from cardiovascular and respiratory diseases, tobacco use, or substance abuse (Olfson et al., 2015). When schizophrenic patients are at risk for self-harm or harm to others, hospitalization is required.

Food and Nutrition Therapies

Oxidative stress or injury and abnormal membrane phospholipid metabolism lead to fatty acid depletion. The short-chain

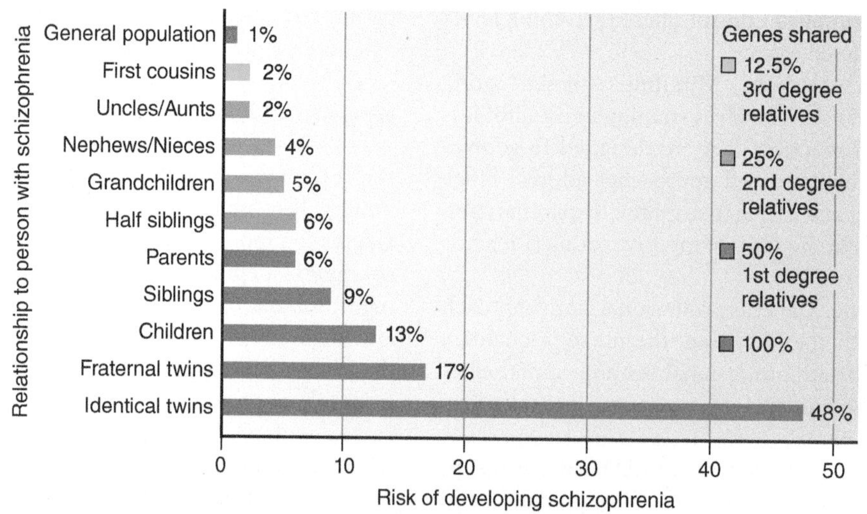

Fig. 19.7 A genogram showing the heritability of schizophrenia. (Data from Schizophrenia.com: Accessed on 19 September, 2020, from http://www.schizophrenia.com/research/hereditygen.htm.)

fatty acids (SCFAs) acetate, butyrate, and propionate are major metabolites derived from fermentation of dietary fibers by gut microbes; their pathways are dysregulated in systemic inflammation (Joseph et al., 2017).

Vitamin D is another factor implicated in the development of SCZ. Low vitamin D availability during pregnancy and infancy interacts with genes and alters brain development. Other important vitamins include folic acid and vitamin B_{12} for DNA to function properly. Thus, a high-fiber, vitamin- and antioxidant-rich Mediterranean diet may improve immune and cardiovascular status in this population.

Application to nursing. Weight gain is an adverse effect of many antipsychotic drugs. Lifestyle intervention and metformin may be suggested for antipsychotic drug–induced weight gain. Nurses play a role in managing patients during psychotic episodes. Psychosocial interventions are important.

Sleep Disorders

Circadian rhythms control sleeping and waking, neurotransmitter secretion, and cellular metabolism. Altered circadian rhythms and short sleep duration may be related to high blood pressure, T2D, depression, obesity, and the metabolic syndrome.

In circadian rhythm sleep disorders, wake–sleep cycles differ from the typical pattern. Primary insomnia occurs in 10% of the population, especially among older adults. Other sleep disorders include obstructive sleep apnea in which breathing halts during sleep, daytime sleepiness (narcolepsy), and restless legs syndrome.

Food and Nutrition Therapies

Melatonin (MT) is formed from L-tryptophan, which plays a major role in sleep and circadian rhythm. Production of MT increases with darkness and drops again with light, including artificial lighting. MT production also decreases with age. Although no specific diet has been identified for use in sleep disorders, light therapy and melatonin supplements have been pilot tested as treatments. Weight loss and avoidance of alcohol and smoking may be used to treat mild sleep apnea.

Application to nursing. Patients with sleep disorders need support and encouragement to try natural therapies before regular use of sleeping pills, in which dependency may occur.

Night shift work has health consequences that are not always recognized. Researchers are studying the effects of "light at night," which disrupts circadian sleep–wake cycles. Disturbed sleep–wake cycles may contribute to excessive body mass index and other medical problems. Melatonin may play a role.

Substance Abuse and Addictions

Addiction is a chronic brain disorder with compulsive and relapsing behavior. The master "pleasure" molecule of addiction is dopamine; it is triggered by heroin, amphetamines, marijuana, alcohol, nicotine, and caffeine. Abnormalities in the metabolism of dopamine, serotonin, and norepinephrine contribute to substance dependency. In some cases, antidepressant medication use alleviates the dependency.

Food and Nutrition Therapies

Addictions share some biologic pathways. Many alcoholics are malnourished, and nutrition intervention is needed to prevent liver disease. Methamphetamine (meth) users often present with poor oral hygiene, xerostomia, rampant caries (meth mouth), and excessive tooth wear. Cocaine users may experience gastrointestinal hemorrhage. Polydrug use may alter food intake, taste preferences, and nutrient metabolism.

Application to nursing. Dysfunctional eating patterns and excessive weight gains have been observed during recovery from drug and alcohol addictions. Patients need reinforcement of new, healthier behaviors.

SUMMARY

- Dietary precursors (tryptophan, tyrosine, and choline) affect nerve functioning and neurotransmitter effectiveness.
- Inflammatory processes, infections, and host immune responses cause chronic neurologic damage in conditions such as Alzheimer's disease, Parkinson's disease, Huntington's disease, and amyotrophic lateral sclerosis (ALS).
- Nutrients that increase the levels of brain catecholamines and protect against oxidative damage include foods rich in omega-3 fatty acids, vitamins C and D and E, zinc, iron, copper, and selenium.
- A Mediterranean diet is useful for brain health. It includes omega-3 fatty acids, light to moderate alcohol use, vegetable oils such as extra-virgin olive oil, nonstarchy vegetables, low-glycemic fruits, and low intake of added sugars.
- Hunger, thirst, and satiety are impaired and lead to weight loss and dehydration in Alzheimer's disease.
- ALS manifests as muscular wasting, atrophy, difficulty speaking, drooling, loss of reflexes, respiratory infections or failure, spastic gait, and weakness. It eventually leads to progressive paralysis and respiratory failure.
- The Glasgow Coma Scale (GCS) is used to assess level of consciousness; a score of 8 or less is usually indicative of coma.
- Patients in a coma or a persistent vegetative state (PVS) require tube feeding.
- Guillain-Barré syndrome (GBS) causes weakness, numbness, pain, and paralysis of the legs, arms, trunk, face, and respiratory muscles, often after infection with a respiratory illness, influenza, or food poisoning. *Campylobacter jejuni*, associated with GBS, is found in contaminated water, undercooked poultry, and unpasteurized milk.
- Huntington's disease (HD) is a progressive, fatal, neurodegenerative disease consisting of chorea, behavioral and psychiatric disturbances, and dementia. Tube feeding is often required.
- Lack of food or sleep; exposure to light; and anxiety, stress, fatigue, or hormonal irregularities can set off a migraine attack. For some people, food allergies may be triggers, and an elimination diet may be beneficial to determine the cause.
- Multiple sclerosis (MS) has a high incidence among Caucasians and affects women two to three times as often as men. Insufficient exposure to sunshine and vitamin D_3 plays a role in MS.
- In myasthenia gravis (MG), symptoms include drooping eyelids (ptosis), double vision (diplopia), weak voice, pneumonia or respiratory arrest, and sleep apnea. Dysphagia is common.
- In Parkinson's disease, loss of dopamine in the brain will occur; levodopa is required, but its long-term use is associated with potentially disabling motor complications. Self-feeding is a problem because of tremors; malnutrition and weight loss are common.
- High intake of red and processed meats, refined grains, sweets, and desserts should be discouraged after a stroke. A plant-based diet or Mediterranean diet high in fruits, vegetables, fish, and whole grains is suggested.
- Anorexia nervosa (AN) is an eating disorder (ED) in which the patient severely rejects food, causing extreme weight loss, low basal metabolic rate, and exhaustion. Emotion acceptance behavior therapy (EABT) is a suggested therapy.
- In avoidant/restrictive food intake disorder (ARFID), restrictive eating is related to emotional problems or gastrointestinal symptoms. Malnutrition is possible.
- Binge-eating disorder (BED) involves recurrent episodes of eating in a discrete period an amount of food larger than most people would eat in the same time, a sense of lack of control over the eating episodes, rapid or secretive eating, guilt, and shame.
- Bulimia nervosa (BN) is an eating disorder with food addiction as the primary coping mechanism. Mindfulness-based eating awareness training (MB-EAT) may be useful.
- Bipolar spectrum involves depression, with varying degrees of excitatory signs and symptoms. Physical and emotional symptoms should be treated. A mixed diet of protein and carbohydrate should provide adequate amounts of tryptophan, the precursor of serotonin.
- Diagnosis of depression is indicated by any four of the following symptoms (remembered by SIGECAPS): *s*leep changes, loss of *i*nterest, inappropriate *g*uilt (hopelessness), *e*nergy decline, *c*oncentration changes, *a*ppetite changes, *p*sychomotor changes, and *s*uicidal thoughts.
- Schizophrenia is a disorder caused by pathogens, genes, and the immune system acting together. A nutritious diet is very important; include vitamin D, omega-3 fatty acids, and other nutrient-dense foods.
- Short sleep duration may be related to high blood pressure, depression, type 2 diabetes, and obesity. Altered circadian rhythms may also lead to the metabolic syndrome. Weight loss and decreased intake of alcohol may help conditions such as sleep apnea.
- Addiction is a chronic brain disorder related to dopamine; it is triggered by substances including heroin, amphetamines, marijuana, alcohol, nicotine, and caffeine.

THE NURSING APPROACH

Clinical Judgment and Next-Generation NCLEX® Examination-Style Questions

Case Study 1

Eating Disorder

Brenda, a 16-year-old junior in high school, came to see the school nurse with complaints of abdominal discomfort. During the interview and examination, the nurse learned that Brenda was concerned about her friend, who had anorexia nervosa. The nurse suspected that Brenda also had some anorexic behaviors. Brenda's school record indicated she weighed 129 pounds 6 months earlier but her current weight was only 109 pounds.

Assessment/Recognize Cues

Subjective (From Patient's Statements)

- "My stomach hurts. I don't have any energy today."
- "I don't remember when my last period was. It probably was a few months ago. I am not sexually active."
- "I have not had any diarrhea or vomiting. I tend to be constipated. No one in my family has been sick."
- "I haven't eaten anything unusual. I frequently skip lunch at school. I would rather spend the time running. I exercise every day."
- "I always feel so fat."
- "I am worried about my friend Sonya, who is in the hospital with anorexia nervosa. Her mother said Sonya just about died 2 days ago. That scares me."

Objective (From Physical Examination)

- Blood pressure: 108/60; temperature: 97.4° F; pulse: 68; respirations: 14
- Height 5 feet 6 inches, weight 109 pounds
- Abdomen tender, bowel sounds hypoactive
- Appears thin, pale; skin dry, hair dull

Diagnoses (Nursing)/Analyze Cues

1. Weight loss related to regular exercise and insufficient intake of food as evidenced by 84% ideal body weight, 16% weight loss in 6 months, feels fat, skips meals, abdominal discomfort, loss of menstruation, constipation, fatigue, and dull hair
2. Decreased self-esteem related to body distortion as evidenced by "I always feel so fat"

Planning/Prioritize Hypotheses

Patient Outcomes

Short term (at the end of this visit):

- Brenda will agree to see a physician for a physical examination and laboratory tests.
- Brenda will agree to eat small meals frequently throughout the day and to return to the school nurse once a week to report eating and activity and to check weight.

Long term (in 4 months):

- Gradual weight gain, preferably about 1 pound per week
- Develop a regular eating pattern
- Return of menstrual periods, energy, shiny hair
- No abdominal pain and no constipation

Nursing Interventions/Generate Solutions

1. Express concern for Brenda's friend, and state observations that Brenda has some danger signs of poor nutrition.
2. Contact parents regarding the need for Brenda to get follow-up medical care and professional care.

Implementation/Take Action

1. Expressed concern for Brenda and her friend. Conveyed a nonjudgmental attitude and praised Brenda for seeking help from the school nurse.
   Establishing trust facilitates open discussion about health concerns.
2. Assessed Brenda's knowledge of possible consequences of anorexia nervosa and its treatment, and then corrected misunderstandings.
   Fear may be a motivating factor for behavioral changes. Full information may lead to wiser choices.
3. Told Brenda that she needs to see a physician to determine the cause of her discomfort and evaluate her general health.
   A medical doctor can assess her health, determine a diagnosis, and prescribe care.
4. Related the nurse's observations of Brenda's health to poor nutrition and emphasized benefits of healthy eating.
   It is common for people with anorexia nervosa to deny eating problems and to not associate health difficulties with poor nutrition. Striving for desirable physical characteristics (e.g., shiny hair) and comfort (e.g., lack of constipation) may motivate behavior changes.
5. Gave her a chart indicating normal weights for adolescents her height and showed her how her weight was much lower than expected.
   An individual who has distorted body image may see a more accurate picture of personal weight when comparing own weight to the expected weight on the chart.
6. Helped Brenda set goals to avoid further weight loss and helped her identify possible changes she could make in her lifestyle.
   Involving the individual in planning contributes to empowerment and a sense of control. Small steps may be needed to reach desired changes.
7. Suggested eating small portions of nutrient-dense foods more frequently, including whole grains, milk, fruits, and vegetables.
   Low intake of calories may initially be necessary to prevent refeeding syndrome. Because of early satiety, food intake should be spread throughout the day. These foods will provide nutrients needed for normal metabolism and function, and fiber and adequate water will help reduce constipation. Quantities may be increased gradually.
8. Asked Brenda to visit the nurse once a week for several weeks. Asked her to keep a food and activity record for the next week and to bring it to the school nurse.
   Frequent monitoring of weight helps track improvement (or lack of improvement) and helps an individual to be accountable. Food records can be used for praise of positive eating when accompanied by stable weight or weight gain. Imbalance of activity versus food may aid discussion and further planning.
9. Telephoned Brenda's parents to invite them to come for a discussion of possible health problems for Brenda and to advise them of the need for medical follow-up and counseling.
   Parents have the responsibility to protect the health of their children and seek medical care as needed. They may not be aware of eating problems. Should the physician diagnose anorexia nervosa, a referral can be made for counseling.

Evaluation/Evaluate Outcomes

Short term (at the end of the visit):

- Brenda said she would see a doctor.
- She reluctantly agreed to record her food intake and activity for 1 week and return to see the school nurse each week for a few weeks.

Short-term goals met.

Discussion Questions

1. What foods might be acceptable to Brenda for frequent small meals?
2. How can the nurse know whether Brenda's food diary is an honest recording of food and fluids she actually consumed?
3. What would be a reasonable weight gain for Brenda at the end of 1 month?

Continued

THE NURSING APPROACH—cont'd

Case Study 2

The intensive care unit (ICU) nurse is mentoring a new graduate nurse in the unit. The nurse is caring for a 25-year-old adult male who was admitted to the ICU with a diagnosis of Guillain-Barré syndrome (GBS). He had been on ventilatory assistance for about a week but is now off the ventilator. The patient has lost more than 10 pounds and a feeding tube was inserted because of issues related to dysphagia. The night nurse reported that the patient's urinary catheter was removed last night.

Complete the statements below using Options 1 for the first statement and Options 2 for the second statement. **Mark an X in boxes.**

The primary nurse notes that the disorder usually shows up after ____________ or ____________.

Sources often associated with this disorder can include ____________, ____________, and ____________.

Options 1	Options 2
Cholecystitis	Contaminated water
Mild upper respiratory infection	Cooked meat
Blood infection	Garden vegetables
Skin infection	Campylobacter in undercooked poultry
Gastroenteritis	Close contact with infected person
Encephalitis	Unpasteurized milk
Pancreatitis	Illegal drugs
Lymphadenitis	Raw fish

CRITICAL THINKING

Clinical Applications

Alzheimer's Disease

Joe, age 70 years, was diagnosed with Alzheimer's disease 5 years ago and is currently residing with his daughter Joni. Joni recently noticed that her father has lost 5 pounds unintentionally in the past month. She is worried about her father's health and decides to bring him in for an examination. Joni reports that Joe is distracted at mealtimes, forgets to eat, and often paces around the house. Joe is 5 feet 9 inches and weighs 185 pounds.

1. What can Joni do to decrease distractions during meals?
2. What suggestions do you have to prevent further weight loss?
3. Joni is worried that she may develop Alzheimer's disease. What foods may protect against this disease?

WEBSITES OF INTEREST

Alzheimer's Association
www.alz.org
Provides background and tips for managing dementias; research advances; publications and resources.

National Alliance on Mental Illness (NAMI)
www.nami.org
The nonprofit, grassroots mental health education, advocacy, and support organization for mental illness in the United States.

National Eating Disorders Association
www.nationaleatingdisorders.org
Devoted to providing information, education, and research to and assistance for individuals and family members of those suffering from eating disorders.

National Institute of Mental Health (NIMH)
www.nimh.nih.gov/health/index.shtml
The largest scientific organization in the United States for prevention of mental disorders and the promotion of mental health.

REFERENCES

Abate, G., et al. (2017). Nutrition and AGE-ing: focusing on Alzheimer's disease. *Oxidative Medicine and Cellular Longevity, 2017*, 7039816.

Armstrong, M. J., & Okun, M. S. (2020). Diagnosis and treatment of Parkinson disease: A review. *The Journal of the American Medical Association, 323*, 548–560.

Baskaran, C., et al. (2017). Effects of anorexia nervosa on the endocrine system. *Pediatric endocrinology reviews: PER, 14*, 302–311.

Bienenstock, J., et al. (2015). Microbiota and the gut-brain axis. *Nutrition Reviews, 73*, S28–S31.

Biglione, B., et al. (2020). Aspirin in the treatment and prevention of migraine headaches: possible additional clinical options for primary healthcare providers. *The American Journal of Medicine, 133*, 412–416.

Binge Eating Disorders. *Patient demographics*. Accessed 19 September, 2020, from https://www.bingeeatingdisorder.com/hcp/patient-demographics

Burgos, R., et al. (2017). ESPEN guideline clinical nutrition in neurology. *Clinical Nutrition, 37*, 354–396.

Byun, K., et al. (2017). Advanced glycation end-products produced systemically and by macrophages: A common contributor to inflammation and degenerative diseases. *Pharmacology & Therapeutics, 177*, 44–55.

Carroll, J. B., et al. (2015). Treating the whole body in Huntington's disease. *Lancet neurology, 14*, 1135–1142.

Dobson, R., & Giovannoni, G. (2019). Multiple sclerosis – a review. *European Journal of Neurology, 26*, 27–40.

Ebrahim Soltani, Z., et al. (2019). Autoimmunity and cytokines in Guillain-Barré syndrome revisited: review of pathomechanisms with an eye on therapeutic options. *European Cytokine Network, 30*, 1–14.

Fisher, M. M., et al. (2014). Characteristics of avoidant/restrictive food intake disorder in children and adolescents: a "new disorder" in DSM-5. *The Journal of Adolescent Health, 55*, 49–52.

Fraser, L. A., et al. (2015). Enzyme-inducing antiepileptic drugs and fractures in people with epilepsy: A systematic review. *Epilepsy Research, 116*, 59–66.

Gazerani, P. (2019). Probiotics for Parkinson's disease. *International Journal of Molecular Sciences, 20*, 4121.
Hay, P. J., et al. (2015). Individual psychological therapy in the outpatient treatment of adults with anorexia nervosa. *Cochrane Database of Systematic Reviews, 7*, CD003909.
Holder, S. D. (2017). Psychotic and bipolar disorders: bipolar disorder. *FP Essent, 455*, 30–35.
Johns Hopkins Medicine, *Frequently Asked Questions About Eating Disorders*. From http://www.hopkinsmedicine.org/psychiatry/specialty_areas/eating_disorders/faq.html. Accessed 19 September, 2020.
Joseph, J., et al. (2017). Modified Mediterranean diet for enrichment of short chain fatty acids: potential adjunctive therapeutic to target immune and metabolic dysfunction in schizophrenia? *Frontiers in Neuroscience, 11*, 155.
Kak, M., et al. (2017). Gastrostomy tube placement is safe in advanced amyotrophic lateral sclerosis. *Neurological Research, 39*, 16–22.
Martin-McGill, et al. (2020). Ketogenic diets for drug-resistant epilepsy. *Cochrane Database of Systematic Reviews, 6*(6), CD001903. Jun 24.
Menon, D., et al. (2020). Novel treatments in myasthenia gravis. *Frontiers in Neurology, 11*, 538.
Millstine, D., et al. (2017). Complementary and integrative medicine in the management of headache. *BMJ 357*, 1805.
Moorhouse, B., & Fisher, C. A. (2016). Long-term use of modified diets in Huntington's disease: a descriptive clinical practice analysis on improving dietary enjoyment. *J Huntingtons Dis, 5*, 15–17.
Olfson, M., et al. (2015). Premature mortality among adults with schizophrenia in the United States. *JAMA Psychiatry, 72*, 1172–1181.
Parks, N. E., et al. (2020). Dietary interventions for multiple sclerosis-related outcomes. *Cochrane Database of Systematic Reviews, 5*(5), CD004192. May 19.
Qi, S. Y., et al. (2016). Early enteral and parenteral nutrition on immune functions of neurocritically ill patients. *Journal of Biological Regulators and Homeostatic Agents, 30*, 227–232.
Richards, P. S., et al. (2017). Can patients with eating disorders learn to eat intuitively? A 2-year pilot study. *Eating disorders, 25*, 99–113.
Salehi, B., et al. (2020). Curcumin's nanomedicine formulations for therapeutic application in neurological diseases. *Journal of Clinical Medicine, 9*, 430.
Strandjord, S. E., et al. (2015). Avoidant/restrictive food intake disorder: illness and hospital course in patients hospitalized for nutritional insufficiency. *The Journal of Adolescent Health, 57*, 673–678.
Sun, J., et al. (2017). Association between malnutrition and hyperhomocysteine in Alzheimer's disease patients and diet intervention of betaine. *Journal of Clinical Laboratory Analysis, 31*, e22090.
Sylvia, L. G., et al. (2015). Medical burden in bipolar disorder: findings from the clinical and health outcomes initiative in comparative effectiveness for bipolar disorder study (Bipolar CHOICE). *Bipolar Disorders, 17*, 212–223.
Tomic, S., et al. (2017). What increases the risk of malnutrition in Parkinson's disease? *Journal of the Neurological Sciences, 375*, 235–238.
Westwood, H., et al. (2018). Assessing ASD in adolescent females with anorexia nervosa using clinical and developmental measures: a preliminary investigation. *Journal of Abnormal Child Psychology, 46*, 183–192.
Yahfoufi, N., et al. (2018). The immunomodulatory and anti-inflammatory role of polyphenols. *Nutrients, 10*, 1618.

20

Nutrition in Cancer and Human Immunodeficiency Virus/Acquired Immunodeficiency Syndrome

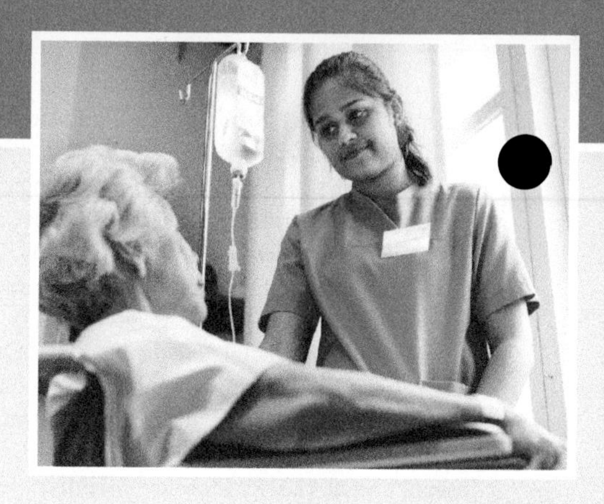

The nutritional status of patients with cancer, human immunodeficiency virus (HIV), and acquired immunodeficiency syndrome (AIDS) is challenged by manifestations not only of the disease but also by the ramifications of treatment.

http://evolve.elsevier.com/GRODNER/FOUNDATIONS

LEARNING OBJECTIVES

- Describe common characteristics of cancer and human immunodeficiency virus/acquired immunodeficiency syndrome (HIV/AIDS) in terms of their effects on the gastrointestinal (GI) tract, on which nutrition therapy focuses.
- List local or systemic effects of cancer that increase risk of malnutrition or cancer cachexia.
- Discuss the individualized nature of nutrition support in the management of cancer and the benefits that may result.
- Summarize the multiple factors that lead to malnutrition in HIV/AIDS.
- Explain the basis of interventions to achieve the goals of HIV nutrition therapy.
- Identify indicators that are key to effective nutrition support and related medical therapies for cancer and HIV/AIDS.

MEDICAL STRESS AND WELLNESS

The nutritional status of patients with cancer or human immunodeficiency virus/acquired immunodeficiency syndrome (HIV/AIDS) can be decimated by the diseases and the myriad complex treatments. Nutrition therapy focuses on reducing these effects and supporting patients through the treatments. The goal of maintaining good nutritional status is to improve survival rates, reduce treatment side effects, and improve the quality of life.

Consider the effects of these disorders on the dimensions of health. The physical health dimension challenge is to halt or minimize the malnutrition and wasting that are often associated with symptoms or treatments. A person must maintain optimal nutrient intake while also dealing with serious illness, requiring intellectual health to comprehend the many different treatment options. Facing the possibility of death stresses emotional health of patients and their families. Social health may be compromised because prejudice or fear of HIV/AIDS and cancer can affect personal and professional relationships. Spirituality and deep faith can provide the inner strength to fight the disease and to heal. Environmental health is implicated because patients who have cancer or HIV infection are at high risk for foodborne illness and superimposed infections.

NUTRITION ASSESSMENT IN CANCER AND HUMAN IMMUNODEFICIENCY VIRUS/ ACQUIRED IMMUNODEFICIENCY SYNDROME

The initial step in assessing nutritional risk for cancer or HIV/AIDS is to evaluate anthropometric data. Comparison of current body weight with usual body weight is more crucial than comparison with an "ideal" body weight. Any unexplained weight loss should be noted, but weight loss greater than 10% in 6 months is considered to put the client at risk. Calculation of body mass index (BMI) also estimates nutrition risk. A calculated BMI of less than 18 is associated with malnutrition and may be associated with increased mortality. Muscle depletion is also significant.

Note that using only weight loss in the assessment may be misleading. Bioelectrical impedance analysis (BIA) has been successfully used to evaluate changes in lean body mass. If BIA is not available, a calculation of upper-arm muscle area can be useful in providing a baseline measurement with which the client can be monitored over time. Other measures such as transferrin value are not applicable because of possible bone marrow suppression.

Dietary assessment may be evaluated by 24-hour recall, food frequency, or food diary. Careful attention should be given to

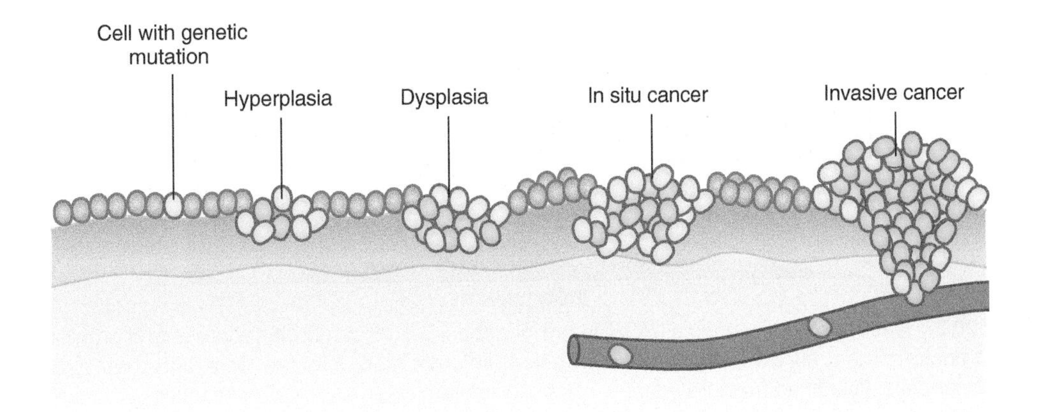

Fig. 20.1 The four stages of carcinogenesis. Stage 0 cancer cells are completely contained in its originating area and have not spread; Stage 1 cancerous cells are still contained within the originating area, showing no significant growth within the area or organ; Stage 2 cancer cells are usually still contained in the originating area but have grown in size; Stage 3 cancerous growth has grown quite large and may have depth; the cancer may have moved into other parts of nearby tissues or to lymph nodes; Stage 4 cancerous growth has become advanced and spread (metastasized) to other parts of the body and or organs. (Modified from Increased Insight: *Understanding the four stages of cancer* https://www.increasedinsight.com/4-stages-of-cancer/. Accessed 20 September, 2020.)

gastrointestinal (GI) function, the presence of steatorrhea and diarrhea, and any other physical symptoms that might interfere with adequate oral intake. In addition, vitamin and mineral status should be monitored closely. Deficiencies may evolve not only from suppressed oral intake but also the increased requirements for certain micronutrients.

Nutrient supplementation has not demonstrated specific benefits. The message continues to be "choose nutritious foods rather than supplements." Whole foods are better choices than refined and highly processed foods.

CO-INFECTION WITH COVID-19

COVID-19 is caused by the airborne coronavirus SARS-CoV-2. COVID-19 is easily spread between people in close contact, through respiratory droplets. People who are immunocompromised from cancer or HIV-infection are at high risk for severe complications. They must take serious precautions to limit contact with others, stay safe, and report any symptoms immediately to their health provider.

CANCER

Cancer cells differ from normal cells in several ways. These characteristics may involve the following: (1) uncontrolled cellular reproduction in which cells become independent of normal growth signals; (2) cells contain an abnormal nucleus and cytoplasm; and (3) increased rate of mitosis. The nuclei of the cells may be abnormally shaped and have clearly altered chromosomes. This process is called carcinogenesis.

The abnormalities in cell replication occur in four stages: initiation, promotion, progression, and malignant conversion (Fig. 20.1). Initiation of the cancer process causes mutation of deoxyribonucleic acid (DNA). Chronic inflammation, physical and chemical agents, or exposure to microorganisms cause the mutation in a genetically susceptible individual. A series of gene modifications, epigenetic changes, and transcription and translation changes will happen based on signaling pathway disorder (Zhang & Xu, 2017). The initiation phase is irreversible.

In the second phase, replication of the mutated cell is promoted with rapid abnormal cell growth. Promoters include estrogen, testosterone, nitrates, cigarette smoke, endocrine disrupters, bisphenol A (BPA), and alcohol. "Promoter" foods are those that are high in saturated fat, refined sugars, and salt and low in fiber, phytochemicals, vitamins, and minerals. The promotion phase is reversible.

The third stage is the progression of the abnormal cells outside the original location of the cell. Progression requires further mutations from genetic (chromosomal) instability during promotion and recruitment of inflammatory immune cells to the tumor. Agents include inflammation, asbestos fibers, benzene, benzoyl peroxide, other peroxides, and oxidative stress.

Progression is an irreversible process and gradually leads to metastasis.

When the cancer has spread to other parts of the body, it is called metastatic cancer. The liver, lungs, lymph nodes, and bones are common areas of spread, but the cancer is still named after the area of the body where it started.

The rate of tumor growth depends on characteristics of both the host and the tumor. Host factors may include age, sex, genetics, nutritional status, the presence of other diseases, hormone production, and immune function. Tumor factors include where the tumor is located and its access to adequate blood supply. The increased blood supply is referred to as a form of angiogenesis.

Cancer remains a leading cause of mortality in the United States. Cancer is the second leading cause of death, accounting for more than 550,000 deaths each year. Most diagnoses of cancer occur in older individuals, with almost two-thirds in people older than 65 years. The most common types of cancer are breast, lung, prostate, and colorectal. Scientists estimate that 50% to 75% of all cancer deaths can be linked to human behaviors and lifestyle factors (Box 20.1).

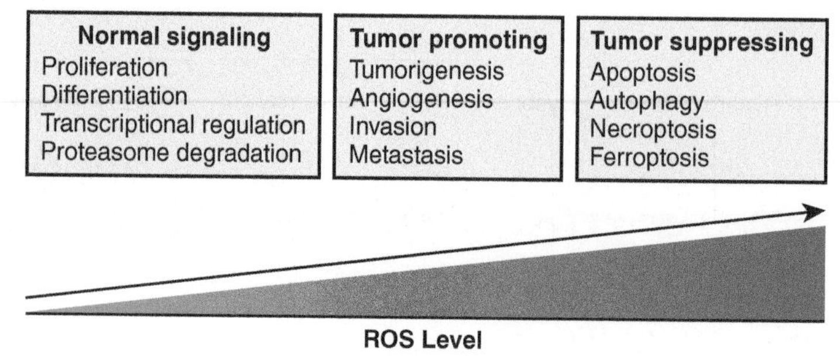

Fig. 20.2 Reactive oxygen species (*ROS*) in tumorigenesis. ROS can both suppress and promote the transformation, survival, proliferation, invasion, inflammation, angiogenesis, and metastasis of tumor cells. (Modified from Galadari, S., et al. Reactive oxygen species and cancer paradox: To promote or to suppress? *Free Radical Biology and Medicine* 104:144–164, 2017.)

BOX 20.1 Risk Factors for Cancer

- **Factors that are known to increase the risk of cancer**
  - Cigarette smoking and tobacco use
  - Infections
  - Radiation
  - Immunosuppressive medicines
- **Factors that may affect the risk of cancer**
  - Alcohol
  - Physical activity
  - Obesity
  - Diabetes
  - Environmental risk factors

(From National Cancer Institute: Causes and prevention. Accessed 20 September, 2020, from https://www.cancer.gov/about-cancer/causes-prevention/patient-prevention-overview-pdq#section/_199.)

Reactive oxygen species (ROS) are produced in the body and play a major role in various cell-signaling pathways. Stress, tobacco, environmental pollutants, radiation, viral infection, diet, and bacterial infection are promoters. ROS have both cancer-suppressing and cancer-promoting actions, making them a paradox (Fig. 20.2).

Nutrition and Cancer Prevention

Nutrition is one of the important environmental and lifestyle factors in the etiology and prevention of cancer. Cancer protection evolves from a metabolic environment that promotes healthy cell replication and tissue integrity: avoiding excess weight, an active way of life, avoiding sedentary behaviors, and choosing healthy dietary patterns rich in plant foods (legumes, wholegrains, pulses, vegetables, and fruits), with modest meat, fish, and dairy, low in alcohol and salt preserved foods (Wiseman, 2019). It is important to choose whole foods over supplements. For example, dietary antioxidants protect cells from DNA mutation, but supplements can be problematic (see the *Critical Thinking* box Food as a Pharmaceutical Agent?).

Nutrition guidelines for cancer prevention are the same as for preventing heart disease, neurologic decline, and T2D. Several general guidelines can help reduce cancer risk with food choices:

- Limit intake of solid fats, sugar-sweetened foods, and empty-calorie snack foods.
- Choose the Mediterranean diet for life.
- Eat 2 to 3 cups of fruits and vegetables every day; cruciferous vegetables are especially protective (broccoli, cauliflower, cabbage, Brussels sprouts).
- Season foods with plenty of herbs and spices, such as turmeric (curcumin).
- Choose whole grains and beans/legumes on most days of the week.
- Try a variety of recipes for mixed dishes; most phytochemicals work best together.
- Enjoy protein foods in moderation; choose fish and lean meat or poultry and cut down on processed and red meats.
- Get recommended intake levels of calcium, vitamin D, and other micronutrients from food.
- Consume fewer salt-cured, salt-pickled or salt-preserved foods.
- Limit alcohol intake to one drink per day for women, two for men. Choose red wine for the benefits of resveratrol.

CRITICAL THINKING

Food as a Pharmaceutical Agent?

Over the past 20 years, epidemiologic researchers have consistently found that people who eat greater amounts of whole grains, fruits, and vegetables have lower rates of cancer. These foods contain hundreds of phytochemicals (plant chemicals) that are not strictly nutrients. Some families of plants have more than others, but phytochemicals are only found in plant foods, not animal foods.

Most health professionals believe that the whole plant is probably more important than the sum of its nutrients and chemical components. More benefits are derived from nutrients and phytochemicals by eating foods rather than swallowing supplements. Clients may ask why they cannot just take specialized phytochemical pills if we know their actions. Here are some issues to consider:

1. Where do these foods fit in the phytochemical categories: Blueberries? Onions and garlic? Green tea? Citrus fruits? Broccoli? Check out websites to see what your patients find when they search.
2. How will you explain the benefits of fruits and vegetables to your patients?
3. What foods will you begin to include in your own diet?
4. No one food causes cancer, and no one food can prevent it. Describe a cancer-preventive diet that could be accepted by children, teens, adults, and seniors. Include several days of menus, with a breakfast, lunch, and dinner option.

Cancer Diagnosis and Cachexia

With more than 100 variations, cancer affects many individuals in the United States. The physiologic response to malignancy is different for each specific tumor type, but there are general nutrition risk factors that may apply. Physical impairment because of the location of the tumor, the extent of tumor involvement, metabolic changes, and the use of cancer drugs all put the patient at increased risk for malnutrition or wasting syndrome.

Cancer cachexia is a complex syndrome, with anorexia, severe wasting of lean body mass, and weight loss. Cytokines are proteins that, in small amounts, assist in the communication between cells of the immune system. These cytokines, such as interleukins, interferons, and tumor necrosis factor (TNF), drive the weight loss, anorexia, hypermetabolism, wasting of skeletal muscle mass, and increased levels of lipid breakdown. Cachexia may be present at the beginning stages of tumor development, even before actual weight loss is observed.

The best treatment of cachexia is a multifactorial approach, with appetite stimulants, cytokine inhibitors, steroids, and nonsteroidal antiinflammatory drugs. Aggressive nutrition support is a major component of medical care. It is also essential to gain the support of family and friends during this time (see the *Personal Perspectives* box Behind the Cancer Headlines).

PERSONAL PERSPECTIVES

Behind the Cancer Headlines

News about the latest cancer therapies is often in the headlines. Information about cancer is readily available on the Internet. What are not as easily accessible are the experiences of individuals whose lives are touched by cancer. Following is a compilation of comments from individuals of varying ages in my life or people whom I've met.

- My mother was in the late stages of a malignant brain tumor, but my brother just couldn't bear the thought of putting "his mother" in a nursing home. Instead, he had her stay with him and his family, setting up a bed in their family room. Within a few days, when she could no longer control her bowels, he found himself sponge bathing his 75-year-old mother, who hardly knew where she was. He then understood that he could no longer care for her.
- My friend Karen fought the good fight against breast cancer. For 9 years she battled but lost. When she was first diagnosed, she came to see each of us (her neighbors) to tell us in person. I felt honored. I think it was her way of making it real, of announcing it to the world. She learned everything there was to know about every kind of treatment. Several times she traveled to the Dominican Republic for controversial stem cell treatments, riding through the countryside in a rickety van with others in search of medical miracles. The cancer spread, but so did Karen's spirit. Perhaps the miracle of Karen's spirit was to show us how to struggle against disease while still enjoying life.
- Barbara said she didn't want to hold her newborn grandson because she was too weak, but I think it was because she knew that her cancer had spread and she didn't want to become too attached to the baby.
- My uncle's case was complicated. What with inoperable bladder and prostate cancer, high blood pressure, anemia, and advancing Parkinson's disease, there was a lot to consider. One day his oncologist told him that "there are no more treatments available for your cancer" and that he (the oncologist) was going on vacation for 2 weeks. Fortunately, my uncle, guided by my aunt, immediately found a new oncologist, who prescribed a different treatment protocol. My uncle is now in remission.

Michele Grodner
Montclair, NJ

Nutrition and Cancer Treatments

Clinical guidelines suggest (1) screening of all patients with cancer for nutritional risk early in the course of their care, regardless of body mass index and weight history; (2) expand nutrition-related assessment to include measures of anorexia, body composition, inflammatory biomarkers, resting energy expenditure, and physical function; (3) individualize plans to increase nutritional intake while lessening inflammation and hypermetabolic stress (Arends et al., 2017).

The comprehensive goals of nutrition during cancer treatment are to:

- Decrease the risk of surgical complications.
- Ensure that patients meet increased energy and protein requirements.
- Help repair and rebuild normal tissues damaged by antineoplastic therapy.
- Promote an increased tolerance to therapy.
- Assist in promoting an enhanced quality of life.

Surgery

Treatment for most solid tumors includes surgical resection. This route of treatment can allow for diagnosis, resecting a solid tumor, preventing metastasis, or reducing the size of the tumor to alleviate pain. The nutritional consequences of surgery depend on the type and extent of the surgical resection. Resections of any portion of the GI tract can alter nutrition intake and nutrient absorption.

Energy and protein requirements may need to be increased to promote optimal wound healing postoperatively. Malabsorption tends to be the primary nutritional problem with procedures involving the GI tract. Unless small bowel resection is extensive, the adaptability of the small intestine may prevent the occurrence of major clinical problems. Many patients with cancer enter surgery already experiencing malnutrition, raising the risk for complications. For example, more than 60% of patients with malignancies affecting the head and neck enter surgery malnourished. Additionally, any problems associated with surgery (Table 20.1) will be further complicated if the patient receives subsequent radiation therapy and chemotherapy.

TABLE 20.1 Nutritional Side Effects of Cancer Surgery

Site of Surgery	Side Effect
Head and neck	Impaired chewing and swallowing
Esophagectomy	Diarrhea, steatorrhea, esophageal stenosis
Vagotomy	Gastric stasis, diarrhea, fat malabsorption
Gastrectomy	Dumping syndrome; hypoglycemia; malabsorption; possible deficiencies of iron, calcium, vitamin B_{12}, and fat-soluble vitamins
Pancreatectomy	T1D mellitus; possible malabsorption of fats, protein, fat-soluble vitamins, minerals
Small bowel resection	Possible malabsorption of many nutrients; depends on extent and site of surgery
Ileostomy	Sodium and water losses, vitamin B_{12}, malabsorption, fat malabsorption, bile salt diarrhea

(Data from Academy of Nutrition and Dietetics: *The complete resource kit for oncology nutrition (online access)*, n.d. Accessed 20 September, 2020, from http://www.oncologynutrition.org/erfc/eating-well-when-unwell/surgery/.)

Chemotherapy

Most chemotherapy protocols involve a combination of agents. Chemotherapy agents include alkylating agents, antimetabolites (folate antagonists), purine/pyrimidine antagonists, anthracyclines, platinum antitumor compounds, antibiotics, nitrosoureas, mitotic inhibitors, cytokines, biologic response modifiers, monoclonal antibodies, immunotherapeutic agents, hormones, and enzymes. These agents act by inhibiting one or more steps of DNA synthesis in the rapidly proliferating cells that are characteristic of the malignant cell or by enhancing the host's immune system to improve the response to therapy. Using a combination of medications that interrupt the cancer process in different ways allows for maximum effect with the fewest side effects.

Cells of the bone marrow and those lining the GI tract tend to be susceptible to damage from chemotherapy because of their rapid turnover rate. The effect on these cells accounts for many of the side effects: nausea, vomiting, diarrhea, inflamed mucous membranes of the mouth (mucositis), hair loss, and immunosuppression. The severity and manifestation of the side effects depend on the specific chemotherapy agent, dosage, duration of treatment, rates of metabolism, accompanying drugs, and individual tolerance. These symptoms can lead to malnutrition through a variety of mechanisms: anorexia; nausea; vomiting; mucositis; cardiac, renal, or liver injury (toxicity); and new food aversions. Nutritional implications of chemotherapeutic agents are summarized in Table 20.2.

Radiation Therapy

Radiation therapy uses ionizing radiation to kill cells by altering the DNA of the malignant cells. This alteration interferes with the factors controlling replication. Irradiation is used to treat tumors that are sensitive to radiation exposure or cannot be surgically resected. Irradiation also can be used to reduce tumor size so that a successful surgical resection can occur. Although technology has allowed for significant specificity in the use of radiation therapy, some normal cells within the treatment range may also be damaged, causing hair loss, mucositis, or vomiting and diarrhea.

Nutritional problems vary according to the region or area of the body irradiated, dose, and whether radiation therapy is used in combination with surgery or chemotherapy. Complications may develop during radiation treatment or may become chronic and progress even after treatment is completed.

Irradiation sites that usually lead to nutrition problems include the head, neck, abdomen, pelvis, and the central nervous system (CNS). Irradiation at any of these sites may cause anorexia, nausea, and vomiting. In the head and neck, problems include difficulty with ingestion, stomatitis, esophageal mucositis, loss of taste sensation, and changes in saliva production. Radiation to the abdomen and pelvis causes radiation enteritis with diarrhea, steatorrhea, malabsorption, ulceration, bowel damage, or obstruction.

Bone Marrow or Stem Cell Transplantation

Bone marrow or stem cell transplantation is used to treat certain hematologic malignancies (acute and chronic leukemia and some forms of lymphoma), as well as in adjunct therapy for solid tumors such as breast cancer.

When bone marrow transplantation (BMT) is used as the treatment of a solid tumor, the patient's own bone marrow is harvested and saved before the initiation of chemotherapy or radiation therapy. The patient then receives high-dose chemotherapy and possibly total body irradiation to eradicate the cancer. The patient's bone marrow is then infused as an autologous "rescue" from the effects of both chemotherapy and irradiation.

TABLE 20.2 Nutritional Implications of Chemotherapeutic Agents

Drug Classification	Selected Examples	Actions	Nutritional Implications
Alkylating agents	Cisplatin Hexamethylmelamine Dacarbazine	React with susceptible deoxyribonucleic acid (DNA) sites	Anorexia, nausea, vomiting, mucositis/stomatitis
Antibiotics	Bleomycin Doxorubicin Dactinomycin	Bind to DNA and inhibit cell division, interfere with ribonucleic acid (RNA) transcription	Anorexia, nausea, mucositis/stomatitis, diarrhea; some may cause decreased calcium and iron absorption
Antimetabolites	Methotrexate 5-Fluorodeoxyuridine 5-Fluorouracil	Inhibit a stage of DNA synthesis	Anorexia, nausea, vomiting, diarrhea, mucositis, abdominal pain, intestinal ulceration; some may cause decreased absorption of vitamin B_{12}, fat, and xylose
Hormones	Prednisone Tamoxifen Diethylstilbestrol	Alter cell metabolism to cause unfavorable tumor growth	Corticosteroids: sodium and fluid retention, hyperglycemia, gastrointestinal upset, osteoporosis (calcium losses), negative nitrogen balance Estrogens: nausea, vomiting, anorexia, hypercalcemia
Enzymes	Asparaginase	Delay DNA and RNA synthesis by inhibiting protein synthesis (deprive cells of asparagine)	Anorexia, nausea, hyperglycemia, pancreatitis, azotemia (uremia), weight loss
Plant alkaloids	Vinblastine Vincristine	Inhibit mitosis	Nausea, vomiting, constipation, diarrhea, abdominal pain
Biologic response modifiers	Interferon Interleukin	Modify host biologic response to tumor	Nausea, vomiting, anorexia, weight change (increase or decrease)

(Data from Academy of Nutrition and Dietetics: *The complete resource kit for oncology nutrition (online access)*, n.d. Accessed 20 September, 2020, from http://www.oncologynutrition.org/erfc/eating-well-when-unwell/chemotherapy/.)

For hematologic malignancies, a patient receives bone marrow from a genetically matched (allogeneic) donor or in some cases from a twin (syngeneic) donor. In a stem cell transplantation, stem cells are removed from a newborn baby's umbilical cord immediately after birth and are stored until needed for a transplant.

The ability to maintain adequate oral intake is difficult because of the nausea, vomiting, and mucositis that are associated with these high-dose therapies. Parenteral nutrition is a standard protocol but use of minimal oral or enteral nutrition is important to promote health of the small intestine.

Immunosuppression from antineoplastic regimens and BMT puts the patient at high risk for infection by bacterial and fungal pathogens. Pathogens can be commonly found in the environment, including fresh fruits and vegetables that ordinarily do not present a hazard to healthy persons (Box 20.2). A low-bacteria, "neutropenic" diet is rarely used in health care facilities, but some of the principles are useful: avoiding undercooked meats and eggs, ensuring that raw fruits and vegetables are washed well and/or are peeled (including salads and garnishes), and following sanitation guidelines for food preparation and storage. Frequent monitoring and encouragement of nutritional intake are essential in the care of immunosuppressed patients (Box 20.3).

A major complication that may occur with an allogeneic BMT is graft-versus-host disease (GVHD), which is a form of

BOX 20.2 Food Safety for Immunocompromised Patients

Advise not to eat:

Raw or undercooked meat or poultry

Raw fish, partially cooked seafood (such as shrimp and crab), and refrigerated smoked seafood

Raw shellfish (including oysters, clams, mussels, and scallops) and their juices

Unpasteurized (raw) milk and products made with raw milk, like yogurt and cheese

Soft cheeses made from unpasteurized milk, such as feta, brie, Camembert, blue-veined, and Mexican-style cheeses (such as such as queso fresco, panela, asadero, and queso blanco)

Raw or undercooked eggs or foods containing raw or undercooked eggs, including certain homemade salad dressings (such as Caesar salad dressing), homemade cookie dough and cake batters, and homemade eggnog. Note that most premade foods from grocery stores, such as Caesar dressing, premade cookie dough, and packaged eggnog are made with pasteurized eggs.

Unwashed fresh vegetables, including lettuce/salads

Unpasteurized fruit or vegetable juices (these juices will carry a warning label)

Hot dogs, luncheon meats (cold cuts), fermented and dry sausage, and other deli-style meats, poultry products, and smoked fish—unless they are reheated until steaming hot

Salads (without added preservatives) prepared on site in a deli-type establishment, such as ham salad, chicken salad, or seafood salad

Unpasteurized, refrigerated pâtés or meat spreads

Raw sprouts (alfalfa, bean, or any other sprout)

(U.S. Food and Drug Association. Food Safety: Importance for At-Risk Groups. Accessed 20 September, 2020 from https://www.fda.gov/food/people-risk-foodborne-illness/food-safety-older-adults-and-people-cancer-diabetes-hivaids-organ-transplants-and-autoimmune.)

BOX 20.3 Nutritional Risk Levels of Acquired Immunodeficiency Syndrome

I. High risk (see a Registered Dietitian [RD] within 1 week).
  A. Poorly controlled diabetes mellitus.
  B. Pregnancy (mother's nutrition; infant: artificial infant formula).
  C. Poor growth, lack of weight gain, or failure to thrive in pediatric patients.
  D. More than 10% unintentional weight loss over 4–6 months.
  E. More than 5% unintentional weight loss within 4 weeks or in conjunction with
    1. Chronic oral [or esophageal] thrush.
    2. Dental problems.
    3. Dysphagia.
    4. Chronic nausea or vomiting.
    5. Chronic diarrhea.
    6. Central nervous system (CNS) disease.
    7. Intercurrent illness or active opportunistic infection.
  F. Severe dysphagia.
  G. Enteral or parenteral feedings.
  H. Two or more medical comorbidities, or dialysis.
  I. Complicated food-drug-nutrient interactions.
  J. Severely dysfunctional psychosocial situation (especially in children).
II. Moderate risk (see RD within 1 month).
  A. Obesity.
  B. Evidence for body fat redistribution.
  C. Elevated cholesterol (>200 mg/dL) or triglycerides (>250 mg/dL), or cholesterol <100 mg/dL.
  D. Osteoporosis.
  E. Diabetes mellitus, controlled or new diagnosis.
  F. Hypertension.
  G. Evidence of hypervitaminoses or excessive supplement intake.
  H. Inappropriate use of diet pills, laxatives, or other over-the-counter medications.
  I. Substance abuse in the recovery phase.
  J. Possible food-drug-nutrient interactions.
  K. Food allergies and intolerance.
  L. Single medical comorbidity.
  M. Oral thrush.
  N. Dental problems.
  O. Chronic nausea or vomiting.
  P. Chronic diarrhea.
  Q. CNS disease resulting in a decrease in functional capacity.
  R. Chronic pain other than oral/gastrointestinal tract source.
  S. Eating disorder.
  T. Evidence for sedentary lifestyle or excessive exercise regimen.
  U. Unstable psychosocial situation (especially in children).
III. Low risk (see RD as needed).
  A. Stable weight.
  B. Appropriate weight gain, growth, and weight-for-height in pediatric patients.
  C. Adequate and balanced diet.
  D. Normal levels of cholesterol, triglycerides, albumin, and glucose.
  E. Stable human immunodeficiency virus disease (with no active intercurrent infections).
  F. Regular exercise regimen.
  G. Normal hepatic and renal function.
  H. Psychosocial issues stable (especially in children).

(From Norad, J., et al.: General nutrition management in patients infected with human immunodeficiency virus, *Clinical Infectious Diseases* 36: S52–S62, 2003. Accessed 10 February, 2021, from https://doi.org/10.1086/367559.)

reverse rejection. In this case, the grafted tissue or organ recognizes the host's cells as foreign and attacks them. GVHD may result in multiple organ damage, but the skin, GI tract, and liver are most sensitive. The nutritional management for GVHD may require intense therapy for several years after transplantation.

Food and Nutrition Therapies

Patients with cancer are at high risk for malnutrition; thus, recognition of the clinical signs and symptoms and early treatment is important. The Patient-Generated Subjective Global Assessment (PG-SGA) screening tool allows for early identification of patients who have a nutrition deficit or who are at risk for one when treatment is initiated (Jager-Wittenaar and Ottery, 2017, Fig. 20.3). Because nutrition should be an essential component of every treatment plan, the following are reasonable goals:

- Maintenance of weight and lean body mass within the established goal range through consumption of adequate energy and protein or with appropriate nutritional support
- Adequate hydration, as measured by clinical and physical assessment
- Adequate energy and protein intakes to perform activities of daily living
- Use of appropriate and safe complementary nutrition therapies

Interventions should be tailored to support the energy and protein needs of the patient. As symptoms arise, interventions can be introduced to maximize nutritional intake (Table 20.3).

Altered Taste

Many cancer patients describe taste alterations with their treatments. These alterations relate to changes in or destruction of the oral mucosa, the systemic presence of tumor byproducts, changes in the quantity or quality of saliva, inadequate mouth care, or drugs. It is appropriate for patients with cancer to avoid those foods that taste bad to them. However, alternate food choices may be required to maintain adequate nutrient intake. Eating foods that are cold, tart or spicy may enhance overall intake.

Anorexia

Anorexia is loss of appetite, generally caused by changes in taste and smell, decreased transit time and subsequent early satiety, opportunistic infections, therapy and medication side effects, pain, and emotional and psychologic effects. Early patient education on the role of nutrition in treatment is essential to promote adequate nutritional intake. The nutrient density of food must be stressed. Small, frequent meals, the use of high-calorie supplements, and a pleasant eating environment can help.

Nausea and Vomiting

Nausea and vomiting may result from delayed transit time, hypercalcemia or CNS involvement, medications, or anxiety. Cold foods without odor tend to be better tolerated.

Hormonal Cancers

Diets rich in vegetable fiber may reduce the risk for breast and prostate cancers. Alcoholic beverages, smoked and barbequed meats, and red meat should be restricted. For both cancers, weight reduction is recommended in patients who are overweight.

Lung, Renal, and Urinary Tract Cancers

Nutritional supplements for beta carotene and single vitamins should be avoided. Otherwise, a healthy cancer-preventive diet is the main recommendation.

Vitamin D and Skin Cancer

Melanins in animals and flavonoids in plants are antioxidant pigments, acting as free radical scavenging mechanisms. Both are phenols synthesized and enhanced after exposure to ultraviolet (UV) rays. Excessive UV radiation damages lipids, nucleic acids, and proteins; alters metabolic functions; and generates free radical damage. Living under high UV radiation near the equator, ancestral Homo sapiens had skin rich in eumelanin, protecting against deleterious effects of UV radiation while allowing UVB-dependent photosynthesis of vitamin D_3.

The proper dose of UVB radiation releases approximately 20,000 IU vitamin D_3 into the circulation within 24 hours. For proper synthesis, exposure to midday sun (10 AM to 3 PM) is required in spring, summer, and fall, 20 minutes per day for a light-skinned person, 60 minutes per day for individual of medium skin tone and 120 minutes/day for a dark-skinned person. Essentially 100% of women of color are vitamin D insufficient during pregnancy, and breastfed infants are also at risk for low vitamin D intake.

The sunlight–vitamin D–cancer relationship is a complex one. Vitamin D affects the expression of many genes and pathways that affect cancer. Humans need sufficient sun exposure, but excess leads to UV damage. Natural sunscreens are found in several polyphenol-rich foods. Soy genistein, resveratrol from grape skins and berries, green tea catechins (EGCG), grape seed proanthocyanidins, rosmarinic acid from lemon balm, lycopene, and fig latex protect against melanoma and keratinocyte cancers (Tong & Young, 2014). Keratinocyte cancer is the new term for basal cell carcinoma and squamous cell carcinoma, previously known as nonmelanoma skin cancers (Sanchez et al., 2016).

Application to nursing. Patients with cancer must receive individualized support. The medical prognosis should be considered to appropriately adjust the aggressiveness of interventions (supportive, adjunctive, and definitive).

Incurable cancer profoundly affects the patient's physical and psychosocial well-being; palliative care is initiated early in the disease trajectory and improves quality of life overall (Haun et al., 2017). Quality of life and patient choices are important considerations. Patients on home parenteral nutrition (HPN) have overall improvements in their quality of life, physical role, and emotional functioning, even with advanced cancer treatments (Bao et al., 2018). Palliative chemotherapy improves quality of life for patients with end-stage cancer, but not when the patient is near death (Prigerson et al., 2015).

Above all, nurses play a key role in helping patients cope with their cancer treatments. Patients should be educated on what to expect from their treatment regimen to decrease fear and anxiety. Nausea and vomiting require adequate and aggressive antiemetic therapy 60 to 90 minutes before meals to ensure

Subjective Global Assessment Rating Form

Patient Name: ____________ ID#: ________ Date: ____________

History

	Rate 1–7
Weight/Weight Change ***(Included in K/DOQI SGA)*** 1. Baseline weight: ________ (Dry weight from 6 months ago) Current weight: ________ (Dry weight today) Actual weight loss/past 6 mo: ________ % loss ________ (actual loss from baseline or last SGA) 2. Weight change over past two weeks: ________ No change ________ Increase ________ Decrease	
Dietary Intake No Change ________ (Adequate) No Change ________ (Inadequate) 1. Change: Suboptimal intake: ________ Protein ________ Kcal ________ Duration ________ Full liquid: ________ Hypocaloric liquid ________ Starvation ________	
Gastrointestinal Symptoms ***(Included in K/DOQI SGA-anorexia or causes of anorexia)*** Symptom: Frequency: Duration: ☐ None ________ ________ ☐ Anorexia ________ ________ ☐ Nausea ________ ________ ☐ Vomiting ________ ________ ☐ Diarrhea ________ ________ Never; daily; 2–3 times/wk; 1–2 times/wk >2 weeks; <2 weeks	
Functional Capacity Description Duration: ☐ No dysfunction ________ ☐ Change in function ________ ☐ Difficulty with ambulation ________ ☐ Difficulty with activity (Patient specific "normal") ________ ☐ Light activity ________ ☐ Bed/chair ridden with little or no activity ________ ☐ Improvement in function ________	
Disease State/Comorbidities as Related to Nutritional Needs Primary Diagnosis ________ Comorbidities ________ ☐ Normal requirements ☐ Increased requirements ☐ Decreased requirements Acute metabolic stress: ☐ None ☐ Low ☐ Moderate ☐ High	

Physical Exam

☐ Loss of subcutaneous fat (Below eye, triceps, biceps, chest) ***(Included in K/DOQI SGA)*** ☐ Some areas ☐ All areas ☐ Muscle wasting (Temple, clavicle, scapula, ribs, quadriceps, calf, knee, interosseous) ***(Included in K/DOQI SGA)*** ☐ Some areas ☐ All areas ☐ Edema (related to undernutrition/use to evaluate weight change)	

Overall SGA Rating

Very mild risk to well-nourished = 6 or 7 most categories or significant, continued improvement. **Mild–moderate** = 3, 4, or 5 ratings. No clear sign of normal status or severe malnutrition. **Severely Malnourished** = 1 or 2 ratings in most categories/significant physical signs of malnutrition.	

Fig. 20.3 The 7-point scale Subjective Global Assessment (*SGA*) form. (Modified from Download Scientific Diagram [researchgate.net]; Jager-Wittenaar, H., & Ottery, F. D. (2017). Assessing nutritional status in cancer: Role of the patient-generated subjective global assessment. *Current Opinion in Clinical Nutrition & Metabolic Care*, 20(5), 322–329.)

effectiveness. Patients are at risk for dehydration, so fluid intake should be encouraged.

Behavioral strategies such as guided imagery and relaxation techniques are useful for many individuals. For anorexia, megestrol (Megace) and dronabinol (Marinol) help to stimulate appetite. Excellent mouth care is another consideration. Indeed, individualization and humane care are the foundations of nursing interventions for cancer.

TABLE 20.3 Nutritional Approaches to Nutrition-Related Problems in Cancer and Cancer Therapy

Problem	Recommendations
Loss of appetite/early satiety	Eat frequent small meals, increase kcal/protein content of foods, use high-protein/high-kcal supplements, eat foods cool or at room temperature, avoid excess fat, exercise regularly if tolerated, limit liquids at mealtime; appetite may be best in the morning
Diarrhea[a]	Eat frequent small meals, eat foods cool or at room temperature, increase fluid intake, eat and drink slowly, decrease fiber intake, avoid excess fat, avoid gas-forming foods, limit liquids at mealtime, avoid highly seasoned foods, limit beverages containing caffeine and alcohol; trial avoidance of lactose may be helpful; take antidiarrheal medication per physician order
Nausea and vomiting	Eat frequent small meals, avoid strong odors, eat foods cool or at room temperature, increase fluid intake, eat and drink slowly, avoid excess fat, limit liquids at mealtime, avoid highly seasoned foods, rest after meals with head elevated, take antiemetic medication per physician order
Chewing and swallowing difficulties	Eat frequent small meals, increase kcal/protein content of foods, use high-protein/high-kcal supplements, eat food cool or at room temperature, increase fluid intake, eat and drink slowly, add sauces and gravy to soften and moisten foods, avoid highly seasoned foods, alcohol, tobacco, and commercial mouthwashes; coarse-textured and acidic foods may irritate
Constipation	Increase fluid intake, increase fiber intake, exercise regularly if tolerated; stool softener and/or laxative may be necessary
Abdominal gas	Eat and drink slowly, decrease fiber intake, avoid excess fat, avoid gas-forming foods, exercise regularly if tolerated, limit lactose if not tolerated
Dry mouth	Increase fluid intake, add sauces and gravy to soften and moisten foods, try using tart foods or sugar-free hard candy to stimulate saliva, avoid alcohol, tobacco, and commercial mouthwash
Taste/smell alterations	Eat food cool or at room temperature, increase fluid intake, use seasonings to enhance flavors, avoid cooking odors, try alternative protein sources for meat aversion

[a]Diarrhea secondary to malabsorption, dumping syndrome, or other causes may require different treatment.
(Data from Academy of Nutrition and Dietetics: *The complete resource kit for oncology nutrition (online access)*, n.d. Accessed 10 February, 2021, from Complete Resource Kit for Oncology Nutrition (Online) (eatrightstore.org).)

BOX 20.4 Food Safety for Immunosuppressed Patients

Safe food handling can help to decrease a person's risk of foodborne illness. People with weakened immune systems must use extra caution to avoid putting themselves at risk of becoming infected by a foodborne pathogen. The following precautions help avoid such infections:

Shopping

- Shop for groceries when you can take food home right away; do not leave food sitting in the car.
- Avoid cans of food that are dented, leaking, or bulging.
- Do not purchase food in cracked glass jars.
- Ensure that safety buttons on metal lids are down and do not make a clicking noise when pushed. Make sure that tamper-resistant safety seals are intact.
- Avoid food in torn or punctured packaging.
- Pick up perishable foods (e.g., meat, eggs, milk) last.
- Place packaged meat, poultry, or fish in separate plastic bags to prevent meat juices from dripping onto other groceries or other meats.
- Make sure the "sell by" or "use by" date has not passed.
- Do not buy any food that has been displayed in any unclean or unsafe manner (e.g., meat allowed to sit outside refrigeration, cooked shrimp displayed next to raw shrimp).
- When ordering in the deli department, make sure the clerk washes their hands between handling raw food and cooked food.

Storage

- Keep your refrigerator and freezer clean.
- Use a refrigerator thermometer to make sure the temperature inside is ≤40°F.
- Make sure the temperature inside the freezer is 0°F.
- On arriving home from the store, immediately refrigerate and freeze appropriate foods.
- Leave eggs in their carton; do not place in refrigerator door.
- Store raw meat, poultry, and fish on the bottom shelf of the refrigerator; prevent their juices from dripping onto other foods. Raw ground meat, poultry, and fish may be stored for 1 or 2 days; other red meat may be stored for 3 to 5 days.
- Store canned foods and other shelf-stable products in a cool, dry place. Avoid hot garages and damp basements.

Preparation

- Wash hands before, during, and after food preparation and service.
- Use plastic or glass surfaces for cutting raw meat and poultry. Use a separate cutting board for preparing other foods, such as fruits, vegetables, and bread.
- Wash cutting boards with hot, soapy water after each use. All cutting boards (except those that are made with laminated wood) can be washed in the dishwasher.
- After handling raw meat, poultry, and fish, wash hands, work surfaces, and utensils with hot, soapy water.
- Wash all fruits and vegetables before cutting, cooking, or eating them raw.
- Defrost frozen food in a bowl in the refrigerator or microwave it. Cook food immediately after thawing.
- Use different utensils and dishes for cooked foods from those used for raw foods.
- Wash kitchen towels and cloths often in hot water in a washing machine.
- A sanitizing solution can be made with one teaspoon of liquid chlorine bleach mixed with one quart of water. Use solution on countertops and other work surfaces. Do not rinse. Allow surface to air-dry.

Cooking

- Keep hot foods hot at ≥140°F and cold foods cold at ≤40°F.
- Do not leave perishable foods out for more than 2 hours.

Continued

BOX 20.4 Food Safety for Immunosuppressed Patients—cont'd

- Promptly refrigerate or freeze leftovers in shallow containers or wrapped tightly in bags.
- Use leftovers within 3 or 4 days.
- When reheating foods in the microwave, cover and rotate or stir foods once or twice during cooking. The food should be steaming hot.
- Do not eat foods past their expiration date.
- Follow the handling and preparation instructions on product labels to ensure top quality and safety.

Meat, Poultry, and Fish
- Do not eat raw or undercooked meat.
- Cook all meat and poultry until it is no longer pink in the middle.
- Fish should be cooked until flaky, not rubbery.
- The temperature inside the meat should be >165°F.
- Cook poultry to an internal temperature of 180° to 185°F.
- Cook fish to 160°F.
- Do not eat stuffing cooked inside poultry. Instead, cook stuffing separately to 165°F.
- Cook only shellfish that are closed. Discard any shellfish that do not open during cooking.

Dairy
- Eat or drink only pasteurized milk or dairy products.

Eggs
- Cook eggs until the yolk and white are solid, not runny.
- Do not eat foods that may contain raw eggs, such as Caesar salad dressing and raw cookie dough.
- If eating fried eggs, be sure eggs are fried on both sides.

Fruits and Vegetables
- Raw fruits and vegetables are generally safe to eat if washed carefully first.
- Discard any fruits or vegetables with mold.
- Wash fruits and vegetables under cool running water.
- Do not let cut fruits or vegetables sit unrefrigerated.
- Discard the outermost leaves of a head of lettuce or cabbage.

Water
- Do not drink water straight from lakes, rivers, streams, or springs.
- Always check with your local health department and water company to learn whether they have issued any special notices for people with weakened immune systems.
- Water bottles and ice trays should be cleaned with soap and water before use.

Other
- Home canned foods: Use within 1 year of canning. Cook food for 10 minutes before eating.
- Commercially canned foods: Safe to eat without any further cooking.
- Condiments: Use a clean utensil when dipping into jars. Keep jars refrigerated. Do not use homemade mayonnaise.
- Baby food: Use a clean utensil to remove amount needed from jar. Store opened jars in the refrigerator.

Dining Away from Home
- Avoid the same foods that you would at home (e.g., raw meats, undercooked eggs).
- If the food arrives undercooked, send it back.
- Avoid foods that may contain raw eggs, such as Caesar salad dressing and uncooked sauces such as Hollandaise.
- If you are not sure about the ingredients in a dish, ask your waiter before you order.
- Do not order any raw or lightly steamed fish or shellfish, such as oysters, clams, mussels, sushi, or sashimi.

Traveling
- Do not eat uncooked fruits and vegetables unless you can peel them.
- Avoid salads.
- Eat cooked foods while they are still hot.
- Boil all water before drinking it.
- Drink only canned or bottled drinks or beverages made with boiled water.
- Steaming hot foods, fruits you peel yourself, bottled and canned processed drinks, and hot coffee or tea should be safe.
- Talk with your health care provider about other advice on travel abroad.

(Modified from Caring4cancer: *Food safety during cancer treatment*, 2010. Accessed 1 October, 2013, from https://www.cancer.org/treatment/survivorship-during-and-after-treatment/staying-active/nutrition/weak-immune-system.html.)

HUMAN IMMUNODEFICIENCY VIRUS INFECTION AND ACQUIRED IMMUNODEFICIENCY SYNDROME

In 1983 the human immunodeficiency virus (HIV) was isolated as the cause for acquired immunodeficiency syndrome (AIDS). A retrovirus injects its ribonucleic acid (RNA) into the target cell and then transcribes the RNA into DNA using a reverse transcriptase enzyme. Target cells for HIV include the T4 or CD4 lymphocytes, B lymphocytes, monocytes, macrophages, and other cells of the immune system. Currently, there are two major strains of HIV. HIV-1 is commonly found in the United States, whereas HIV-2 is the strain found on the African continent.

HIV is a bloodborne infection. It is transmitted through contact with contaminated blood, semen, vaginal secretions, and breast milk. HIV also crosses the placenta from the mother to the baby. Approximately 40 million people throughout the world have HIV infection, concentrated in southern and eastern African countries. In sub-Saharan Africa, AIDS is the leading cause of death. In the United States, nearly 1.2 million people live with HIV infection, primarily minority populations, women, and youth (U.S. Statistics, 2020).

The initial infection with HIV may involve symptoms such as fever and malaise. Antibodies are produced against the virus and are detectable within 2 to 4 months of exposure. Screening technology with enzyme-linked immunosorbent assay (ELISA) allows for rapid testing for HIV infection; follow-up tests are needed to confirm the presence of HIV antibodies.

As many as 1 billion copies of HIV can be made in 1 day, and several generations can exist in just hours. The replication of the infected cell results in a steady depletion of the CD4 cell count, causing a severe depression of immunity, and increasing the risk for opportunistic infections and malignancies (Box 20.4).

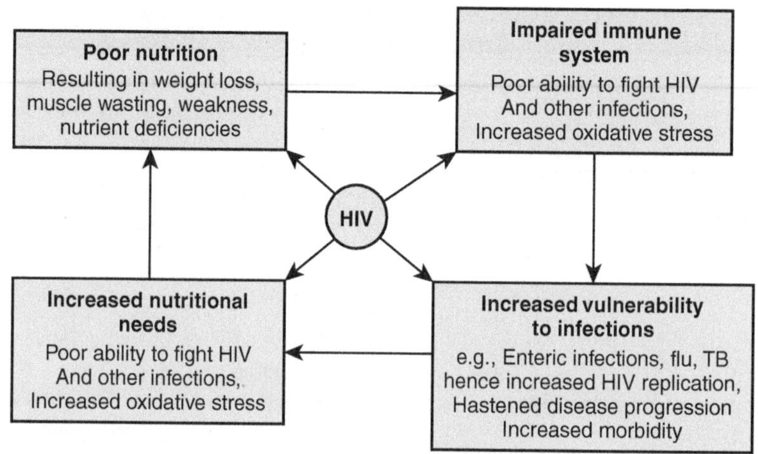

Fig. 20.4 Vicious circle of malnutrition and acquired immunodeficiency syndrome. *HIV*, Human immunodeficiency virus; *TB*, tuberculosis.. (Research Gate. Modified from The Vicious Cycle of Malnutrition and HIV. Accessed 20 September, 2020. https://www.researchgate.net/figure/The-vicious-cycle-of-malnutrition-and-HIV-Source_fig2_317731802.)

The progression from HIV to AIDS varies for each person and may not be evident for several years. The two major prognostic factors for HIV are the CD4 cell count and the measurement of plasma HIV RNA (viral load for HIV). The diagnosis of AIDS includes the positive antibody test result for HIV, a CD4 cell count of less than 200/mm^3 or less than 14% of the total white blood cell count, and the clinical diagnosis of 1 of 25 AIDS-defining diseases.

There has been significant progress in treatment of HIV and AIDS over the past decade with the use of drug combinations for highly active antiretroviral therapy (HAART). The goal of these treatment regimens is to maintain a low viral load.

Malnutrition in Human Immunodeficiency Virus/Acquired Immunodeficiency Syndrome

Impaired nutrient absorption occurs during infection. Energy requirements are 10% to 15% above normal; protein needs are 50% to 100% greater than normal. Malnutrition has been documented in all stages of HIV infection. Most nutritional problems coincide with the incidence of high viral loads, opportunistic infections, and the development of viral resistance.

With the evolution of HAART, nutritional problems have shifted to include more chronic disease issues, such as hyperlipidemia, insulin resistance, and diabetes mellitus. In infected individuals who do not have access to these medication regimens and in people who choose not to use them, malnutrition is still common.

AIDS-related wasting syndrome consists of involuntary weight loss of greater than 10% of body weight in 1 month with the presence of chronic diarrhea, weakness, or fever for more than 30 days in the absence of a concurrent illness or condition. Malnutrition in HIV and AIDS is multifactorial, as shown in Fig. 20.4. Altered nutrient intake, weight loss and body composition changes, physical impairment, endocrine disorders, metabolic changes, malabsorption, the presence of opportunistic infections, psychosocial issues, and economic conditions all contribute.

Malnutrition and weight loss are important predictors of both morbidity and mortality from AIDS. Thus, nutrition is a crucial element of medical care, not simply an alternative or adjunct therapy. Nutrition is one area in which clients can exert some control over their medical care. It is critical to begin interventions early. The first step should be education about the role of nutrition. Emphasizing the benefits of maintaining nutritional status is important, such as repair and building of tissue, preserving lean body mass and GI function, minimizing fatigue, and improving quality of life (see the *Teaching Tool* box Maximizing Food Intake in Human Immunodeficiency Virus/Acquired Immunodeficiency Syndrome).

TEACHING TOOL

Maximizing Food Intake in Human Immunodeficiency Virus/Acquired Immunodeficiency Syndrome

The following strategies improve calories and protein intake without necessarily increasing the volume of food:

- Substitute nutrient-dense, high-calorie foods and beverages for low- or no-kcal foods and beverages: milk or shakes instead of coffee or tea; 100% fruit juice for sugar-free drinks.
- Offer five or six small meals/snacks.
- Fortify foods with high-calorie, protein-containing ingredients. Add skim milk or whey protein powder to milk, shakes, gravies, mashed potatoes, hot cereals.
- Use high-calorie condiments. Add butter/margarine to hot cereals, vegetables, and starches.
- Modify diet according to tolerances. Try cold or room-temperature foods, bland or salty foods; avoid greasy and sweet foods and liquids between meals.
- Offer supplements between meals, such as Carnation Instant Breakfast or milkshakes.
- Drink liquids often to avoid dehydration. Cut back on alcoholic beverages.
- Avoid caffeine during periods of diarrhea. Consume yogurt with active cultures.
- For mouth pain, cut back on citrus and spicy foods; drink beverages with a straw; choose foods at room temperature or cooler.

More tips are available at these websites:

WebMD https://www.webmd.com/hiv-aids/guide/nutrition-hiv-aids-enhancing-quality-life

USDA https://www.nutrition.gov/topics/diet-and-health-conditions/aidshiv

Food and Nutrition Therapies

Altered Nutrient Intake

Anorexia, or loss of appetite, is a common symptom of altered nutrient intake. Economic availability of adequate food supplies cannot be forgotten and often may be the most difficult problem to solve. Strategies for coping with loss of appetite are listed in Table 20.3.

Body Composition and Weight Changes

Patients with HIV/AIDS may experience weight loss and changes in body composition. Weight loss appears to occur not only from fat stores but also from lean body mass. This phenomenon is not as easily explained. Acute weight loss differs from chronic weight loss, not only in its etiology but also in the type of energy stores that are depleted. Chronic weight loss from malnutrition is often accompanied by a decrease in metabolic rate and a reliance on fat stores for energy. Acute weight loss, such as seen in stress, is accompanied by an increase in metabolic rate, a reliance on glucose as fuel, and a depletion of lean body mass. These changes in body composition and weight loss are commonly seen in the wasting syndrome and often coincide with increases in viral load. Regular checkups are important to evaluate changes in status (Fig. 20.5).

Endocrine and Metabolic Disorders

Hypogonadism is common with this disease and leads to fatigue, decreased libido, loss of muscle mass, muscle weakness, impotence, and loss of body hair. The associated fatigue contributes not only to decreased appetite but also to impaired ability to prepare and consume meals. Loss of lean body mass is a primary feature. Adrenal insufficiency may contribute to changes in appetite, loss of fuel storage, and alterations in metabolism.

Exercise

Regular aerobic exercise and resistance training assist with lipid abnormalities, the fat redistribution syndrome, and other body composition changes. Recommendations should be individualized and initiated slowly after receiving a physician's approval. Benefits may include the following:

- Increased muscle volume, strength, functional capacity, and quality of life
- Decreased abdominal fat
- Prevention of glucose abnormalities and reduced insulin sensitivity
- Better circulation
- Improved bone density

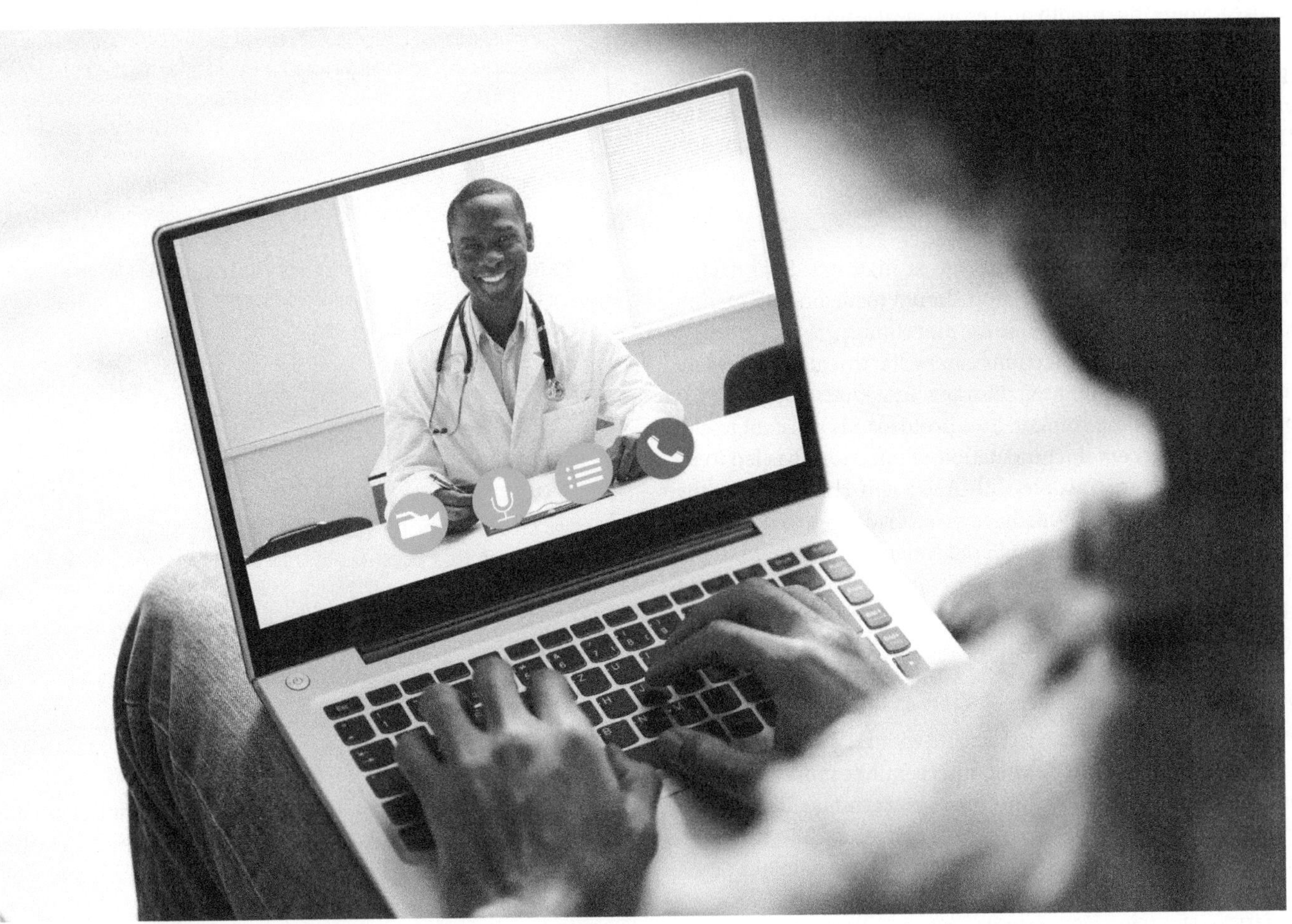

Fig. 20.5 Telehealth is beneficial for managing human immunodeficiency virus/acquired immunodeficiency syndrome (HIV/AIDS). (From © iStock Photo; Credit: AndreyPopov.)

Fat Redistribution Syndrome (Lipodystrophy)

HIV-associated lipodystrophy syndrome (HALS) is a known side effect of HAART. HALS is associated with both body composition changes (lipoatrophy, lipohypertrophy) and metabolic alterations (dyslipidemia, glucose intolerance, diabetes, hypertension, endothelial dysfunction, and atherosclerosis). A Mediterranean-style diet and supplementation with omega-3 fatty acids is recommended.

Malabsorption

Malabsorption can be a result of (1) opportunistic infections that damage the GI tract, (2) the effects of malnutrition on villus height and enterocyte function, and (3) the disease itself. In patients with HIV-related diarrhea, steatorrhea has been noted. Treatment of the underlying cause, if possible, is crucial.

Restriction of fat and lactose is common. Lactose-free supplements and supplements containing medium-chain triglycerides (Advera, Alitraq, Peptamen, Lipisorb) are commonly prescribed. Additionally, probiotics and prebiotics, as well as glutamine and arginine, either in enteral products or given separately, have been used to assist in malabsorption syndrome and diarrhea. Careful attention must be given to ensure adequate caloric and protein intake when fat and lactose, important energy and protein sources, must be restricted.

Physical Impairment

Nausea, vomiting, mouth and esophageal lesions, and impaired dentition are common problems. They may be a result of candidiasis and gingivitis, or they may be side effects of antiretroviral therapy, prophylactic treatments, and pain medication. Determining the cause of impaired intake is important for a successful intervention (see Table 20.3).

Prevention of Food Poisoning

As CD4 cell counts fall, clients are at high risk for infections from foods. Nutrition education should focus on safe methods for food purchasing, preparation, and storage.

Cryptosporidium infections can be life threatening and may lead to chronic, debilitating diarrhea. Infectious outbreaks have been linked to water sources. This protozoan is resistant to chlorination, and recent documentation of infections has led to recommendations that people with AIDS and HIV monitor their water sources. Suggestions have been made to avoid all public tap water and to drink only filtered water or water that has been boiled for 1 minute (Box 20.5). Fruits and vegetables can be cleaned with a mixture of 20 drops of 2% iodine in 1 gallon of water to prevent contamination.

Wasting and Malnutrition—A Vicious Circle

Wasting and malnutrition in patients with HIV and AIDS create a vicious circle that can be fatal. Interventions must be provided early. Research has shown promise concerning the efficacy of nutrition interventions. Conducting nutrition assessment and providing counseling have enabled patients to maintain or gain weight. Health care teams can treat the nutritional problems of HIV and AIDS with multiple and complementary modes of therapy (Box 20.6).

BOX 20.5 Safe Water for Immunosuppressed Patients

Immune system functioning may be diminished because of the effects of chemotherapy drugs, drugs used to prevent organ-transplant rejection, and human immunodeficiency virus/acquired immunodeficiency syndrome (HIV/AIDS). Because public water quality and treatment vary throughout the United States, always check with the local health department and water utility for any special notices about the use of tap water by immunocompromised persons. Heating water at a rolling boil for 1 minute kills *Cryptosporidium*. After the boiled water cools, put it in a clean bottle or pitcher with a lid, and store it in the refrigerator. Use the water for drinking, cooking, or making ice. Water bottles and ice trays should be cleaned with soap and water before use. Additional measures include filtering water or using commercially bottled water.

When traveling to developing nations, poor water treatment and food sanitation are a consideration. Raw fruits and vegetables, tap water, ice made from tap water, unpasteurized milk or dairy products, and items purchased from street vendors might be contaminated. Processed carbonated (bubbly) drinks in cans or bottles are probably safe, but drinks made at a fountain might not be because they are made with tap water.

(Modified from Centers for Disease Control and Prevention, accessed 6 August, 2017 at http://www.cdc.gov/parasites/crypto/gen_info/prevent_ic.html.)

BOX 20.6 Evaluation of Complementary and Alternative Therapies

Because currently there are no cures for some cancers and human immunodeficiency virus/acquired immunodeficiency syndrome (HIV/AIDS), patients with these diseases are potential victims for unproven or fraudulent health and nutrition therapies. High doses of vitamins and minerals can result in toxicities that are potentially harmful. Complementary and alternative therapies not only may be extremely costly, but also may interfere with current medical treatments, putting the patient at even more risk. For example, microbial growth in herbal supplements may pose a risk of opportunistic infections in immunosuppressed patients.

The National Center for Complementary and Alternative Medicine (NCCAM) at the National Institutes of Health provides the structure for evaluating complementary and alternative therapies. Currently, clinical studies have been or are being conducted to assess the value of complementary and alternative therapies for disorders such as cancer and HIV/AIDS. Questionable practices or products may be reported to the following sources:

- Federal Trade Commission (FTC) Bureau of Consumer Protection; regional FTC office; chief postal inspector, US Postal Service; editor or station manager of media outlet where advertisement appeared; regional U.S. Food and Drug Administration (FDA) office; state attorney general; state health department; local Better Business Bureau; congressional representative; local or state professional society; local hospital (if practitioner is a staff member); state licensing board; local district attorney
- National Council Against Health Fraud (www.ncahf.org); Consumer Health Information Research Institute; local, state, or national professional or voluntary health groups.

Application to nursing. Prevention of dehydration and effective monitoring of intake and output are required in patients with HIV/AIDS. Fluid losses may be high in the patient with diarrhea.

Highly active antiretroviral therapy (HAART) uses combinations of fusion inhibitors, integrase inhibitors, nucleoside/nucleotide reverse transcriptase inhibitors, nonnucleoside reverse transcriptase inhibitors, and protease inhibitors. Adherence to the regimen is difficult because of the number and the complexity of medications that must be taken daily. Drug resistance can develop if adherence is not maintained. Side effects of these medications include nausea, vomiting, diarrhea, and other metabolic changes.

Depression, loneliness, fear, anxiety, and other psychosocial issues can play a significant role in the client's desire to eat. Physical impairment from mucositis, esophagitis, pain, nausea, and vomiting affects the client's ability to ingest adequate nutrients. Anorexia may be caused by the HIV infection, the presence of other opportunistic infections, fatigue, or fever or may be a medication side effect.

Medications can be prescribed to assist with anorexia and body composition changes. Megestrol acetate (Megace), dronabinol (Marinol), oxandrolone (Oxandrin) or oxymetholone, testosterone, dehydroepiandrosterone (DHEA), and recombinant human growth hormone (r-hGH) have all been used with this population. Dronabinol has been shown to improve appetite, mood, and nausea, resulting in weight maintenance. Side effects include euphoria, dizziness, and impaired thinking. Oxandrolone is an oral analog of testosterone that increases lean body mass, elevates mood, and improves libido. DHEA and human growth hormone (r-hGH) have been used to improve lean body mass with a decrease in abdominal adiposity.

The ingestion of food along with certain medications may affect the absorption of the drugs and vice versa. Examples are as follows:

Efavirenz (Sustiva): Avoid taking with high-fat meals.

Lopinavir (Kaletra) + ritonavir (Norvir): Moderate-fat meals increase availability of capsules; take with food.

Saquinavir (Invirase): Take this protease inhibitor within 2 hours of a meal containing high-fat foods or a large snack containing carbohydrate, protein, or fat.

Ritonavir (Norvir): If this protease inhibitor is consumed with a meal, it may decrease the abdominal cramping and diarrhea that is common when this drug is initially prescribed. These symptoms usually disappear within 8 weeks.

Indinavir (Crixivan): This protease inhibitor should be taken on an empty stomach. A meal can be eaten 1 hour after the drug is taken or 2 hours before. Some patients may find it necessary to eat a small snack with the drug, but fat should be avoided.

Effective treatment requires a multidisciplinary approach based on collaboration of all health care team members, including the nurse, dietitian, social worker and pharmacist. Early recognition and intervention of nutritional risk are vital (see the *Cultural Diversity and Nutrition* box Human Immunodeficiency Virus/Acquired Immunodeficiency Syndrome and Ethnic Issues in Healing and Medicine: Lessons From Tuskegee).

CULTURAL DIVERSITY AND NUTRITION

Human Immunodeficiency Virus/Acquired Immunodeficiency Syndrome and Ethnic Issues in Healing and Medicine: Lessons From Tuskegee

As we attempt to "heal" our patients, we need to understand history to fully comprehend the perspective of the patients with whom we work. During the middle of the twentieth century (1932–1972), a medical study called the Tuskegee Experiment followed the course of syphilis among Black American men from a poor county in Georgia. When the study began, there was no known cure for syphilis, but shortly into the study, penicillin was recognized as an effective drug against the ravages of this sexually transmitted disease. Nonetheless, such treatment was withheld from the men participating in this study, and most were followed to their deaths, which may or may not have been from syphilis-related causes. The study did not end until the 1970s after the men, their wives, and children suffered the consequences of a serious systemic disease that could have been cured with inexpensive penicillin. Many people believe that the reason such an unethical protocol was allowed was because the participants were poor Black American.

In 1973 a class action lawsuit for the individuals and family members affected by the study was filed by the National Association for the Advancement of Colored People (NAACP). A $9 million settlement was awarded and distributed among those affected. In 1997, President Clinton issued a formal apology on behalf of the U.S. government.

Application to Nursing

Knowledge of such mistreatment provides an understanding of current bias against government-sponsored medical treatment. By understanding history, we can educate clients about the ethical medical treatments available now.

(Data from Chadwick A: *Remembering Tuskegee*, Washington, DC, 25 July, 2002, National Public Radio. Accessed 20 September, 2020, from www.npr.org/templates/story/story.php?storyId=1147234.)

SUMMARY

- Cancer and human immunodeficiency virus/acquired immunodeficiency syndrome (HIV/AIDS) often involve wasting and malnutrition, caused by the effect of the disorders or the secondary consequences of treatment on the gastrointestinal tract.
- Nutrition therapy focuses on identifying at-risk patients, preventing malnutrition, and reducing the effects of treatment.
- Local or systemic effects of the cancer combined with antineoplastic therapy put the cancer patient at risk for malnutrition or cancer cachexia through a variety of mechanisms: anorexia, nausea, vomiting, mucositis, organ injury (toxicity), and learned food aversions.
- Nutrition support must be individualized and is an essential component of the total management of cancer.
- With the provision of adequate nutritional support, patients with cancer may have a decreased risk of surgical complications.
- Nutrients are needed to rebuild normal tissues that have been affected by antineoplastic therapy, in order to have a higher tolerance to therapies.
- AIDS, caused by the retrovirus HIV, leads to the breakdown of the immune system, opportunistic infections, or enteropathy.
- Malnutrition in HIV/AIDS is multifactorial and includes decreased nutrient (food) intake, malabsorption, and altered metabolism.
- Goals of HIV nutrition therapy are individualized, and interventions are based on nutritional status, causes of malnutrition, infections, and complications.
- Early recognition of and intervention for HIV nutritional risk factors and indicators are keys to effective nutrition support and related medical therapies.

THE NURSING APPROACH

Clinical Judgment and Next-Generation NCLEX® Examination-Style Questions

Case Study 1

Cancer and Chemotherapy

Sophia, age 35 years, is visiting the nurse practitioner for a follow-up related to her breast cancer treatment. She has been receiving chemotherapy and radiation therapy for the past month after having a lumpectomy of the right breast.

Assessment/Recognize Cues

Subjective (From Patient Statements)

- "I've been really sick from the chemotherapy. It makes me feel nauseated all the time, and often I vomit right after the treatment."
- "I've lost 5 pounds since starting the chemotherapy and radiation treatments."
- "It's hard to eat very much because my mouth is sore and nothing tastes good anyway."
- "I'm too tired to do any cooking."

Objective (From Physical Examination)

- Height 5 feet 6 inches, weight 119 pounds
- Temperature 98.8° F
- Mouth inflamed, tongue appears red and raw; white raised patches on tongue and oral mucosa
- White blood cell (WBC) count 3000/mm^3

Diagnoses (Nursing)/Analyze Cues

1. Weight loss related to nausea, fatigue, and impaired taste and oral mucous membranes, as evidenced by the loss of 5 pounds in the past month
2. Potential for infection related to immunosuppression secondary to chemotherapy as evidence by WBC 3000/mm^3

Planning/Prioritize Hypotheses

Patient Outcomes

Short term (by end of this visit):

- Sophia will describe ways she can improve her overall comfort and increase her food intake.
- She will agree to obtain resources about coping with chemotherapy from American Cancer Society.

Long term (by follow-up visit in 1 month):

- Lesions in mouth will be diminished, and Sophia will be able to eat with less discomfort.
- Sophia will maintain or increase weight.
- There will be no signs of infection.

Nursing Interventions/Generate Solutions

1. Discuss measures to improve comfort and increase food intake.
2. Provide Sophia with resources for information about cancer and chemotherapy.

Implementation/Take Action

1. Recommended small, frequent meals rather than large meals.
   Small meals are usually easier to tolerate than large meals when the gastrointestinal system is altered. Antineoplastic medications kill cancer cells because they divide rapidly. However, chemotherapy also kills normal cells that divide rapidly, involving the gastrointestinal system, bone marrow, and hair. Commercial nutritional supplements should be consumed between meals rather than with meals to reduce satiety at mealtime.
2. Discussed ways to reduce nausea and vomiting.
   It is best to avoid foods with strong odors. If that is not possible, staying out of the kitchen and having someone else do the cooking may reduce nausea. Room deodorizers also may be helpful. Fried foods are harder to digest, so they should be avoided or minimized.
3. Stressed the importance of eating a well-balanced diet, using nutrient-dense foods. Also suggested eating favorite foods and taking a vitamin supplement.
   A well-balanced diet, including high-protein and high-kcal foods, will provide nourishment and energy to fight cancer, enable better toleration of chemotherapy, promote healing, and prevent infection. Choosing favorite foods may stimulate appetite.
4. Encouraged Sophia to prioritize her activities and to rest before meals.
   When energy is limited, an individual should do the most important activities first. When rested, a patient is more willing to expend energy to eat.
5. Encouraged Sophia to ask for help with shopping and meal preparation.
   Family members, friends, or church groups may provide assistance so that the patient's energy can be conserved and healing can take place.

Continued

THE NURSING APPROACH—cont'd

6. Discussed oral care and treatment for mouth sores.
   Stomatitis (inflammation of the mouth) is a common side effect of chemotherapy. Good oral care with a soft toothbrush and flossing will reduce infection and the likelihood of damage to the oral mucosa. Frequent mouthwashing with baking soda and water helps sores heal by shifting the pH to a less acidic environment. Mouthwashes with alcohol should be avoided because they irritate the mucosa.
7. Administered viscous lidocaine and Nystatin swish-and-swallow as prescribed.
   Use of viscous lidocaine before eating may numb the sore mouth, decreasing discomfort and allowing the patient to eat. When immunosuppression is present, infection from Candida albicans (yeast infection, called thrush) often occurs; Nystatin swish-and-swallow may be prescribed for treatment.
8. Discussed bacterial precautions regarding food.
   Chemotherapy often causes a low white blood cell count, so the patient or food preparer should wash hands thoroughly with soap and water before preparing food and before eating. Cutting boards for meats should be designated and kept separate from cutting boards for other foods.
   No raw fruits and vegetables should be consumed, and commercially bottled water is safer than tap water. Foods need to be well cooked and must be kept hot until eaten. Leftovers need refrigeration and should be eaten within 24 hours.
9. Wrote some suggestions for improving eating while Sophia is receiving chemotherapy.
   When the patient has a sore mouth, soft, bland, cool, or lukewarm food and drinks should be consumed. Avoid tart, salty, acidic (citrus fruits and tomatoes), spicy, coarse, dry, and scratchy foods. Also avoid caffeine, alcohol, and tobacco. Such foods could cause irritation of the mucous membranes, adding to the damage done by the chemotherapy.
10. Encouraged Sophia to download patient information about nutrition from the American *Cancer Society (at* https://www.cancer.org/treatment/survivorship-during-and-after-treatment/staying-active/nutrition/nutrition-during-treatment.html*). Education promotes empowerment.*

Evaluation/Evaluate Outcomes

Short term (by the end of this visit):

- Sophia committed to try methods designed to increase her comfort and food intake.
- She agreed to get resources from American Cancer Society.

Goals met.

Discussion Questions

At a follow-up visit in 1 month, Sophia said her mouth was feeling better and she was able to eat somewhat more easily. She said that she still had problems with nausea and no energy. Her weight was stable, and she had no signs of infection. She said the information from American Cancer Society had been very helpful.

1. How could the nurse encourage Sophia and help her to set some small, realistic goals?
2. What high-calorie and nutrient-dense foods would you recommend for Sophia?

Case Study 2

Maximizing Food Intake in Human Immunodeficiency Virus/Acquired Immunodeficiency Syndrome (HIV/AIDS) Patients

The nurse is caring for an HIV/AIDS patient who is suffering from wasting and malnutrition. What are some nutritional strategies to help improve calories and protein intake without necessarily increasing the volume of food for patients with HIV/AIDS?

Use an X to mark the strategies that improve calorie and protein intake for patients with HIV/AIDS.

Number	Strategy
1.	Offer six to eight small meals/snacks daily.
2.	Limit liquids to increase food consumption.
3.	Avoid caffeine during periods of diarrhea. Consume yogurt with active cultures.
4.	Fortify foods with high-calorie, protein-containing ingredients.
5.	Modify diet according to tolerances. Avoid cold or room-temperature foods and bland or salty foods. Encourage sweet foods.
6.	Use high-calorie condiments. Add butter/margarine to hot cereals, vegetables, and starches.
7.	Offer supplements between meals, such as popcorn and crackers.
8.	Substitute nutrient-dense, high-calorie foods and beverages for low- or no-kcal foods and beverages.

CRITICAL THINKING

Clinical Applications

Minnie, age 20 years, is a college student with an uneventful medical history and no significant illness. After finals, she came down with the flu and has felt run down ever since. She has also had a persistent low-grade fever since the flu. She was admitted to the hospital for dehydration and fever of unknown origin. Laboratory tests show that she has gonorrhea. Minnie confides in you that she has recently started having unprotected sex with a new male partner. She agrees to be screened for human immunodeficiency virus (HIV). The results show that she is HIV positive, and the doctor immediately starts her on a combination of highly active antiretroviral therapy (HAART). She is 5 feet 6 inches tall and weighs 120 pounds on admission. Her usual weight is 130 pounds.

1. What side effects from HAART might Minnie encounter?
2. How will they affect her nutritional status?
3. What suggestions do you have to help Minnie prevent further weight loss?

WEBSITES OF INTEREST

American Institute for Cancer Research

http://www.aicr.org

Offers excellent resources and reviews of research regarding nutrition and cancer prevention.

HIV/AIDS Dietetic Practice Group (Academy of Nutrition and Dietetics)

http://www.hivaidsdpg.org

Provides excellent links for information on HIV/AIDS, caregivers, and organizations offering medical nutrition therapy and food outreach programs.

National Cancer Institute (NCI)

www.cancer.gov

Makes available CancerNet (a cancer database on treatment, screening, prevention, and clinical trials), cancer Trials (clinical trials information center), and CANCERLIT (a bibliographic database).

REFERENCES

Arends, J., et al. (2017). ESPEN expert group recommendations for action against cancer-related malnutrition. *Clinical Nutrition, 36*, 1187–1196.

Bao, Y., et al. (2018). Chemotherapy use, end-of-life care, and costs of care among patients diagnosed with stage IV pancreatic cancer. *Journal of Pain and Symptom Management, 55*(4), 1113–1121.

Haun, M. W., et al. (2017). Early palliative care for adults with advanced cancer. *Cochrane Database of Systematic Reviews,* (6), CD011129.

Jager-Wittenaar, H., & Ottery, F. D. (2017). Assessing nutritional status in cancer: Role of the patient-generated subjective global assessment. *Current Opinion in Clinical Nutrition & Metabolic Care, 20*(5), 322–329.

Prigerson, H. G., et al. (2015). Chemotherapy use, performance status, and quality of life at the end of life. *JAMA Oncology, 1*, 778–784.

Sanchez, G., et al. (2016). Sun protection for preventing basal cell and squamous cell skin cancers. *Cochrane Database of Systematic Reviews,* (7), CD011161.

Tong, L. X., & Young, L. C. (2014). Nutrition: the future of melanoma prevention? *Journal of the American Academy of Dermatology, 71*(1), 151–160.

U.S. Statistics: *Living with HIV*. At https://www.hiv.gov/hiv-basics/overview/data-and-trends/statistics. (Accessed 20 September, 2020)

Wiseman, M. (2019). Nutrition and cancer: prevention and survival. *British Journal of Nutrition, 122*, 481–487.

Zhang, H., & Xu, X. (2017). Mutation-promoting molecular networks of uncontrolled inflammation. *Tumor Biology, 39,* 1010428317701310.

GLOSSARY

A

absorption the process by which substances pass through the intestinal mucosa into the blood or lymph

Academy of Nutrition and Dietetics formerly known as the American Dietetic Association; sets standards of education and expectations for registered dietitians/nutritionists (RDN) and for dietetic technicians, registered (DTRs). The new credential for registration may be stated as RD or RDN, as selected by the individual practitioner

acanthosis nigricans hyperpigmentation and thickening of the skin into velvety irregular folds in the neck and flexural areas

Acceptable Macronutrient Distribution Range (AMDR) intake range for an energy source associated with reducing chronic disease risk while supplying adequate essential nutrients

acesulfame K a synthetically produced nonnutritive sweetener

acetyl coenzyme A (acetyl CoA) important intermediate byproduct in metabolism formed from the breakdown of glucose, fatty acids, and certain amino acids

acupuncture the use of fine needles to open blockages of the flow of Qi, or life force, and thus restore balance

acute respiratory failure (ARF) sudden absence of respirations, with confusion or unresponsiveness caused by obstructive airflow or failure of the pulmonary gas exchange mechanism

acute tubular necrosis (ATN) sudden death of cells in the small tubules of the kidneys as a result of disease or injury

adaptive thermogenesis energy (or heat released) used by the body to adjust to changing physical and biologic environments

adenosine triphosphate (ATP) an energy-rich compound used for all energy-requiring processes in the body

adequate intake (AI) the approximate level of an average nutrient intake, determined by observation of or experimentation with a particular group or population that appears to maintain good health

adipocytes cells specialized for storage of fat

adipose tissue stored form of fat (mainly triglycerides) in the body

ADIME acronym for *a*ssessment, nutrition *d*iagnosis, *i*mplementation, and *m*onitoring-*e*valuation

adrenocorticotropic hormone (ACTH) an adrenal cortex hormone that stimulates secretion of more hormones

aerobic glycolysis the conversion of glucose to ATP for energy when oxygen is available

aerobic pathway a form of energy production that depends on oxygen and increases the use of fat

alcoholic cirrhosis associated with chronic alcohol abuse; accounts for 50% of all cases; also called Laënnec's cirrhosis

aldosterone a hormone secreted by the adrenal gland in response to sodium levels in the kidneys; affects kidneys to balance fluid levels as needed

allogeneic transplant between different individuals who are not genetically identical

alternative medicine healing practices that replace conventional medical treatment

alternative sweeteners nonnutritive sweeteners (or artificial sweeteners) synthetically produced to be sweet tasting but to provide no nutrients and few, if any, kcal; aspartame, saccharin, acesulfame K, and sucralose are alternative sweeteners

Alzheimer's disease a progressive, degenerative disorder that attacks the brain's nerve cells or neurons, resulting in loss of memory, thinking and language skills, and behavioral changes

amenorrhea absence of a menstrual period in a woman of reproductive age; a condition that may occur with anorexia nervosa

amino acid pool the assortment of amino acids available to cells

amino acid score a simple measure of an amino acid composition of a food as compared with a reference protein; based on the limiting amino acid

amino acids organic compounds containing carbon, hydrogen, oxygen, and nitrogen

aminopeptidase an intestinal peptidase that releases free amino acids from the amino end of short-chain peptides

amyloidosis a disorder characterized by accumulation of waxy, starchlike glycoprotein (amyloid) in organs and tissues, affecting their function

anaerobic glycolysis the conversion of glucose to pyruvate to provide energy in the absence of oxygen

anaerobic pathway a form of energy production that does not require oxygen

anaphylaxis a severe immune system response to an allergen

anencephaly a congenital defect in which the brain does not develop; death may occur shortly after birth

angina pectoris chest pain that often radiates down the left arm and is often accompanied by a feeling of suffocation and impending death

anorexia nervosa a mental disorder characterized by self-imposed starvation; may include binge-eating episodes associated with bulimic behaviors

antidiuretic hormone (ADH) a hormone secreted by the pituitary gland in response to low fluid levels; affects kidneys to decrease excretion of water; also called vasopressin

antineoplastic therapy substance, procedure, or measure that prevents the proliferation of malignant cells; usually chemotherapy, radiation therapy, surgery, biologic response modifiers, or bone marrow transplantation

antioxidant a compound that guards other compounds from damaging oxidation

anuria excretion of less than 250 mL urine every 24 hours

appetite desire for food

ariboflavinosis a group of symptoms associated with riboflavin deficiency

aromatherapy use of extracts or essences of herbs, flowers, and trees in the form of essential oils to support health and well-being

arteriosclerosis thickening, loss of elasticity, and calcification of arterial walls, resulting in decreased blood supply to tissues

ascites abnormal intraperitoneal accumulation of fluid containing large amounts of protein and electrolytes, usually resulting in abdominal swelling, hemodilution, edema, and/or decreased urinary output

aspartame a nonnutritive sweetener formed by the bonding of the amino acids phenylalanine and aspartic acid

asthma a chronic respiratory disorder characterized by airway obstruction due to excessive mucus production and respiratory mucosal edema; may be triggered by infection, cold air, vigorous exercise, stress, or inhalation of environmental allergens or pollutants

ataxia muscle weakness and loss of coordination

atherosclerosis development of lesions (also called fatty streaks) in the intima of arteries; during aging the lesions develop into fibrous plaques that project into the vessel lumen and begin to disturb blood flow

athetoid purposeless weaving motions of the body or extremities

atonic lacking normal muscle tone

autoantibodies self-antibodies produced in the pancreas; these include autoantibodies to islet cells, to insulin, and to glutamic acid decarboxylase (GAD65)

autologous transplantation in which the organ or tissue is from the same individual (oneself)

Ayurveda a system of healing focusing on diet and herbal remedies that emphasizes the use of body, mind, and spirit to prevent and treat disorders

B

basal metabolism the amount of energy required to maintain life-sustaining activities for a specific period

beikost *(BYE-cost)* supplemental or weaning foods

beriberi a severe chronic deficiency of thiamine characterized by muscle weakness and pain, anorexia, mental disorientation, and tachycardia

beta cells insulin-producing cells situated in the islets of Langerhans of the pancreas
bezoars physical obstacles created by tangles of fibrous material in the gastrointestinal (GI) tract that may cause dangerous obstructions of the tract
bile a substance that emulsifies fats to aid the digestion of lipids; produced by the liver and stored in the gallbladder
biliary atresia a congenital condition in which the major bile duct is blocked, limiting the availability of bile for fat digestion
biliary cirrhosis cirrhosis associated with obstruction of biliary drainage or biliary disorders; accounts for 15% of all cases of the disease
binge-eating disorder (BED) a mental disorder characterized by frequent binge-eating behaviors, not accompanied by purging or compensatory behaviors; commonly called compulsive overeating
bingeing losing control when eating, resulting in the consumption of excessive amounts of food; often stress-related
bioelectric impedance analysis (BIA) a method using a mild electric charge to estimate lean body mass to determine body fat composition
biofeedback the use of special devices to convey physiologic information to enable a person to learn how to consciously control medically important functions
biologic value a method to determine the quality of food protein by measuring the amount of nitrogen kept in the body after digestion, absorption, and excretion
body mass index (BMI) a measure that describes relative weight for height and is significantly correlated with total body fat content
bolus a masticated lump or ball of food ready to be swallowed
branched-chain amino acids (BCAAs) leucine, isoleucine, and valine; important in metabolism of lean body mass
bulimia nervosa a mental disorder characterized as the binge-and-purge syndrome; includes experiencing repetitive food binges accompanied by purging or compensatory behaviors

C

cachexia general ill health and malnutrition, marked by weakness and emaciation
calcitonin a hormone that reacts in response to high blood levels of calcium; released by the special C cells of the thyroid gland
calcitriol active vitamin D hormone that raises blood calcium levels
calcium rigor a condition of hardness or stiffness of muscles when blood calcium levels are too high
calcium tetany a condition of spasms and nerve excitability when blood calcium levels are too low
cancer uncontrolled growth of cells that tend to invade surrounding tissue and metastasize to distant body sites
carbohydrates organic compounds composed of carbon, hydrogen, and oxygen
carboxypeptidase a pancreatic protease that hydrolyzes polypeptides and dipeptides into amino acids
cardiac cachexia unintentional severe weight loss caused by heart disease
carcinogenesis the process of cancer production
cardiac decompensation impaired cardiac output (reasons not entirely understood)
cardiovascular endurance the ability of the body to take in, deliver, and use oxygen for physical work
cerebrovascular conditions affecting the blood supply of the brain; *cerebrovascular accident* is another term for stroke
cheilosis inflammation of the mucous membrane of the mouth and lips (angular stomatitis) caused by deficiencies of riboflavin and other B vitamins
chemical digestion the chemical altering effects of digestive secretions, gastric juices, and enzymes on food substance composition
chiropractic manipulation a manipulation modality addressing the ties between body structure (particularly of the spine) and function and how those ties affect the maintenance and return to health
cholecystectomy surgical removal of the gallbladder, performed to treat cholelithiasis and cholecystitis
cholecystitis acute inflammation of the gallbladder associated with pain, tenderness, and fever
cholecystokinin (CCK) a hormone secreted by the small intestine that initiates pancreatic exocrine secretions, acts against gastrin, and activates the gallbladder to release bile
choledocholithiasis gallstones in the common bile duct
cholelithiasis presence of stones in the gallbladder
chronic dieting syndrome a lifestyle inhibited or controlled by a constant concern about food intake, body shape, or weight that affects an individual's physical and mental health status
chronic hunger a continual experience of undernutrition, often related to food insecurity
chronic obstructive pulmonary disease (COPD) a progressive and irreversible condition identified by obstruction of airflow, chronic bronchitis, asthma, and emphysema (also called chronic obstructive lung disease)
chylomicrons the first lipoproteins formed after absorption of lipids from food
chyme a semiliquid mixture of food mass
chymotrypsin a pancreatic protease that hydrolyzes polypeptides into dipeptides
***cis* fatty acids** *cis* indicates the configuration of the double bond in a natural oil
coenzyme a substance that activates an enzyme
colic sharp visceral pain
colostomy surgical creation of an artificial anus on the abdominal wall by incising the colon and bringing it out to the surface; may be single-barreled (one opening) or double-barreled (distal and proximal loops open onto the abdomen)
colostrum the fluid secreted from the breast during late pregnancy and the first few days postpartum; contains immunologically active substances (maternal antibodies) and essential nutrients
complementary and alternative medicine (CAM) a cluster of medical and health care approaches, methods, and items not associated with conventional medicine; also called integrative medicine
complementary medicine non-Western healing approaches used at the same time as conventional medicine
complete protein protein containing all nine essential amino acids
complex carbohydrates polysaccharides of starch and fiber
component pureeing each food item is pureed separately (food thickeners may be added to help maintain consistency) and presented in a manner that resembles the original product (e.g., a pork chop can be pureed and molded into a pork chop shape and served)
comprehensive nutritional assessment a procedure conducted by dietetic professionals to determine appropriate medical nutrition therapy based on the identified needs of the patient
congestive heart failure (CHF) circulatory congestion resulting in the heart's inability to maintain blood supply adequate to meet oxygen demands
constipation straining to pass hard, dry stools; slow movement of feces through colon
conventional insulin therapy consists of (1) one or two daily injections of insulin, including mixed intermediate and rapid-acting insulins; (2) daily self-monitoring of urine or blood glucose; and (3) education about diet and exercise
cor pulmonale an abnormal cardiac condition characterized by hypertrophy of the right ventricle as a result of hypertension of the pulmonary circulation
coronary artery disease (CAD) term used for several abnormal conditions that may affect the arteries of the heart and have various pathologic effects, especially reduction in flow of oxygen and nutrients to the cardiac tissue
Crohn's disease an inflammatory disorder that involves all layers of the wall of the small or large intestine or both; is associated with stricture formation, fistulous tracts, and abscesses
cystic fibrosis a genetic disorder in which excessive mucus is produced, primarily affecting respiratory airways; also limits fat absorption in the digestive system; most common among white populations

D

daily values (DVs) a system for food labeling composed of two sets of reference values: reference daily intakes (RDIs) and daily reference values

deamination a process through which an amino acid group breaks off from an amino acid molecule, resulting in molecules of ammonia and keto acid
denatured a change in the shape of protein structures caused by heat, light, acids, alcohol, or mechanical actions
densitometry underwater weighing
diabetes mellitus a disorder of carbohydrate metabolism characterized by hyperglycemia and caused by either defective or deficient insulin
diabetic ketoacidosis (DKA) a potentially life-threatening complication in patients with diabetes mellitus (usually type 1) resulting from a shortage of insulin and producing acidic ketone bodies
dialysate dialysis solution
dialysis a procedure that involves diffusion of particles from an area of high to lower concentration, osmosis of fluid across the membrane from an area of lesser to greater concentration of particles, and the ultrafiltration or movement of fluid across the membrane as a result of an artificially created pressure differential
diarrhea frequent passing of loose, watery bowel movements
diet-induced thermogenesis/thermic effect of food (TEF) an increase of cellular activity when food is eaten
diet manual the reference (usually in a three-ring binder or on computer) that describes the rationale and indications for using a specific diet, lists the allowed and restricted foods, and provides sample menus
dietary fiber carbohydrates (polysaccharides) and lignin in plant foods that cannot be digested by humans
Dietary Reference Intakes (DRIs) dietary standards, including estimated average requirement (EAR), recommended dietary allowance (RDA), adequate intake (AI), and Tolerable Upper Intake Level (UL)
dietary standards a guide to adequate nutrient intake levels against which to compare the nutrient values of foods consumed
dietary supplements substances consumed orally as an addition to dietary intake
dietetic technicians, registered (DTRs) technicians trained in food and nutrition who are an integral part of the health care and foodservice management teams. DTRs have met the following criteria: completion of at least a 2-year degree from an accredited institution, supervised practice, and a national examination through the Accreditation Council for Education in Nutrition and Dietetics (ACEND) of the Academy of Nutrition and Dietetics
digestion the process through which foods are broken down into smaller and smaller units to prepare nutrients for absorption
digestive system a series of organs that functions to prepare ingested nutrients for digestion and absorption
dipeptidase an intestinal peptidase that completes the hydrolysis of proteins to amino acids
disaccharides a sugar formed by two single carbohydrate units bound together; sucrose, maltose, and lactose are disaccharides
disease prevention the recognition of a danger to health that could be reduced or alleviated through specific actions or changes in lifestyle behaviors
diverticula pouchlike herniations protruding from the muscular layer of the colon
diverticulitis inflammation of one or more diverticula
diverticulosis the presence of diverticula
dry beriberi thiamine deficiency affecting the nervous system that produces paralysis and extreme muscle wasting
dumping syndrome contents from the stomach empty too rapidly into the duodenum, causing symptoms of profuse sweating, nausea, dizziness, and weakness
durable power of attorney a legal document in which a competent adult authorizes another competent adult to make decisions for them in the event of incapacitation
dyslipidemia an abnormal amount of lipid (cholesterol, fatty acids) in the blood
dysphagia the inability to swallow normally or freely or to transfer liquid or solid foods from the oral cavity to the stomach; may be caused by an underlying central neurologic or isolated mechanical dysfunction

E

eating disorders a group of behaviors fueled by unresolved emotional conflicts, symptomatized by altered food consumption
edema excess accumulation of fluid in interstitial spaces caused by seepage from the circulatory system
edentulous toothless
eicosapentaenoic acid (EPA) the main omega-3 fatty acid in fish
elemental formulas solutions that provide ready-to-absorb basic nutrients, requiring minimal digestion
emetic substance that causes vomiting
emulsifier a substance that works by being soluble in water and fat at the same time
endogenous originating from within the body or produced internally
endometrium mucous membrane of the uterus
end-stage renal disease (ESRD) the kidneys can no longer function properly; also known as the fifth or final stage in chronic kidney disease
enrichment returning nutrients that were lost during processing to their original levels in foods
enteral nutrition administration of nourishment via the gastrointestinal tract
enteritis infection of the small intestine caused by a virus, bacteria, or protozoa
enzyme-linked immunosorbent assay (ELISA) a test that uses color change and antibodies to detect the presence of a substance, usually an allergen, in the bloodstream
ergogenic aids drugs and dietary regimens believed by some (but not proven) to increase strength, power, and endurance
esophageal varices large and swollen veins at the lower end of the esophagus that are especially vulnerable to ulceration and hemorrhage, usually the result of portal hypertension
esophagitis inflammation of the lower esophagus
essential amino acids (EAAs) amino acids that cannot be manufactured by the human body
essential fat certain components of body fat that are essential for life
essential fatty acids (EFAs) polyunsaturated fatty acids that cannot be made in the body and must be consumed in the diet
essential or primary hypertension elevated blood pressure for which the cause is unknown
estimated average requirement (EAR) the amount of a nutrient needed to meet the basic requirements of half the individuals in a specific group; the basis for setting the RDAs
estimated energy requirement (EER) dietary energy intake predicted to maintain energy balance in a healthy adult of a defined age, weight, and level of physical activity consistent with good health
exocrine glands glands that secrete chemicals into ducts that release into a cavity or to the surface of the body, such as salivary glands (mouth) and the liver (gallbladder)
exogenous originating outside the body or produced from external sources
extracellular fluids all fluids outside cells, including interstitial fluid, plasma, and watery components of body organs and substances

F

faith healing healing by invoking divine intervention without the use of conventional or surgical therapy
fatty infiltration accumulation of fat (triglycerides) in the liver
feeding relationship the interactions or patterns of behaviors that surround food preparation and consumption within a family
fetal alcohol syndrome (FAS)/fetal alcohol spectrum disorder (FASD) a disorder caused by maternal alcohol consumption during pregnancy that produces a range of specific anatomic and central nervous system defects in the fetus
flatus intestinal gas
flexibility the ability to move muscles to their full extent without injury
fluid volume deficit (FVD) the state in which a person experiences vascular, cellular, or intracellular dehydration
fluid volume excess the state in which a person experiences increased fluid retention and edema
fluorosis a condition of mottling or brown spotting of the tooth enamel caused by excessive intake of fluoride
food allergy the overreaction to a food protein or other large molecule that produces an immune response
food choice the specific foods that are convenient to choose when we are actually ready to eat

food intolerance an adverse reaction to a food that does not involve the immune system

food preferences the foods we choose to eat when all foods are available at the same time and in the same quantity

fractionation administration of radiation therapy in smaller doses over time rather than in a single large dose; minimizes tissue damage

functional foods foods or ingredients in a food that have potentially positive health effects beyond basic nutrition

G

galactosemia an autosomal recessive disorder resulting in an inability to metabolize galactose and lactose milk products

gastrin a hormone secreted by stomach mucosa that increases the release of gastric juices

gastroesophageal reflux (GER) return of gastric contents into the esophagus that results in a severe burning sensation under the sternum; commonly called heartburn

gastroesophageal reflux disease (GERD) a syndrome of chronic or recurrent return of gastric contents into the esophagus that results in a severe burning sensation under the sternum and possibly nausea, belching, cough, or hoarseness

gastrointestinal (GI) tract the main organs of the digestive system that form a tube that runs from the mouth to the anus

gerontology the study of aging

gestational diabetes mellitus (GDM) a form of diabetes occurring most commonly after the 20th week of gestation

glomerulonephritis inflammation of the glomerulus of the kidney, characterized by proteinuria, hematuria, decreased urine production, and edema

glossitis inflammation of the tongue

glucagon a pancreatic hormone that releases glycogen from the liver

glucocorticoid an adrenal cortex hormone that affects food metabolism

gluconeogenesis the process of producing glucose from fat and protein

glycemic index the level to which a food raises blood glucose levels compared with a reference food

glycemic load the total glycemic index effect of a mixed meal or dietary plan; calculated by the sum of products of the glycemic index for each of the foods multiplied by the amount of carbohydrate in each food

glycogen carbohydrate energy stored in the liver and muscles

glycogenesis the process of converting glucose to glycogen

glycogenolysis the process of converting glycogen back to glucose

glycolysis the conversion of glucose to carbon compounds

glycosylated hemoglobin (A_{1c}) a substance (glycohemoglobin) formed when hemoglobin combines with some of the glucose in the bloodstream

goiter enlargement of the thyroid gland caused by iodine deficiency

graft-versus-host disease (GVHD) a complication that can occur after a stem cell or bone marrow transplantation in which the newly transplanted donor cells attack the transplant recipient's body as if it were a foreign substance; GVHD is more common in transplants where the donor and recipient are unrelated

H

hard water water containing high amounts of minerals, such as calcium and magnesium

health the merging and balancing of five physical and psychological dimensions of health: physical, mental, emotional, social, and spiritual

health literacy the ability to understand basic health concepts and apply them to one's own health decisions

health promotion strategies used to increase the level of health of individuals, families, groups, and communities

healthy weight weight that allows comfortable physical movement, without undue food restrictions, excessive exercise, or experience of weight-related associative disorders

heme iron dietary iron found in animal foods of meat, fish, and poultry

hemochromatosis a hereditary disorder of iron metabolism characterized by excessive dietary iron absorption and deposition of iron in body tissues

hemodialysis a procedure to remove impurities or wastes from the blood in treating renal insufficiency by shunting the blood from the body through a machine for diffusion and ultrafiltration and then returning it to the patient's circulation

hemodilution dilution of the blood

hemoglobin oxygen-transporting protein in red blood cells

hemosiderosis a condition in which too much iron is stored in the body

heparinized use of an antithrombin factor to prevent intravascular clotting

hepatic coma neurophysiologic symptom of extensive liver damage caused by chronic or acute liver disease

hepatic encephalopathy a type of brain damage caused by liver disease and consequent ammonia intoxication

hepatotoxic potentially destructive to liver cells

hiatal hernia herniation of a portion of the stomach into the chest through the esophageal hiatus of the diaphragm

high-density lipoproteins (HDLs) lipoproteins that carry fats and cholesterol from body cells to the liver and are made of large proportions of proteins

high-fructose corn syrup (HFCS) corn syrup processed to contain an increased proportion of fructose, producing sweetness similar to or higher than that of sugar (sucrose)

high-quality protein a food containing the best balance and assortment of essential and nonessential amino acids for protein synthesis

homeopathic medicine an alternative medical system through which a small amount of a diluted substance is prescribed to relieve symptoms for which the same substance, given in larger amounts, will cause the same symptoms

homeostasis a state of physiologic equilibrium produced by a balance of functions and of chemical composition within an organism

hormones substances that act as messengers between organs to cause the release of needed secretions

hunger a physiologic need for food

hydrogenation breaking a double bond on a fatty acid carbon chain and saturating it with hydrogen

hydroxyapatite a natural mineral structure of bones and teeth

hyperbilirubinemia a neonatal condition of excessively high levels of bilirubin (red bile pigment) leading to jaundice, in which bile is deposited in tissues throughout the body

hypercaloric containing more than 1 kcal/mL

hypercholesterolemia total blood cholesterol levels greater than 200 mg/dL; greater than normal amounts of cholesterol in the blood; may be reduced or prevented by avoiding saturated fats

hyperemesis gravidarum severe and unrelenting vomiting in the second trimester of pregnancy or vomiting that severely interferes with the mother's life; a serious condition usually requiring intravenous replacement of nutrients and fluids

hyperglycemia elevated blood glucose level (>120 mg/dL)

hyperosmolar abnormally increased osmolarity

hyperplasia an increase in the number of cells occurring during the growth spurts accompanying normal development

hypertension (HTN) an average systolic blood pressure >140 mm Hg or a diastolic pressure >90 mm Hg (or both)

hypertonic having greater concentration of solute than another solution

hypertrophy an increase in the size of cells

hypoglycemia blood glucose levels that are below normal values

hypogonadism a deficiency in the secretory activity of the ovary or testis

hyponatremia low blood sodium level

hypophosphatemia low serum phosphorus level

hyporeflexia a neurologic condition characterized by weakened reflex reactions

hypoxia lack of oxygen to the cells

I

iatrogenic inadvertently caused by treatment or diagnostic procedures

idiopathic steatorrhea fat malabsorption caused by unknown causes

ileostomy in a patient with entire colon and rectum removed, surgical formation of an opening of the ileum onto the surface of the abdomen, through which fecal matter is emptied

incidental (indirect) food additives substances that inadvertently contaminate processed foods

incomplete protein proteins lacking one or more of the essential amino acids
insensible perspiration water lost invisibly through evaporation from the lungs and skin
insoluble dietary fibers dietary fibers that do not dissolve in fluids
insulin a hormone produced by the pancreas that regulates blood glucose levels
integrative medicine merging of conventional medical therapies with complementary and alternative medicine (CAM) modalities for which safety and efficacy, based on scientific data, have been demonstrated
intensive insulin therapy consists of (1) administration of insulin more than three times daily (injection or pump) with dosage adjusted according to results of self-monitoring of blood glucose performed at least four times daily, (2) dietary intake, and (3) anticipated exercise
intentional (direct) food additives substances purposely added during manufacturing to food products
interstitial fluid fluid between the cells containing concentrations of sodium and chloride
intracellular fluid fluid within the cells composed of water plus concentrations of potassium and phosphates
intrinsic factor a substance produced by stomach mucosa that is required for vitamin B_{12} absorption
irradiation a procedure by which food is exposed to radiation that destroys microorganisms, insect growth, and parasites that could spoil food or cause illness
ischemic deficient supply of blood to a body part (as the heart or brain) that is due to obstruction of the inflow of arterial blood
isotonic having the same concentration of solute as another solution, therefore exerting the same amount of osmotic pressure as that solution

K

keratomalacia a condition caused by vitamin A deficiency in which the cornea becomes dry and thickens from the formation of hard protein tissue
ketone bodies a breakdown product of fatty acid catabolism
ketosis a condition in which the absence of plasma glucose results in partial oxidation of fatty acids and the formation of excessive amounts of ketones
Kt/V a calculation used to quantify hemodialysis and peritoneal dialysis treatment adequacy. K = dialyzer clearance of urea; t = dialysis time; V = volume of distribution of urea, approximately equal to patient's total body water
kwashiorkor malnutrition in children caused by a lack of protein in spite of adequate energy consumption

L

lactation the production of breast milk
lacto-vegetarian dietary pattern a food plan consisting of only plant foods plus dairy products
lifestyle a pattern of behaviors
limiting amino acid the essential amino acid or amino acids that incomplete proteins lack
linoleic acid an essential polyunsaturated fatty acid with the first double bond located at the sixth carbon atom from the omega end
linolenic acid an essential polyunsaturated fatty acid with the first double bond located at the third carbon atom from the omega end
lipogenesis anabolism (synthesis) of lipids
lithotripsy extracorporeal shock wave lithotripsy (ESWL), a noninvasive technique whereby high-intensity shock waves cause fragmentation of gallstones from a device outside the body
locus of control the perception of one's ability to control life events and experiences
low birth weight weighing less than 5.5 pounds (2500 g) at birth
low-density lipoproteins (LDLs) lipoproteins that carry fats and cholesterol to body cells and that are made of large proportions of cholesterol

M

macrophages cells that are able to surround, engulf, and digest microorganisms and cellular debris; big scavenger cells
macrosomia abnormally large body size in a newborn infant
macrovascular pertaining to larger blood vessels found in the aorta, coronary arteries, limbs, and brain
major minerals essential nutrient minerals required daily in amounts of 100 mg or higher
malnutrition an imbalanced nutrient and/or energy intake
marasmus malnutrition in children caused by a severe lack of energy (kcal) intake
MCT fats (oils) specialized modular formulas made of medium-chain triglycerides that do not require pancreatic lipase or bile for digestion and absorption; they are absorbed directly into the portal vein (like amino acids and monosaccharides) rather than through the lymphatic system like other lipids
mechanical digestion the crushing and twisting effects of teeth and peristalsis that divide foods into smaller pieces
medical nutrition the use of specific nutrition services to treat an illness, injury, or condition
medical nutrition therapy legal definition of nutrition therapy provided by a registered dietitian for Medicare clients (pre-renal failure, diabetes only)
meditation a self-directed technique of relaxing the body and calming the mind
megacolon massive, abnormal dilation of the colon that may be congenital, toxic, or acquired
menopause the end of menstruation due to the cessation of ovarian and follicular function
metabolism a set of processes through which absorbed nutrients are used by the body for energy and to form and maintain body structures and functions
metastasis the spread of malignant cells to other sites from the original tumor location
microcephaly abnormal smallness of head with brain underdevelopment
monosaccharides a sugar composed of a single carbohydrate unit; glucose, fructose, and galactose are monosaccharides
monounsaturated fatty acid a fatty acid containing a carbon chain with one unsaturated double bond
mucosa the inside gastrointestinal muscle tissue layer composed of mucous membrane
mucositis inflammation of mucous membranes
multifactorial phenotype a characteristic that is the product of numerous genetic and environmental factors
multiple organ dysfunction syndrome (MODS) the progressive failure of two or more organ systems (e.g., the renal, hepatic, cardiac, or respiratory systems) at the same time
muscular strength and endurance the ability of the muscles to perform hard or prolonged work
muscularis a thick layer of muscle tissue surrounding the submucosa
myocardial infarction (MI) occlusion of a coronary artery; sometimes called heart attack
myoglobin oxygen-transporting protein in muscle

N

naturopathic medicine the use of the body's natural healing forces to recover from disease and to achieve wellness; it incorporates techniques from Eastern and Western traditions
nephrosclerosis necrosis of the renal arterioles; associated with hypertension
nephrotoxic toxic or destructive to a kidney
night blindness the inability of the eyes to readjust from bright to dim light caused by vitamin A deficiency
nitrogen-balance studies measurement of the amount of nitrogen entering the body compared with the amount excreted
nocturia excessive urination at night
nonessential amino acids (NEAAs) amino acids manufactured by the human body
nonheme iron dietary iron found in plant foods
nutrients substances in foods required by the body for energy, growth, maintenance, and repair
nutrition the study of essential nutrients and the processes by which nutrients are used by the body
nutritional genomics a science studying the relationship among the human genome, nutrition, and health; how food affects genes and how genetic differences affect response to dietary intakes
Nutrition Care Process a systematic approach to providing high-quality nutrition care by registered dietitians; includes steps of assessment, nutrition diagnosis, intervention, monitoring, and evaluation
nutrition therapy the provision of nutrient, dietary, and nutrition education needs based on a comprehensive nutritional assessment to

treat an illness, injury, or condition; definition may be dictated by state laws licensing registered dietitians (RDs)

nutritional risk the potential to become malnourished because of primary (inadequate intake of nutrients) or secondary (causes by disease or iatrogenic effects) factors

nutritional support although commonly used in reference to enteral and parenteral nutrition delivery systems, can refer to any nutrition intervention used to minimize patient morbidity, mortality, and complications

nutritionist a professional who has completed a master's or doctoral degree in foods and nutrition

O

oliguria less than 400 mL urine excretion every 24 hours

osmolality concentration of electrically charged particles per kilogram of solution

osmotic diarrhea diarrhea-associated water retention in the large intestine resulting from an accumulation of nonabsorbable water-soluble solutes

osteodystrophy defective bone development associated with disturbances in calcium and phosphorus metabolism and renal insufficiency

osteomalacia an adult disorder caused by vitamin D or calcium deficiency and characterized by soft, demineralized bones

osteopathic medicine an approach based on the assumption that the systems of the body function together and that diseases stem from the musculoskeletal system

osteoporosis a multifactorial disorder in which bone density is reduced and remaining bone is brittle, breaking easily

overnutrition consumption of too many nutrients and too much energy in comparison with Dietary Reference Intake levels

ovo-lacto vegetarian dietary pattern a food plan consisting of only plant foods plus dairy products and eggs

oxygen debt the amount of oxygen required to clear lactic acid buildup from the body

oxytocin a hormone that initiates the uterine contractions of labor and has a role in the ejection of milk in lactation

P

pancreatitis inflammation of the pancreas; may be acute or chronic

parathormone a hormone that raises blood calcium levels; secreted by the parathyroid gland in response to low blood calcium levels

parenteral nutrition administration of nutrients by a route other than the gastrointestinal (GI) tract, usually intravenous

pellagra the deficiency disorder of niacin characterized by diarrhea, dermatitis, and dementia

pepsin a gastric protease

pepsinogen the inactive form of pepsin

percutaneous endoscopic placement (PEG) placing a feeding tube into the stomach via the esophagus and then drawing it through the abdominal skin using a stab incision

perimenopause the time before menopause during which hormonal, biologic, and clinical changes begin to occur

peripheral vascular disease (PVD) condition affecting blood vessels outside the heart, characterized by a variety of signs and symptoms such as numbness, pain, pallor, elevated blood pressure, and impaired arterial pulsations. Causative factors include obesity, cigarette smoking, stress, sedentary occupations, and numerous metabolic disorders

peristalsis the rhythmic contractions of muscles causing wavelike motions that move food down the gastrointestinal tract

peritoneal dialysis (PD) a dialysis procedure performed to correct an imbalance of fluid or electrolytes in the blood or other wastes by using the peritoneum as the diffusible membrane

pernicious anemia inadequate red blood cell formation caused by a lack of intrinsic factor in the stomach with which to absorb vitamin B_{12}

phenylketonuria (PKU) a genetic disorder in which the body cannot break down excess phenylalanine

phospholipids lipid compounds that form part of cell walls and act as fat emulsifiers

physical activity any body movement produced by skeletal muscles that results in energy expenditure

physical fitness the limits on the actions that the body is capable of making

phytochemicals nonnutritive substances in plant-based foods that appear to have disease-fighting properties

pica a condition characterized by a hunger and appetite for nonfood substances

plaque deposits of fatty substances, including cholesterol, that attach to arterial walls

polydipsia excessive thirst

polymeric formulas solutions that provide intact nutrients (e.g., whole proteins and long-chain triglycerides) that require a normally functioning gastrointestinal tract

polyphagia excessive hunger and eating

polysaccharide a carbohydrate consisting of many units of monosaccharides joined together; starch and fiber are food sources, and glycogen is a storage form in the liver and muscles

polyunsaturated fatty acid (PUFA) a fatty acid containing two or more double bonds on the carbon chain

polyuria excessive urination

portal hypertension increased blood pressure in the portal circulation caused by compression or occlusion in the portal or hepatic vascular system

postischemic injury after decreased blood supply to a body organ or part

postnecrotic cirrhosis associated with history of viral hepatitis, improperly treated hepatitis, or hepatic damage from toxic chemicals

postprandial occurring after a meal

preeclampsia a sudden rise in arterial blood pressure accompanied by rapid weight gain and marked edema during pregnancy; also known as pregnancy-induced hypertension

primary or essential hypertension elevated blood pressure for which the cause is unknown; often a genetic component

prolactin a hormone responsible for milk synthesis

proteases protein enzymes

protein efficiency ratio (PER) a method to determine the quality of food protein by comparing weight gain with protein intake

protein-energy malnutrition (PEM) malnutrition caused by the lack of protein, of energy, or both

proteins organic compounds formed from chains of amino acids

Q

Qi gong a modality of traditional Chinese medicine that merges breathing regulation, movement, and meditation to increase the flow of Qi, or life force, in the body

quality of life (QOL) the general well-being of an individual

R

reactant a substance that enters into and is altered during a chemical reaction

reactive oxygen species chemically active compounds containing oxygen; they may cause chronic inflammation and tissue damage over time

recombinant erythropoietin (EPO) recombinant human erythropoietin; drug used to treat anemia by replacing erythropoietin for patients with chronic renal failure who do not produce this hormone in adequate amounts

recommended dietary allowance (RDA) the level of nutrient intake sufficient to meet the needs of almost all healthy individuals of a life stage and gender group

recumbent measures measurements taken while the subject is lying down or reclining

refeeding syndrome physiologic and metabolic complications associated with reintroducing nutrition (refeeding) too rapidly to a person with protein-energy malnutrition; can include malabsorption, cardiac insufficiency, congestive heart failure, respiratory distress, convulsions, coma, and perhaps death

refined grains grains that contain only some of the edible kernel

regional enteritis a form of inflammatory bowel disease more commonly called Crohn's disease

registered dietitian/nutritionist (RDN) a professional trained in foods and the management of diets (dietetics) who is credentialed by the Commission on Dietetic Registration of the Academy of Nutrition and Dietetics; credentialing is based on completing a Bachelor of Science degree from a U.S. accredited program, receiving clinical and administrative supervised practice, and passing the national registration examination

reiki an energy therapy based on the belief that healing the patient's spirit also heals the physical body

renal transplantation the transfer of a kidney from one person to another

respiratory distress syndrome (RDS) a respiratory disorder identified by insufficient respiration and abnormally low levels of circulating oxygen in the blood

respiratory quotient (RQ) ratio of CO_2 exhaled to O_2 inhaled; depending on the net metabolic needs of the body, the ratio ranges from 0.7 to 1 and averages around 0.8; carbohydrate metabolism produces an RQ of 1; protein metabolism, an RQ of 0.8; and fat metabolism, an RQ of 0.7

retrovirus a ribonucleic acid (RNA) virus that becomes integrated into the deoxyribonucleic acid (DNA) of a host cell during replication; human immunodeficiency virus (HIV) is a retrovirus

rickets a childhood disorder caused by vitamin D or calcium deficiency and leads to insufficient mineralization of bone and tooth matrix

S

saccharin a nonnutritive sweetener

saliva the secretions of the salivary glands of the mouth

saturated fatty acid a fatty acid with carbon chains completely saturated or filled with hydrogen

scurvy extreme vitamin C deficiency disorder characterized by inflammation of connective tissues, gingivitis, muscle degeneration, bruising, and hemorrhaging as the vascular system weakens

secondary hypertension elevated blood pressure for which the cause can be identified

secretin a hormone secreted by the small intestine that causes the pancreas to release bicarbonate to the small intestine

segmentation the forward and backward muscular action that assists in controlling food mass movement through the gastrointestinal tract

senescence older adulthood

sepsis systemic infection

serosa the outermost layer of the gastrointestinal wall; made of serous membrane

set point a natural level (of some characteristic) that the body regulates or defends

simple carbohydrates monosaccharides and disaccharides

sleep apnea disorder in which breathing stops for short periods during sleep

small for gestational age (SGA) having a lower birth weight than expected for the length of gestation

soft water water filtered to replace some of the minerals with sodium

soluble dietary fibers dietary fibers that dissolve in fluids

solute a substance dissolved in another substance

solvent the liquid in which another substance (the solute) is dissolved to form a solution

somatic protein skeletal muscle protein

somatostatin a hormone produced by the pancreas and hypothalamus that inhibits insulin and glucagon

spina bifida a congenital neural-tube defect caused by the incomplete closure of the fetus's spine during early pregnancy; may involve incomplete development of brain, spinal cord, and/or their protective coverings, resulting in a range of disabilities

steatorrhea presence of excess fat in the feces

stem cell transplantation a procedure that replaces a person's faulty stem cells with healthy ones from blood or bone marrow

sterols fatlike class of lipids that serve vital functions in the body

stomatitis inflammation of mucous membranes of the mouth

storage fat layers and cushions of fat providing stored energy and protection from extremes of environmental temperatures; also protects internal organs against physical trauma

submucosa a layer of connective muscle tissue under the mucosa

sucralose a nonnutritive sweetener, suitable for cooking, that provides no energy

sugar alcohols nutritive sweeteners related to carbohydrates that provide 2 to 3 kcal/g; sorbitol, mannitol, and xylitol are sugar alcohols, also called sugar replacers

syngeneic genetically and immunologically compatible transplant from an identical twin

systemic lupus erythematosus (SLE) a chronic autoimmune inflammatory disease affecting many systems of the body; pathophysiology includes severe vasculitis, renal involvement, and lesions of the skin and nervous system

T

tachycardia rapid beating of the heart

teratogen an agent capable of producing a malformation or a defect in the unborn fetus

The Joint Commission (TJC) a United States–based nonprofit organization that accredits more than 20,000 health care organizations using a peer review process for quality of care

therapeutic touch an energy therapy based on facilitating energy flow in and around the body

thermic effect of food (TEF)/diet-induced thermogenesis an increase of cellular activity when food is eaten

third space (third spacing) a condition in which fluid shifts from the blood into a body cavity or tissue from which it is no longer available as circulating fluid

thrombosis an abnormal vascular condition in which a blood clot (thrombus) develops within a blood vessel

thrombus blood clot

thyrotoxicosis iodine-induced goiter

Tolerable Upper Intake Level (UL) the level of nutrient intake that should not be exceeded to prevent adverse health risks

trace minerals essential nutrient minerals required daily in amounts of 20 mg or less

***trans* fatty acids** fatty acids with unusual double-bond structures caused by hydrogenated unsaturated oils

tricarboxylic acid (TCA) cycle cellular reactions that liberate energy from fragments of carbohydrates, fats, and protein; also called the Krebs cycle

triglycerides the largest class of lipids found in food and body fat; composed of three fatty acids and one glycerol molecule

trypsin the primary pancreatic protease

T1D mellitus (T1DM) a form of diabetes mellitus in which the pancreas produces no insulin at all

T2D mellitus (T2DM) a form of diabetes mellitus in which the pancreas produces some insulin that is defective and unable to serve the complete needs of the body

U

ulcerative colitis (UC) an inflammatory bowel disease confined to the mucosa of any or all of the large intestine

undernutrition consumption of insufficient energy or nutrients based on Dietary Reference Intake values

unrefined grains grains prepared for consumption containing all edible portions of kernels; also known as whole grains

urea product of ammonia conversion produced during deamination

uremia excessive amounts of urea and other nitrogenous waste products in the blood

uremic toxicity buildup of toxic waste products (urea and other nitrogenous waste products) in the blood; symptoms include anorexia, nausea, metallic taste in the mouth, irritability, confusion, lethargy, restlessness, and pruritus (itching)

V

vegan dietary pattern a food plan consisting of only plant foods

very low-calorie diets (VLCDs) usually defined as diets containing 800 kcal/day or less

very low-density lipoproteins (VLDLs) lipoproteins that carry fats and cholesterol to body cells and are made of the largest proportions of cholesterol

villi fingerlike projections on the walls of the small intestine that increase the mucosal surface area

visceral fat fat that is within the abdominal cavity

visceral proteins proteins other than muscle tissue; for example, internal organs and blood

vitamins essential organic molecules needed in very small amounts for cellular metabolism

vomiting reverse peristalsis

W

wasting syndrome an involuntary weight loss of more than 10% in 1 month, with the presence of either chronic diarrhea, weakness, or fever for more than 30 days in the absence of a concurrent illness or condition

wellness a lifestyle enhancing our level of health

Wernicke-Korsakoff syndrome cerebral form of beriberi that affects the central nervous system

wet beriberi thiamine deficiency with edema affecting cardiac function by weakening of heart muscle and vascular system

whole-grain products food items made using unrefined grains

Wilson's disease a rare, inherited disorder of copper metabolism in which copper accumulates slowly in the liver and is then released and taken up in other parts of the body; as copper accumulates in red blood cells, hemolysis and hemolytic anemia occur

X

xerophthalmia a condition caused by vitamin A deficiency with symptoms ranging from night blindness to keratomalacia; may result in complete blindness

INDEX

Page numbers followed by "*f*" indicate figures, "*t*" indicate tables, and "*b*" indicate boxes.

R

S